LHRH
and Its Analogs
Contraceptive and Therapeutic Applications
Part 2

LHRH
and Its Analogs
Contraceptive and Therapeutic Applications
Part 2

Edited by
B. H. Vickery and J. J. Nestor Jr.

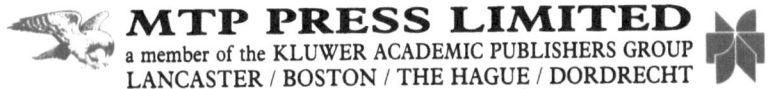
MTP PRESS LIMITED
a member of the KLUWER ACADEMIC PUBLISHERS GROUP
LANCASTER / BOSTON / THE HAGUE / DORDRECHT

Published in the UK and Europe by
MTP Press Limited
Falcon House
Lancaster, England

British Library Cataloguing in Publication Data

LHRH and its analogs : contraceptive and
    therapeutic applications
    Part 2
    1. Generative organs -- Diseases --
    Chemotherapy 2. Luteinizing hormone
    releasing hormone -- Therapeutic use
    I. Vickery, B.H. II. Nestor, J.J.
    615'.766   RC877

ISBN 978-94-010-7949-5   ISBN 978-94-009-3229-6 (eBook)
DOI 10.1007/978-94-009-3229-6

Published in the USA by
MTP Press
A division of Kluwer Academic Publishers
101 Philip Drive
Norwell, MA 02061, USA

Contents

Contents

*Published separately

Foreword

Since the discovery of LHRH in 1971, research into the physiology and therapeutics of this compound can be divided into three distinctly different phases.

In the first phase, attention was paid chiefly to the natural sequence hormone; efforts were channeled to explore its diagnostic use; and nearly all the clinical investigations were coordinated by a single pharmaceutical company. The successes in this area were quite limited and the interest in the promise of this agent as a diagnostic test has long since waned. This phase of research consumed roughly the first seven years of clinical testing after the isolation and characterization of the compound by the two groups involved in the Nobel effort.

With the appearance of long-acting LHRH agonists, the second phase of research on LHRH began in the late '70's. LHRH agonists were the only compounds available during this period of research and paradoxical desensitization was the predominant therapeutic basis for the discoveries. An ever-widening number of therapeutic applications using this approach were unearthed. A second theme which emerged during this second 5-7 year period was that the pulsatile administration of the natural sequence LHRH could be used to treat LHRH deficiency in men and women. However, by far the greatest amount of literature was related to the diverse therapeutic aspects of LHRH agonists which have now found niches in the treatment of several disorders including precocious puberty, prostate cancer, and a wide variety of reproductive disorders. Thus, a natural diversification of therapeutic efforts became apparent during this second phase and the spectrum of applications of these compounds will continue to have far-reaching and diverse opportunities to suppress reproductive function in a safe, effective, and reversible manner.

The third phase of research on LHRH and its analogs encompasses the most recent efforts in which investigation is still ongoing, having built upon the well-established therapeutic advances mentioned above. Present research is primarily focusing upon the combination of LHRH analogs with other agents. For example, the ability to use LHRH agonists to forestall puberty while adding other newly-developed growth-promoting agents such as growth hormone and somatomedin C is but one new application employing LHRH analogs as an adjuvant to other therapies. A similar approach is now emerging in prostate cancer in which a combination of LHRH agonists and anti-androgens appear quite promising. Similar efforts are now planned in breast cancer, with anti-estrogens and LHRH combinations. The possibilities of using the stimulatory phase of LHRH agonist administration to synchronize other therapies have yet to be explored.

The alternative theme which is emerging in the present phase of LHRH research is the identification of potent LHRH antagonists. Although encountering some early difficulties with a histamine-release side effect, several LHRH antagonists are now reported which have some therapeutic value and will combine the completeness of blockade of LHRH agonists with the immediacy of onset of the antagonists.

It is to this third phase of LHRH research that Dr Vickery and his colleagues have turned their efforts in this present volume. This work, representing a very timely update of their previous efforts, should permit the reader to have insight into the present state-of-the-art of LHRH research and to obtain valuable insights into the future directions of this field. All of the authors are knowledgeable in their area of expertise and the editors are to be congratulated on assembling a volume which will guide the reader through this ever-expanding maze of applications of LHRH therapeutic manipulation.

William F Crowley, Jr
Massachusetts General Hospital
May 11, 1987

List of Contributors

Dr R. Abbasi
Department of Obstetrics
and Gynecology
Brooke Army Medical
Center
Fort Sam Houston
San Antonio
TX 78234-6200, USA

Dr L.A. Adams
Veterans Administration
Medical Center (III)
1660 South Columbian Way
Seattle, WA 98108, USA

Dr J.L. Andreyko
Reproductive
Endocrinology Center
Department of Obstetrics,
Gynaecology and
Reproductive Sciences
University of California
San Francisco
CA 94143, USA

Dr A.L. Barkan
Division of Endocrinology
and Metabolism
Department of Internal
Medicine
University of Michigan
Hospital and VA
Medical Center
University of Michigan
Ann Arbor
MI 48109-0368, USA

Dr S. Bhasin
Division of Endocrinology
Harbor-UCLA Medical
Center
1000 Carson Street
Torrance, CA 90509, USA

Dr C. Bishop
Research Laboratories
Ortho Pharmaceutical
Corporation
Raritan, NJ 08869, USA

Dr C. Bowers
Endocrine Unit
Tulane University School
of Medicine
New Orleans
LA 70112, USA

Dr T.A. Bramley
Department of Obstetrics
and Gynecology
Centre for Reproductive
Biology
37 Chalmers Street
Edinburgh EH3 9EW
Scotland

Dr W.J. Bremner
Division of Endocrinology
Veterans Administration
Hospital
4435 Beacon Avenue South
Seattle, WA 98108, USA

Dr R.J. Capetola
Research Laboratories
Ortho Pharmaceutical
Corporation
Raritan, NJ 08869, USA

Dr R.L. Chan
Bioanalytical and
Metabolic Research
Syntex Research
Palo Alto
CA 94304, USA

Dr N.C. Chaturvedi
Department of
Biochemistry
Indiana University School
of Medicine
Indianapolis
IN 46223, USA

Dr P.M. Conn
Department of
Pharmacology
University of Iowa
Iowa City, IA 52242, USA

Dr D.H. Coy
Peptide Research
Laboratories
Department of Medicine
Tulane University Medical
Center
New Orleans
LA 70112, USA

Dr I. Craft
Humana Hospital
Wellington
Wellington Place
London NW8, England

Dr L.W. Crim
Memorial University of
Newfoundland
Marine Sciences Research
Laboratory
St. John's, Newfoundland
Canada A1C 5S7

Dr T. de Chalain
Department of Obstetrics
and Gynecology
University of Cape Town
Medical School
Groote Schuur Hospital
7925 Observatory
Cape Town, South Africa

Dr D.M. de Kretser
Department of Anatomy
Monash University
Clayton, Melbourne
Victoria 3168, Australia,

Dr R.J. Donnelly
Clinical Research
Department
Imperial Chemical
Industries plc
Macclesfield
Cheshire SK10 4TG
England

Dr A. Eshel
The Middlesex Hospital
Medical School and
University College London
Mortimer Street
London W1N 8AA, England

Dr N. Faure
Endocrinologie de la
Reproduction
Hôpital Saint-Françoise
d'Assise
10 Rue de l'Espinay
Québec, Canada G1L 3L5

Dr D.-M. Feng
Institute for Biomedical
Research
The University of Texas
at Austin
Austin, TX 78712, USA

Dr K. Folkers
Institute for Biomedical
Research
The University of Texas
at Austin
Austin, TX 78712, USA

Dr H.M. Fraser
MRC Reproductive Biology
Unit
Centre for Reproductive
Biology
37 Chalmers Street
Edinburgh EH3 9EW
Scotland

Dr M.B. Garnick
Dana-Farber Cancer
Institute
Boston, MA 02115, USA

Dr H.A. Garverick
Dept Dairy Science
111 Animal Sciences
Center
University of Missouri-
Columbia
Columbia, MO 65211, USA

Dr L.M. Glode
University of Colorado
Medical Center
Denver, CO 80262, USA

Dr J.C. Goodpasture
Institute of Biological
Sciences
Syntex Research, R7-241
3401 Hillview Avenue
Palo Alto, CA 94304, USA

Dr D.W. Hahn
Reproductive Research
Section
Ortho Pharmaceutical
Corporation
Route 202
Raritan, NJ 08869, USA

Dr F. Hardie
Department of Obstetrics
and Gynecology
University of Cape Town
Medical School
Groote Schuur Hospital
7925 Observatory
Cape Town, South Africa

Dr H.A. Harvey
Hershey Medical Center
Hershey, PA 17033, USA

Dr M.P. Hedger
Gamete Biology Section
Laboratory of
Reproductive and
Developmental
Toxicology
National Institute of
Environmental Health
Sciences
Research Triangle Park
NC 27709, USA

Dr M.R. Henzl
Institute of Clinical
Medicine
Syntex Research, A3-288
3401 Hillview Avenue
Palo Alto, CA 94304, USA

Dr G. Hodgen
Eastern Virginia Medical
School
Norfolk, VA 23501, USA

Dr P. Hoffman
Institute of Clinical
Medicine
Syntex Research, A3-288
3401 Hillview Avenue
Palo Alto, CA 94304, USA

Dr W.A. Hook
Clinical Immunology
Section
Laboratory of
Microbiology and
Immunology
National Institute of
Dental Research
National Institutes of
Health
Bethesda, MD 20892, USA

Dr T. Hrinyo-Pavlina
Department of
Biochemistry
Indiana University School
of Medicine
Indianapolis
IN 46223, USA

Dr H.S. Jacobs
Cobbold Laboratories
Middlesex Hospital
London W1N 8AA, England

Dr R.B. Jaffe
Department of
Obstetrics/Gynecology,
M-1480
University of California
San Francisco
CA 94143, USA

Dr H. Kaplan
Department of Obstetrics
and Gynecology and
University of Cape Town
Medical School
Groote Schuur Hospital
7925 Observatory
Cape Town , South Africa

Dr M.J. Karten
National Institute of
Child Health and Human
Development
Landow Building, Room
7A04
7910 Woodmont Avenue
Bethesda, MD 20205, USA

Dr D. Kenigsberg
Dept. of Obstetrics and
Gynecology
Stony Brook
NY 11794, USA

Dr J.A. King
Medical Research Council
Regulatory Peptides
Research Unit
Department of Chemical
Pathology
University of Cape Town
Medical School
Observatory 7925
Cape Town, South Africa

Dr J. Kirkland
Department of Pediatrics
Baylor College of
Medicine
1200 Moursund Avenue
Houston, TX 77030, USA

Dr W.J. Kovacs
Division of Endocrinology
Department of Medicine
Vanderbilt University
AA-4206
Medical Center North
Nashville, TN 37232, USA

Dr M. Kowalczuk
Department of
Biochemistry
Indiana University School
of Medicine
Indianapolis
IN 46223, USA

Dr G. van der Kraak
Department of Zoology
University of Alberta
Edmonton
Alberta, Canada T6G 2E9

Prof. A. Lemay
Université Laval
Endocrinologie de la
Reproduction
Hôpital Saint-François
d'Assise
10, Rue de l'Espinay
Québec, Canada G1L 3L5

Dr T.H. Lin
Department of Pediatrics
Baylor College of
Medicine
Houston, TX 77030, USA

Dr A. Lipton
Hershey Medical Center
Hershey, PA 17033, USA

Dr A. Ljunqqvist
Institute for Biomedical
Research
The University of Texas
at Austin
Austin, TX 78712, USA

Dr J.C. Marshall
Division of Endocrinology
Department of Internal
    Medicine and
    Pediatrics
University of Michigan
Ann Arbor, MI 48109, USA

Dr D.T. Max
Abbott Laboratories
North Chicago
IL 60064, USA

Dr C.A. McArdle
Department of
    Pharmacology
The University of Iowa
    College of Medicine
Iowa City, IA 52242, USA

Dr J.L. McGuire
Research Laboratories
Ortho Pharmaceutical
    Corporation
Route 202
Raritan, NJ 08869, USA

G.I. McRae
·Department of Physiology
Institute of Biological
    Sciences
Syntex Research
3401 Hillview Avenue
Palo Alto
CA 94304, USA

Dr R.P. Millar
Medical Research Council
    Regulatory Peptides
    Research Unit
Department of Chemical
    Pathology
University of Cape Town
    Medical School
Observatory 7925
Cape Town, South Africa

Dr R.A.V. Milsted
ICI Pharmaceuticals
    Division
Alderley Park
Macclesfield, SK10 4TG
England

Dr S.E. Monroe
Reproductive
    Endocrinology Center
Department of Obstetrics
    Gynecology and
    Reproductive Sciences
University of California
San Francisco
CA 94143, USA

Dr C.A. Nerenberg
Bioanalytical and
    Metabolic Research
Syntex Research
Palo Alto
CA 94304, USA

Dr J.J. Nestor
Department of Peptide
    Research
Institute of Bio-Organic
    Chemistry
Syntex Research
3401 Hillview Avenue
Palo Alto, CA 94304, USA

Dr K. Nikolics
Genentech, Inc.
Department of
    Developmental Biology
460 Point San Bruno Blvd
South San Francisco
CA 94080, USA

Dr T. Okamoto
Institute for Biomedical
    Research
The University of Texas
    at Austin
Austin, TX 78712, USA

Dr S.J. Ory
Section of Reproductive
    Endocrinology
Mayo Clinic
Rochester, MN 55905, USA

Dr S.N. Pavlou
Division of Endocrinology
School of Medicine
Vanderbilt University
Nashville, TN 37232, USA

Dr R.E. Peter
Department of Zoology
University of Alberta
Edmonton
Alberta, Canada T6G 2E9

Dr A. Phillips
Research Laboratories
Ortho Pharmaceutical
    Corporation
Raritan, NJ 08869, USA

Dr L. Pillay
Department of Obstetrics
    and Gynecology
University of Cape Town
    Medical School
Groote Schuur Hospital
7925 Observatory
Cape Town, South Africa

Dr C.G. Pitt
Research Triangle
    Institute
PO Box 12194
Research Triangle Park
NC 27709, USA

Dr R. Porter
The Middlesex Hospital
    Medical School and
    University College
    London
Mortimer Street
London W1N 8AA, England

Dr W. von Rechenberg
Hoechst AG
Pharmacology H 821
D-6230 Frankfurt 80
Federal Republic of
    Germany

Dr R.L. Reid
Etherington Hall
Queens University
Kingston, Ontario
Canada K7L 3N6

Dr J.E. Rivier
Clayton Foundation
Laboratories for Peptide
    Biology
The Salk Institute
La Jolla, CA 92037, USA

Dr D.M. Robertson
Department of Anatomy
Monash University
Melbourne
Victoria 3168, Australia

Dr R.W. Roeske
Indiana University
School of Medicine
Indianapolis
IN 46223, USA

Dr J. Sandow
Department of
    Pharmacology
Hoechst-AG
6230 Frankfurt 80
Federal Republic of
    Germany

Dr K Nikolics
Department of Molecular
    Biology
Genentech, Inc.
460 Point San Bruno Blvd.
South San Francisco
CA 94080, USA

Dr T. Siler-Khodr
University of Texas
Health Science Center at
    San Antonio
7703 Floyd Curl Drive
San Antonio
TX 78284, USA

Dr R.P. Siraganian
Clinical Immunology
    Section
Laboratory of
    Microbiology and
    Immunology
National Institute of
    Dental Research
National Institutes of
    Health
Bethesda, MD 20892, USA

Dr J.A. Smith
The University of Utah
    Medical Center
Salt Lake City
UT 84132, USA

Dr Z.M. van der Spuy
Department of Obstetrics
    and Gynecology
University of Cape Town
    Medical School
Groote Schuur Hospital
7925 Observatory
Cape Town, South Africa

Dr B.S. Steiner
Division of Endocrinology
Harbor-UCLA Medical
    Center
Torrance, CA 90509, USA

Dr R.A. Steiner
Veterans Administration
    Medical Center (III)
1660 South Columbian Way
Seattle, WA 98108, USA

Dr J.S. Stevenson
Dept. Animal Sciences and
    Ind.
Call Hall
Kansas State University
Manhattan, KS 66506, USA

Dr R.S. Swerdloff
Division of Endocrinology
Harbor-UCLA Medical
    Center
Torrance, CA 90509, USA

Dr P.-F.L. Tang
Institute for Biomedical
    Research
The University of Texas
    at Austin
Austin, TX 78712, USA

Dr B.H. Vickery
Department of Physiology
Institute of Biological
    Sciences
Syntex Research
3401 Hillview Avenue
Palo Alto, CA 94304, USA

Dr G.B. Wakefield
Division of Endocrinology
Department of Medicine
Vanderbilt University
AA-4206
Medical Center North
Nashville, TN 37232, USA

Dr M. van der Watt
Department of Obstetrics
    and Gynecology
University of Cape Town
    Medical School
Groote Schuur Hospital
7925 Observatory
Cape Town, South Africa

Dr J. Waxman
St. Bartholomew's
    Hospital and
The Institute of Urology
London EC1 7BE, England

Dr S.S.C. Yen
Division of Reproductive
    Endocrinology
Department of
    Reproductive Medicine
University of California
La Jolla, CA 92093, USA

Dr Y. Zhang
Institute for Biomedical
    Research
The University of Texas
    at Austin
Austin, TX 78712, USA

Introduction

J.J. NESTOR, Jr. and B.H. VICKERY

Institutes of Bio-Organic Chemistry and Biological Sciences,
Syntex Research, Palo Alto, CA 94304, USA

The scope of research related to luteinizing hormone/follicle stimulating hormone-releasing hormone (LHRH; GnRH) is very broad, spanning peptide chemistry, physiology, pharmacology, biochemistry, novel delivery systems and clinical studies for applications in human and veterinary medicine. Part 1 of this book attempted to cover this breadth of research with invited chapters summarizing the state-of-the-art in 1983 (see Table of Contents for Part 1).

In the three years which have elapsed since the publication of Part 1 of this series there have been several important changes in the scope and direction of LHRH research. The use of LHRH agonists for treatment of metastatic prostate cancer is no longer a theoretical possibility being studied in clinical trials. Three compounds are now available on prescription in several countries for this indication and one (tryptorelin) is also indicated for treatment of precocious puberty in Europe (Table 1). The registration of several additional compounds/formulations for prostatic cancer is rapidly approaching. The applicability of LHRH agonists for the treatment of gynecological disorders such as endometriosis is also the subject of wide-spread clinical trials; registrations for sale are expected in 1987.

Although a number of small scale, single dose studies have been performed with LHRH antagonists over the years, the low potency and short duration of action of the earlier classes of antagonists were major problems. The substantial advances which have been achieved in the chemistry and pharmacology of the antagonists are now allowing the initiation of larger, definitive, multiple dose studies of this class of compounds. Problems still remain with the LHRH antagonists, however, since the most potent compounds synthesized, until recently, suffered from side-reactions resulting from their ability to cause mast cell degranulation.

CHEMISTRY/PHARMACOLOGY

Although the increased knowledge about the structures of gonadotropin releasing hormone in lower vertebrates (Chapter 5)

Table I. LHRH analogs in clinical development or clinical study (adapted from [1])

Compound	USAN	Indication/level of study	Dosage form	Company/sponsor
Agonist				
LHRH	gonadorelin	diagnostic (marketed in United States)	injection	Ayerst
LHRH	cystorelin	cystic ovaries in cattle (marketed, United States/Europe)	injection	Hoechst
LHRH	cryptorelin	Cryptorchidism (marketed in Europe)	injection	Hoechst
$[D-Leu^6,Pro^9NEt]LHRH$	leuprorelin	Prostatic cancer (marketed in United States/Europe)	daily injection	TAP/Abbott
$[D-Trp^6]LHRH$	tryptorelin	Prostatic cancer, precocious puberty (marketed Europe, Brazil)	injectable polymer/1 x mouth	DeBiopharm
$[D-Trp^6,Pro^9NEt]LHRH$		Clinical trial, various indications	injection	Salk Institute
$[D-Trp^6,NMeLeu^7,Pro^9NEt]LHRH$	lutrelin	Clinical trial	injection	Wyeth
$[D-Ser(tBu)^6,Pro^9NEt]LHRH$	buserelin	Prostatic cancer (marketed in Europe) Advanced clinical trial, various indications	Daily injection, followed by nasal	Hoechst
$[D-Ser(tBu)^6,Aza-Gly^{10}]LHRH$	goserelin	Prostatic cancer, breast cancer	Polymer implant, 1 x month	ICI Ltd.
$[D-His(Bzl)^6,Pro^9-NEt]LHRH$	histrelin	Clinical trial, endometriosis	daily injection, nasal	Population Council/Ortho
$[D-Nal(2)^6]LHRH$	nafarelin	Advanced clinical trial, various indications	Nasal/injectable polymer	Syntex
$[D-Nal(2)^6,Aza-Gly^{10}]LHRH$		Veterinary trials, various indications	Silastic implant	Syntex
Antagonist				
$[N-Ac-D-pCl-Phe^1,D-pCl-Phe^2,D-Trp^3,D-Arg^6,D-Ala^{10}]LHRH$		Clinical pharmacology	Injection	Organon
$[N-Ac-D-Nal(2)^1,D-pCl-Phe^2,D-Trp^3,D-hArg(Et_2)^6,D-Ala^{10}]LHRH$	detirelix	Clinical pharmacology	Injection	Syntex
$[N-Ac-D-Nal(2)^1,D-pCl-Phe^2,D-Pal(3)^3,Arg^5,D-Glu(AA)^6,D-Ala^{10}]LHRH$		Clinical pharmacology	Injection	NICHHD-CDB/Population Council

has led to a group of interesting chimeric analogs [3], no new LHRH agonists have entered human clinical development since 1983. The azagly derivative of nafarelin ([D-Nal(2)^6,Aza-Gly^{10}]-LHRH) has been the subject of extensive veterinary study (Chapter 34). A series of agonistic analogs containing unnatural amino acids designed for phospholipid membrane binding yielded a very potent new class of relatively hydrophilic analogs (e.g. [D-hArg(Et$_2$)^6,Pro^9-NHEt] LHRH; 140 x LHRH potency, _in_ _vivo_ [4]). These analogs lend further support to the concept that affinity for cell membranes may be an important property for neuropeptides (Chapter 1).

Toxicology studies on the "D-Arg^6 class" of LHRH antagonists, the preclinical development of which was discussed in Part 1 of this series (see also Chapter 1), revealed that they caused a serious side effect, anaphylactoid responses (Chapters 11, 12, 13). New classes of compounds designed to avoid this side effect are reported in Chapters 2 and 3. Reproductive pharmacology of LHRH antagonists has been studied in male (Chapter 14) and female (Chapter 15) primates, and the overall animal pharmacology has been summarized in Chapter 13. Specific applications for the LHRH antagonists which do not necessarily overlap with those of the agonists are now being suggested (Table 2).

Table 2. Suggested therapeutic applications of LHRH antagonist analogs (modified from [2])

Indication	
Human	
Diagnostic; predicting osteoporosis	Interception
Suppression of ovulation	Premenstrual syndrome
Luteal suppression	Male contraception
Gonadal hormone dependent tumors	
Veterinary	
Interruption of heat	Pregnancy termination

LHRH effects and mechanism of action were reviewed at both a cellular (Chapters 6 and 7) and a tissue level (Chapters 8-10). Investigation of the biosynthesis of LHRH has uncovered a cosecreted product which also may have a profertility role as a suppressor of prolaction secretion (Chapter 4).

CLINICAL STUDIES

The initial results from clinical trials with the newer, more potent LHRH antagonists are described in Chapters 17-19. A possible diagnostic application for antagonists is discussed on the basis of a primate study (Chapter 31).

The clinical status of the principal LHRH agonists has now reached a mature state (Table 1) and is reviewed in a series of chapters (21-28). A new focus here is on gynecological appli-cations of the LHRH agonists (Chapters 17, 22, 26, 27). An interesting new concept deserves to be highlighted. Chapter 20 discusses the use of LHRH agonists to suppress endogenous gonadotropin production while adding carefully controlled doses of exogenous gonadotropins for in vitro fertilization/egg transfer protocols and for increased in vivo fertility in poor prognoses such as polycystic ovarian disease. This therapy also is being applied in oligomenorrhea and premature menopause induced by chemotherapy [5,6]. Table 3 lists a range of suggested indica-tions for agonists. Pilot clinical studies for several of these applications are reported in Chapter 17.

Table 3. Suggested therapeutic applications of LHRH agonist analogs (modified from [2])

Indication	
Human	
Ovulation inhibition	Acute intermittent porphyria
Cancer (prostate, ovary, breast)	Cyclic luteal deafness
In vitro fertilization	Cryptorchidism
Endometriosis	Fibrocystic breast disease
Polycystic ovarian disease	Premenstrual syndrome
Fertility after chemotherapy	BPH
Interception	Acne
Luteal suppression	Male contraception
Hirsutism	Precocious puberty
Dysfunctional uterine bleeding	Protection from gonadal or
Uterine leiomyoma	bone marrow toxicity of
Anorexia nervosa	chemotherapy
Veterinary	
Cystic ovaries in heifers	Tumors (breast, anal, prostate)
Cycle suppression in heifers	Cystic hyperplasia, prostate
Suppression of heat in pets	

Although it had been expected that the suppression of gameto-genesis through the use of an LHRH agonist would offer protection from the sterilizing effects of chemotherapy, results from a clinical trial (Chapter 30) and animal studies (Chapter 29) appear to rule out this hope. These results should not be taken as indicating that a regimen employing the more rapidly acting antagonists would not be effective, however.

Veterinary issues (Chapters 32-34) range from induced spawning in fish, in which down regulation does not appear to result from high dose agonist treatment, to use of both agonist and antagonist analogs for different contraceptive possibilities in pets.

A critical issue for the acceptance of peptide drugs is the development of appropriate formulations. Chapters 35 and 36 discuss advanced approaches for enhanced nasal absorption and controlled release implants/injections, respectively.

Part 2 of this series extends but does not replace the previous volume. The breadth of coverage of the previous volume has been maintained and the chapters cover the progress in specific fields of research up to late 1986. The particular focus in this volume has been on the latest developments in the chemistry, physiology and clinical studies with LHRH antagonists as well as overviews of the clinical studies of the principal LHRH agonists. In order to provide for the most rapid possible publication of this volume, the contributing authors were asked to provide camera-ready manuscripts, a significantly increased effort on their part which we acknowledge and for which we thank them.

REFERENCES

1. Vickery, B.H. Comparison of the potential for therapeutic utilities with gonadotropin-releasing hormone agonists and antagonists. Endocr. Rev., 7, 115 (1986).

2. Vickery, B.H. and Nestor, J.J. Jr. LHRH analogues: development and mechanism of action. Sem. Reprod. Endocrinol. (1987) in press.

3. Folkers, K., Bowers, C.Y., Tang, P.-F.L. and Kabota, M. Decapeptides as effective agonists from L-amino acids biologically equivalent to the luteinizing hormone-releasing hormone. Proc. Natl. Acad. Sci. USA, 82, 1070 (1985).

4. Nestor, J.J. Jr., Tahilramani, R., Ho, T.L., McRae, G.I. and Vickery, B.H. Potent LHRH agonists containing N^G, $N^{G'}$-dialkyl-D-homoarginines. In "Peptides: Structure and Function". C.M. Deber, V.J. Hruby, and K.D. Kopple (Eds), Pierce Chemical Co., Rockford, IL., 1985, p. 557.

5. Fleming, R., Adam, A.H., Barlow, D.H., Black, W.P., Macnaughton, M.C., and Coutts, J.R.T. A new systematic treatment for infertile women with abnormal hormonal profiles. Brit. J. Obstet. Gynaecol., 89, 80 (1982).

6. Fleming, R., Hamilton, M.P.R., Barlow, D.H., Cordiner, J.W. and Coutts, J.R.T. Pregnancy after ovulation induction in a patient with menopausal gonadotropin levels after chemotherapy. Lancet, 1, 399 (1984).

SECTION 1

CHEMISTRY

1
Development of LHRH Antagonists

J.J. NESTOR, Jr

Institute of Bio-Organic Chemistry, Syntex Research, Palo Alto, CA 94304, USA

INTRODUCTION

Soon after the first syntheses [1,2] of LHRH ($<$Glu^1-His^2-Trp^3-Ser^4-Tyr^5-Gly^6-Leu^7-Arg^8-Pro^9-Gly^{10}-NH$_2$), the first LHRH antagonist was discovered [3]. Analogs which block the stimulation of gonadotropin release by LHRH originally were sought for anti-fertility applications. Although potent LHRH agonists were found to accomplish a reversible "medical gonadectomy" during continued treatment [4], through a receptor overload-desensitization mechanism [5,6], potent LHRH antagonists are still desired because of their immediate and profound suppression of gonadotropin secretion [7,8].

Since LHRH is secreted in a pulsatile manner throughout the day [9] and as little as 10% receptor occupancy may stimulate gonadotropin secretion [10], an effective competitive receptor antagonist must possess high receptor affinity and a prolonged duration of action [11]. These requirements have led to analogs containing modifications which provide protection from proteolysis and good pharmacokinetics. It is reasonable to assume that an antagonist must merely interact in or near the receptor binding site and does not need to have the specific receptor contacts which stimulate the signal transduction process (e.g., by specific allosteric conformational change of the receptor, direct interaction with guanine nucleotide regulatory proteins, etc.). Therefore a greater latitude in acceptable structural modification might be expected relative to the agonists. In accord with this concept, the most potent LHRH agonists contain only one or two substitutions while the most recent LHRH antagonists (Chapters 2, 3, 13) have as many as seven of the ten residues replaced by amino acids with novel side chains and/or a D-configuration.

The development of the current generation of highly modified LHRH antagonists with potential clinical utility has been a complicated, frequently empirical process, resulting from stepwise increases in potency from many analog studies. This review provides a simplified introduction and overview of this development. More exhaustive reviews of the chemistry and applications of LHRH antagonists are available [8,11-14].

ANTAGONIST DESIGN

Initial directions

The importance of position 2 for antagonist design became evident from the observation that [des-His[2]]LHRH had weak antagonistic activity in vitro [15]. However, mere removal of the side chain (e.g., [Gly[2]]LHRH) or replacement by other aromatic amino acid side chains [16] gave analogs with residual agonistic activity as demonstrated in vitro by LH secretion [15-17] or at the level of the intracellular second messenger system [18]. As observed with the LHRH agonists [19], incorporation of a D-Ala[6] residue (which inhibits proteolysis and increases receptor affinity) resulted in increased inhibitory potency for [des-His[2],D-Ala[6]]LHRH. An impor- tant lead for further antagonist development resulted from the observation that replacement of His[2] by D-aromatic amino acids [17], coupled with D-amino acid substitution in position 6 [20,21], resulted in remarkable increases in antagonistic potency. Thus [D-Phe[2],D-Ala[6]]LHRH was the first analog to block normal ovula- tion in the rat, albeit at the high dose of 6 x 1 mg [20].
  The incorporation of hydrophobic 6-position substitutions, so effective in the LHRH agonists, initially did not result in increased potency in the antagonists [21]. That removal of the aromatic side chain of His[2] did not completely destroy agonistic activity [15] might be taken to suggest a partial role for the aromatic Trp[3] side chain in stimulus-response coupling. Replace- ment of Trp[3] by Phe[3] [22], Pro[3] [23], and especially D-Trp[3] [24] caused significant potency increases (Table 1). Thus [D-Phe[2,6], D-Trp[3]]LHRH inhibited ovulation at a 1 mg dose (noon, proestrus) [25] and provided a substitution pattern for later modifications.
  The initial potency increases from position 1 substitutions [26] followed energy minimization calculations [27] which predicted that the orientation of the <Glu[1] residue in LHRH would be most closely mimicked by a D-<Glu[1] residue in the antagonist struc- tures described above. While one of the resulting structures ([D-<Glu[1],D-Phe[2],D-Trp[3,6]]LHRH) was more potent [26], later studies showed that Ac-Pro[1] [28,29], Ac-D-hydrophobic amino acid[1] [30], Ac-Δ[3]-Pro[1] [31] or even Ac-Gly[1] [32] could result in highly potent analogs. It may be that such substitutions primarily affect the enzymatic degradation rate and/or global hydrophobicity of the molecule.

Hydrophobic antagonists

Increasingly hydrophobic analogs were explored with the combi- nation of substitutions at positions 1, 2, 3, and 6. The incorpo- ration of the most hydrophobic natural amino acid (Trp) in posi- tions 3 and 6, coupled with a hydrophobic N-terminus, produced [N-Ac-D-Phe[1],D-Phe[2],D-Trp[3,6]]LHRH, which blocked ovulation at a single dose of 250 µg/rat [33]. Replacement of D-Phe[2] by the more hydrophobic D-pCl-Phe yielded [Ac-D-Phe[1],D-pCl-Phe[2],D-Trp[3,6]]LHRH, which was substantially more potent [33]. The 3-(2-naphthyl)-D-

4

Table 1. Early LHRH antagonists

Compound[a]	Approximate ED_{50}[b] (µg) Noon of Proestrus (vehicle--corn oil)	
1 [des-His^2]LHRH	---c	[15]
2 [des-His^2,D-Ala^6]LHRH	---c	[19]
3 [D-pF-Phe^2,D-Ala^6]LHRH	6x1000	[21]
4 [D-Phe^2,Pro^3,D-Trp^6]LHRH	<750	[23]
5 [D-Phe^{2,6},D-Trp^3]LHRH	<350	[25]
6 [N-Ac-Pro^1,D-Phe^2,D-Trp^{3,6}]LHRH	<250	[28]
7 [N-Ac-D-Phe^1,D-pCl-Phe^2,D-Trp^{3,6}]LHRH	<15	[33]
8 [N-Ac-Δ^3-Pro^1,D-pF-Phe^2,D-Nal(2)^{3,6}]LHRH	2.8	[35]
9 [N-Ac-Pro^1,D-pF-Phe^2,D-Nal(2)^{3,6}]LHRH	3.3	[29]

[a]Superscript denotes the position of substitution within the LHRH (<Glu^1-His^2-Trp^3-Ser^4-Tyr^5-Gly^6-Leu^7-Arg^8-Pro^9-Gly^{10}-NH$_2$) structure. Unnatural amino acids are: pF-Phe, para-fluorophenylalanine; pCl-Phe, para-chlorophenylalanine; Δ^3-Pro, $\Delta^{3,4}$-dehydroproline; Nal(2), 3-(2-naphthyl)-alanine. [b]ED_{50} is given as "less than" a value which was reported to be >50% effective at that dose. [c]Weak antagonistic activity in vitro.

alanine residue [D-Nal(2)] had previously been used in position 6 of LHRH agonists to yield very potent and long-acting analogs [11, 34], probably due to its ability to cause hydrophobic depoting in the body. Its use in the antagonist series resulted in the extremely hydrophobic and extensively studied analogs [N-Ac-Δ^3-Pro^1,D-pF-Phe^2,D-Nal(2)^{3,6}]LHRH [35,36] and [N-Ac-Pro^1,D-pF-Phe^2,D-Nal(2)^{3,6}]LHRH [29,37], both with ED_{50} ~3 µg/rat for ovulation inhibition. These latter structures can be looked at as the end of this phase of LHRH antagonist development, which focused on hydrophobic substitutions.

Hydrophilic antagonists

The very low water solubility of the hydrophobic antagonists which resulted from the earlier synthetic directions prompted a reexamination of position 6 substitutions using polar amino acids [38]. Although the most active analogs prior to this point had the very hydrophobic Trp or Nal(2) residue in position 6, in this study the analogs with hydrophilic, positively charged side chains in this position (Lys, Arg) retained surprisingly high potency [38] and a more prolonged duration of action (Table 2) [39]. Thus while [N-Ac-Pro^1,D-pF-Phe^2,D-Nal(2)^{3,6}]LHRH has an ED_{50} ~3 µg/rat when administered at noon on proestrus, the ED_{50} is ~40 fold higher (140 µg/rat) if it is administered 24 hr earlier on diestrus II (D_{II}). In contrast, [N-Ac-D-pCl-Phe^1,D-pCl-Phe^2,D-Trp^3,D-Arg^6,D-Ala^{10}]LHRH

[38] has an ED_{50} of ~5 µg when administered on D_{II} [39], which is only a 4 fold higher ED_{50} than that on proestrus.

Some balancing of the hydrophobic character of the molecule appeared to be necessary since very hydrophobic 1-position substitutions were required for highest potency [29,40,41]. Thus [N-Ac-D-Nal(2)[1],D-pF-Phe[2],D-Trp[3],D-Arg[6]]LHRH [29,40] and [N-Ac-D-Nal(2)[1],D-pCl-Phe[2],D-Trp[3],D-Arg[6],D-Ala[10]]LHRH [41] are representative models of this phase of antagonist development and have been the subject of clinical studies [42,43]. The latter analog has five substitutions and derives increased potency from a D-Ala[10] residue [44] which may protect the C-terminus from proteolysis [45]. While D-amino acid[10] substitution did not cause increased potency in the agonist series, the Pro[9]-NHEt and aza-Gly[10] substitutions which were important in that series [46,47] have been less useful in the antagonist series [29,40,48,49].

Further potency increases resulted from substitutions in positions 3 and 7. Based on the observation that the more hydrophobic Trp is present in the chicken II gonadotropin releasing hormone instead of the Leu[7] in LHRH, studies of analogs with substitutions in position 7 resulted in [N-Ac-D-Nal(2)[1],D-pCl-Phe[2],D-Pal(3)[3], D-Arg[6],Trp[7],D-Ala[10]]LHRH [50] and [N-Ac-D-Nal(1)[1],D-pCl-Phe[2], D-Trp[3],D-Arg[6],Phe[7],D-Ala[10]]LHRH [51] as the most potent members of the series. The use of 3-(3-pyridyl)-D-alanine [Pal(3)], which combines aromatic, basic and hydrophilic character, as a replacement for D-Trp[3], produced a potency enhancement in an earlier hydrophobic series [52]. This relatively hydrophilic substitution is paired most effectively here with the Trp[7] modification [50]. In contrast, the D-Trp[3] substitution gave the most potent analog when paired with the less hydrophobic Phe[7] [51]. These observations again point to the modulation of the global hydrophobicity as an important consideration in analog design.

Antagonists designed for membrane binding

The surprisingly prolonged duration of action of 10 may be due to depoting in the body by binding to cell membranes. This may take place through an electrostatic interaction between the positively charged Arg and the negatively charged phospholipid head group [11]. A series of unnatural amino acids was designed for enhanced membrane binding by the incorporation of alkyl substitutions on the guanidine function [11,39]. This class of amino acids, the $N^G,N^{G'}$-dialkylhomoarginines [hArg(R_2)], therefore combines the positive charge of Arg (electrostatic) with further stabilization of the membrane binding by interaction of the alkyl groups with hydrophobic portions of the phospholipid (Figure 1). Detirelix (RS-68439; [N-Ac-D-Nal(2)[1],D-pCl-Phe[2],D-Trp[3],D-hArg(Et$_2$)[6],D-Ala[10]]-LHRH) was the most potent analog produced in that series and had an even more prolonged duration of action than 10 in laboratory animals [13,39,52-54] and in man ($t_{1/2}$ >48 hr [Chapter 18]).

A similar line of reasoning [Chapter 3] independently led to the synthesis of N^ϵ-isopropyl-Lys and its incorporation into antagonists (see below).

6

Table 2. Hydrophilic antagonists

Compound[a]	Approximate ED$_{50}$[b] (µg)		
	Proestrus (vehicle—corn oil)	Diestrus II	
9 $[N\text{-}Ac\text{-}Pro^1,\underline{D}\text{-}pF\text{-}Phe^2,\underline{D}\text{-}Nal(2)^{3,6}]LHRH$	3.3	140	[29]
10 $[N\text{-}Ac\text{-}\underline{D}\text{-}pCl\text{-}Phe^1,\underline{D}\text{-}pCl\text{-}Phe^2,\underline{D}\text{-}Trp^3,\underline{D}\text{-}Arg^6,\underline{D}\text{-}Ala^{10}]LHRH$	1.8[c]	5	[38]
11 $[N\text{-}Ac\text{-}\underline{D}\text{-}Nal(2)^1,\underline{D}\text{-}pF\text{-}Phe^2,\underline{D}\text{-}Trp^3,\underline{D}\text{-}Arg^6]LHRH$	2.4[c]	9	[40]
12 $[N\text{-}Ac\text{-}\underline{D}\text{-}Nal(2)^1,\underline{D}\text{-}pCl\text{-}Phe^2,\underline{D}\text{-}Trp^3,\underline{D}\text{-}Arg^6,\underline{D}\text{-}Ala^{10}]LHRH$	<1[c]		[41]
13 $[N\text{-}Ac\text{-}\underline{D}\text{-}Nal(2)^1,\underline{D}\text{-}pCl\text{-}Phe^2,\underline{D}\text{-}Pal(3)^3,\underline{D}\text{-}Arg^6,Trp^7,\underline{D}\text{-}Ala^{10}]LHRH$	<0.25		[50]
14 $[N\text{-}Ac\text{-}\underline{D}\text{-}Nal(2)^1,\underline{D}\text{-}pCl\text{-}Phe^2,\underline{D}\text{-}Trp^3,\underline{D}\text{-}Arg^6,Phe^7,\underline{D}\text{-}Ala^{10}]LHRH$	<0.5		[51]
15 $[N\text{-}Ac\text{-}\underline{D}\text{-}Nal(2)^1,\underline{D}\text{-}pCl\text{-}Phe^2,\underline{D}\text{-}Trp^3,\underline{D}\text{-}hArg(Et_2)^6,\underline{D}\text{-}Ala^{10}]LHRH$	0.5	2.5	[39]
16 $[N\text{-}Ac\text{-}\underline{D}\text{-}Nal(2)^1,\underline{D}\text{-}\alpha\text{-}Me,pCl\text{-}Phe^2,\underline{D}\text{-}Trp^3,Arg^5,\underline{D}\text{-}Tyr^6,\underline{D}\text{-}Ala^{10}]LHRH$	<1		[74]
17 $[N\text{-}Ac\text{-}\underline{D}\text{-}Nal(2)^1,\underline{D}\text{-}pCl\text{-}Phe^2,\underline{D}\text{-}Pal(3)^3,Arg^5,\underline{D}\text{-}Trp(For)^6,\underline{D}\text{-}Ala^{10}]LHRH$	0.5		[56]
18 $[N\text{-}Ac\text{-}\underline{D}\text{-}Nal(2)^1,\underline{D}\text{-}pCl\text{-}Phe^2,\underline{D}\text{-}Pal(3)^3,Arg^5,\underline{D}\text{-}Glu(\text{-}\phi\text{-}OCH_3),\underline{D}\text{-}Ala^{10}]LHRH$	<1.4[d]		[56]
19 $[N\text{-}Ac\text{-}\underline{D}\text{-}Nal(2)^1,\underline{D}\text{-}pCl\text{-}Phe^2,\underline{D}\text{-}Pal(3)^{3,6},Pal(3)^5,\underline{D}\text{-}Ala^{10}]LHRH$	<1		[75]
20 $[N\text{-}Ac\text{-}\underline{D}\text{-}Nal(2)^1,\underline{D}\text{-}pCl\text{-}Phe^2,\underline{D}\text{-}Pal(3)^{3,6},Arg^5,\underline{D}\text{-}Ala^{10}]LHRH$	<0.13		[75]
21 $[N\text{-}Ac\text{-}\underline{D}\text{-}Nal(2)^1,\underline{D}\text{-}\alpha\text{-}Me,pCl\text{-}Phe^2,\underline{D}\text{-}Pal(3)^3,\underline{D}\text{-}Arg^6,Lys(iPr)^8,\underline{D}\text{-}Ala^{10}]LHRH$	<0.5		[e]
22 $[N\text{-}Ac\text{-}\underline{D}\text{-}Nal(2)^1,\underline{D}\text{-}\alpha\text{-}Me,pCl\text{-}Phe^2,\underline{D}\text{-}Pal(3)^3,\underline{D}\text{-}Lys(iPr)^6,Lys(iPr)^8,\underline{D}\text{-}Ala^{10}]LHRH$	<0.5		[e]
23 $[N\text{-}Ac\text{-}\underline{D}\text{-}Nal(2)^1,\underline{D}\text{-}\alpha\text{-}Me,pCl\text{-}Phe^2,\underline{D}\text{-}Pal(3)^3,\underline{D}\text{-}Arg^6,\underline{D}\text{-}hArg(Et_2)^8,\underline{D}\text{-}Ala^{10}]LHRH$	<1		[e]

[a]The compound names are given in standard form where the superscript denotes the position of substitution within the LHRH (pGlu^1-His^2-Trp^3-Ser^4-Tyr^5-Gly^6-Leu^7-Arg^8-Pro^9-Gly^{10}-NH$_2$) structure. The standard three letter code is given for the proteinogenic amino acids. Unnatural amino acids are: pF-Phe, para-fluorophenylalanine; pCl-Phe, para-chlorophenylalanine; Δ^3-Pro, $\Delta^{3,4}$-dehydroproline; Nal(2), 3-(2-naphthyl)-alanine; hArg(Et$_2$), N^G,N$^{G'}$-diethylhomo-arginine; α-Me,pCl-Phe, C-alpha-methyl-pCl-phenylalanine; Glu($\text{-}\phi\text{-}$OCH$_3$), 4-(p-methoxybenzoyl)-2-aminobutyric acid; Pal(3), 3-(3-pyridyl)alanine. [b]In cases where a true ED$_{50}$ value is not available, an approximate value is given as "less than" a value which was reported to be more than 50% effective at that dose. [c]Vehicle—50% propylene glycol-saline; see [39] [d]Vehicle—saline. [e]Chapter 2.

7

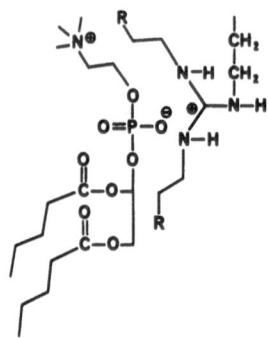

Figure 1.   Hypothesized   interaction   between   hArg(R_2) and phospho-
             lipid membranes.

FACTORS AFFECTING POTENCY

The potency of a compound in vivo is the result of a series of
interacting factors, including receptor affinity, intrinsic
agonistic activity (stimulus-response coupling), tissue distribution and biological half-life ($t_{1/2}$). For competitive antagonists,
very high receptor affinity and a long duration of action are
critical factors.   While receptor binding data are not always
reported for antagonists (see, however, [40,55,56]), many of the
most potent analogs do have receptor affinities equal to the best
of the LHRH agonists (5-20x that of LHRH).   Receptor kinetics
studies showed also that the LHRH antagonists as a class had much
slower off-rates than LHRH [57,58]. Unfortunately, the receptor
affinity of antagonists does not correlate well with in vivo
potency [40,55,56].   Beyond a certain level of receptor affinity
receptor kinetics, distribution, and pharmacokinetic distribution
may become overriding factors.
     Attempts to increase the duration of action of peptide hormone
analogs have frequently focused on blocking sites of proteolysis.
The most potent antagonists studied recently have D-amino acids
blocking the N- and C-termini as well as the known sites of attack
by endoproteases (bonds 1-2, 3-4, 5-6, 9-10).   Protection from
proteolysis alone is not sufficient to provide analogs with very
long duration of action [59], however, since small molecules may
still be cleared rapidly by glomerular filtration.
     The overall hydrophobicity of drugs frequently plays a role in
their distribution and pharmacokinetics [60].   Studies with LHRH
agonists showed that potency could be correlated with hydrophobicity, both qualitatively [11,61] and in quantitative structure-
activity relationships [62,63]. In early studies of LHRH agonists,
increased hydrophobicity was suggested to cause a prolonged duration of action due to hydrophobic depoting in the body [11,34].
This could be due to binding to hydrophobic sites in plasma (serum
albumin [64]) and on cell membranes [P. Felgner, unpublished].
     Until recently, the most potent LHRH antagonists were very
hydrophobic molecules. A hydrophilic type of depoting which relies

8

on electrostatic attraction between positively charged residues and negatively charged cell membranes has been hypothesized [11,65] and used in the design of LHRH agonists and antagonists [11,65,66]. The most potent LHRH antagonists contain both very hydrophobic and positively charged residues. Such analogs are expected to show very high affinity for cell membranes and hydrophobic spaces in the body. These analogs should spend little time in the body in a free state, and therefore be unavailable for proteolysis and renal filtration. The combination of high membrane affinity and polycationic nature seems ideally suited for mast cell degranulation.

Hydrophobicity also has been correlated with increased receptor affinity [67]. Schwyzer hypothesized that peptide ligands must interact with cell membranes prior to receptor loading [68]. This suggests [65] that changes which facilitate membrane interaction, such as increased hydrophobicity (to a point), may increase receptor affinity [69]. Overall _in vivo_ potency therefore probably reflects changes in both $t_{1/2}$ and receptor affinity.

SIDE EFFECTS

Mast cell degranulation

Toxicological study of the "D-Arg^6" class of antagonists uncovered their ability to cause mast cell degranulation and anaphylactoid effects [70]. Many neuropeptides, including LHRH itself, cause mast cell degranulation [71,72], but the "D-Arg^6" antagonists are particularly potent in this regard with ED_{50}'s for this action of $<10^{-6}M$ _in vitro_ [73; Chapters 11,12]. _In vitro_ studies are not always good predictors of the _in vivo_ histamine response, however, and rate of entry of the compound into the body seems important. Although 11 and the more hydrophobic detirelix (15) have similar _in vitro_ histamine releasing potencies, the former causes a systemic histamine release (edema) when given subcutaneously (sc) to rats at 1.25 mg/kg [71] while detirelix only shows this systemic effect when massive doses (20 mg/kg or more) are given sc [Chapter 14]. By rapid intravenous administration, however, detirelix will cause some edema at doses less than 1 mg/kg [Chapter 14]. The difference may be caused by an increased ability of detirelix to form a depot in the body and be more slowly released to the circulation.

Compounds which have high membrane affinity and two or more positive charges are frequently good mast cell degranulators [71]. Peptide hormones are thought to have membrane affinity in order to interact efficiently with membrane bound receptors [68], and this may explain why many neuropeptides are histamine releasers [72].

Analogs with reduced histamine release

The fact that side reactions were seen in toxicology studies [70, 73; Chapters 11,12,14] and mild side reactions (wheal and flare; urticaria; flushing) were observed intermittently in man [42; Chapter 18] with these agents led much of the recent work in this

9

area to be devoted to the design of analogs with reduced histamine release [Chapters 2,3,11,12]. Initial studies focused on increasing the distance between the Arg[8] of the native LHRH sequence and the D-Arg[6] substitution which gave increased duration of action [75]. [Ac-D-Nal(2)[1],D-α-Me,pCl-Phe[2],D-Trp[3],Arg[5],D-Tyr[6],D-Ala[10]]-LHRH was 37x less potent for histamine release but was only diminished slightly in its antiovulatory potency. A similar series of analogs [56], employing Pal(3)[3] and focusing on 6-position substitution, provided analogs such as 17 and 18, which combined high potency and lowered histamine releasing potency compared to 11. Compound 18 contains a hydrophobic substitution in position 6 which arose as a byproduct during synthesis (addition of anisole to Glu in strong acid) and was chosen for possible clinical studies.

When the Pal residue is used in position 6, high antiovulatory potency is achieved [75] with only moderate histamine release (compounds 19, 20). Compound 20 is currently the most potent LHRH antagonist reported, achieving a 60% suppression of ovulation at a 0.125 µg dose (ED$_{100}$ 0.5 µg). The Pal(3) residue has resulted in potency increases in several analog studies and might be functioning as a moderately basic, membrane binding component.

A series of compounds which were designed for enhanced membrane interaction (see above; Chapter 3) containing N$^\epsilon$-alkyl-Lys residues (compounds 21, 22) also showed diminished histamine release relative to compound 11. Compound 22 is particularly interesting since the Arg[8] of LHRH has been replaced in this analog, resulting in a significant fall in histamine release but high antiovulatory potency. A frequently seen sequence in the neuropeptides which release histamine is Arg-Pro [76]. This suggests an involvement of Arg[8] of LHRH in histamine release, in accord with the results of Lys(iPr)[8] substitution. The decreased histamine release of 21 is unlikely to be due to the reduced basicity of the Lys(iPr) versus Arg since 23, containing the strongly basic hArg(Et$_2$) residue, behaves similarly. Shielding of the charge on the residue in position 8 is a more likely explanation and will undoubtably receive further study. The incorporation of amino acids in position 8 which have increased shielding or a further reduced basicity, but which retain an electrostatic attraction for the negatively charged membrane, is an attractive strategy for the design of analogs with reduced histamine releasing potency.

CONCLUDING REMARKS

The synthetic studies with LHRH antagonists follow from the observation that His[2] and possibly Trp[3] were involved in the stimulus-response coupling of the receptor. The development process has involved a stepwise introduction of residues (generally hydrophobic) which block proteolysis, increase receptor affinity and prolong the pharmacokinetics of the molecule, possibly by depoting in the body. More recently, the introduction of additional positively charged residues into LHRH antagonists has resulted in increased potency and duration of action, but at the cost of increased mast cell degranulating activity. Current analog synthesis studies are focused on retention of high antiovulatory potency with reduced histamine-releasing potency.

Laboratory animal models and preliminary clinical studies have demonstrated the superiority of the early LHRH antagonists to the LHRH agonists for rapidity of action in gonadal suppression. The ongoing detailed clinical studies with the present generation of more potent, longer acting LHRH antagonists are expected to provide further support for the eventual commercial development of a drug candidate, particularly if the reduced capacity to induce release of mast cell mediators noted in vitro and in animal models holds true in clinical evaluation.

REFERENCES

1. Matsuo, H., Arimura, A., Nair, R.M.G. and Schally, A.V. Synthesis of the porcine LH- and FSH-releasing hormone by the solid-phase method. Biochem. Biophys. Res. Commun., 45, 822 (1971).
2. Burgus, R., Butcher, M., Amoss, M., Ling, N., Monahan, M.W., Rivier, J. and Fellows, R. Primary structure of the ovine hypothalamic luteinizing hormone-releasing factor (LRF). Proc. Natl. Acad. Sci. USA, 69, 278 (1972).
3. Monahan, M.W., Rivier, J., Vale, W., Guillemin, R. and Burgus, R. [Gly^2]LRF and des-His^2-LRF. The synthesis, purification, and characterization of two LRF analogues antagonistic to LRF. Biochem. Biophys. Res. Commun., 47, 551 (1972).
4. Corbin, A. and Beattie, C.W. Inhibition of the preovulatory proestrus gonadotropin surge, ovulation and pregnancy with a peptide analog of luteinizing hormone-releasing hormone. Endocr. Res. Commun., 2, 1 (1975).
5. Loumaye, E. and Catt, K.J. Homologous regulation of gonadotropin-releasing hormone receptors in cultured pituitary cells. Science, 215, 983 (1982).
6. Keri, G., Nikolics, K., Teplan, I. and Molnar, J. Desensitization of luteinizing hormone release in cultured pituitary cells by gonadotropin-releasing hormone. Mol. Cell. Endocrinol., 30, 109 (1983).
7. Rivier, C., Vale, W. and Rivier, J. Effects of gonadotropin releasing hormone agonists and antagonists on reproductive functions. J. Med. Chem., 26, 1545 (1983).
8. a. Vickery, B.H. Pharmacology of LHRH antagonists. In "Pharmacology and Clinical Uses of Inhibitors of Hormone Secretion and Action", B.J.A. Furr and A. Wakeling (Eds.), Bailliere Tindall, London, 1986, p. 385. b. Vickery, B.H. Comparison of the potential for therapeutic utilities with gonadotropin-releasing hormone agonists and antagonists. Endocr. Rev., 7, 115 (1986).
9. Belchetz, P.E., Plant, T.M., Nakai, Y., Keogh, E.J. and Knobil, E. Hypophyseal responses to continuous and intermittent delivery of hypothalamic gonadotropin-releasing hormone. Science, 202, 631 (1978).
10. Clayton, R.N. Gonadotropin-releasing hormone modulation of its own pituitary receptors: evidence for biphasic regulation. Endocrinology, 111, 152 (1982).

11. Nestor, J.J. Jr., Ho, T.L., Tahilramani, R., Horner, B.L., Simpson, R.A., Jones, G.H., McRae, G.I. and Vickery, B.H. LHRH agonists and antagonists containing very hydrophobic amino acids. In "LHRH and Its Analogs: Contraceptive and Therapeutic Applications", B.H. Vickery, J.J. Nestor, Jr., and E.S.E. Hafez (Eds.), MTP Press, Boston, 1984, p. 23.

12. Karten, M.J. and Rivier, J.E. Gonadotropin-releasing hormone analog design. Structure-function studies toward the development of agonists and antagonists: rationale and perspectives. Endocr. Rev., 7, 44 (1986).

13. Nekola, M.V. and Coy, D.H. LHRH antagonists in females. In "LHRH and Its Analogs: Contraceptive and Therapeutic Applications", B.H. Vickery, J.J. Nestor, Jr. and E.S.E. Hafez (Eds.), MTP Press, Boston, 1984, p. 125.

14. Vickery, B.H. and Nestor, J.J. Jr. LHRH analogues: development and mechanism of action. Sem. Reprod. Endocrinol., in press (1986).

15. Vale, W., Grant, G., Rivier, J., Monahan, M., Amoss, M., Blackwell, R., Burgus, R. and Guillemin, R. Synthetic polypeptide antagonists of the hypothalamic luteinizing hormone releasing factor. Science, 176, 933 (1972).

16. Grant, G.F. and Vale, W. Hypothalamic control of anterior pituitary hormone secretion-characterized hypothalamic-hypophysiotropic peptides. In "Current Topics in Experimental Endocrinology", V.H.T. James and L. Martini (Eds.), Academic Press, New York, 1974, p. 38.

17. Rees, R.W.A., Foell, T.J., Chai, S-Y. and Grant, N. Synthesis and biological activities of analogs of the luteinizing hormone-releasing hormone (LH-RH) modified in position 2. J. Med. Chem., 17, 1016 (1974).

18. Strulovici, B. and Nestor, J.J. Jr. Gonadotropin releasing hormone induces the phosphorylation of specific pituitary proteins: direct involvement of protein kinase C. VIth International Conference on Cyclic Nucleotides, Calcium and Protein Phosphorylation, Bethesda, MD, September 1986, Abstract 191.

19. Monahan, M.W., Amoss, M.S., Anderson, H.A. and Vale, W. Synthetic analogs of the hypothalamic luteinizing hormone releasing factor with increased agonist or antagonist properties. Biochemistry, 12, 4616 (1973).

20. Yardley, J.P., Foell, T.J., Beattie, C.W. and Grant, N.H. Antagonism of luteinizing hormone release and of ovulation by an analog of the luteinizing hormone-releasing hormone. J. Med. Chem., 18, 1244 (1975).

21. Beattie, C.W., Corbin, A., Foell, T.J., Garsky, V., McKinley, W.A., Rees, R.W.A., Sarantakis, D. and Yardley, J.P. Luteinizing hormone-releasing hormone. Antiovulation activity of analogs substituted in position 2 and 6. J. Med. Chem., 18, 1247 (1975).

22. De la Cruz, A., Coy, D.H., Vilchez-Martinez, J.A., Arimura, A. and Schally, A.V. Blockade of ovulation in rats by inhibitory analogs of luteinizing hormone-releasing hormone. Science, 191, 195 (1976).

23. Humphries, J., Wan, Y.P., Folkers, K. and Bowers, C.Y. Presence of proline in position 3 for potent inhibition of the

activity of the luteinizing hormone-releasing hormone and of ovulation. Biochem. Biophys. Res. Commun., 72, 939 (1976).

24. Coy, D.H., Vilchez-Martinez, J.A. and Schally, A.V. Structure-function studies on LRF. In "Peptides 1976", A. Loffet (Ed.), Editions de l'Université de Bruxelles, 1977, p. 463.

25. Seprodi, J., Coy, D.H., Vilchez-Martinez, J.A., Pedroza, E. and Schally, A.V. Branched-chain analogues of luteinizing hormone-releasing hormone. J. Med. Chem., 21, 276 (1982).

26. Rivier, J.E. and Vale, W.W. [D-pGlu[1],D-Phe[2],D-Trp[3,6]]LRF: A potent luteinizing hormone-releasing factor antagonist in vitro and inhibitor of ovulation in the rat. Life Sci., 23, 869 (1978).

27. Momany, F.A. Conformational analysis of the molecule luteinizing hormone-releasing hormone. 3. Analog inhibitors and antagonists. J. Med. Chem., 21, 63 (1978).

28. Humphries, J., Wisiak, T., Wan, Y-P. and Folkers, K. An antiovulatory decapeptide of higher potency which has an L-amino acid (Ac-Pro) in position 1. Biochem. Biophys. Res. Commun., 85, 709 (1978).

29. Nestor, J.J. Jr., Tahilramani, R., Ho, T.L., McRae, G.I. and Vickery, B.H. Luteinizing hormone-releasing hormone antagonists containing very hydrophobic amino acids. J. Med. Chem., 27, 1170 (1984).

30. Channabasavaiah, K. and Stewart, J.M. New analogs of luliberin which inhibit ovulation in the rat. Biochem. Biophys. Res. Commun., 86, 1266 (1979).

31. Rivier, J., Rivier, C., Perrin, M., Porter, J. and Vale, W.W. GnRH analogs: Structure activity relationships. In "LHRH Peptides as Female and Male Contraceptives", G.I. Zatuchni, J.D. Shelton and J.J. Sciarra (Eds.), Harper & Row, Philadelphia, 1981, p. 13.

32. Spatola, A.F. and Agarwal, N.S. A highly potent antiovulatory LH-RH analogue with no 1-position side chain. Biochem. Biophys. Res. Commun., 97, 1571 (1980).

33. Coy, D.H., Mezo, I., Pedroza, E., Nekola, M.V., Vilchez-Martinez, J.A., Piyachaturawat, P., Schally, A.V., Seprodi, J. and Teplan, I. LHRH antagonists with potent antiovulatory activity. In "Peptides: Structure and Biological Function", E. Gross and J. Meienhofer (Eds.), Pierce Chemical Co., Rockford, IL, 1979, p. 775.

34. Nestor, J.J. Jr., Ho, T.L., Simpson, R.A., Horner, B.L., Jones, G.H., McRae, G.I. and Vickery, B.H. The synthesis and biological activity of some very hydrophobic analogs of luteinizing hormone-releasing hormone. J. Med. Chem., 25, 795 (1982).

35. Rivier, C., Rivier, J., Perrin, M. and Vale, W. Comparison of the effect of several gonadotropin releasing hormone antagonists on luteinizing hormone secretion, receptor binding and ovulation. Biol. Reprod., 29, 374 (1983).

36. Cetel, N.S., Rivier, J., Vale, W. and Yen, S.S.C. The dynamics of gonadotropin inhibition in women induced by an antagonistic analog of gonadotropin-releasing hormone. J. Clin. Endocrinol. Metab., 57, 62 (1983).

37. McRae, G.I., Vickery, B.H., Nestor, J.J. Jr., Bremner, W.J.

and Badger, T.M. Biological activity of a highly potent LHRH antagonist. In "LHRH and Its Analogs: Contraceptive and Therapeutic Applications", B.H. Vickery, J.J. Nestor, Jr. and E.S.E. Hafez (Eds.), MTP Press, Boston, 1984, p. 137.

38. Coy, D.H., Horvath, A., Nekola, M.V., Coy, E.J., Erchegyi, J. and Schally, A.V. Peptide antagonists of LH-RH: large increases in antiovulatory activities produced by basic D-amino acids in the six position. Endocrinology, 110, 1445 (1982).

39. Nestor, J.J. Jr., Tahilramani, R., Ho, T.L., McRae, G.I., Vickery, B.H. and Bremner, W.J. New luteinizing hormone-releasing factor antagonists. In "Peptides: Structure and Function", V.J. Hruby and D.H. Rich (Eds.), Pierce Chemical Co., Rockford, IL, 1983, p. 861.

40. Rivier, J., Rivier, C., Perrin, M., Porter, J. and Vale, W. LHRH analogs as antiovulatory agents. In "LHRH and Its Analogs--Contraceptive and Therapeutic Applications", B.H. Vickery, J.J. Nestor, Jr. and E.S.E. Hafez (Eds.), MTP Press, Boston, 1984, p. 11.

41. Horvath, A., Coy, D.H., Nekola, M.V., Coy, E.J., Schally, A.V. and Teplan, I. Synthesis and biological activity of LH-RH antagonists modified in position 1. Peptides, 3, 969 (1982).

42. Hall, J.E., Brodie, T.D., Rivier, J., Vale, W, Badger, T.M. and Crowley, W.F. Jr. Use of a gonadotropin releasing hormone antagonist in the early follicular phase of the menstrual cycle. Clin. Res., 34, 425A (1986).

43. Vickery, B.H., McRae, G.I., Sanders, L.M., Hoffman, P., Pavlou, S.N. Studies with nafarelin and a long-acting LHRH antagonist. In "Proceedings of the International Symposium on Hormonal Manipulation of Cancer: Peptides, Growth Factors and New (Anti) Steroidal Agents", J.G.M. Klijn (Ed.), 1986, in press.

44. Erchegyi, J., Coy, D.H., Nekola, M.V., Coy, E.J., Schally, A.V., Mezo, I. and Teplan, I. Luteinizing hormone-releasing hormone analogs with increased anti-ovulatory activity. Biochem. Biophys. Res. Commun., 100, 915 (1981).

45. Marks, N. and Stern, F. Enzymatic mechanisms for the inactivation of luteinizing hormone-releasing hormone (LHRH). Biochem. Biophys. Res. Commun., 61, 1458 (1974).

46. Fujino, M., Shinagawa, S., Yamazuki, I., Kobayashi, S., Obayashi, M., Fukuda, T., Nakayama, R., White, W.F. and Rippel, R.H. [Des-Gly-NH$_2$[10],Pro-ethylamide[9]]-LH-RH: A highly potent analog of luteinizing hormone-releasing hormone. Arch. Biochem. Biophys., 154, 488 (1973).

47. Dutta, A.S., Furr, B.J.A., Giles, M.B., Valcaccia, B. and Walpole, A.L. Potent agonist and antagonist analogues of luliberin containing an azaglycine residue in position 10. Biochem. Biophys. Res. Commun., 81, 382 (1978).

48. Folkers, K., Bowers, C.Y., Stepinski, J., Placinsky, T., Sakagami, M. and Kubiak, T. Analogs of the luteinizing hormone releasing hormone having the azagly[10] moiety with antiovulatory activity. Z. Naturforsch., 39b, 528 (1984).

49. Vilchez-Martinez, J.A., Schally, A.V., Coy, D.H., Coy, E.J., Miller, C.M. and Arimura, A. An in vivo assay for anti-LH-RH

14

and anti-FSH-RH activity of inhibitory analogues of LHRH. Endocrinology, 96, 1130 (1975).

50. Folkers, K., Bowers, C.Y., Shieh, H-M., Yin-Zeng, L., Shao-Bo, X., Tang, P-F.L. and Ji-Yu, C. Antagonists of the luteinizing hormone releasing hormone (LHRH) with emphasis on the Trp[7] of the salmon and chicken II LHRH's. Biochem. Biophys. Res. Commun., 123, 1221 (1984).

51. Hocart, S.J., Nekola, M.V. and Coy, D.H. Improved antagonists of luteinizing hormone-releasing hormone modified in position 7. J. Med. Chem., 28, 967 (1985).

52. Folkers, K., Bowers, C.Y., Kubiak, T. and Stepinski, J. Antagonists of the luteinizing hormone releasing hormone with pyridyl-alanines which completely inhibit ovulation at nanogram dosage. Biochem. Biophys. Res. Commun., 111, 1089 (1983).

53. Weinbauer, G.F., Surmann, F.J., Akhtar, F.B., Shah, G.V., Vickery, B.H. and Nieschlag, E. Reversible inhibition of testicular function by a gonadotropin hormone-releasing hormone antagonist in monkeys (Macaca fascicularis). Fertil. Steril., 42, 906 (1985).

54. Adams, L.A., Bremner, W.J., Nestor, J.J. Jr., Vickery, B.H. and Steiner, R.A. Suppression of plasma gonadotropins and testosterone in adult male monkeys (Macaca fascicularis) by a potent inhibitory analog of gonadotropin-releasing hormone. J. Clin. Endocrinol. Metab., 62, 58 (1986).

55. Perrin, M., Rivier, J. and Vale, W. Radioligand assay for gonadotropin-releasing hormone: relative potencies of agonists and antagonists. Endocrinology, 106, 1289 (1980).

56. Rivier, J.E., Porter, J., Rivier, C.L., Perrin, M., Corrigan, A., Hook, W.A., Siraganian, R.P. and Vale, W.W. New effective gonadotropin releasing hormone antagonists with minimal potency for histamine release in vitro. J. Med. Chem., 29, 1846 (1986).

57. Heber, D., Dodson, R., Swerdloff, R.S., Channabasavaiah, K. and Stewart, J.M. Pituitary receptor site blockade by a gonadotropin-releasing hormone antagonist in vivo: mechanism of action. Science, 216, 420 (1982).

58. Loumaye, E., Wynn, P.C., Coy, D. and Catt, K.J. Receptor-binding properties of gonadotropin-releasing hormone derivatives. J. Biol. Chem., 259, 12663 (1984).

59. Rudinger, J. The design of peptide hormone analogs. In "Drug Design, Vol. II", E.J. Ariens (Ed.), Academic Press, New York, NY, 1971, p. 319.

60. Gillette, J.R. Overview of drug-protein binding. Ann. N.Y. Acad. Sci., 226, 6 (1973).

61. Rivier, J., Brown, M., Rivier, C., Ling, N. and Vale, W. Hypothalamic hypophysiotropic hormones. In "Peptides 1976", A. Loffet (Ed.), Editions de l'Université de Bruxelles, Brussels, 1977, p. 427.

62. Nadasdi, L. and Medzihradszky, K. A study of the applicability of QSAR calculation for peptide hormones. Biochem. Biophys. Res. Commun., 99, 451 (1981).

63. Zeelen, F.J. The strategy of the development of peptide drugs. Chemtech, 419 (1983).

64. Chan, R.L. and Chaplin, M.D. Plasma binding of LHRH and nafarelin acetate. Biochem. Biophys. Res. Commun., 127, 673 (1985).

65. Nestor, J.J. Jr. Luteinizing hormone-releasing hormone agonists and antagonists as drugs. In "Third SCI-RSC Medicinal Chemistry Symposium, Special Publication No. 55", R.W. Lambert (Ed.), The Royal Society of Chemistry, London, 1986, p. 362.

66. Nestor, J.J. Jr., Tahilramani, R., Ho, T.L., McRae, G.I. and Vickery, B.H. Potent LHRH agonists containing $N^G, N^{G'}$-dialkyl-D-homoarginines. In "Peptides--Structure and Function", C.M. Deber, V.J. Hruby and K. Koppel (Eds.), Pierce Chemical Co., Rockford, IL, 1985, p. 557.

67. Geiger, R. Design and synthesis of LHRH agonists and antagonists. In "LHRH and Its Analogues--Basic and Clinical Aspects", F. Labrie, A. Belanger and A. Dupont (Eds.), Elsevier Science Publishers, NY, 1984, p. 36.

68. Schwyzer, R., Gremlich, H-U., Gysin, B., Sargent, D.F. and Fringeli, U-P. Specific interactions between peptide hormones and artificial lipid membranes. In "Peptides: Structure and Function", V.J. Hruby and D.H. Rich (Eds.), Pierce Chemical Co., Rockford, IL, 1983, p. 657.

69. Nestor, J.J. Jr., Newman, S.R., DeLustro, B.M. and Schreiber, A.B. Antagonistic analogs of human transforming growth factor alpha. In "Peptides--Structure and Function", C.M. Deber, V.J. Hruby and K. Koppel (Eds.), Pierce Chemical Co., Rockford, IL, 1985, p. 39.

70. Schmidt, F., Sundaram, K., Thau, R.B. and Bardin, C.W. [Ac-D-Nal(2)^1,4FD-Phe^2,D-Trp^3,D-Arg^6]-LHRH, a potent antagonist of LHRH, produces transient edema and behavioral changes in rats. Contraception, 29, 283 (1984).

71. Lagunoff, D., Martin, T.W. and Read, G. Agents that release histamine from mast cells. Ann. Rev. Pharmacol. Toxicol., 23, 331 (1983).

72. Foreman, J. and Jordan, C. Histamine release and vascular changes induced by neuropeptides. Agents and Actions, 13, 105 (1983).

73. Morgan, J.E., O'Neil, C.E., Coy, D.H., Hocart, S.J. and Nekola, M.V. Antagonistic analogs of luteinizing hormone-releasing hormone are mast cell secretagogues. Int. Arch. Allergy Appl. Immunol., 80, 70 (1986).

74. Roeske, R.W., Chaturvedi, N.C., Rivier, J., Vale, W., Porter, J. and Perrin, M. Substitution of Arg^5 for Tyr^5 in GNRH antagonists. In "Peptides: Structure and Function", C.M. Deber, V.J. Hruby and K.D. Kopple (Eds.), Pierce Chemical Co., Rockford, IL, 1985, p. 561.

75. Folkers, K., Bowers, C., Shao-bo, X., Tang, P-F.L. and Kubota, M. Increased potency of antagonists of the luteinizing hormone releasing hormone which have D-3-Pal in position 6. Biochem. Biophys. Res. Commun., 137, 709 (1986).

76. Sydbom, A. and Terenius, L. The histamine-releasing effect of dynorphin and other peptides possessing Arg-Pro sequences. Agents and Actions, 16, 269 (1985).

2
LHRH Antagonists with Low Histamine Releasing Activity

R.W. ROESKE, N.C. CHATURVEDI, T. HRINYO-PAVLINA and M. KOWALCZUK

Department of Biochemistry, Indiana University School of Medicine, Indianapolis, IN 46223, USA

INTRODUCTION

Many synthetic antagonists of LHRH having pituitary receptor binding affinities of 10 to 20 times that of LHRH itself have been made. Generally, the best antagonists have an ED_{50} of about one microgram per animal in the rat antiovulatory assay. Most of these highly effective antagonists have a D-arginine residue in position 6 which, with the L-arginine[8] of the native molecule and with a hydrophobic cluster of residues in the N-terminal part of the molecule, appears to be a potent combination for the release of histamine from mast cells.

As a result of the observation by Schmidt et al. [1] of an inflammatory reaction in rats that had received subcutaneous injections of various potent LHRH antagonists, attention has been focused for several years on modifying the structures of antagonists in order to minimize histamine releasing potency while maintaining or improving antiovulatory activity (Chapter 11). This chapter summarizes progress toward that end.

TRANSPOSITION OF RESIDUES 5 AND 6

The structural requirements for potent histamine releasing activity in peptides are not well defined but almost always include two or more Lys or Arg residues adjacent to each other or not far removed in the sequence. A change in the configuration of one of the residues, presumably leading to a different conformational relationship of the ends of the basic side chains may change the histamine releasing activity. Thus, the histamine releasing activity of somatostatin, H-Ala-Gly-Cys-Lys-Asn-Phe-Phe-Trp-Lys-Thr-Phe-Thr-Ser-Cys-OH, is reduced by 80% by a D-Lys[4] substitution, but increased 4-fold by a D-Lys[9] [2]. In a pair of LHRH antagonists, the Arg[6,8] combination of residues is 20% as effective in releasing histamine as is the D-Arg[6], Arg[8] pattern (Chapter 11), but the former has much lower antiovulatory activity.

By transposing residues 5 and 6 in an LHRH antagonist (compare 1 and 2; Tyr[5], D-Arg[6] --> Arg[5], D-Tyr[6]) we found that the histamine releasing activity was reduced to about 3% that of the original analog and the antiovulatory activity was reduced by about 50% [3]. This was a serendipitous finding, since we were led to make the switch for a different reason. The presence of a β-turn involving residues 5-8 of LHRH was predicted by conformational energy calculations [4]. Good evidence for such a turn was provided since the use of a δ-lactam conformational constraint in place of residues 6 and 7 to form a constrained molecule simulating a β-turn was more active than the native hormone [5]. Since a D-residue in position 6, which also stabilizes the β-turn, improves both agonist and antagonist activity, the presence of a 5-8 β-turn in both agonist and antagonist molecules was a reasonable assumption. It seemed likely to us that in the receptor-antagonist complex, the side chain of residue 6 is not in contact with a specific group, but interacts with components of the cell membrane, either the negatively-charged head groups or the hydrocarbon chains of the lipids. This would explain the high activity of either a large hydrophobic residue or of a positively-charged residue in position 6 and the low activity of an antagonist having D-Glu[6]. Nestor et al. [6,7] have used the same concept to design long-acting antagonists modified in position 6. In order to determine whether the side chain of residue 5 was in a similar environment, we synthesized a series of antagonists having Arg[5] or Lys[5] with a hydrophobic D-residue in position 6. Many substitutions for Tyr[5] had been made earlier, but none had a basic side chain. Compound 2 was the best of the series. Rivier et al. [8] explored the 5,6-transposition further with a series of D-Pal[3], Arg[5], D-hydrophobic[6]-containing analogs, e.g. 3-6, 8-10 and found that none had substantially lower histamine releasing potency than 2.

Similarly, Folkers et al. [9], in synthesizing a series of D-Pal[6] antagonists, found the Arg[5], D-Pal[6] combination 8, to have the highest AO activity. Histamine release was determined by measuring wheal area in vivo and is difficult to compare with the in vitro assay. However, it was established that D-Pal[6] analogs release somewhat less histamine than the comparable D-Arg[6] compounds.

In general, Arg[5], D-(hydrophobic residue)[6] analogs have slightly lower antiovulatory potency than the corresponding Tyr[5], D-Arg[6] compounds, but are only 3 to 5% as active in releasing histamine. This favorable separation of activities in the transposition analogs was explored further using alkylated basic side chains.

ALKYLATED AMINES IN POSITIONS 5, 6 AND 8

Another class of peptides that has provided separation of anti-ovulatory and histamine releasing activity is characterized by one or more residues having alkyl groups on the nitrogen atoms of basic side chains, e.g. diethylhomoarginine, hArg(Et$_2$), N$^\epsilon$-isopropyl lysine, Lys(iPr), N$^\delta$-isopropyl ornithine, Orn(iPr), N$^\epsilon$-trimethyl lysine, Lys(Me$_3$), and N-methyl-3-pyridinium alanine, Me-Pal. As in the 5,6-transposition series, the lowered histamine-releasing activity was a fortuitous finding; initially the rationale for making the compounds was not related to histamine release.

Diethylhomoarginine, prepared by reaction of lysine with diethylcarbodiimide, was introduced by Nestor et al. [6] as a hydrophobic derivative of arginine, to prolong the activity of agonists and antagonists by increasing their affinity for cell membranes. We first used Orn(iPr) and Lys(iPr) as residues that approximated the conformation of arginine [10] and might enhance oral activity of peptides by facilitating their diffusion through the intestinal wall.

Residue 8 appears to be a more important determinant of histamine release than residue 6. Although substitution of D-Arg^6 by D-hArg(Et$_2$) lowers histamine release only slightly (compare 1 and 11), substitution of Arg^8 by hArg(Et$_2$), 12, or by Lys(iPr), 13, is much more effective. In comparing 12 and 13 with 1, the effect of the C-α-methyl group on histamine release is probably quite small, but the D-Pal^3 residue may contribute somewhat more to reduced potency. Replacing both D-Arg^6 and Arg^8 by D- and L-Lys(iPr), respectively, gives 14, having less than 2% of the histamine releasing potency of 1, without any loss of antiovulatory activity. The Lys(iPr)^5, D-Tyr^6, Lys(iPr)^8 combination, 15, is about half as effective as 14 and the Lys(iPr)^5, D-Trp^6, Arg^8 array, 16, is about one-third as effective in reducing histamine release. The D-Lys(iPr)^6, Lys(iPr)^8 compound was improved by substitution of Tyr^5 by Ile^5 to give 17, further reducing the histamine releasing activity to an ED$_{50}$ of 9.9, approximately 1% that of the standard compound 1, while retaining very high anti-ovulatory activity. There is some earlier evidence that aromatic residues enhance histamine release more than aliphatic residues of comparable hydrophobicity [11]. Thus, replacing a D-Phe by D-Leu in the cyclic octapeptide polymyxin B, which contains four basic residues, lowers histamine release by a factor of 50.

In searching for an explanation of the efficacy of Lys(iPr) and hArg(Et$_2$) residues, we postulated that alkyl groups obstruct the formation of hydrogen bonds between the amino groups and the histamine-release receptor. These bonds probably are not required for a good (electrostatic) interaction with the LHRH receptor in the pituitary, since antiovulatory activity and binding constants are not changed appreciably by the substitutions in positions 5, 6 and 8. If this is valid, Lys(Me$_3$) residues should be at least as effective as Lys(iPr) in lowering histamine release, since they cannot participate in hydrogen bonding. But when 18 was synthesized and tested, the ugly facts were that the ED$_{50}$ for histamine release was 1.10 μg/ml, about 1/6 that of the analogous Lys(iPr) compound 14, and that the antiovulatory activity was also lower. This postulate was abandoned.

Another residue, Me-Pal, also devoid of hydrogen bonding possibilities, was more effective than Lys(Me$_3$) but less effective than Lys(iPr) when it was used in both positions 6 and 8 in the same molecule (compare 14, 18 and 19).

When the different basic residues are used in the same molecule, in positions 5 or 6 and 8, the results are less clear. Ranking various combinations in decreasing order of effectiveness in lowering histamine release gives the following sequence:

Table 1. Histamine releasing potency and antiovulatory potency of LHRH analogs

Analog	In Vitro Histamine Release (ug/ml) ED$_{50}$	Ovulation Inhibition[b] (ug/rat) Corn Oil ED$_{100}$
1. [N-Ac-D-Nal(2)[1],D-pCl-Phe[2],D-Trp[3],D-Arg[6],D-Ala[10]]LHRH	0.10	1.0
2. [N-Ac-D-Nal(2)[1],D-C-α-Me-pCl-Phe[2],D-Trp[3],Arg[5],D-Tyr[6], D-Ala[10]]LHRH	3.7	2.5
3. [N-Ac-D-Nal(2)[1],D-pCl-Phe[2],D-Pal(3)[3],Arg[5],D-Tyr[6],D-Ala[10]]LHRH	3.7	>1.0
4. [N-Ac-D-Nal(2)[1],D-pCl-Phe[2],D-Pal(3)[3],Arg[5],D-Nal(2)[6],D-Ala[10]]LHRH	1.9	>1.0
5. [N-Ac-D-Nal(2)[1],D-pCl-Phe[2],D-Pal(3)[3],Arg[5],D-Trp[6],D-Ala[10]]LHRH	2.1	1.0
6. [N-AC-D-NAL(2)[1],D-pCl-Phe[2],D-Pal(3)[3],Arg[5],D-Glu[6],D-Ala[10]]LHRH	17	>>10.0
7. [N-Ac-D-Nal(2)[1],D-pCl-Phe[2],D-Trp[3],Lys[5],D-Nal(2)[6],D-Ala[10]]LHRH	—	10.0
8. [N-Ac-D-Nal(2)[1],D-pCl-Phe[2],D-Pal(3)[3],Arg[5],D-Pal(3)[6],D-Ala[10]]LHRH	2.9	1.0
9. [N-Ac-D-Nal(2)[1],D-pCl-Phe[2],D-Pal(3)[3],Arg[5],D-Trp(CHO)[6],D-Ala[10]]LHRH	3.4	>0.5
10. [N-Ac-D-Nal(2)[1],D-pCl-Phe[2],D-Pal(3)[3],Arg[5],D-His(Bzl)[6],D-Ala[10]]LHRH	4.4	>0.5
11. [N-Ac-D-Nal(2)[1],D-pF-Phe[2],D-Trp[3],D-hArg(Et[2])[6],D-Ala[10]]LHRH	0.29	>1.5
12. [N-Ac-D-Nal(2)[1],D-C-α-Me-pCl-Phe[2],D-Pal(3)[3],D-Arg[6],hArg(Et[2])[8],D-Ala[10]]LHRH	4.9	1.0
13. [N-Ac-D-Nal(2)[1],D-C-α-Me-pCl-Phe[2],D-Pal(3)[3],D-Arg[6],Lys(iPr)[8],D-Ala[10]]LHRH	4.0	1.0
14. [N-Ac-D-Nal(2)[1],D-pCl-Phe[2],D-Trp[3],D-Lys(iPr)[6],Lys(iPr)[8],D-Ala[10]]LHRH	6.6	1.0
15. [N-Ac-D-C-α-Me-pCl-Phe[2],D-Pal(3)[3],Lys(iPr)[5],D-Tyr[6],Lys(iPr)[8],D-Ala[10]]LHRH	3.2	1.0
16. [N-Ac-D-Nal(2)[1],D-pCl-Phe[2],D-Pal(3)[3],Lys(iPr)[5],D-Tyr[6],D-Ala[10]]LHRH	1.97	1.0
17. [N-Ac-D-Nal(2)[1],D-pCl-Phe[2],D-Pal(3)[3],Ile[5],D-Lys(iPr)[6],Lys(iPr)[8],D-Ala[10]]LHRH	9.92	>0.5
18. [N-Ac-D-Nal(2)[1],D-pCl-Phe[2],D-Trp[3]-D-Lys(Me[3])[6],Lys(Me[3])[8],D-Ala[10]]LHRH	1.10	2.0
19. [N-Ac-D-Nal(2)[1],D-pCl-Phe[2],D-Trp[3],D-MePal[6],MePal[8],D-Ala[10]]LHRH	3.45	>>0.5
20. [N-Ac-D-Nal(2)[1],D-pCl-Phe[2],D-Pal(3)[3],D-MePal[6],Lys(iPr)[8],D-Ala[10]]LHRH	7.1	
21. [N-Ac-D-Nal(2)[1],D-pCl-Phe[2],D-Pal(3)[3],MePal[5],D-Tyr[6],Lys(Me[3])[8],D-Ala[10]]LHRH	5.62	
22. [N-Ac-D-Nal(2)[1],D-pCl-Phe[2],D-Pal(3)[3],MePal[5],D-Trp[6],Lys(iPr)[8],D-Ala[10]]LHRH	4.33	>0.5
23. [N-Ac-D-Nal(2)[1],D-pCl-Phe[2],D-Pal(3)[3],D-MePal[6],Lys(Me[3])[8],D-Ala[10]]LHRH	2.63	1.0

Table 1. (Continued)

24.	[N-Ac-D-Nal(2)^1,D-pCl-Phe^2,D-Pal(3)^3,Lys(iPr)^5,D-Trp^6,D-Ala^{10}]LHRH	1.97	>1.0
25.	[N-Ac-D-Nal(2)^1,D-pCl-Phe^2,D-Pal(3)^3,Lys(iPr)^5,D-MePal^6,Lys(iPr)^8,D-Ala^{10}]LHRH	9.72	>>0.5
26.	[N-Ac-D-Nal(2)^1,D-pCl-Phe^2,D-Pal(3)^3,MePal^5,D-Lys(iPr)^6,Lys(iPr)^8,D-Ala^{10}]LHRH	7.9	>>0.5
27.	[N-Ac-Δ^3Pro^1,D-pF-Phe^2,D-Nal(2)^3,Lys(iPr)^5,D-Nal(2)^6,Lys(iPr)^8]LHRH	17.3	>5.0
28.	[N-Ac-Δ^3Pro^1,D-pF-Phe^2,D-Nal(2)^3,D-Nal(2)^6,Lys(iPr)^8]LHRH	10.7	5.0
29.	[N-Ac-D-Nal(2)^1,D-pCl-Phe^2,D-Trp^3,Glu^5,D-Arg^6,D-Ala^{10}]LHRH	—	>>25

[a] Histamine release determinations were performed by Dr. W. A. Hook of the National Institute of Dental Research, in duplicate or triplicate using mast cells from a minimum of three individual rats.
[b] Standard antiovulatory assays [13] were conducted by Drs. Rehan Naqvi and Marjorie Lindberg of EG&G Mason Research Institute.
[c] The symbol (>) denotes the fact that there was a statistically significant reduction in the number of rats ovulating compared to the control although an ED$_{100}$ value was not achieved at the dose indicated.
[d] The symbols (>>) indicated that, at the dose tested, the analog was inactive.
[e] Analogs 1 and 3 were made in the laboratory of D. Coy and K. Folkers, respectively; 4, 5, 6, 9 and 11 are in ref. 8; 8 is in ref. 9; 2, 7 and 29 are in ref. 3; 11 was made under NIH contract with the Salk Institute; the remaining analogs were made by the authors.

D-Me Pal[6], Lys(iPr)[8] > D-Lys(iPr)[6], Lys(iPr)[8] > Me-Pal[5], Lys(Me$_3$)[8] > D-Arg[6], hArg(Et$_2$)[8] > Me-Pal[5], Lys(iPr)[8] > D-Arg[6], Lys(iPr)[8] > D-Me-Pal[6], Me-Pal[8] > Lys(iPr)[5], Lys(iPr)[8] > D-Me- Pal[6], Lys(Me$_3$)[8] > Lys(iPr)[5], Arg[8] > D-Lys(Me$_3$)[6], Lys(Me$_3$)[8]. Although there are minor variations in the remaining residues, such as D-Trp[6] or D-Tyr[6], D-Pal[3] or D-Trp[3], in general the ranking is valid. One anomaly stands out: the combination of Me-Pal[5], Lys(Me$_3$)[8] is more effective than would be expected considering the low rank of Lys(Me$_3$) in other combinations.

Two of the most effective compounds, 25 and 26, have three positively-charged side chains. Thus, both the D-Lys(iPr)[6], Lys(iPr)[8] and the Lys(iPr)[5,8] combinations are improved by the substitution of a Me-Pal residue for Tyr in positions 5 and 6, respectively. The effectiveness of a Me-Pal[5] is about the same as Ile[5] (compare 17 and 25).

REDUCTION OF HYDROPHOBICITY AT POSITION 1

It is well established that the combination of several basic residues and several hydrophobic, preferably aromatic, residues leads to high histamine releasing activity. Position 1 appears to be an important determinant of histamine release. Replacing Ac-D-Nal[1] by Ac-Δ^3-Pro[1] in a Lys(iPr)[5,8] compound, even while increasing hydrophobicity at positions 3 and 6, lowered histamine release by about 4-fold (compound 27), but the antiovulatory activity also decreased by about the same degree. A similar result was obtained with 28, having only one basic residue.

INTRODUCTION OF AN ACIDIC AMINO ACID RESIDUE

Both Jasanai et al. [11] and Stanworth et al. [12] have observed that the presence of a carboxylate group in peptides lowers histamine release considerably, compared to the analogous ester or amide, and that an aspartic or glutamic residue near the cluster of basic residues has a similar effect. Indeed, compound 6, containing D-Glu[6], has quite low histamine releasing activity but also sharply reduced antiovulatory activity. A Glu[5] analog, 29, [3] is inactive in the AO assay at a dose of 25 μg but it has not been tested in the mast cell assay. In spite of these negative results, synthesis of antagonists having negatively charged residues in other positions would seem to be worth pursuing as part of a search for separation in activities.

CONCLUDING REMARKS

Histamine-releasing activity of LHRH antagonists, which was a strong deterrent to their clinical investigation, has been reduced considerably by several approaches. Some progress was made initially by changing the positions of basic amino acid residues from 6, 8 to 5, 8, which lowered histamine release by at least a factor of ten and also confirmed our hypothesis that the side chain of residue 5, as well as that of residue 6, can be either hydrophobic or positively-charged.

Marked improvement in the degree of separation of antiovulatory activity and histamine releasing activity was made by using N^{ϵ}-isopropyl lysine residues in positions 6 and 8 or 5 and 8. This residue is remarkably effective in lowering histamine release while maintaining high antiovulatory activity. We are continuing our investigation of alkylated basic side chains in order to establish the limits of effectiveness of these residues.

REFERENCES

1. Schmidt, F., Sundaram, K., Thau, R.B. and Bardin, C. W. [Ac-D-Nal(2)[1], 4F-D-Phe[2],D-Trp[3], D-Arg[6]]-LHRH, a potent antagonist of LHRH, produces transient edema and behavioral changes in rats. Contraception, 29, 283 (1984).
2. Theoharides, T.C. and Douglas, W.W. Mast cell histamine secretion in response to somatostatin analogues: structural considerations. Eur. J. Pharmacol., 73, 131 (1981).
3. Roeske, R.W., Chaturvedi, N., Rivier, J., Vale, W., Porter, J. and Perrin, M. Substitution of Arg[5] for Tyr[5] in GnRH antagonists. In: "Peptides: Structure and Function." C.M. Deber, V.J. Hruby and K.D. Kopple (Eds.), Pierce Chemical Co., Rockford, IL, 1985, p. 561.
4. Momany, F.A. Conformational energy analysis of the molecule, luteinizing hormone-releasing hormone. 1. Native decapeptide. J. Am. Chem. Soc., 98, 2990 (1976).
5. Freidinger, R.M., Veber, D.F., Perlow, D.S., Brooks, J.R. and Saperstein, R. Bioactive conformation of luteinizing hormone-releasing hormone: Evidence from a conformationally constrained analog. Science, 210, 656 (1980).
6. Nestor, J.J., Jr., Ho, T.L., Tahilramani, R., McRae, G.E. and Vickery, B.H. Long-acting LHRH agonists and antagonists. In: "LHRH and Its Analogues," F. Labrie, A. Belanger, A. Dupont (Eds). Elsevier, Amsterdam, 1984, p. 24.
7. Nestor, J.J., Jr., Ho, T.L., Tahilramani, R., Horner, B.L., Simpson, R.A., Jones, G.H., McRae, G.I. and Vickery, B.H. LHRH agonists and antagonists containing very hydrophobic amino acids. In: "LHRH and Its Analogs: Contraceptive and Therapeutic Applications," B.H. Vickery, J.J. Nestor, Jr. and E.S.E. Hafez (Eds.), MTP Press, Boston, 1984, p. 23.
8. Rivier, J.E., Porter, J., Rivier, C.L., Perrin, M., Corrigan, A., Hook, W.A., Siraganian, R.P. and Vale, W.W. New effective gonadotropin releasing hormone antagonists with minimal potency for histamine release in vitro. J. Med. Chem., 29, 1846 (1986).
9. Folkers, K., Bowers, C., Shao-bo, X., Tang, P. and Kubota, M. Increased potency of antagonists of the luteinizing hormone releasing hormone which have D-3-Pal in position 6. Biochem. Biophys. Res. Comm., 137, 709 (1986).

10. Prasad, K.U., Roeske, R. W., Weitl, F. L., Vilchez-Martinez, J.H. and Schally, A.V. Structure–activity relationships in luteinizing hormone–releasing hormone. J. Med. Chem., _19_, 492 (1976).

11. Jasani, B., Kreil, G., Mackler, B.F. and Stanworth, D.R. Further studies on the structural requirements for poly-peptide-mediated histamine release from rat mast cells. Biochem. J. _181_, 623 (1979).

12. Stanworth, D.R., Kings, M., Roy, P., Moran, J. and Moran, D. Synthetic peptides comprising sequences of the human immunoglobulin E heavy chain capable of releasing histamine. Biochem. J., _180_, 665 (1979).

13. Corbin, A. and Beattie, C.W. Inhibition of the pre-ovulatory proestrous gonadotropin surge, ovulation and pregnancy with a peptide analogue of luteinizing hormone releasing hormone. Endocr. Res. Commun., _2_, 1 (1975).

3

Specificity of Design to Achieve Antagonists of LHRH of Increasing Effectiveness in Therapeutic Activity

*K. FOLKERS, **C. BOWERS, *P.-F. L. TANG, *D. FENG,
*T. OKAMOTO, *Y. ZHANG and *A. LJUNGQVIST
*Institute for Biomedical Research, The University of Texas at Austin,
Austin, TX 78712. **Endocrine Unit, Tulane University School of
Medicine, New Orleans, LA 70112, USA

INTRODUCTION

The pioneering work on TRH [1-4] inspired the staff of the Institute for Biomedical Research of the University of Texas at Austin to isolate concentrates of LHRH from tissue and conduct chemical and enzymic inactivation experiments toward determining certain amino acids in LHRH. These studies [5] resulted in the crucial conclusion that LHRH is a decapeptide rather than a nonapeptide [6]. These inactivation experiments not only provided accurate structural information, but were the basis for the synthesis of <Glu-Tyr-Arg-Trp-NH$_2$ [7], the first reported synthetic LHRH agonist. These early successes on TRH and LHRH were the basis for K. Folkers and C. Bowers to join in the transition to antagonists of LHRH.

Periodic increases in the antiovulatory potency (AOA) of antagonists were achieved with new analog designs. During 1976-78, potencies of less than 100% (AOA) were observed at dosages of 100 µg in the rat. By 1982-84, potencies of 100% AOA were being observed at dosages of 250 ng. In 1986, the goals of design were reoriented toward negligible release of histamine while maintaining AOA potency.

Although empiricism was not absent, the stepwise achievement of increased effectiveness of antagonists resulted largely from intellectual inputs from peptide sequence-activity relationships, substantial input from classical medicinal chemistry methods, and the ongoing data.

During 1972-74, designs with emphasis of substitutions in positions 2, 3 and 6 of LHRH gave antagonists of increasing AOA potency. The importance of introducing aromatic residues in positions 2 and 3 and D-residues in position 6 was elucidated, and such substitutions are maintained in 1986.

In 1977, the N-terminal acetyl group was introduced and is a structural feature maintained in 1986. In 1981-82, the synthesis and introduction of unnatural basic and aromatic alanines yielded superior antagonists, a feature which is also maintained in 1986. 3-(3-Pyridyl)-D-alanine and 3-(3-quinolyl)-D-alanine were exceptional contributors to these potency increases. In 1983-84, the introduction of Trp[7] and the transfer of D-Arg[6] to L-Arg[5] with D-Pal(3)[6] gave antagonists which had 100% AOA at 250 ng.

Of the 10 amino acids in LHRH, only Ser[4] and Pro[9] are frequently maintained without change in the best antagonists. Of all the L-amino acids of LHRH, the best antagonists of 1986 have D-amino acids in positions 1, 2, 3, 6 and 10.

The principal contributions of Folkers-Bowers and their associates during 1972-1986 toward achieving effective antagonists of LHRH have been summarized.

CONTRIBUTIONS TO THE DESIGN OF EFFECTIVE LHRH INHIBITORS

The contributions from Texas and Tulane during the years 1973-86 are chronologically organized and are summarized with concern for significance and perspective rather than detail. The years cited are those in which the contributions were made under the NICHD contracts. The references show the years of publication.

Substitutions in positions 2, 3 and 6. In 1973 interest focused upon His[2] of LHRH, because [des-His[2]]LHRH [8] showed no agonistic activity and reduced the secretion rate of LH in dispersed rat pituitary cells. The presumption that His[2] of LHRH was required for receptor recognition and LHRH activity was ambiguous, because [Trp[2]]LHRH was 40% as potent as LHRH, in vitro. [Des-His[2]]LHRH appeared to be the only deletion analog to have antagonistic activity [8].

Since Trp is functional, His[2]-Trp[3] appeared to be a significant sequence of LHRH to alter for enhanced inhibition. Replacement of these moieties with the aliphatic Leu[2],Leu[3]-sequence was background peptide chemistry. Consequently, [Leu[2,3]]LHRH was designed and found to inhibit the LHRH-induced release of LH and FSH, in vitro, [9]. In 1974 we synthesized [Leu[2,3],D-Ala[6]]LHRH and [Val[2],Leu[3],D-Ala[6]]LHRH which inhibited, in vitro, at a dosage of 10 µg/ml and had a ratio of inhibitor:LHRH of 30,000:1. [Leu[2,3],D-Ala[6]]LHRH completely inhibited the LHRH-induced release of LH and FSH at 1/10 the inhibitory dosage of [Leu[2,3]]LHRH [10]. The introduction of D-Ala[6] was an influence from agonist analogs.

In 1986, His[2],Trp[3] of LHRH are still replaced, but with the D configurations of unnatural aromatic amino acids. The early recognition of the essentiality of replacement of His[2],Trp[3] was valid. Replacement with unnatural aromatic amino acids was more effective than with aliphatic combinations like Leu[2],Leu[3]. Even in 1986, a D-amino acid in position 6 is still of high priority for high antagonist activity.

Irreversible LHRH antagonism. Baker [11] had reviewed the design of active-site-directed irreversible inhibitors which was a unique approach to enzyme inhibition which might also be applicable to an antagonist of LHRH. The nitrogen mustard, chlorambucil, (Chl), contains a chemically reactive group that can form a covalent bond with nucleophilic sites. Consequently, <Glu[1] of LHRH was replaced with Chl[1] in an analog to provide [Chl[1],Leu[2,3], D-Ala[6]]LHRH. Levels of 3-50 µg of [Chl[1],Leu[2,3], D-Ala[6]]LHRH inhibited 0.3 ng of LHRH, in vitro [12]. However, this Chl analog had definite LH and FSH releasing activity in vitro [12] and effective antagonists of LHRH have not arisen from the concepts of Baker on active-site-directed irreversible inhibition.

Substitution with Pro[3]. In 1976 Humphries et al. [14] reported that [D-Phe[2],Pro[3],D-Trp[6]]LHRH completely inhibited the release of LH and FSH by LHRH from isolated rat pituitaries in a ratio of analog:LHRH of 50:1. This analog had no agonistic activity. The Pro[3]-analog completely inhibited ovulation in rats at a single sc injection of 750 µg. The Leu[3]-analogs gave complete inhibition of ovulation at 750 µg with D-Phe[6] and at 1.5 mg with D-Trp[6].

Importance of the N-terminal acetyl group. In 1977 Humphries et al. [16] designed an antiovulatory decapeptide which had a high potency and an L-amino acid (Ac-Pro) in position 1. The structure of an acetylated Pro residue is related to the <Glu-structure in that the cyclic amide carbonyl of <Glu has been displaced from a rigid five-membered ring and relocated as a side chain substituent on the ring of Pro. This eliminates the alpha-NH group of residue 1 to yield a tertiary amide in which the -CO- would be expected to have more rotational freedom. The Ac-D-Pro[1] analog was much less active than the Ac-Pro[1] analog. This difference may indicate a configurational preference for the L-form in position 1 for this particular substitution.

[Ac-Pro[1],D-Phe[2],D-Trp[3,6]]LHRH completely inhibited ovulation in cycling rats at 200 µg/rat and is comparable in activity to the corresponding D-<Glu[1]-analog. This Ac-Pro[1]-analog was the most potent antiovulatory peptide known at that time having an L-amino acid in position 1. This result emphasized that for the design of potent inhibitors of ovulation, a D-amino acid residue is not essential for position 1, although for many analogs a D-amino acid in position 1 can be superior. The corresponding Ac-D-Pro[1]- and Kic[1] analogs completely inhibited ovulation at 750 µg/rat, but not at 200 µg/rat. The Cpc[1]-analog was inactive at these dosages.

The introduction of the N-terminal acetyl group turned out to be a very significant structural feature of antagonists. Even in 1986, the best antagonists have an N-terminal acetyl group.

Analogs having more than ten residues. In 1978 a linear analog of LHRH longer than a decapeptide was described which, for the first time, was equivalent in potency to the best known inhibitors of ovulation (200 µg/rat). This undecapeptide, [(<Glu-Pro)[1], D-Phe[2],D-Trp[3,6]]LHRH caused 100% inhibition of ovulation at 200 µg/rat [17]. The two related analogs, [(<Glu-Gly)[1],

27

D-Phe[2],D-Trp[3,6]]LHRH and [(Gly-Pro)[1],D-Phe[2],D-Trp[3,6]]-
LHRH, were less active in vivo. All of these undecapeptides
inhibited the action of 0.6 ng/ml of LHRH by greater than 50% at
the very low level of 10 ng/ml.

In spite of the promise of such undecapeptides, the most
potent known inhibitors of ovulation in 1986 are decapeptides.
This may well be because the conformations of LHRH and that of the
most effective antagonists are not simulated by antagonists with
more than ten amino acids.

Aza-Gly[10] antagonists. In 1979 we began a study of the possible
advantage of the aza-Gly[10] moiety to minimize C-terminal
degradation in vivo. Folkers et al. [18] described 7 new analogs
having a aza-Gly[10] moiety and 3 corresponding Gly[10] analogs
for comparison of inhibitory potency. Three procedures were
studied to achieve a synthesis of aza-Gly[10] peptides, and the
reaction of cyanate ion with hydrazides was the most favorable.
The data from the antiovulatory assays showed that the aza-Gly[10]
moiety may not depress activity and may allow equal or higher
activity than the Gly[10] moiety, depending upon the analog.
[N-Ac-D-Thr[1],D-pCl-Phe[2],D-Trp[3,6],aza-Gly[10]]LHRH was more
inhibitory than the corresponding Gly[10] analog. It is
considered that in an ultimate clinical use of an antagonist of
LHRH to block ovulation, the aza-Gly[10] moiety could be advantageous for limiting enzymatic degradation. The synthetic
difficulties of preparing the aza-Gly[10] analogs and the finding
that such analogs were not significantly more potent than the
corresponding Gly[10] analogs discouraged their investigation.
Ultimately, the introduction of D-Ala[10] became widely used and
replaced aza-Gly[10].

Folkers et al. [20] designed 24 new analogs of LHRH which were
bioassayed for antiovulatory activity in rats. [N-Ac-Δ[3]-
Pro[1],pF-D-Phe[2],D-Trp[3,6],aza-Gly[10]]LHRH completely
inhibited ovulation at 6 µg and was the most potent of the 24
analogs. Of these analogs, D-Arg[6] was better than D-Trp[6], and
pCl-D-Phe[6] was superior to D-Trp[6]. D-Trp[3,6] was superior to
D-Nal(2)[3,6] and D-His[3,6].

Antagonists with a high number of D-amino acids. [N-Ac-Thr[1],
D-Phe[2],D-Trp[3,6]]LHRH was the model antagonist which was the
basis for the design, synthesis and bioassay in 1980 of 7 peptides
having 4, 5 and 6 D-amino acids. It was thought that antagonists
with D-amino acids might have prolonged action and oral activity
in addition to potency.

[N-Ac-Thr[1],D-Phe[2],D-Trp[3],D-Ser[4],D-Tyr[5],D-Trp[6],
D-Arg[8]]LHRH with 6 D-amino acids had antiovulatory activity
which was higher than that of the model antagonist, i.e. 70%
antiovulatory activity at 25 µg/rat compared with 50% activity
at 50 µg/rat, respectively [19]. Empirical energy calculations
gave a conformational structure for this antagonist with 6 D-amino
acids which is similar to that calculated for the previous potent
antagonists. These results were considered a basis for new

designs for antagonists having up to ten D-amino acids toward parenteral and particularly oral activity. The effective antagonists of 1986 frequently have 5 or more D-amino acids.

Introduction of 3-(3-quinolyl)-D-alanine. By 1981, as the first decade of the international research on antagonists of LHRH continued, more unnatural amino acids were synthesized and introduced into new analogs. From time to time, certain of these new unnatural amino acids resulted in superior antagonists.

Analogs of LHRH containing 3-(3-quinolyl)-D-alanine (Qal) were synthesized toward more effective inhibitors of ovulation. [N-Ac-pCl-D-Phe[1,2],D--Pal(3)[3],D-Qal(3)[6],D-Ala[10]]LHRH was the most effective and had an antiovulatory activity of 40% at 1 µg/rat. D-Qal(3)[6] was as effective as D-Trp[6] in combination with [N-Ac-Δ[3]-Pro,pF-D-Phe[2],D-Trp[3]] [21].

Superior antagonists with pyridyl-alanines. Partly on the basis of the success of introducing D-Qal(3)[6] in antagonists, 3-(3-pyridyl)-D-alanine [Pal(3)] was synthesized to provide a basic version of Phe. In retrospect, D-Qal(3) was a basic version of the 3-(2-naphthyl)-D-alanine of Nestor et al. [22].

[N-Ac-D-Nal(2)[1],D-pCl-Phe[2],D-Pal(3)[3],D-Arg[6],D-Ala[10]]-LHRH caused 100% and 57% inhibition of ovulation in rats, sc, at 500 and 250 ng, respectively, and 56% per os at 500 µg. [N-Ac-3,4--diCl-D-Phe[1],pCl-D-Phe[2],D-Pal(3)[3],D-Arg[6], D-Ala[10]]LHRH inhibited ovulation, sc, 82% at 500 ng, and 63%, per os at 500 µg [23]. These analogs were the most effective reported inhibitors of ovulation at the time. Pyridyl-alanine appeared to be a superior substituent, and its use was extended from 1982 to 1986.

D--Pal(3)[3] was superior to D-Pal(2)[3] and D-Pal(4)[3]. D-Arg[6] was superior to D-Pal(3)[6], and D-Pal(4)[6] was superior by two-fold to D-Arg[6].

Introduction of Trp[7] based upon avian LHRH-II. The sequences of four naturally occurring luteinizing hormone releasing hormones differ only in positions 5, 7 and 8. The salmon and chicken II LHRH's have Trp[7]. In 1983 we synthesized thirteen antagonists having Trp[7] and 8 antagonists with other substitutions in position 7 [24]. One of these thirteen antagonists with the natural Trp[7], [N-Ac-D-Nal(2)[1],D-pCl-Phe[2],D-Pal(3)[3], D-Arg[6],Trp[7],D-Ala[10]]LHRH, not only maintained activity, but had increased potency by ca. 58%; the antiovulatory activity was 90% at 250 ng in rats in comparison with a companion analog with the natural Leu[7] of the mammalian LHRH's.

Introduction of Arg[5] and D-Pal(3)[6]. Folkers et al. [25] achieved an antiovulatory potency of 100% in the rat at 250 ng by [N-Ac--D-Nal(2)[1],D-pCl-Phe[2],D-Pal(3)[3,6],Ile[5],D-Ala[10]]-NH2. When D-Arg[6] was replaced with D-Pal(3)[6], an

antiovulatory activity of 85% at 250 ng was found for [N-Ac-D-Nal(2)[1],D-pCl-Phe[2],D-Pal(3)[3,6],Arg[5],D-Ala[10]]-NH$_2$.
This peptide with D-Pal(3)[6] caused 60% inhibition at 125 ng and appeared to be the most potent antagonist described up to that time. The strategies of design were replacement of D-Arg[6] with D-Pal(3)[6] and of Tyr[5] with Arg[5] [26].

In the design and synthesis of 26 decapeptides with emphasis on Lys[8] and Arg[8] and various substitutions in positions 3, 5, 6, 7 and 8 by Folkers et al. [25], two antagonists emerged which showed 80-85% antiovulatory activity at 250 ng in the rat. These two peptides were [N-Ac-D-Nal(2)[1],D-pCl-Phe[2],D-Pal(3)[3], D-Arg[6],Lys[8],D-Ala[10]]LHRH and [N-Ac-D-Nal(2)[1],D-pCl-Phe[2], D-Pal(3)[3],Arg[5],D-Pal(3)[6],D-Ala[10]]LHRH.

Of four pairs of analogs with Arg[8] and Lys[8], respectively, two pairs favored Lys[8] over Arg[8] for potency. One pair showed negligible difference and another pair favored Arg[8] over Lys[8].

TOWARD ANALOGS WITH REDUCED HISTAMINE RELEASE

Schmidt et al. [27] observed that [Ac-D-Nal(2)[1],D-pF-Phe[2], D-Trp[3],D-Trp[6]]LHRH caused a transient edema of the face and extremities when it was administered sc to rats. In 1986 Karten and Rivier [28] reviewed the design of analogs, summarized rationale, perspective and structure-function studies, and emphasized that the reorientation of the goal of an effective antagonist was necessary. The reorientation called for the reduction of activity to release histamine to a negligible level. In their review [28] of the release of histamine by diverse peptides and particularly by antagonists of LHRH, Karten and Rivier proposed that the essential structural features for histamine release are the presence in close proximity of two moieties of arginine and/or lysine as well as the presence of a cluster (perhaps three amino acids) of hydrophobic amino acids at the N-terminal end of the peptide.

Folkers et al. [29] designed 40 analogs with one emphasis on positions 1, 5 and 6, and another emphasis on positions 1, 2 and 3. The most potent analog of the 40 analogs was [N-D-Nal(2)[1], pCl-D-Phe[2],D-Pal(3)[3],D-Arg[6],D-Ala[10]]-NH$_2$ which had a 57% AOA at 250 ng and 100% AOA at 500 ng. The wheal area for histamine release of this analog was 184 $\pm$ 35 mm. Other analogs showed wheal areas as high as 140 $\pm$ 7 mm, and the analog causing this level of histamine release had D-His[6] rather than D-Arg[6] ([N-Ac-D-Nal(2)[1],D-pCl-Phe[2],D-Pal(3)[3],Arg[5],D-His[6], D-Ala[10]]LHRH).

ACHIEVEMENT OF AN ANTAGONIST WHICH RELEASES INSIGNIFICANT HISTAMINE

Some of the best antagonists presently known have Arg (L or D) in positions 5 or 6 as well as Arg in position 8. In the apparent absence of knowledge on the specific chemical reactions that are taking place in the mast cell which allow the release of histamine, one can speculate on alternatives. It is known that

Table 1. LHRH Antagonists Providing Significant Potency Advances

Compound	Antiovulatory Potency[a] (AOA)		
	Dose (µg/animal)	% Inhibition of Ovulation	
[Leu2,3,D-Ala6]LHRH	b	b	[10]
[D-Phe2,Pro3,D-Trp6]LHRH	750	100	[14]
[N-Ac-Pro1,D-Phe2,D-Trp3,6]LHRH	200	100	[16]
[N-Ac-D-Thr1,pCl-D-Phe2,D-Trp3,6,aza-Gly10]LHRH	25	100	[18]
[N-Ac-Thr1,D-Phe2,D-Trp3,D-Ser4,D-Tyr5,D-Trp6,D-Arg8]LHRH	25	70	[19]
[N-Ac-pCl-D-Phe1,2,D-Pal(3)3,D-Qal(3)6,D-Ala10]LHRH	1	40	[21]
[N-Ac-D-Nal(2)1,pCl-D-Phe2,D-Pal(3)3,D-Arg6,D-Ala10]LHRH	0.5	100	[23]
[N-Ac-D-Nal(2)1,pCl-D-Phe2,D-Pal(3)3,D-Arg6,Trp7,D-Ala10]LHRH	0.25	90	[24]
[N-Ac-D-Nal(2)1,pCl-D-Phe2,D-Pal(3)3,6,Arg5,D-Ala10]LHRH	0.125	60	[26]
[N-Ac-D-Nal(2)1,pCl-D-Phe2,D-Pal(3)3,Lys(Nic)5,D-Lys(Nic)6, Lys(iPr)8,D-Ala10]LHRH	1	100	

aBioassays were performed as described [24]. bED100 for inhibition of LH release _in vitro_ was 10 µg/ml.

histamine results from the decarboxylation of histidine as catalyzed by the coenzyme of the vitamin B_6 group, pyridoxal 5'-phosphate. It seemed possible that the chemical reactions involving Arg and Lys in histamine release are because Arg and Lys are functional.

Katayama et al. [30] demonstrated that the apoenzyme of the transaminase GOT in mitochondria has 401 amino acids in each subunit. There is organic structural proof that pyridoxal 5'-phosphate becomes attached to Lys in position 250 of this enzyme. If an antagonist of LHRH has the Lys moiety, it seemed possible that this antagonist might compete for Lys in the complex multi-enzyme system and release histamine. If so, acylation or alkylation of a Lys-antagonist might prevent histamine release. Although acylation or alkylation of Arg in an antagonist is conceivable, it seemed more likely that an Arg containing antagonist might cause histamine release through an ionic mechanism involving interaction of the protonated guanidino group of Arg with the phosphate group of the coenzyme in the complex multi-enzyme system. In such a case, elimination of the Arg moiety from an antagonist and its replacement by a modified Lys might be a good approach to avoid histamine release. Roeske et al. [31] had introduced Lys(iPr)[8] with some reduction of histamine release.

N^ϵ-Nicotinyl-lysine [Lys(Nic)] was synthesized in both the L and D forms on the basis that Lys(Nic) would not have the functionality of Lys but would have basicity because of the pyridine nucleus.

From the ongoing synthesis and bioassay of peptides containing acylated and alkylated Lys in one or more of the three positions, 5, 6 and 8, a peptide was found which was still relatively potent for AOA and which released an insignificant level of histamine. The ED_{50} (µg/ml) for in vitro histamine release was >300 ([N-Ac-D-Nal(2)[1],pCl-D-Phe[2],D-Pal(3)[3],Lys(Nic)[5],D-Lys(Nic)[6], Lys(iPr)[8],D-Ala[10]]LHRH). In comparison, the ED_{50} value for LHRH was 205, that for the superagonist [D-Trp[6],Pro[9]-NHEt]LHRH was 32 and the ED_{50} for the reference antagonist [N-Ac-D-Nal(2)[1],pF-D-Phe[2],D-Trp[3],D-Arg[6]]LHRH) was 0.11 µg/ml (data provided by Dr. Marvin Karten). The AOA of this antagonist was 100% at 1 µg in our assay and 100% at 3 µg in an assay reported to us by Dr. Marvin Karten. This antagonist is about 50% as potent as its parent antagonist having Tyr[5],D-Arg[6],Arg[8], which showed 100% AOA at 500 ng.

A closely related antagonist, which contains Tyr[5], D-Lys(Nic)[6],Lys(iPr)[8], showed an ED_{50} of 133 µg/ml which is superior to that of a superagonist currently in widespread clinical use and fulfills the goal of an antagonist which releases insignificant levels of histamine. Therefore, it may not be necessary to replace Tyr[5] but only to modify positions 6 and 8 through the elimination of unsubstituted or unmodified Lys and/or Arg. The future challenge now in November, 1986, is to achieve new designs which maintain insignificant release of histamine, but have increased AOA, better than 100% at 500 ng.

CONCLUDING REMARKS

There have probably never been more extensive international programs in medicinal chemistry and endocrinology by multi-groups to achieve clinically useful peptides than those on antagonists of LHRH during the last fifteen years. These programs were supported by governmental agencies and the pharmaceutical industry at budgetary levels of millions of dollars resulting in well over 2,000 peptides. This extraordinary research will surely serve as a model for programs to achieve antagonists of other peptide hormones. The achievement of antagonists of Substance P has been facilitated by this enormous background of research on LHRH antagonists.

The first meaningful guideline which appeared in the early years was that an effective antagonist of LHRH must have zero agonistic activity. Many of the early peptides reported to be antagonists actually released LH at some dosage. It may well be a generally applicable guideline that an effective antagonist has zero agonistic activity. Another guideline which eventually evolved was the recognition that the D forms of the amino acids used in the synthesis of projected antagonists were essential. This guideline was also productive in research on antagonists of Substance P.

In the early years, most groups made substitutions of the 10 amino acids of LHRH by using the naturally occurring and commercially available amino acids. Ultimately, it became evident that the synthesis and introduction of unnatural amino acids closely related to the natural amino acids allowed improvements in activity and potency with the elimination of all agonistic activity. The design and synthesis of unnatural amino acids for introduction into the decapeptides became perhaps the most important strategy for achievement.

One example of the most potent currently known antagonists is [N-Ac-D-Nal(2)[1],pCl-D-Phe[2],D-Pal(3)[3,6],Arg[5],D-Ala[10]]-LHRH. This antagonist contains five unnatural and/or D-amino acids. No one surmised in the early years that potent antagonists would have so many unnatural and D-amino acids. These D-forms presumably contribute to enzymic stability _in vivo_. This also presumably reflects some conformational relationship to the superagonists which also have a D-amino acid in position 6.

The presently known state of achievement is based on decapeptides. Although peptides which have a lower or higher number of amino acids, which are cyclic, or which have some of the other structural departures have been explored, they have not been as effective.

Presumably the requirements for effective receptor binding of an antagonist are restrictive, yet they allow for the replacement of <Glu[1] in LHRH by N-Ac-D-Nal(2)[1] in an antagonist. The retention of pCl-D-Phe[2],D-Pal(3)[3] as aromatic and heterocyclic replacements for His[2],Trp[3] of LHRH may reflect traditional medicinal chemistry. The retention of Ser[4],Leu[7],Pro[9] provides some overlap with LHRH but the introduction of a D-amino acid in position 6 in place of the Gly[6] of LHRH is a crucial, essential feature.

Whether the ultimately desired higher potency will result from "fine-tuning" of the present best antagonists or will result from a radical change in design is now the challenge.

ACKNOWLEDGEMENT

Appreciation is expressed to Dr. Marvin Karten and to the Contraceptive Development Branch of the National Institute of Child Health and Human Development under contract N01-HD-4-2831, and to the Robert E. Welch Foundation for their support of this research.

The following postdoctorates conducted the synthesis of the LHRH antagonists and evolved successful designs, during 1972-1986:

Dong-mei Feng   Yin-Zeng Liu   Georg Rampold   Janusz Stepinski
Klaus Friebel   Anders Ljungqvist   Masanori Sakagami P. Louisa Tang
John Humphries   Wilson Lutz   Bernhard Schircks Y.P. Wan
Teresa Kubiak   Tomasz Plucinski   Hong-Ming Shieh   Tadeusz Wasiak
Minoru Kubota

REFERENCES

1. Folkers, K., Enzmann, F. and Boler, J. Discovery of modification of the synthetic tripeptide-sequence of the thyrotropin releasing hormone having activity. Biochem. Biophys. Res. Commun., 37, 123 (1969).
2. Enzmann, F., Boler, J., Folkers, K., Bowers, C.Y., and Schally, A.V. Structure and synthesis of the thyrotropin releasing hormone. J. Med. Chem., 14, 469 (1971).
3. Boler, J., Enzmann, F. and Folkers, K., Bowers, C.Y. and Schally, A.V. The identity of chemical and hormonal properties of the thyrotropin releasing hormone and pyroglutamyl-histidyl-proline amide. Biochem. Biophys. Res. Commun., 37, 705 (1969).
4. Boler, J. Chang, J.-K., Enzmann, F. and Folkers, K. Synthesis of the thyrotropin releasing hormone. J. Med. Chem., 14, 475 (1971).
5. Bogentoft, C., Currie, B.L., Sievertsson, H., Chang, J.-K., Folkers, K. and Bowers, C.Y. On the structure of the hypothalamic luteinizing releasing hormone. Evidence for the presence of arginine, tyrosine, and tryptophan by inactivation. Biochem. Biophys. Res. Commun., 44, 403 (1971).
6. Schally, A.V., Baba, Y., Arimura, A., Rodding, T.W. and White, W.F. Evidence for peptide nature of LH and FSH-releasing hormones. Biochem. Biophys. Res. Commun., 42, 50 (1971).
7. Chang, J.-K., Sievertsson, H., Bogentoft, C., Currie, B.L. and Folkers, K. Discovery of a new synthetic tetrapeptide having luteinizing releasing hormone (LRH) activity. Biochem. Biophys. Res. Commun., 44, 409 (1971).

8. Vale, W., Grant, G., Rivier, J., Monahan, M., Amoss, M., Blackwell, R., Burgus, R. and Guillemin, R. Synthetic polypeptide antagonists of the hypothalamic luteinizing hormone releasing factor. Science, 176, 933 (1972).

9. Humphries, J., Fisher, G., Wan, Y.P., Folkers, K. and Bowers, C.Y. Analogs of the luteinizing hormone-releasing hormone to study conformational aspects of the aromatic amino acid moieties and inhibition. J. Med. Chem., 17, 569 (1974).

10. Wan, Y.P., Humphries, J., Fisher, G., Folkers, K. and Bowers, C.Y. Inhibitors of the luteinizing hormone-releasing hormone based upon modifications in the 2, 3 and 6 positions. J. Med. Chem., 19 199 (1976).

11. Baker, B.R., "Design of active-site-directed irreversible enzyme inhibitors," John Wiley and Sons, Inc., New York, 1967.

12. Bowers, C.Y., Wan, Y.P., Humphries, J. and Folkers, K. Studies on inhibition of the luteinizing hormone-releasing hormone by an irreversible inhibitor at the receptor site. Biochem. Biophys. Res. Commun., 61, 698 (1974).

13. Bowers, C.Y., Humphries, J., Wan, Y.P. and Folkers, K. LHRH analog antagonists. Fed. Proc. Abstracts, 34, 240 (1975).

14. Humphries, J., Wan, Y.P., Folkers, K. and Bowers, C.Y. Presence of proline in position 3 for potent inhibition of the activity of the luteinizing hormone releasing hormone and of ovulation. Biochem. Biophys. Res. Commun., 72, 939 (1976).

15. Bowers, C.Y. and Folkers, K. Contraception and inhibition of ovulation by minipump infusion of the luteinizing hormone releasing hormone, active analogs and antagonists. Biochem. Biophys. Res. Commun., 72, 1003 (1976).

16. Humphries, J., Wasiak, T., Wan, Y.P., Folkers, K. and Bowers, C.Y. An antiovulatory decapeptide of higher potency which has an L-amino acid (Ac-Pro) in position 1. Biochem. Biophys. Res. Commun., 85, 709 (1978).

17. Wasiak, T., Humphries, J., Folkers, K. and Bowers, C.Y. A new category of ovulation inhibitors. Linear LHRH analogues having more than ten amino acids. Biochem. Biophys. Res. Commun., 86, 843 (1979).

18. Folkers, K., Bowers, C.Y., Lutz, W., Friebel, K., Kubiak, T., Schircks, B. and Rampold, G. Synthesis and bioassay of antagonists of the luteinizing hormone releasing hormone having the Azagly[10] moiety. Z. Naturforsch., 37b, 1075 (1982).

19. Folkers, K., Bowers, C.Y., Momany, F., Friebel, K., Kubiak, T. and Maher, J. Antiovulatory potency and conformation of an antagonist of the luteinizing hormone-releasing hormone having six D-amino acids. Z. Naturforsch., 37b, 872 (1982).

20. Folkers, K., Bowers, C.Y., Stepinski, J., Pluchinski, T., Sakagami, M. and Kubiak, T. Analogs of the luteinizing hormone releasing hormone having the Azagly[10] moiety with antiovulatory activity. Z. Naturforsch., 39b, 528 (1984).

21. Folkers, K., Bowers, C.Y., Kubiak, T. and Stepinski, J. Synthesis and antiovulatory activities in rats of analogs of

the luteinizing hormone releasing hormone having a moiety of β-(3-quinolyl)-D-α-alanine in position 3 and 6. Z. Naturforsch., 38b, 1253 (1983).

22. Nestor, J.J. Jr., Ho, T., Simpson, R.A., Horner, B.L., Jones, G.H., McRae, G.I. and Vickery, B.H. Synthesis and biological activity of some very hydrophobic superagonist analogues of luteinizing hormone-releasing hormone. J. Med. Chem., 25, 795 (1982).

23. Folkers, K., Bowers, C.Y., Kubiak, T. and Stepinski, J. Antagonists of the luteinizing hormone releasing hormone with pyridyl-alanines which completely inhibit ovulation at nanogram dosage. Biochem. Biophys. Res. Commun., 111, 1089 (1983).

24. Folkers, K., Bowers, C.Y., Shieh, H-M, Liu, Y-Z, Xiao, S-B, Tang, L. and Chu, J-Y. Antagonist of the luteinizing hormone releasing hormone (LHRH) with emphasis on the Trp[1] of the salmon and chicken II LHRH's. Biochem. Biophys. Res. Commun., 123, 1221 (1984).

25. Folkers, K., Bowers, C.Y., Tang, P-F. L., Kubota, J., Xiao, S.-B., Bender, W. and Liu, Y.-Z. Relative potencies of antagonists of the luteinizing hormone releasing hormone with Lys[8] and Arg[8] and substitutions in positions 3, 5, 6, 7 and 8. Z. Naturforsch., in press (1986).

26. Folkers, K., Bowers, C.Y., Xiao, S-B, Tang, P-F.L. and Kubota, M. Increased potency of antagonists of the luteinizing hormone releasing hormone which have D-Pal(3) in position 6. Biochem. Biophys. Res. Commun., 137, 709 (1986).

27. Schmidt, F., Sundaram, K., Thau, R.B. and Bardin, C.W. [Ac-D-Nal(2)[1],4-FD-Phe[2],D-Trp[3],D-Arg[6]]-LHRH, a potent antagonist of LHRH, produces transient edema and behavioral changes in rats. Contraception, 29, 283 (1984).

28. Karten, M.J. and Rivier,J.E. Gonadotropin-releasing hormone analog design. Structure-function studies toward the development of agonists and antagonists: rationale and perspectives. Endocr. Rev., 7, 44 (1986).

29. Folkers, K., Bowers, C.Y., Xiao, S-B, Tang, P-F.L., Kubota, J., Stepinski, J. and Kubiak, T. Activities of antagonists of the luteinizing hormone releasing hormone with emphasis on positions 1, 5 and 6 and on positions 1, 2 and 3. Z. Naturforsch., in press (1986).

30. Katayama, Y. and North, R.A. Nature, 274, 387 (1978).

31. Roeske, R.W., Chaturvedi, N.C., Rivier, J., Vale, W., Porter, J. and Perrin, M. Substitution of Arg[5] for Tyr[5] in GnRH antagonists. In "Peptides: Structure and Function" Proceedings of the Ninth American Peptide Symposium. C.M. Deber, V.J. Hruby, and K.D. Kopple (Eds.), Pierce Chemical Co., Rockford, IL, 1985, p. 561.

4

Biosynthesis of LHRH

K. NIKOLICS and P.H. SEEBURG

Genentech, Inc., Department of Developmental Biology,
460 Point San Bruno Blvd, South San Francisco, CA 94080, USA

INTRODUCTION

Mammalian reproduction is controlled by humoral factors of the central nervous system, a fact recognized by G. Harris [1]. The key hypothalamic factor regulating luteinizing hormone (LH) and follicle stimulating hormone (FSH) secretion from pituitary gonadotrophs was isolated, purified and its structure determined as the decapeptide luteinizing hormone-releasing hormone, LHRH, 15 years ago by A.V. Schally's laboratory [2,3]. LH and FSH regulate gonadal function in both sexes which in response produce compounds that act as feedback signals for the hypothalamus and the pituitary gland. Homeostasis of this system, as other endocrine systems, is maintained by controlling mechanisms. The action of hypothalamic releasing and release- inhibiting hormones can be controlled through their biosynthesis, processing and secretion as well as at their target, the pituitary gland.

After thyrotropin-releasing hormone, TRH, a tripeptide [4,5], the LHRH decapeptide was only the second hypothalamic regulatory peptide to be structurally characterized. Progress toward understanding the biosynthesis of LHRH has been difficult. The peptide is present in the central nervous system (CNS) in extremely low concentrations and cells producing it are located in a relatively diffuse area putting the existing most sensitive and specific methods to the test. In addition to these technical problems, understanding of peptide biosynthetic processes was incomplete, a fact reflected in earlier work.

Because of the small size of the first hypothalamic peptides discovered, it was assumed that hypothalamic neurosecretory cells did not have the protein synthetic ability peripheral endocrine glands do. Based on analogy with other small biologically active peptides which are assembled by enzyme-directed synthesis [6,7], early studies of LHRH biosynthesis focused on possible non-ribosomal biosynthesis, without clear conclusions [8,9]. *In vivo* biosynthesis of LHRH in mammalian hypothalamus was shown only recently by injecting radiolabeled amino acids into the third ventricle or the preoptic area. The demonstration of incorporation of the label into the decapeptide clearly suggested ribosomal mRNA-directed synthesis of LHRH [10,11].

In certain vertebrate species including fish and chicken, two separate forms of LHRH were found and sequenced [12-16]. These peptides have structural differences but both show gonadotropin-releasing activity [14].

The existence of two different forms of LHRH within one species implies that related genes encode these peptides.

Studies of LHRH biosynthesis and that of other peptide hormones have been based on the characterization, isolation and localization of either the <u>peptide</u> itself or the <u>nucleic acids</u> encoding and translating the peptide. We will also review earlier and current data accordingly.

ISOLATION, CHARACTERIZATION AND LOCALIZATION OF LHRH-LIKE PEPTIDES

High-molecular weight immunoreactive forms of LHRH

Studies of mRNA-directed biosynthesis of peptide precursors and their intracellular secretory pathways increased our knowledge in the area of peptide hormone biosynthesis. In addition, during the 1970s, high molecular weight forms of known biologically active peptides were detected and isolated. Many of these were identified as precursors of peptide hormones ("preprohormones" and "prohormones") which are cleaved by processing enzymes to generate the biologically active hormones [reviewed in 17-20].

Using antisera generated against synthetic LHRH, high molecular weight immunoreactive (HMW-IR) forms of the hormone were detected in extracts of the hypothalami of several mammalian species including rat, sheep and pig. Different isolation studies reported extremely different sizes of such putative precursor forms, which ranged from 1.8 to 70 kilodaltons [21-28]. Most of the size estimates were based on gel filtration under non-denaturing conditions and therefore cannot be considered accurate. Furthermore, in some of these studies the possibility of macromolecule-bound LHRH or aggregates of the decapeptide or its prohormone cannot be excluded. These studies relied on the specificity of polyclonal antibodies, often even on a single antiserum, which may have introduced artefacts. In addition, the influence of proteases present in hypothalamic tissue extracts might have caused additional unexpected modifications of the isolated HMW-IR LHRH fractions. Even today, with our knowledge of the correct LHRH precursor structure, it is difficult to interpret some of these earlier results.

In two studies [25,28] using several antibodies specific for the middle region of the decapeptide or postulated extended peptides, three peaks of LHRH-immunoreactivity were found: a high MW form (26 kD in one study [28], and >5 kD in the other [25]), one component only slightly larger than the decapeptide (1.8 kD) and finally LHRH itself. The HMW-IR material was shown to generate LHRH upon tryptic and aminopeptidase cleavage [26].

To characterize the processing of the HMW-IR peak, the putative prohormone, in different parts of the hypothalamus, a combination of two antibodies specific for processed and unprocessed LHRH were used. As expected, the median eminence contained primarily processed decapeptide, whereas the supraoptic chiasmatic area contained primarily unprocessed HMW-IR LHRH [26]. The 26 kD material was found mainly in axo/cytoplasmic supernatants of hypothalamic tissue homogenates whereas the 1.8 kD form and LHRH itself were found in the synaptosomal fraction corresponding to nerve endings [28]. These studies

38

seemed to support the ribosomal biosynthesis of LHRH in cells of the preoptic area and consecutive enzymatic processing of the prohormone during transport to the median eminence.

Analogy with other peptide precursors suggested that the precursor form of LHRH might be extended at either its N- or C-terminus, or both. pGlu was found to be formed from Gln by spontaneous cyclization in gastrin and other peptides [29] suggesting a similar mechanism for the formation of the N-terminus of LHRH. The discovery of a C-terminal amidating enzyme [30] suggested that in the LHRH precursor an additional glycine follows the decapeptide sequence.

The 26 and 1.8 kD materials were also found in placental extracts where LHRH is known to be synthesized [28]. However, only relatively low concentrations of the decapeptide compared to the HMW forms were found [31], suggesting tissue-specific differences in precursor processing between hypothalamus and placenta. Rat testis is also known to contain LHRH- immunoassayable material [32-34]. The processed decapeptide and higher MW forms were shown to be present in testicular tissue extracts, although only in very low amounts [34].

Immunohistochemical studies of LHRH biosynthesis

Immunohistochemical studies and radioimmunoassays of well characterized brain nuclei in different species revealed the sites of production of LHRH [reviewed in 35-38]. Combinations of LHRH antisera specific for different structural regions of the decapeptide proved to be extremely useful to localize the production in perikarya, axonal transport and processing of LHRH [39-41]. The decapeptide shows a wide tissue distribution. Cells that synthesize LHRH destined for secretion from neurovascular terminals into portal blood and thus regulate gonadotropin release, reside in the diagonal band of Broca, the septal preoptic area and the organum vasculosum of the lamina terminalis. Further locations of interest are extrahypothalamic CNS regions including the olfactory bulb, the cortex and the pineal. Mammalian forebrain contains a total of only 1000 cells producing LHRH-immunoreactive material resulting in the very low abundance of the peptide in the CNS [46]. LHRH was shown to be involved in the regulation of mating behaviour in mammals [42,43]. The mechanism of this action is not known. However, LHRH was found to be a neurotransmitter in frog sympathetic ganglia [44,45]. Whether LHRH regulates reproductive behaviour by acting as a neurotransmitter in mammalian brain, remains to be demonstrated.

The gonads, lactating mammary tissue and placenta also contain LHRH or LHRH-like immunoreactive material [28,31-34,47]. The physiological role of LHRH in those tissues has not been clearly established although receptor binding has been demonstrated and some functions have been recognized [48-52].

Immunohistochemical studies in mammalian brain with antisera raised against LHRH conjugated via the C-terminus stained perikarya and axons preferentially [35]. This finding seemed to support that LHRH is extended at its C-terminus or at both of its termini. "Conformational" antisera which recognize the spatially close ends of the decapeptide (with pGlu and Gly-NH$_2$ ends) showed intense staining of nerve terminals in the median eminence and only little or no staining of perikarya [39], however, another similar antiserum stained perikarya and axons with similar intensity [41]. These studies provided evidence for prohormone processing in perikarya and during axonal transport,which, however, seems to be different in different species [39-41].

Cellular pathways of biosynthesis and processing could be visualized by electron microscopic immunohistochemistry which provided further support for the ribosomal synthesis of an LHRH precursor. LHRH-immunostaining was evident in the rough endoplasmic reticulum, the Golgi apparatus and in secretory vesicles [39,53].

ISOLATION, CHARACTERIZATION AND LOCALIZATION OF NUCLEIC ACIDS INVOLVED IN LHRH BIOSYNTHESIS

Methods allowing for the isolation and characterization of DNA and mRNA encoding peptide precursors were developed during the late 1970s and provided an alternative to study mRNA-directed synthesis of peptides and proteins [reviewed in 54,55].

Cell-free translation of hypothalamic RNA

Cell-free translation of rat and sheep hypothalamic poly(A^+) RNA in the presence of labeled amino acids followed by immunoprecipitation and gel electrophoresis was used to characterize the size of the LHRH precursor [56-60]. One study utilizing several antisera including middle-specific antisera ideal for precursor recognition, failed to detect possible precursor forms of LHRH. Such failure suggested that the mRNA species is less than a millionth of total hypothalamic mRNA [56]. However, in another study using a single antiserum a major 28 kD form was described as a putative LHRH prohormone [57]. This 28 kD protein was absent in RNA from hypogonadal mice deficient in LHRH [58]. A recent characterization of the antiserum (HC-6) used in this study showed that it is highly specific for the modified ends of the decapeptide, pGlu and Gly-NH_2, and insensitive to changes in the middle region, suggesting that this antiserum could not have detected the prohormonal form of LHRH [59]. In a similar approach using cell-free translation a 60 kD protein was immunoprecipitated with a single antiserum [60]. Both of these studies illustrate the limitations of this methodology.

Cloning of LHRH precursor cDNA

Whereas the use of antibodies can reveal structural determinants of proteins and peptides the cloning and analysis of coding sequences for these proteins will reveal their complete primary structure. The usefulness of the recombinant DNA approach lies in the fact that very large cDNA libraries can be generated starting from any given tissue. These libraries can be screened with radiolabeled oligonucleotides for the presence of cloned sequences encoding peptides of interest. The large size of the libraries guarantees that even rare mRNA species are represented as cloned cDNAs and will yield their sequences, once found with the use of the appropriate probe. Alternatively, sequences of interest can also be isolated from genomic libraries. Since most genes have a mosaic structure such that coding sequences are interrupted by intronic DNA, it is not possible to predict protein structures by gene analysis alone. A gene segment can be used, however, to screen a cDNA library for the cloned cDNA that is derived from the genome. Knowledge of the cDNA sequence in turn is essential to determine the number of exons and their location within the genomic DNA.

Signal peptide: LHRH: Cleavage site:

```
MKPIQKLLAGLILLTSCVEGCSS        QHWSYGLRPG      GKR
METIPKLMAAVVLLTVCLEGCSS        QHWSYGLRPG      GKR
```

GAP (GnRH/LHRH-associated peptide):

```
DAENLIDSFQEIVKEVGQLAETQRFECTTHQPRSPLRDLKGALESLIEEETGQKKI
NTEHLVDSFQEMGKEEDQMAEPQNFECTVHWPRSPLRDLRGALERLIEEEAGQKKM
```

Figure 1   Amino acid sequence of human (top) and rat (bottom) preproLHRH in the one-letter code as deduced from the cDNA sequences [66,67].

During the past decade the cDNA sequences of several biologically active peptide precursors have been determined, among them those of known hypothalamic hormones. These included precursors of somatostatin [61], corticotropin releasing hormone [62], growth hormone releasing hormone [63], enkephalins [64,65], LHRH (as discussed below in detail) [66,67] and thyrotropin releasing hormone [68].

To determine the structure of the LHRH precursor by recombinant DNA methods a combination of approaches based on genomic and cDNA libraries was used [66]. Oligonucleotide probes were constructed to encode a hypothetical peptide containing the decapeptide structure extended at its N-terminus by a -Lys-Arg- enzymatic processing site and an additional glycine residue at the C-terminus to serve as amide donor. These oligonucleotides proved sufficiently homologous to identify one human genomic clone which contained the LHRH gene. A 600-base pair DNA restriction fragment of the genomic clone was used to isolate the corresponding cDNA from a human placental cDNA library [66]. Subsequently, a hypothalamic cDNA was also isolated and sequenced [67]. The hypothalamic precursor structure is completely identical with the placental one. The human and rat sequences are shown in Fig. 1.

In the precursor a 23-amino acid signal sequence precedes the LHRH decapeptide which, in turn, is followed by a -Gly-Lys-Arg- processing and amidation site and a 56-amino acid peptide which we call GAP (GnRH-associated peptide). The C-terminus of GAP is -Lys-Lys-Ile in the human sequence whereas in the rat and mouse it is -Lys-Lys-Met, which may represent a further cleavage site.

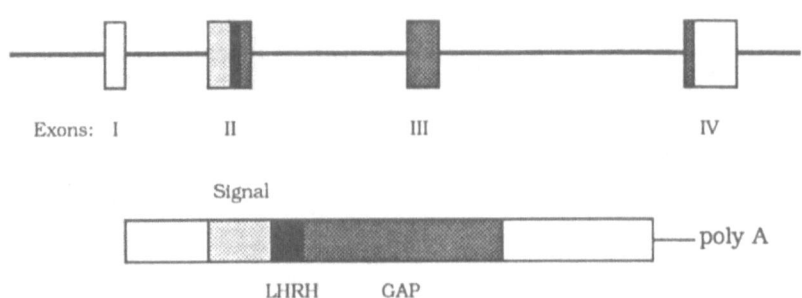

Exons: I   II   III   IV

Signal

poly A

LHRH   GAP

Figure 2 Schematic structure of the mammalian LHRH gene and cDNA [67]. The two scales are not proportional.

The LHRH gene in human, rat and mouse consists of four exons and three introns (Fig. 2). The identity in coding and 3' untranslated regions of the placental and hypothalamic cDNAs suggested the expression of the same gene in both tissues, as confirmed by Southern analysis and chromosomal localization [67,69]. Interestingly, this single LHRH gene is translated differently in hypothalamus and placenta such that mRNAs are generated which differ in the structure of their 5' untranslated regions. Thus, this mRNA region retains the sequence of the first intron in all but neural tissues where it is removed by an additional splicing event. Furthermore, different promoters control transcription in neural and peripheral tissues (Joel S. Hayflick and Peter H. Seeburg, unpublished).

The isolation and sequence determination of the LHRH precursor cDNA provided the basis of a variety of studies at the nucleic acid and the peptide level. We will review the currently available data.

STUDIES BASED ON THE PRECURSOR STRUCTURE

Localization of LHRH cells by *in situ* hybridization

In situ hybridization histochemistry has become a powerful method to study the location of peptide hormone biosynthesis. This technique based on hybridization of cDNA or synthetic cDNA fragments with mRNA in tissue preparations is able to measure mRNA levels in individual cells [reviewed in 70]. Using a synthetic oligonucleotide based on the human cDNA sequence (corresponding to amino acids -5 to 15) [66] to probe rat forebrain sections, the LHRH mRNA-containing cells could be identified [71]. However, a probe corresponding to amino acids 33 to 52 of the human prohormone failed to hybridize with rat brain LHRH mRNA [71] probably due to differences between the human and rat sequences (17 differences/60 total vs. 6/59 for the other probe). Using oligonucleotide probes corresponding to amino acids 9 to 24 and 54 to 69 of the mouse precursor, cells producing LHRH could be clearly visualized in mouse brain sections (Fig.3) [72,73].

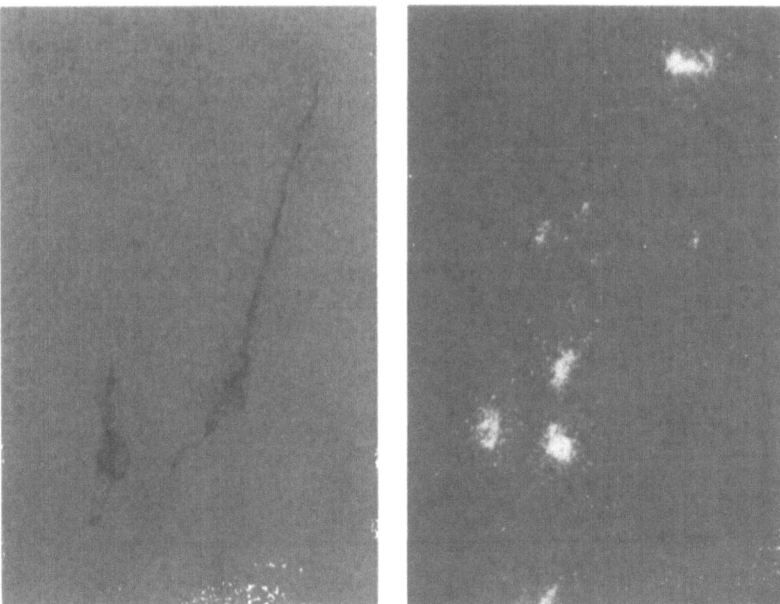

Figure 3 Immunohistochemical (left) and *in situ* (right) localization of proLHRH in the preoptic area of mouse brain. Antiserum against rat GAP-20-43 (prohormone 33-56) and an oligo- nucleotide corresponding to amino acids 9-24 of the mouse prohormone were used, respectively. (courtesy of J.N. Wilcox).

Immunohistochemical localization of pro-LHRH

Specific antibodies were produced against synthetic fragments of the GAP portion of the LHRH prohormone and were used for immunohistochemical localization of the prohormone products and the development of radioimmunoassays to study tissue distribution and secretion of these peptides [74]. An RIA based on an antibody raised against the middle 14 amino acids of GAP (27-40) detected the presence of GAP-like antigen in rat hypothalamic extracts. The same antibody was also used for the immunocytochemical colocalization of LHRH and GAP in the septo-preoptic region and other areas of rat brain [74]. Similar results were obtained with other antisera raised against different peptide fragments corresponding to the human and rat 56-amino acid peptides. Primate brain showed identical CNS distribution of LHRH and GAP in all regions examined [75]. Extrahypothalamic peripheral tissues also contained both peptides in identical cell types [76]. In mice, no significant difference between hypothalamic and gonadal processing of the prohormone was found [73]. These findings further support the existence of a single functional gene of LHRH in mammals since the decapeptide is always accompanied by GAP. Obviously, the possibility of a structurally different precursor containing a different GAP cannot be excluded at this time.

Both products of the LHRH prohormone could be detected along axons projecting to the median eminence [74]. Electron microscopic localization of GAP-like immunoreactivity revealed dense-cored vesicles in terminal and preterminal varicosities representative of secretory vesicles.

Secretion and pituitary effects of pro-LHRH products

In mammals LHRH is secreted into the hypothalamo-pituitary portal circulation in a characteristic pulsatile manner necessary for normal reproductive function [77]. Using RIAs based on antisera generated against GAP regions we found that GAP is also secreted into hypophyseal portal blood in sheep and the pattern of secretion is very similar to that of LHRH in individual animals using frequent sampling (Fig.4) [78].

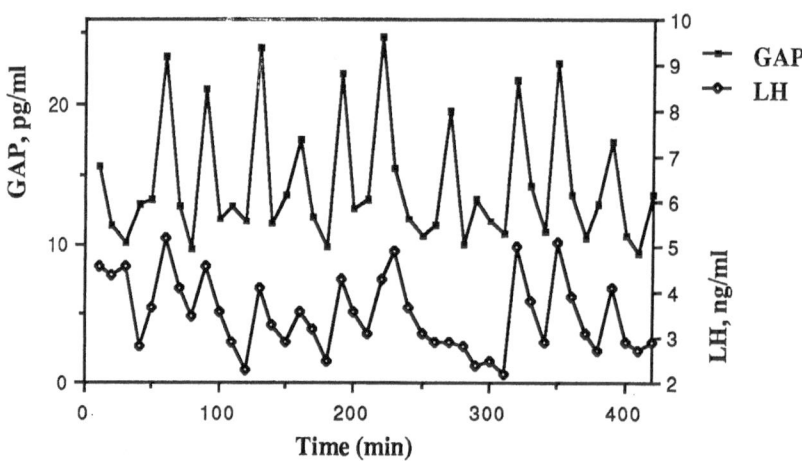

Figure 4 Secretion of GAP into portal blood (■) and LH into peripheral blood (◊) of an ovariectomized sheep using simultaneous sampling at 10 min intervals [data from 78].

The fact that GAP reaches the anterior pituitary via portal circulation suggested that the 56-amino acid peptide might exert an effect on pituitary hormone secretion. GAP produced by recombinant DNA methods was tested in rat anterior pituitary cell cultures *in vitro* and it was found to inhibit basal prolactin secretion and stimulate gonadotropin secretion [79]. This finding was confirmed using chemically synthesized GAP [80]. *In vivo,* the peptide inhibited suckling-induced prolactin secretion in rats [80]. Hypogonadal (hpg) mice which lack hypothalamic LHRH [81] were treated with multiple daily injections of GAP for two weeks. As a result, serum prolactin levels decreased in both males and females with a simultaneous increase in pituitary prolactin content [80,82]. Rabbits immunized with GAP-related synthetic antigens had greatly elevated prolactin levels which correlated with increasing GAP antibody titers [79]. However, GAP had no effect on serum prolactin levels in several experimental paradigms including normal and steroid-treated rats and sheep [80]. Partial N-terminal peptide fragments of GAP were reported to have gonadotropin-releasing activity *in vitro* [83] and therefore the possiblity of further processing of GAP cannot be excluded. The fact that LHRH and GAP both have pituitary effects opens new aspects of the integration of pituitary hormone secretion. The isolation of GAP or GAP fragments from natural sources and tests of their activity will provide more information on the possible physiological role(s) of the peptide in extrahypothalamic tissues.

Genetic deficiency of LHRH

The infertile hypogonadal (hpg) mouse was demonstrated to lack detectable amounts of LHRH and believed to have a defect in either its biosynthetic or processing mechanisms [81]. The defect can be partly corrected by LHRH replacement therapy [84] or by transplantation of normal brain tissue [85,86].

Analysis of the hpg mouse LHRH gene revealed a deletion of part of the gene which, however, does not remove the LHRH coding sequence but only that of GAP [72]. Although a defective mRNA is transcribed, the decapeptide is not processed from the translation product of the defective mRNA.

Introduction of the complete LHRH-GAP gene into transgenic hpg homozygous mice reversed the phenotypic defects: the transgenic animals had virtually normal levels of LHRH, GAP, gonadotropins and prolactin and animals of both sexes were found to be fertile [73]. This result supports the idea that expression of this single gene determines LHRH synthesis and is pivotal for mammalian reproduction.

CONCLUSIONS AND PERSPECTIVES

After a long search for the biosynthetic protein precursor of LHRH by methods of peptide chemistry and immunology, its structure was predicted by recombinant DNA methods [69,70]. The precursor generates two peptides, LHRH and GAP, although the existence of further processed fragments cannot be excluded at this time. In the prohormone, LHRH is only extended through its C-terminus. Thus, some of the earlier results on LHRH biosynthesis can be explained whereas others cannot. There is a "HMW form" of LHRH (~7.5 kD as monomer or ~15 kD as a disulfide-linked dimer) and possibly a slightly larger form (LHRH-Gly-Lys-Arg). However, the steps and kinetics of prohormone cleavage are not known yet. Tryptic cleavage generates LHRH from the prohormone but exopeptidases do not.

Knowledge of a polyprotein precursor structure opens up a whole spectrum of further investigations. In the case of the LHRH precursor, several exciting questions will be answered using the information provided by the DNA and peptide sequences. LHRH is regulated by steroid feedback signals but the level of regulation is not known. By analogy with other steroid-regulated mechanisms it is anticipated that transcription is controlled [87] although posttranslational processing can also be regulated [88].

Expression of the gene in the CNS and in peripheral tissues can be studied based on the sequences. The cloned cDNA will be used to chart all body tissues using *in situ* hybridization for expression of the LHRH gene. Similarly, immunohistochemistry using antibodies against different regions of the LHRH prohormone can be used for localization of expression, to follow posttranslational processing and transport of processed products. Possible differences in splicing, expression, translation and posttranslational processing in different tissues can be investigated. It will be a task for the future to analyze the physiology of LHRH and GAP in extrahypothalamic tissues.

A further fascinating issue that still remains to be addressed is the possible multiplicity of LHRH genes. Lower vertebrate species have different genes encoding different forms of the decapeptide whereas mammals have a single gene of reproductive significance. The possible existence of a second variant gene in mammals cannot be excluded at this time but evidence summarized above suggests that in mammals the gene described is the one that is essential in the control of reproduction.

REFERENCES

1. Harris, G.W. Neural control of the pituitary gland. Physiol. Rev. **28**, 139 (1948)
2. Schally, A.V., Arimura, A., Baba, Y., Nair, R.M.G., Matsuo, H., Redding, T.W., Debeljuk, L. and White W.F. Isolation and properties of the FSH and LH-releasing hormone. Biochem. Biophys. Res. Commun. **43**, 393 (1971)
3. Matsuo, H., Baba, Y., Nair, R.M.G., Arimura, A. and Schally, A.V. Structure of the porcine LH and FSH releasing hormone I. Proposed amino acid sequence. Biochem. Biophys. Res. Commun. **43**, 1334 (1971)
4. Burgus, R., Dunn, T.F., Desiderio, D., Ward, D.N., Vale, W. and Guillemin, R. Characterization of ovine hypothalamic hypophysiotropic TSH-releasing factor. Nature **226**, 321 (1970)
5. Nair, R.M.G., Barrett, J.F., Bowers, C.Y., Schally, A.V. Structure of porcine thyrotropin-releasing hormone. Biochemistry **9**, 1103 (1970)
6. Mooz, E.D. and Meister, A. Tripeptide (glutathione) synthetase. Purification, properties and mechanism of action. Biochemistry **6**, 1722 (1967)
7. Kurahashi, K. Biosynthesis of small peptides. Ann. Rev. Biochem. **43**, 445 (1974)
8. Reichlin, S. and Mitnick. Enzymatic synthesis of growth hormone releasing factor (GH-RF) by rat incubates and by extracts of rat and porcine hypothalamic tissue. Proc. Soc. Exp. Biol. Med. **142**, 497 (1973)
9. Johansson, K.N.G., Currie, B.L. and Folkers, K. Biosynthesis of the luteinizing hormone releasing hormone in mitochondrial

preparations and by a possible pantetheine-template mechanism. Biochem.Biophys. Res. Commun. 53, 502 (1973)

10. Kochman, K., Kerdelhue, B., Ostrowska, A., Chomicka, L., Domanski, E. and Jutisz, M. Biosynthesis *in vivo* of gonadotropin-releasing hormone in the hypothalamus of normal and ovariectomized female rats. Mol. Cell. Endocrinol. 25, 193 (1982)

11. Krause, J.E., Advis, J.P. and McKelvy, J.F. *In vivo* biosynthesis of hypothalamic luteinizing hormone-releasing hormone in individual free-running female rats. Endocrinology 111, 344 (1982)

12. King, J.A. and Millar, R.P. Structure of chicken hypothalamic luteinizing hormone-releasing hormone II. Isolation and characterization. J. Biol. Chem. 257, 10729 (1982)

13. Miyamoto, K., Hasegawa Y., Minegishi, T., Nomura, M., Takahashi, Y., Igarashi, M., Kangawa, Y. and Matsuo, H. Isolation and characterization of chicken hypothalamic luteinizing hormone-releasing hormone. Biochem. Biophys. Res. Commun. 107, 820 (1982)

14. Miyamoto, K., Hasegawa Y., Nomura M., Igarashi, M., Kangawa, Y. and Matsuo, H. Identification of the second gonadotropin-releasing hormone in chicken hypothalamus: evidence that gonadotropin secretion is probably controlled by two distinct gonadotropin-releasing hormones in avianspecies. Proc. Natl. Acad. Sci. USA 81, 3874 (1984)

15. Sherwood, N.M., Eiden, L., Brownstein, M., Spiess, J., Rivier, J. and Vale, W. Characterization of a teleost gonadotropin-releasing hormone. Proc. Natl. Acad. Sci. USA 80, 2794 (1983)

16. Sherwood, N.M., Sower, S.A., Marshak, D.R., Fraser B.A. and Brownstein, M.J. Primary structure of gonadotropin-releasing hormone from lamprey brain. J. Biol. Chem. 261, 4812 (1986)

17. Docherty, K. and Steiner, D.F. Posttranslational proteolysis in polypeptide hormone biosynthesis. Ann. Rev. Physiol. 44, 625 (1982)

18. Eipper, B.A. and Mains, R.E. Structure and biosynthesis of pro-adrenocorticotropin/endorphin and related peptides. Endocrine Rev. 1, 1 (1980)

19. Brownstein, M.J., Russell, J.T. and Gainer, H. Synthesis, transport and release of posterior pituitary hormones. Science 207, 373 (1980)

20. Lingappa, V.R. and Blobel, G. Early events in the biosynthesis of secretory and membrane proteins: the signal hypothesis. Rec. Prog. Horm. Res. 36, 451 (1980)

21. Kerdelhue, B, Jutisz, M., Gillessen, D. and Studer, R.O. Obtention of antisera against a hypothalamic decapeptide (LH/FSH-RH) which stimulates the release of pituitary gonadotropins and development of its radioimmunoassay. Biochim. Biophys. Acta 297, 540 (1973)

22. Fawcett, C.P., Beezley, E.A. and Wheaton, J.E. Detection of a second form of luteinizing hormone releasing factor. J. Int. Res. Commun. 2, 1663 (1974)

23. Barnea, A. and Porter, J.C. Demonstration of a macromolecule cross-reacting with antibodies to luteinizing hormone releasing hormone and its tissue distribution. Biochem. Biophys. Res. Commun. 67, 1346 (1975)

24. Fawcett, C.P., Beezley, E.A. and Wheaton, J.E. Chromatographic evidence for the existence of another species of luteinizing hormone-releasing factor (LRF). Endocrinology 96, 1311 (1975)

25. Millar, R.P., Aehnelt, C. and Rossier, G. Higher molecular weight

immunoreactive species of luteinizing hormone releasing hormone: possible precursors of the hormone. Biochem. Biophys. Res. Commun. **74**, 720 (1977)

26. Millar, R.P., Denniss, P., Tobler, C., King, J.C., Schally, A.V. and Arimura, A. Presumptive prohormonal forms of hypothalamic peptide hormones. In: Coll. Int. C.N.R.S. 280, Vincent, J.D. and Kordon, C. (eds.), CNRS, Paris, 1977, p. 487

27. Millar, R.P., Wegener, I. and Schally, A.V. Putative prohormonal luteinizing hormone releasing hormone. In: Neuropeptides: Biochemical and Physiological Studies, Millar, R.P. (ed.), Churchill Livingstone, Edinburgh, 1981, p. 111

28. Gautron, J.P., Pattou, E. and Kordon, C. Occurrence of higher molecular forms of LHRH in fractionated extracts from rat hypothalamus, cortex and placenta. Mol. Cell. Endocrinol. **24**, 1 (1981)

29. Gregory, R.A. Grossman, M.I., Tracy, H.J. and Bentley, P.H. Isolation of two "big gastrins" from Zollinger-Ellison tumours. Lancet ii, 797 (1972)

30. Bradbury, A.F., Finnie, M.D.A. and Smyth, D.G. Mechanism of C-terminal amide formation by pituitary enzymes. Nature **298**, 686 (1982)

31. Tan, L. and Rousseau, P. The chemical identity of the immunoreactive LHRH-like peptide biosynthesized in the human placenta. Biochem. Biophys. Res. Commun. **109**, 1061 (1982)

32. Sharpe, R.M., Fraser, H.M., Cooper, I. and Rommerts, F.F.G. Sertoli-Leydig cell communication via an LHRH-like factor. Nature **290**, 785 (1981)

33. Bhasin, S., Heber, D., Peterson, M. and Swerdloff, R. Partial isolation and characterization of testicular GnRH-like factors. Endocrinology **112**, 1144 (1983)

34. Hedger, M.P., Robertson, D.M., Browne, C.A. and de Kretser, D.M. The isolation and measurement of luteinizing hormone-releasing hormone (LHRH) from the rat testis. Mol. Cell. Endocrinol. **42**, 163 (1985)

35. Sternberger, L.A. and Hoffman, G.E. Immunocytology of luteinizing hormone-releasing hormone. Neuroendocrinology **25**, 111 (1978)

36. Krey, L.C. and Silverman, A.J. Luteinizing hormone-releasing hormone. In: Brain Peptides, Krieger, D.T., Brownstein, M.J. and Martin, J.B. (eds.), Wiley, New York, 1983, p. 687

37. Shivers, B.D., Harlan, R.E. and Pfaff, D.W. Reproduction: the central nervous system role of luteinizing hormone releasing hormone. In: *ibid*. p. 389

38. Palkovits, M. Distribution of neuropeptides in the central nervous system: a review of biochemical mapping studies. Prog. Neurobiol. **23**, 151 (1984)

39. King, J.C. and Anthony, E.L.P. Biosynthesis of LHRH: Inferences from immunocytochemical studies. Peptides **4**, 963 (1983)

40. Ellinwood, W.E., Ronnekleiv, O.K., Kelly, M.J. and Resko, J.A. A new antiserum with conformational specificity for LHRH: usefulness for radioimmunoassay and immunocytochemistry. Peptides **6**, 45 (1985)

41. King, J.C., Anthony, E.L.P., Fitzgerald, D.M. and Stopa, E.G. Luteinizing hormone-releasing hormone neurons in human preoptic/hypothalamus: differential intraneuronal localization of immunoreactive forms. J. Clin. Endocrinol. Metab. **60**, 88 (1985)

42. Moss, R.L. and McCann, S.M. Induction of mating behaviour in rats by luteinizing hormone-releasing factor. Science **181**, 177 (1973)
43. Pfaff, D.W. Luteinizing hormone-releasing factor potentiates lordosis behaviour in hypophysectomized, ovariectomized female rats. Science **182**, 1148 (1973)
44. Jan, Y.N., Jan, L.Y. and Kuffler, S.W. A peptide as a possible transmitter in sympathetic ganglia of the frog. Proc. Natl. Acad. Sci. USA **76**, 1501 (1979)
45. Jan, L.Y. and Jan, Y.N. Peptidergic transmission in sympathetic ganglia of the frog. J. Physiol. **327**, 219 (1982)
46. Shivers, B.D., Harlan, R.E., Morrell, J.I. and Pfaff, D.W. Immunocytochemical localization of luteinizing hormone-releasing hormone in male and female rat brains: Quantitative studies on the effect of gonadal steroids. Neuroendocrinology **36**, 1 (1983)
47. Smith, S.S. and Ojeda, S.R. Maternal modulation of infantile ovarian development and available ovarian luteinizing hormone-releasing hormone receptors via milk LHRH. Endocrinology **115**, 1973 (1984)
48. Ekholm, C., Hillensjo, T. and Isaksson, O. Gonadotropin-releasing hormone agonists stimulate oocyte meiosis and ovulation in hypophysectomized rats. Endocrinology **108**, 2022 (1981)
49. Clayton, R.N. and Catt K.J. Gonadotropin-releasing hormone receptors: characterization, physiological regulation and relationship to reproductive function. Endocrine Rev. **2**, 186 (1981)
50. Hsueh, A.J.W. and Jones, P.B.C. Gonadotropin releasing hormone: extrapituitary actions and paracrine control mechanisms. Ann. Rev. Physiol. **45**, 83 (1983)
51. Hsueh, A.J.W., Adashi, E.Y., Jones, P.B.C. and Welsh, T.H. Hormonal control of the differentiation of cultured ovarian granulosa cells. Endocrine Rev. **2**, 437 (1984)
52. Birnbaumer, L., Shahabi, N., Rivier, J. and Vale, W. Evidence for a physiological role of a gonadotropin-releasing hormone (GnRH) or GnRH-like material in the ovary. Endocrinology **116**, 1367 (1985)
53. Krisch, B. Two types of luliberin-immunoreactive perikarya in the preoptic area of the rat. Cell Tissue Res. **212**, 443 (1980)
54. Douglass, J., Civelli, O. and Herbert, E. Polyprotein gene expression: Generation of diversity of neuroendocrine peptides. Ann. Rev. Biochem. **53**, 665 (1984)
55. Mayo, K.E., Evans, R.E. and Rosenfeld, G.M. Genes encoding neuroendocrine peptides: Strategies toward their identification and analysis. Ann. Rev. Physiol. **48**, 431 (1986)
56. Jutisz, M., Counis, R. and Corbani, M. Biosynthesis of gonadotropin releasing hormone (GnRH): present status. Psychoneuroendocrinol. **8**, 251 (1983)
57. Curtis, A. and Fink, G. A high molecular weight precursor of luteinizing hormone releasing hormone from rat hypothalamus Endocrinology **112**, 390 (1983)
58. Curtis, A., Lyons, V. and Fink, G. The human hypothalamic LHRH precursor is the same size as that in rat and mouse hypothalamus. Biochem. Biophys. Res. Commun. **117**, 872 (1983)
59. Curtis, A., Szelke, M. and Fink, G. Detection of a high-molecular-weight LHRH precursor by cell-free translation of mRNA from human, rat and mouse hypothalamus. Meth. Enzymol. **124**, 318 (1986)

60. Charli, J.L., Cohen, S., Diaz de Leon, L., Millar, R.P., Arimura, A. and Joseph-Bravo, P. Molecular weight of a putative LHRH precursor synthesized in a cell-free system. 7th Int. Cong. Endocrinol. Excerpta Medica Int. Cong. Series 652, Abstract 411 (1984)

61. Shen, L.P., Pictet, R.L. and Rutter, W.J. Human somatostatin I: sequence of the cDNA. Proc. Natl. Acad. Sci. USA 79, 4575 (1982)

62. Furutani, Y., Morimoto, Y., Shibahara, S., Noda, M., Takahashi, H., Hirose, T., Asai, M., Inayama, S., Hayashida, H., Miyata, T. and Numa, S. Cloning and sequence analysis of cDNA for ovine corticotropin-releasing factor precursor. Nature 301, 537 (1983)

63. Gubler, U., Monahan, J.J., Lomedico, P.T., Bhatt, R.S., Collier, K.J., Hoffman, B.J., Bohlen, P., Esch, F., Ling, N., Zeytin, F., Brazeau, P., Poonian, M.S. and Gage, L.P. Cloning and sequence analysis of human growth hormone-releasing factor, somatocrinin. Proc. Natl. Acad. Sci. USA 80, 4311 (1983)

64. Noda, M., Furutani, Y., Takahashi, H., Toyosato, M., Hirose, T., Inayama, S., Nakanishi, S. and Numa, S. Cloning and sequence analysis of cDNA for bovine adrenal preproenkephalin. Nature 295, 202 (1982)

65. Gubler, U., Seeburg, P.H., Hoffman, B.J., Gage, L.P. and Udenfriend, S. Molecular cloning establishes proenkephalin as precursor of enkephalin-containing peptides. Nature 295, 206 (1982)

66. Seeburg, P.H. and Adelman, J.P. Characterization of cDNA for precursor of human luteinizing hormone releasing hormone. Nature 311, 666 (1984)

67. Adelman, J.P., Mason, A.J., Hayflick, J.S. and Seeburg, P.H. Isolation of the gene and hypothalamic cDNA for the common precursor of gonadotropin-releasing hormone and prolactin-inhibiting factor in human and rat. Proc. Natl. Acad. Sci. USA 83, 179 (1986)

68. Lechan, R.M., Wu, P., Jackson, I.M.D., Wolf, H., Cooperman, S., Mandel, G. and Goodman, R.H. Thyrotropin-releasing hormone precursor: characterization in rat brain. Science 231, 159 (1986)

69. Yang-Feng, T.L., Seeburg, P.H. and Francke, U. Human luteinizing hormone-releasing hormone gene (LHRH) is located on short arm of chromosome 8 (region 8p11.2-p21). Som. Cell Mol. Genetics 12, 95 (1986)

70. Wilcox, J.N., Gee, C.E. and Roberts, J.L. In situ cDNA:mRNA hybridization development of a technique to measure mRNA levels in individual cells. Meth. Enzymol. 124, 510 (1986)

71. Shivers, B.D., Harlan, R.E., Hejtmancik, J.F., Conn, P.M. and Pfaff, D.W. Localization of cells containing LHRH-like mRNA in rat forebrain using in situ hybridization. Endocrinology 118, 883 (1986)

72. Mason, A.J., Hayflick, J.S., Zoeller, R.T., Young, W.S., Phillips, H.S., Nikolics, K. and Seeburg, P.H. A deletion truncating the GnRH gene is responsible for hypogonadism in the hpg mouse. Science, in press (1986)

73. Mason, A.J., Pitts, S., Nikolics, K., Szonyi, E., Wilcox, J.N., Seeburg, P.H. and Stewart, T. The hypogonadal mouse: reproductive functions restored by gene therapy. Science, in press (1986)

74. Phillips, H.S., Nikolics, K., Branton, D. and Seeburg, P.H. Immunocytochemical localization in rat brain of a prolactin release-inhibiting sequence of gonadotropin-releasing hormone prohormone. Nature 316, 542 (1985)

75. Song, T., Nikolics, K., Seeburg, P.H. and Goldsmith, P.C.

GnRH-prohormone-containing neurons in the primate brain: immunostaining for the GnRH-associated peptide. Peptides, in press

76. Clarke, I.J. and Cummins, J.T. The temporal relationship between gonadotropin releasing hormone (GnRH) and luteinizing hormone (LH) secretion in ovariectomized ewes. Endocrinology **111**, 1737 (1982)

77. Padula, C.A., Nikolics, K., Seeburg, P.H. and Goldsmith, P.C. Evidence for proGnRH in rat peripheral tissues: immunostaining with antibodies against GnRH and the GnRH-associated peptide. 1st Int. Cong. Neuroendocrinol., San Francisco, Abstract #100, (1986)

78. Nikolics, K., Seeburg, P.H. and Clarke, I.J. Secretion of gonadotropin releasing hormone (GnRH) and GnRH-associated peptide (GAP) into the hypothalamo-pituitary portal circulation in sheep. 68th Ann. Meeting Endocrine Soc., Anaheim, Abstract #33. (1986)

79. Nikolics, K., Mason, A.J., Szonyi, E., Ramachandran, J. and Seeburg, P.H. A prolactin-inhibiting factor within the precursor for human gonadotropin-releasing hormone. Nature **316**, 511 (1985)

80. Schally, A.V., Olsen, D.B., Gulyas, J., Szoke, B., Horvath, J., Karashima, T., Ressing, T.W., Nikolics, K. and Seeburg, P.H. 68th Ann. Meeting Endocrine Soc., Anaheim, Abstract #8. (1986)

81. Cattanach, B.M., Iddon, C.A., Charlton, H.M., Chiappa,S.A. and Fink, G. Gonadotrophin releasing hormone deficiency in a mutant mouse with hypogonadism. Nature **269**, 338 1977

82. Nikolics, K., Szonyi, E., Ramachandran, J. and Seeburg, P.H., in preparation

83. Millar, R.P., Wormald, P.J. and Milton, R.C. de L. Stimulation of gonadotropin release by a non-GnRH peptide sequence of the GnRH precursor. Science **232**, 68 (1986)

84. Charlton, H.M., Halpin, D.M.G., Iddon, C., Rosie, R., Levy, G., McDowell, I.F.W., Megson, A., Morris, J.F., Bramwell, A., Speight, A., Ward, B.J., Broadhead, J., Davey-Smith, G. and Fink, G. The effects of daily administration of single and multiple injections of gonadotropin-releasing hormone on pituitary and gonadal function in the hypogonadal (hpg) mouse. Endocrinology **113**, 535 (1983)

85. Krieger, D.T., Perlow, M.J., Gibson, M.J., Davies, T.F., Zimmermann, E.A., Ferin, M. and Charlton, H.M. Brain grafts reverse hypogonadism of gonadotrophin releasing hormone deficiency. Nature **310**, 61 (1982)

86. Charlton, H.M. Use of neural transplants to study neuroendocrine mechanisms. In: "Frontiers of Neuroendocrinology", vol 9., Ganong, W.F. and Martini, L., eds. Raven Press, New York, 1986, p.77

87. Birnberg, N., Lissitzki, J.C., Hinman, M. and Herbert, E. Glucocorticoids regulate POMC gene expression in vivo at the level of transcription and translation. Proc. Natl. Acad. Sci. USA **80**, 6982 (1983)

88. Funder, J.W., Smith, A.I., Morgan, F.J., Fullerton, M., Clarke, I.J. and Engler, D. Post-translational processing of CRF in the ovine median eminence. 1st Int. Cong. Neuroendocrinol., San Francisco, Abstract #349 (1986)

5
Phylogenetic Diversity of LHRH

J. A. KING and R. P. MILLAR
Medical Research Council Regulatory Peptides Research Unit, Department of
Chemical Pathology, University of Cape Town Medical School, Observatory 7925,
Cape Town, South Africa

INTRODUCTION

Early studies suggested mammalian hypothalamic luteinizing hormone-
releasing hormone (here referred to as gonadotropin-releasing hormone
(GnRH)) was a unique molecular form, but research over the past eight
years established that there is considerable diversity in the structure of the corresponding releasing hormone in other species. Structural variations in hypothalamic GnRH were demonstrated in species
from all the vertebrate classes, and the sequence of four distinct
GnRH molecules was established in nonmammalian vertebrates. Multiple
forms of GnRH within brain tissue of a single species were demonstrated, thus posing the question of different functions of vertebrate
brain GnRHs. Polymorphism of GnRH within individuals of a species
has not been detected. The presence of multiple forms of GnRH, some
of which are common to species in different vertebrate classes, will
assist in establishing the evolutionary origins of the GnRH molecule.
Precursor molecules for GnRH were identified in mammalian brain.
GnRH or GnRH-like peptides which may differ from the mammalian hypothalamic decapeptide were also found in various non-neural tissues
such as gonads, placenta and pancreas.

For many years the only function ascribed to GnRH was the
release of gonadotropins from the pituitary. It is now believed,
however, that GnRH has additional functions since: a) multiple forms
are present in the brain of most species; b) GnRH is present in
extrahypothalamic brain regions; c) GnRHs or GnRH-like molecules
occur in tissues outside the central nervous system; d) specific
receptors for GnRH are present in extrapituitary tissues.

In this chapter we review current knowledge on the molecular
heterogeneity of GnRHs, the biological actions of GnRHs and related
molecules, structure-activity relations of GnRH and analogs in
vertebrates, and the evolution of the hormone.

STRUCTURALLY IDENTIFIED FORMS OF VERTEBRATE GnRHs

The structures of five different GnRH molecules have been established
(Fig. 1). In mammals, the structure of GnRH (LHRH; here designated
mGnRH) is identical in porcine [1] and ovine [2] hypothalamus, and a

GnRH in rat brain has the same amino acid composition [3]. Two GnRHs
were isolated from chicken hypothalamus : [Gln^8]LHRH (chicken GnRH I;
designated cGnRH I) [4-6] and [His^5,Trp^7,Tyr^8]LHRH (chicken GnRH II;
designated cGnRH II) [7]. GnRHs isolated from salmon (Oncorhynchus
keta) brain [8] and lamprey (Petromyzon marinus) brain [9] have the
structures [Trp^7,Leu^8]LHRH (designated sGnRH) and [Tyr^3,Leu^5,Glu^6,
Trp^7,Lys^8] LHRH (designated lGnRH), respectively. Among amphibians,

```
              1  2   3   4   5   6   7   8   9   10

porcine/ovine pGlu-His-Trp-Ser-Tyr-Gly-Leu-Arg-Pro-Gly-NH2

chicken I     ---------------------------- Gln -----------

chicken II    ------------------ His --- Trp-Tyr -----------

salmon        ------------------------ Trp-Leu -----------

lamprey       --------- Tyr --- Leu-Glu-Trp-Lys -----------
```

FIGURE 1   Structures of the five identified forms of GnRH. The
          conserved amino acids are boxed.

a GnRH in bullfrog (Rana catesbeiana) brain has the same amino acid
composition as mGnRH [10]. Certain regions of the molecule have been
highly conserved, while other regions have undergone evolutionary
change. The length of the decapeptide, the NH$_2$-terminal pGlu^1-His^2
and Ser^4, and the COOH-terminal Pro^9-Gly^{10}NH$_2$ have remained unchanged during 500 million years of evolution. The conservation of
the NH$_2$- and COOH-termini suggests these regions are of functional
significance for conformation, receptor binding, resistance to
enzymatic degradation and in receptor-mediated events required for
gonadotropin release.

PHYLOGENETIC DISTRIBUTION OF GnRH MOLECULAR FORMS

In view of the small quantities of GnRH in brain tissue, isolation
and sequence analysis is an arduous task. We and other groups have
used an 'indirect' approach in studies on the nature of GnRHs in
different vertebrates, which utilises reverse phase high performance
liquid chromatography (HPLC) to separate and identify the GnRHs in
conjunction with radioimmunoassay with specific antisera raised
against the known GnRHs. Biological activity of the peptides is
assessed by measuring their ability to release gonadotropins from
dispersed chicken pituitary cells. Chicken pituitary cells are used
rather than mammalian pituitary cells as they respond to greater
structural variation in GnRH than do the mammalian cells [11,12].

Mammals

Hypothalamic GnRH. The hypothalamic GnRH in all mammalian species
studied has identical chromatographic, immunological and biological

properties to mGnRH. Although it was generally believed that mammalian brain contained a single molecular form of GnRH, there is recent evidence for multiple forms. In ovine hypothalamus we demonstrated the presence of an immunoreactive GnRH which was less positively charged than mGnRH [13]. A more thorough study on ovine and rat hypothalamus has revealed three novel forms of GnRH which are clearly distinct from the known vertebrate GnRHs. The peptides differ in HPLC retention time and in their interaction with GnRH antisera, and they stimulate luteinizing hormone (LH) release from chicken pituitary cells [unpublished]. Two or more chromato-graphically distinct peptides with GnRH activity were reported in rat brain and porcine hypothalamus [7]. Although only a single GnRH sequence (mGnRH) was detected in the mammalian genome [14], this may be due to significant structural differences in other form/s which do not hybridize well with the mGnRH probe.

Extrahypothalamic brain GnRHs. Immmunoreactive GnRH is present in extrahypothalamic brain regions, but few studies have investigated the molecular nature of the peptide/s. The ovine pineal gland has a GnRH identical to the hypothalamic peptide, and a second form of similar size to mGnRH but less positively charged [13,15].

Gonadal GnRH. GnRH has direct effects on the gonads of mammals, and high affinity binding sites for GnRH analogs have been demonstrated in the Leydig cells of the testis and in the granulosa cells of the ovary [see reviews 16, 17 and chapter 9]. GnRH-like peptides have been demonstrated in testicular extracts and follicular fluid [see reviews 16, 17 and chapter 10].

GnRH in other tissues. GnRH in the placenta of various mammals has chromatographic, immunological and biological properties identical to the hypothalamic decapeptide [see chapter 11]. Elucidation of the sequence of human placental GnRH cDNA [14], which codes for a 92 amino acid precursor, has confirmed the presence of a GnRH in the placenta with the identical structure of the hypothalamic peptide.

GnRH-like immunoreactive material was demonstrated in the mammalian pancreas, olfactory system, milk, portal blood and in mammary tumours; specific binding sites for GnRH are present in the placenta, adrenal gland and mammary carcinoma tissue [see review 17].

Birds

An early study on bird hypothalamic GnRH suggested an identity [18] of bird GnRH with mammalian GnRH, but others indicated that there were structural differences [19–21]. Chicken and pigeon (Columbia livia) hypothalamic GnRHs had a similar molecular size to the mammalian peptide but were less positively charged and differed immunologically [20,21]. Examination of overlapping sequence requirements of various region-specific antisera indicated that the alteration in this form of chicken hypothalamic GnRH (cGnRH I), resided at Arg^8. The difference was further investigated by noting the interaction with the different antisera after selectively modifying the molecule at constituent amino acid residues of GnRH by chemical and enzymic treatment [22]. These data showed that cGnRH I differed at Arg^8. The difference in isoelectric points of cGnRH I and mGnRH was compatible with a neutral amino acid substitution for Arg^8 of mGnRH. On the basis of evolutionary probability of amino acid interchange for Arg, Gln was a likely candidate. The putative cGnRH I ([Gln^8]LHRH) (Fig. 1) was synthesized and shown to have identical chromatographic, immunological and biological properties to the natural peptide [22].

In concurrent studies, 17 μg of cGnRH I was purified from 250,000 chicken hypothalami using a combination of affinity chromatography, cation exchange HPLC and reverse phase HPLC. Amino acid analysis revealed an absence of Arg and the presence of an additional Glu, compatible with the proposed structure [4,5]. Sequence analysis confirmed the location of Gln as a replacement for Arg in the eight position [5; unpublished]. Another group confirmed the structure of this cGnRH I as [Gln^8]LHRH [6]. Subsequently, a second form of GnRH ([His^5,Trp^7,Tyr^8]LHRH; designated cGnRH II) (Fig. 1) was isolated from chicken hypothalamus [7].

GnRHs have not been isolated from any other species of bird. Recent studies using chromatographic, immunological and bioassay assessment have established the presence of cGnRH I and cGnRH II in ostrich (Struthio camelus) hypothalamus and extrahypothalamic brain [23] (Fig. 2).

Reptiles

Immunoreactive GnRH in extracts of lizard (Mabuya capensis) and tortoise (Chersine angulata) hypothalami exhibited immunological and charge properties different from those of mGnRH [20,21]. Immunological data pointed to alterations in the vicinity of Leu^7 of mGnRH. Since GnRH in these species was less positively charged than mGnRH [20,21], it appears that the basic Arg^8 is also not present in the GnRHs of these reptiles or that a neutral amino acid has been substituted by an acidic residue.

More extensive studies demonstrated that the major form of GnRH in lizard (Cordylis nigra) brain was identical to sGnRH in chromatographic, immunological and biological properties [24] (Fig. 2). Three additional immunoreactive GnRHs were detected. One of these had HPLC properties and LH-releasing activity in the chicken identical to that of cGnRH II. In lizard (Podarcis sicula) brain, three GnRH forms were demonstrated. Two of these had HPLC and immunological properties, and LH-releasing activity, identical to sGnRH and cGnRH I (Fig. 2), while the third is a novel form of GnRH [unpublished]. cGnRH II was demonstrated in skink (Calcides ocellatus) brain using chromatographic, immunological and biological techniques [unpublished] (Fig. 2).

Alligator (Alligator mississipiensis) hypothalamic GnRH was shown to differ immunologically from mGnRH in position eight [25]. Recent HPLC, immunological and biological studies on alligator brain indicated the presence of two GnRHs, cGnRH I and cGnRH II [unpublished] (Fig. 2).

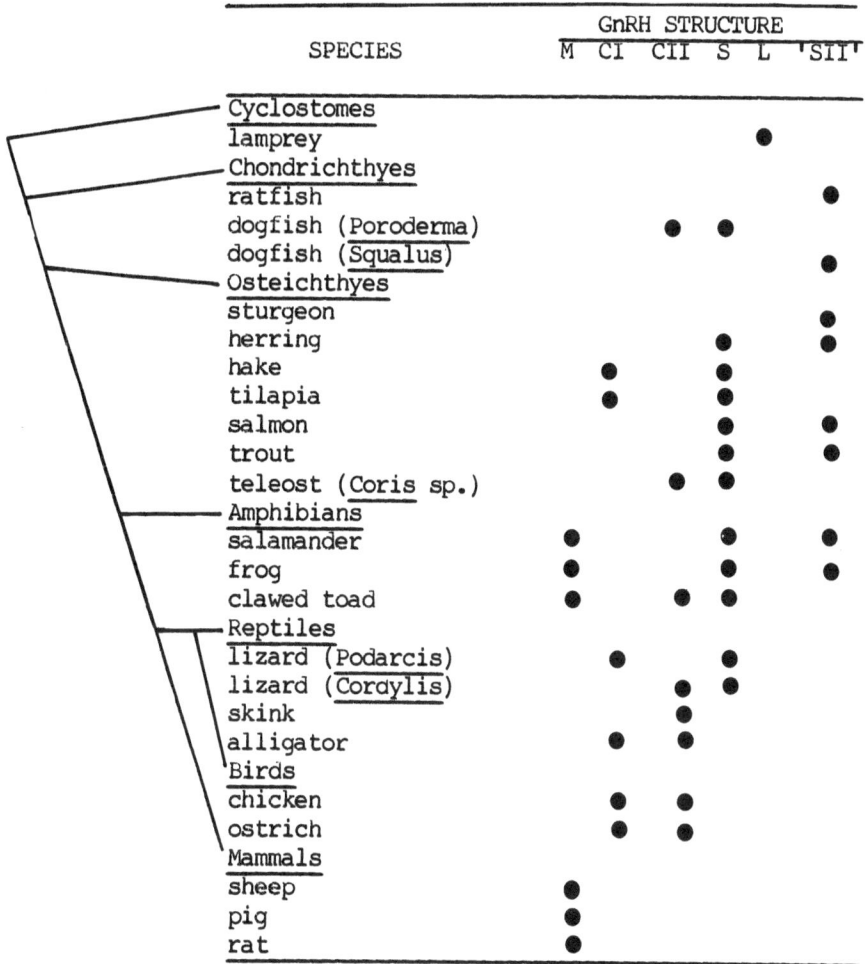

| | GnRH STRUCTURE | | | | | |
SPECIES	M	CI	CII	S	L	'SII'
Cyclostomes						
lamprey					●	
Chondrichthyes						
ratfish						●
dogfish (Poroderma)			●	●		
dogfish (Squalus)						●
Osteichthyes						
sturgeon						●
herring				●		●
hake		●		●		
tilapia		●		●		
salmon				●		●
trout				●		●
teleost (Coris sp.)			●	●		
Amphibians						
salamander	●			●		●
frog	●			●		●
clawed toad	●		●	●		
Reptiles						
lizard (Podarcis)		●		●		
lizard (Cordylis)			●	●		
skink			●			
alligator		●	●			
Birds						
chicken		●	●			
ostrich		●	●			
Mammals						
sheep	●					
pig	●					
rat	●					

FIGURE 2 Phylogenetic distribution of GnRH molecular forms. The classical evolutionary cladogram is represented in diagrammatic form. M, mammalian GnRH; CI, chicken GnRH I; CII, chicken GnRH II; S, salmon GnRH; L, lamprey GnRH; 'SII', 'salmon GnRH II'.

Amphibians

Hypothalamic GnRH in frogs (Rana pipiens, R. catesbeiana) [26–28], clawed toad (Xenopus laevis) [20,21] and toad (Bufo gariepensis) [21] was shown to have identical physicochemical properties to mGnRH. A GnRH with an amino acid composition identical to that of mGnRH was isolated from R. catesbeiana brain [10] (Fig. 2). More recently, two major forms of GnRH, with identical chromatographic, immunological and biological properties to mGnRH and cGnRH II, were identified in X. laevis brain [29] (Fig. 2). A third GnRH, with properties similar to sGnRH, was also identified in this species (Fig. 2). Multiple forms of GnRH were also demonstrated in the brains of other anurans (R. pipiens, Hyla regilla) and in urodeles (Ambystoma gracile and

Taricha granulosa). In all species mGnRH was present as well as sGnRH and/or 'salmon GnRH II' [30] (Fig. 2). 'sGnRH II' may be a novel form/s of GnRH, or it may be identical to cGnRH II [30]. In the light of our recent evidence for cGnRH II in X. laevis brain [29], it is likely the GnRH referred to as 'sGnRH II' [30] is in fact cGnRH II.

Hypothalamic immunoreactive GnRH content in X. laevis [31], toad (Bufo japonicus) [32] and in the newt (T. granulosa) [33] was shown to vary in relation to season and reproductive physiological state. The role of the different forms of GnRH in amphibian reproduction has not been determined.

Immunological and HPLC studies revealed that R. catesbeiana retina extracts have mGnRH in addition to a more hydrophobic GnRH with HPLC properties similar to sGnRH [28]. This additional form of GnRH (thought to be sGnRH) is the major form found in the frog sympathetic ganglion and adrenal gland [28].

The GnRH form found in ganglion (possibly sGnRH) was reported to predominate in brain extracts of metamorphic R. catesbeiana tadpoles, while mGnRH predominated in postmetamorphic frogs and adults [27]. Brain immunoreactive GnRH content increases steadily during metamorphosis, with a rapid rise at postclimax [34]. The functions of the multiple forms of GnRH during metamorphosis remain to be determined.

Gnathostomes

Among osteichthyes, teleost fish (tilapia, Sarotherodon mossambicus) brain GnRH differed from mGnRH in the vicinity of Leu^7 and was less positively charged, suggesting the absence of Arg^8 [20,21]. Similarly, codfish (Gadus morhua morhua) brain GnRH [35] is immunologically different from mGnRH. Sequence analysis of a GnRH from salmon (O. keta) brain revealed the structure $[Trp^7,Leu^8]$LHRH (sGnRH) [8] (Fig. 1).

The salmon brain form of GnRH (sGnRH) is widespread in teleost fish. In all species thus far investigated, the major GnRH molecular form has identical properties to sGnRH (Fig. 2). These species include hake (Merluccius capensis) pituitary gland [36], tilapia (Tilapia sparrmanii) brain [36], Coris julis brain [37], codfish brain [38], mullet (Mugil cephalus), milkfish (Chanos chanos) and trout (Salmo gairdneri) brain [39], herring (Clupea harengus pallasi) brain [40], and trout, goldfish (Carassius auratus) and sole (Solea solea) brain [41].

Multiple forms of GnRH were described in various species of teleost fish and in a chondrostean species [8,35,36,38-40]. In chromatographic and immunological studies, we demonstrated that in addition to sGnRH, hake pituitary gland and tilapia brain also contain cGnRH I [36] (Fig. 2). In herring, milkfish, mullet, salmon, goldfish and trout brain, a second GnRH termed 'sGnRH II' was identified on the basis of HPLC and immunological properties [8,39,40] (Fig. 2). If 'sGnRH II' in fish is the same as 'sGnRH II' in amphibians, then our data indicate that it is in fact cGnRH II. However, isolation and sequence analysis of the peptide will be necessary to clarify this issue. In the only study on a chondrostean species, it was reported that sturgeon (Acipenser transmontanus) brain contains no sGnRH (unlike all the teleost species studied), and that 'sGnRH II' and a novel GnRH are present in this species [40] (Fig. 2). Immunological evidence suggests the novel GnRH differs from mGnRH in the NH_2-terminal residues 2-5 and that the blocked NH_2- and COOH-termini of GnRH are retained [40]. Among holostean fish, bowfin (Amia calva) brain contains immunoreactive GnRH [42].

In chondrichthyes, dogfish (Poroderma africanum) hypothalamic GnRH differed from mGnRH in the vicinity of Leu^7 [21]. Immunoreactive GnRHs were detected in other elasmobranchs, dogfish (Squalus acanthias) [43,44] and shark (Triakis scyllia) [45], and in a holocephalan, the ratfish (Hydrolagus colliei) [43]. More recently, multiple forms of GnRH within a single species were demonstrated. Two forms were identified in P. africanum brain, which had identical HPLC, immunological and biological properties to sGnRH and cGnRH II [37] (Fig. 2). Novel forms of GnRH were also demonstrated in this tissue. In S. acanthias and ratfish brain, 'sGnRH II' and novel GnRHs were identified using HPLC and immunological techniques [40,44] (Fig. 2).

GnRH immunoreactivity was demonstrated in brain areas outside the hypothalamus, but it remains uncertain as to whether there is a differential distribution within the brain of the multiple forms of GnRH. Immunoreactive GnRH was also demonstrated in carp, goldfish and trout retina [46,47], and in eel (Anguilla anguilla) [48] and dogfish (P. africanum) [21] systemic blood.

Cyclostomes

Among cyclostomes, immunoreactive GnRH was demonstrated in lamprey (Entosphenus tridentata [49], Lampetra richardsoni [50], E. japonica [51], Petromyzon marinus [44]) brain. Recently, a unique GnRH was isolated from P. marinus brain and its structure determined as $[Tyr^3,Leu^5,Glu^6,Trp^7,Lys^8]LHRH$ (lGnRH) [9] (Fig. 1). A second form of GnRH was isolated, which differs by three amino acid residues from lGnRH [9]. In hagfish, the presence of GnRHs is not firmly established. The presence of immunoreactive GnRH was reported in Heptatretus hexatrema [21] and Eptatretus stouti [43] brain, while in other studies GnRHs were not detected in hagfish brain [44,49,51]. Hagfish is likely to have a GnRH variant which is sufficiently different from the known GnRHs not to allow detection by available antisera.

Lower organisms

Immunoreactive GnRH was demonstrated in a protochordate (Ciona intestinalis) [52] but not in invertebrates: prawn (Penaeus monodon), liverfluke (Schistosoma mansoni) [40], earthworm (Lumbricus terrestris), snail (Helix sp.) and beetle (Onymachris sp.) [unpublished] tissues. At present there is no conclusive evidence for the presence of GnRHs in any organism lower on the evolutionary scale than cyclostomes.

GnRH-related molecules

In addition to the various GnRHs identified in different vertebrates, there are several peptides which have sequence homology with GnRH [see 17]. Yeast alpha-mating factor has six amino acids in common with mGnRH and lGnRH, five residues in common with cGnRH I, and four in common with cGnRH II and sGnRH. The structural homology of alpha-mating factor with mGnRH allows specific binding to rat pituitary GnRH receptors [53] and stimulation of LH release from rat [53] and chicken [unpublished] gonadotropes. Although there are both structural and functional similarities between the two peptides, their evolutionary relationship is not known. Chicken gastrin-releasing peptide (GRP) has a sequence of five amino acids in common with the COOH-terminal sequence of cGnRH I (including Gly-Gly from which Gly-NH$_2$ is derived). Chicken GRP was more effective than yeast alpha-mating factor in stimulating LH release from chicken pituitary cells and had a similar activity to lGnRH [unpublished]. Ovine prolactin has a series of five amino acids in common with mGnRH [see 17], which may account for the inhibition of gonadotropins by high doses of prolactin. The similar degree of homology between yeast alpha-mating factor, chicken GRP and lGnRH with cGnRH I complicates any interpretation of evolutionary relationships of the molecules and suggests that if they arise from a common ancestral gene the GnRH-like structure has been co-opted for different functions during evolution.

BIOLOGICAL ACTIVITY OF VERTEBRATE GnRHs

Synthetic mammalian GnRH is biologically active at low doses in a variety of mammals, suggesting that GnRH and its receptor are conserved throughout the class Mammalia. cGnRH I has low (1-3% relative to mGnRH) gonadotropin-releasing activity in sheep [12,54] and rat [7,55] pituitary cell bioassays and 2.5% of the potency of mGnRH in a rat pituitary receptor binding assay [56] (Table 1). sGnRH is slightly more active (2-5%) in rat [8] or ovine [12] pituitary cell bioassays (Table 1). cGnRH II exhibits a further enhancement in LH-releasing activity (8%) in ovine pituitary cells [12] and has 32% and 41% respectively, of the potency of mGnRH in stimulating LH and follicle-stimulating hormone (FSH) release from rat pituitary cells [7] (Table 1). lGnRH had no LH-releasing activity in ovine pituitary cells and was ineffective in displacing iodinated mGnRH analog from rat pituitary membrane receptors [unpublished] (Table 1).

In birds, cGnRH I and mGnRH are equipotent in releasing LH from chicken pituitary cells [54], and LH and FSH from quail hemi-pituitaries [57] (Table 1). They are also equipotent in vivo in releasing LH in chickens [58,59], and LH and FSH in quail [57,60]. The two peptides have identical affinities for chicken pituitary GnRH receptors [54]. In contrast, other investigators reported that cGnRH I was more potent than mGnRH in stimulating LH release in avian systems [55,58]. cGnRH II is 5-6 times more potent than cGnRH I in releasing LH from chicken pituitary cells [12,16,17,61] and 14 times

Table 1. Biological activity of vertebrate GnRHs in different vertebrate classes

GnRH type	Species					
	Mammal	Bird	Reptile	Amphibian	Teleost	Cyclostome
Mammalian	++++	+++	++++	++++	++++	++++
Chicken I	+	+++	O	++++	++++	
Chicken II	++	++++			++++	
Salmon	+	+++			++++	++++
Lamprey	O	O			O	++++

Plus signs indicate relative biological activity of GnRH in different vertebrates : ++++, full activity; +++, high activity; ++, intermediate activity; +, low activity; O, no activity.

more potent in releasing FSH in this system [12,16,17] (Table 1). This suggests GnRHs may have differential effects in the regulation of LH and FSH release. In quail the two chicken GnRHs were equipotent in vitro [62]. In vivo studies in chickens and quail indicate that cGnRH II has equal [61,62] or greater [unpublished] potency than cGnRH I in stimulating LH and/or FSH release. sGnRH is 2.5 times more potent than cGnRH I in releasing LH and 1.8 times more potent in releasing FSH from chicken pituitary cells [12] (Table 1). The greater potency of cGnRH II and sGnRH in the chicken system is likely to be due to the presence of the hydrophobic Trp^7 in these GnRHs. lGnRH has little LH-releasing activity in chicken pituitary cells [unpublished] (Table 1).

The pituitary responsiveness to GnRH in the chicken, in terms of calcium-dependence, ED_{50} and biphasic release are similar to those in mammals, but desensitization in the chicken is more rapid and partially calcium-dependent [63].

In early studies on reptiles, low doses of mGnRH increased plasma levels of LH and progesterone in the turtle (Chrysemys picta), while very high doses were required in another species (Chelonia mydas) [64]. mGnRH was ineffective in the turtle (Lepidochelys olivacea) [65], and mGnRH and cGnRH I failed to change plasma LH levels in another turtle (Sternotherus odoratus) [66]. Male C. picta respond to mGnRH in vivo [67], and perifused hemipituitaries from two species of turtle (C. picta and Pseudemys scripta) secreted LH in response to similar doses of mGnRH to those effective in mammals [68]. Among snakes, the cobra (Naja naja) was unresponsive to mGnRH [66]. In contrast, mGnRH stimulated plasma testosterone in male alligators [24] (Table 1). Administration of [His^5,D-Arg^6,Trp^7,Tyr^8] LHRH to female iguanas (Iguana iguana) stimulated plasma estradiol which ellicited reproductive behaviour in males [69].

Regarding the effects of GnRH on gonadotropes in reptiles, prolonged doses of [D-Ser(Bu^t)^6,Pro^9-NHEt]LHRH induced desensitization of the pituitary in lizards in vivo [70]. The sensitivity of turtle (C. picta and P. scripta) pituitaries in vitro is similar to that of mammals [68]. Reptiles are relatively insensitive to exogenously administered GnRH compared to mammals [66,67]. Rapid degradation of GnRH in the circulation [unpublished] may account for the relatively poor activity in vivo.

Among amphibians, mGnRH (a form present in frog hypothalamus) stimulates gonadotropin secretion, steroidogenesis and spawning in anurans [66,71], and stimulates spermatogenesis and ovulation in urodeles [72,73]. cGnRH I is equipotent with mGnRH in stimulating LH and FSH secretion in bullfrogs (R. catesbeiana) in vivo [66] (Table 1). The doses required for gonadotropin release in vivo are considerably higher than those required in mammals. The sensitivity of bullfrog (R. pipiens and R. catesbeiana) pituitaries to GnRH in vitro suggests that the receptor binding affinity is high, as in mammals [74]. We have observed rapid degradation of mGnRH by toad (X. laevis) plasma [unpublished] which may account for the relatively poor activity in vivo. Both in vivo and in vitro studies have demonstrated the phenomenon of self-priming in amphibians, and the frog pituitary shows a greater resistance to desensitization than does the mammalian pituitary [74-76].

In fish, mGnRH and its analogs have poor gonadotropin-releasing activity in vivo compared with doses required in mammals [for reviews, see 77,78 and chapter 42]. In in vitro studies, however, cultured trout (S. gairdneri) pituitaries [79] and perifused goldfish pituitaries [80] had relatively sensitive and clear dose-dependent responses to GnRH. The lack of sensitive in vivo responses might relate to the endogenous gonadotropin release-inhibitory activity of dopamine [81,82]. sGnRH stimulates ovulation in salmon (O. keta) [8] (Table 1). mGnRH and sGnRH are equipotent in stimulating plasma testosterone and 17-beta-estradiol in tilapia (T. sparrmanii) in vivo [83], and in stimulating gonadotropin release from perifused goldfish pituitaries [80] (Table 1). sGnRH, mGnRH, cGnRH I and cGnRH II were equally effective in stimulating gonadotropin secretion in goldfish in vivo [84; unpublished] (Table 1). In contrast to the stimulatory activity of the above GnRHs, lGnRH had no effect on steroidogenesis in salmon (O. kisutch), while it stimulated steroidogenesis and ovulation in the lamprey (P. marinus) [unpublished]. Analogs of mGnRH elevated plasma estradiol and thyroxine levels in P. marinus [85].

The interspecific differences in gonadotropin-releasing activities of vertebrate GnRHs (Table 1) emphasize the high specificity of the mammalian GnRH receptor and a relative nonspecificity ('promiscuity') of the receptor in the nonmammalian vertebrates. This nonspecificity of the GnRH receptor in nonmammalian vertebrates has probably also allowed for greater variation in the structure of GnRH.

Aside from GnRH action in regulating pituitary gonadotropin secretion, novel functions of GnRHs are emerging. In mammals, GnRH or a related molecule might act as a neurotransmitter and directly affect reproductive behaviour [86-89]. The presence of GnRH receptors in mammalian extrapituitary tissues such as the testis, ovary, placenta, adrenal gland and mammary carcinoma [see 16,17], and biological effects of GnRH and analogs on these tissues [see 16,17], points to paracrine or autocrine roles of GnRH-related peptides produced in these tissues. The specificity and molecular size of gonadal GnRH receptors suggests they are identical to the pituitary receptor [90] although other studies have found differences in binding specificity [91]. Testicular GnRH differs structurally from mGnRH [92]. Sequence analysis of human placental GnRH mRNA has confirmed an identity of placental GnRH with the hypothalamic peptide [14]. Low affinity GnRH receptors exist in the placenta, and mGnRH stimulates beta-human chorionic gonadotropin secretion by human placenta in vitro [93]. The functions are not apparent for the GnRH receptors reported in mammalian adrenal gland [94] and mammary carcinoma [95], nor for the presence of GnRH-like peptides in pancreas [96], milk [97] and in mammary tumours [98].

In birds, mGnRH directly affects gonadal steroidogenesis [99] and behaviour [100]. mGnRH and sGnRH stimulate nerve firing in bullfrog sympathetic ganglia [101,102], and a GnRH similar to sGnRH in this tissue [28] is thought to resemble a sympathetic neuro-transmitter [103]. mGnRH was 10-fold more potent than sGnRH in pressor activity in the toad [104]. In fish, a terminal nerve system is thought to be important in the pherohormonal triggering of sexual responses [89]. Certain GnRH neurones in this system send axons to the retina [46,47], and in goldfish sGnRH modulates the electro-physiological response in retinal ganglion cells.

STRUCTURE-ACTIVITY RELATIONS OF GnRHs AND ANALOGS IN VERTEBRATES

The structural requirements of GnRHs for gonadotropin-releasing acti-vity in different vertebrates have been reviewed [17,81], and will be discussed only briefly in this chapter. Structure-activity relations of GnRHs in vertebrates were examined by studying gonadotropin-releasing activity of the naturally-occurring GnRHs and synthetic analogs: a) with amino acid substitutions in those positions which vary in the natural GnRHs; b) agonists; and c) antagonists [16,17; unpublished].

Substitution of Arg^8 in mGnRH with various amino acids reduces activity in ovine pituitary cells while only Glu^8 substitution leads to a substantial loss of activity in chicken pituitary cells. Thus, Arg^8 comprises an integral part of and/or contributes to the con-formation of the binding region of GnRH for the mammalian receptor while this does not pertain in the chicken. The postulate that con-formational stabilization is more important for activity in the mammal than in the chicken was supported by studies showing that a gamma-lactam (Gly-Leu) mGnRH analog with enhanced activity in the mammalian system, did not exhibit enhanced activity in the chicken. The mammalian pituitary GnRH receptor is generally similar to the chicken receptor in its acceptance of substitutions in positions five and seven. It appears that Trp^7 is the major contributing factor to the enhancement in activity of cGnRH II and sGnRH. The relatively greater FSH-releasing activity of cGnRH II compared with cGnRH I suggests that the ratio of the two GnRHs secreted from the hypo-thalamus could have a role in determining relative FSH:LH production. These findings indicate that chicken pituitary GnRH receptors are 'promiscuous' in their binding of a range of structural variants of GnRH. This also appears to be true in amphibians and teleost fish.

Selective processes apparently resulted in the mammalian pituitary GnRH receptor being more discriminatory in order to distinguish between mGnRH and related forms serving other functions.

The structural features for superactivity or antagonistic activity of GnRH analogs are different in mammals compared to birds, amphibians and teleost fish. Agonists with superactivity in nonmammalian vertebrates similar to those developed for mammals have yet to be realised.

EVOLUTION OF GnRH STRUCTURE AND FUNCTION

GnRH structure varies not only between species but also in different tissues within the same species or even within the same tissue. At present five forms of GnRH have been structurally characterized (Fig. 1). Chromatographic, immunological and biological properties indicate the presence of additional, novel forms of GnRH which await characterization.

All of the known GnRHs except lGnRH exhibit gonadotropin-releasing activity, especially in nonmammalian vertebrates. However, GnRHs may have other biological activities, for example the stimulation of growth hormone secretion in fish [T. Marchant and R.E. Peter, personal communication], actions on the placenta, ovary, testis and adrenal gland in certain mammals, and effects in the central and peripheral nervous systems. It appears, therefore, that the basic GnRH structure has been recruited through evolutionary selective processes to serve diverse functions. The specificity of these actions is achieved in a variety of ways. a) Through the evolution of different forms of GnRH and tissue-specific receptors. b) Through paracrine regulation of closely-localized cells (e.g. in the gonads) which does not allow the peptide to enter the general circulation in concentrations sufficient to bind other GnRH receptors. Therefore, the GnRH and receptors in different tissues can be identical. c) Through the existence of a 'private' conducting system (e.g. the hypothalamo-pituitary portal system). d) Through intimate contact between the secretory and target cells as occurs in neuronal communication.

The functional significance of multiple hypothalamic GnRHs in vertebrates has not been established. In the chicken, both forms stimulate secretion of LH and FSH at concentrations appropriate for physiological regulation. Since cGnRH II is more active than cGnRH I in stimulating gonadotropin secretion, it is possible that cGnRH II is the main regulator and that cGnRH I acts as a modulator. The relatively greater FSH-releasing activity of cGnRH II compared with cGnRH I provides a basis for this type of functional relationship. Both GnRHs appear to act on the same gonadotrope type. There is no evidence that the two peptides act through different receptor types.

Pituitary GnRH receptors in nonmammalian species are less discriminating than their mammalian counterparts with regard to GnRH structure. Since amino acids five, seven and eight of GnRH have been subject to substitution during evolution, the lower stringency in structural requirement of this region for biological activity in nonmammalian vertebrates might be anticipated. The high specificity of the mammalian receptor toward position eight substitution may reflect a need to discriminate between mGnRH and a related molecule serving a different function. Although the nonmammalian vertebrates exhibit a greater tolerance of amino acid substitutions in position eight, they are not identical in this regard and display distinct differences. The mammalian pituitary GnRH receptor shows some similarity to the nonmammalian receptors in its tolerance of substitutions in positions five and seven. Distinct differences do exist, however, as is evident in the acceptance of His^5 substitution in mGnRH for activity in the mammal while this change causes a decline in activity in the chicken.

Certain structural features of the GnRH molecule have been well-conserved during evolution. The length of the known GnRHs is constant, and the $pGlu^1-His^2$ at the NH_2-terminus, Ser in position four, and $Pro^9-Gly^{10}NH_2$ at the COOH-terminus, have remained unchanged. The conservation of the NH_2- and COOH-terminal sequences suggests these regions play a vital functional role. Both termini may be important in receptor binding while the NH_2-terminus is responsible for receptor activation. Appropriate amino acid substitutions in the NH_2-terminus produce molecules which bind the receptor but do not activate gonadotropin release (antagonists) [105]. Cross-linking these antagonists by antibodies re-establishes gonadotropin release [106], suggesting that the structural information in the NH_2-terminus of GnRH is associated with receptor aggregation which is required for initiating gonadotropin release. The chicken receptor domain which interacts with the NH_2-terminus of GnRH may differ from that of the mammal, since GnRH antagonists exhibited different properties in mammalian and chicken bioassay systems [unpublished].

From a phylogenetic point of view, in mammals only one of the five known GnRHs (mGnRH) is present. In birds and the alligator (thought to be closely related to birds) cGnRH I and cGnRH II are present, while in 'lower' reptiles one or more of these forms and/or sGnRH is present. Most amphibian species studied have the mammalian-type GnRH together with cGnRH II and sGnRH. Most species of bony and cartilaginous fish studied contain sGnRH, while lGnRH has only been found in lamprey. cGnRH II is most widespread, occurring in species as diverse as birds and cartilaginous fish. This structural variant may represent a primitive form of GnRH.

The presence of multiple forms of GnRH in representative species of all the vertebrate classes suggests that gene duplication occurred early in vertebrate evolution or even preceded the earliest vertebrates. lGnRH is the most different from the other GnRHs since a minimum of six nucleotide changes are required to account for the amino acid changes. cGnRH II is also very different, requiring 3-4 nucleotide changes to account for the amino acid changes in mGnRH, cGnRH I and sGnRH, while mGnRH, cGnRH I and sGnRH require 1-4, 1-4 and 2-3 changes, respectively. Since cGnRH II is very different and is also the most widespread and commonly represented form in vertebrates, it may have arisen early after gene duplication and been highly conserved during evolution.

Trp^7 occurs in three of the known GnRHs (lGnRH, sGnRH and cGnRH II), whereas Leu^7 occurs in mGnRH and cGnRH I. This may indicate how the GnRHs have evolved. lGnRH, sGnRH and cGnRH II may have evolved first as they occur mainly in lower vertebrates while mGnRH and cGnRH

I are characteristic of higher vertebrates. There is an inherent weakness in making such phylogenetic interpretations from the structures of GnRHs in extant vertebrates. The structures of GnRHs in living vertebrate species which separated from a main evolutionary lineage millions of years ago may have changed independently such that they no longer represent the structure present in the ancestral form. To obviate this problem it is necessary to establish conservation of the ancestral molecules by showing the presence of the same structure in different primitive species which diverged from each other early in evolution (e.g. lamprey and hagfish).

The multiplicity of actions of GnRHs in reproduction, acting in the central nervous system to stimulate reproductive behaviour, in the pituitary to stimulate gonadotropins, in the gonad to affect steroidogenesis, in the placenta to affect human chorionic gonadotropin secretion, and possibly also in the lactating breast, appears to be a remarkable conservation of function within a major physiological system. However, GnRHs appear also to have functions unrelated to reproduction, and GnRH-like sequences are present in peptides with nonreproductive functions such as chicken GRP and mammalian prolactin. There appears to be considerable plasticity in the co-option of certain peptide sequences for diverse functions during the course of evolution.

ACKNOWLEDGEMENTS

We thank members of the MRC Regulatory Peptides Research Unit for excellent research assistance, the scientific community for gifts of research materials, and Mrs L. Odes for typing. Unpublished work includes collaborative studies with G. Ciarcia, J.S. Davidson, R.W. Day, M.F. Hassan, V. Lance, P. Licht, D.R. Marshak, R.C.deL. Milton, C. Nahorniak, J.J. Nestor, R.E. Peter, R.C. Powell, R.W. Roeske, P.J. Sharp, N.M. Sherwood, S. Sower, J. Spiess and R.J. Sterling. The research was financed by the South African Medical Research Council and the University of Cape Town.

REFERENCES

1. Matsuo, H., Baba, Y., Nair, R.M.G., Arimura, A. and Schally, A.V. Structure of the porcine LH- and FSH-releasing hormone. I. The proposed amino acid sequence. Biochem. Biophys. Res. Commun. 43, 1334 (1971).
2. Amoss, M., Burgus, R., Blackwell, R., Vale, W., Fellows, R. and Guillemin, R. Purification, amino acid composition and N-terminus of the hypothalamic luteinizing hormone releasing factor (LRF) of ovine origin. Biochem. Biophys. Res. Commun. 44, 205 (1971).
3. Bohlen, P., Castillo, F., Yin, S.Y., Brazeau, P., Baird, A. and Guillemin, R. A general approach to the microisolation of peptides. In "Peptides : Synthesis-Structure-Function", D.H. Rich and E. Gross (Eds.), Pierce Chemical Company, Rockford, IL, 1981, p. 777.
4. King, J.A. and Millar, R.P. Structure of avian hypothalamic

gonadotrophin-releasing hormone. S. Afr. J. Sci. 78, 124 (1982).

5.   King, J.A. and Millar, R.P. Structure of chicken hypothalamic luteinizing hormone-releasing hormone. II. Isolation and characterization. J. Biol. Chem. 257, 10729 (1982).

6.   Miyamoto, K., Hasegawa, Y., Igarashi, M., Chino, N., Sakakibara, S., Kangawa, K. and Matsuo, H. Evidence that chicken hypothalamic luteinizing hormone-releasing hormone is [Gln^8]LH-RH. Life Sci. 32, 1341 (1983).

7.   Miyamoto, K., Hasegawa, Y., Nomura, M., Igarashi, M., Kangawa, K. and Matsuo, H. Identification of the second gonadotropin-releasing hormone in chicken hypothalamus : evidence that gonadotropin secretion is probably controlled by two distinct gonadotropin-releasing hormones in avian species. Proc. Natl. Acad. Sci. USA 81, 3874 (1984).

8.   Sherwood, N., Eiden, L., Brownstein, M., Spiess, J., Rivier, J. and Vale, W. Characterization of a teleost gonadotropin-releasing hormone. Proc. Natl. Acad. Sci. USA 80, 2794 (1983).

9.   Sherwood, N.M., Sower, S.A., Marshak, D.R., Fraser, B.A. and Brownstein, M.J. Primary structure of gonadotropin-releasing hormone from lamprey brain. J. Biol. Chem. 261, 4812 (1986).

10. Rivier, J., Rivier, C., Branton, D., Millar, R., Spiess, J. and Vale, W. HPLC purification of ovine CRF, rat extrahypothalamic brain somatostatin and frog brain GnRH. In "Peptides : Synthesis-Structure-Function", D.H. Rich and E. Gross (Eds.), Pierce Chemical Company, Rockford, IL, 1981, p. 771.

11. Millar, R.P. and King, J.A. Structure-activity relations of LHRH in birds. J. Exp. Zool. 232, 425 (1984).

12. Millar, R.P., Milton, R.C.deL., Follett, B.K. and King, J.A. Receptor binding and gonadotropin-releasing activity of a novel chicken gonadotropin-releasing hormone (GnRH) ([His^5,Trp^7,Tyr^8] GnRH) and a D-Arg^6 analog. Endocrinology 119, 224 (1986).

13. King, J.A. and Millar, R.P. Decapeptide luteinizing hormone-releasing hormone in ovine pineal gland. J. Endocr. 91, 405 (1981).

14. Seeburg, P.H. and Adelman, J.P. Characterization of cDNA for precursor of human luteinizing hormone releasing hormone. Nature 311, 666 (1984).

15. Millar, R.P., Denniss, P., Tobler, C. and Symington, R.B. Immunological, biochemical and functional differences in pineal and hypothalamic luteinizing hormone-releasing hormone. In "Pineal Function", C.D. Matthews and R.F. Seamark (Eds.), Elsevier/North-Holland Biomedical Press, Amsterdam, 1981, p. 151.

16. Millar, R.P., King, J.A., Wegener, I., Tobler, C., Dutlow, C., Roeske, R.W., Day, W.A., Rivier, J.E., Vale, W.W. and Licht, P. Molecular evolution of vertebrate luteinizing hormone-releasing hormone. In "Neuronal Communications", B. Meyer and S. Kramer (Eds.), Balkema Press, Cape Town, 1984, p. 114.

17. Millar, R.P. and King, J.A. Structural and functional evolution of gonadotropin-releasing hormone. Int. Rev. Cytol. 106 (in press, 1986).

18. Jeffcoate, S.L., Sharp, P.J., Fraser, H.M., Holland, D.T. and Gunn, A. Immunochemical and chromatographic similarity of rat, rabbit, chicken and synthetic luteinizing hormone releasing

hormones. J. Endocr. 62, 85 (1974).

19. Jackson, G.L. Comparison of rat and chicken luteinizing hormone-releasing factors. Endocrinology 89, 1460 (1971).

20. King, J.A. and Millar, R.P. Heterogeneity of vertebrate luteinizing hormone-releasing hormone. Science 206, 67 (1979).

21. King, J.A. and Millar, R.P. Comparative aspects of luteinizing hormone-releasing hormone structure and function in vertebrate phylogeny. Endocrinology 106, 707 (1980).

22. King, J.A. and Millar, R.P. Structure of chicken hypothalamic luteinizing hormone-releasing hormone. I. Structural determination on partially purified material. J. Biol. Chem. 257, 10722 (1982).

23. Powell, R.C., Jach, H., Millar, R.P. and King, J.A. Identification of Gln[8]-GnRH and His[5],Trp[7],Tyr[8]-GnRH in the hypothalamus and extrahypothalamic brain of the ostrich (Struthio camelus). Peptides 7 (in press, 1986).

24. Powell, R.C., King, J.A. and Millar, R.P. [Trp[7],Leu[8]]LH-RH in reptilian brain. Peptides 6, 223 (1985).

25. Lance, V.A., Vliet, K.A. and Bolaffi, J.L. Effect of mammalian luteinizing hormone-releasing hormone on plasma testosterone in male alligators, with observations on the nature of alligator hypothalamic gonadotropin-releasing hormone. Gen. Comp. Endocrinol. 60, 138 (1985).

26. Alpert, L.C., Brawer, J.R., Jackson, I.M.D. and Reichlin, S. Localization of LHRH in neurons in frog brain (Rana pipiens and Rana catesbeiana). Endocrinology 98, 910 (1976).

27. Branton, W.D., Jan, L.Y. and Jan, Y.N. Non-mammalian luteinizing hormone-releasing factor (LRF) in tadpole and frog brain. Soc. Neurosci. Abstr. 8, 14 (1982).

28. Eiden, L.E., Loumaye, E., Sherwood, N. and Eskay, R.L. Two chemically and immunologically distinct forms of luteinizing hormone-releasing hormone are differentially expressed in frog neural tissues. Peptides 3, 323 (1982).

29. King, J.A. and Millar, R.P. Identification of His[5],Trp[7],Tyr[8]-GnRH (chicken GnRH II) in amphibian brain. Peptides 7 (in press, 1986).

30. Sherwood, N.M., Zoeller, R.T. and Moore, F.L. Multiple forms of gonadotropin-releasing hormone in amphibian brains. Gen. Comp. Endocrinol. 61, 313 (1986).

31. King, J.A. and Millar, R.P. Hypothalamic luteinizing hormone-releasing hormone content in relation to the seasonal reproductive cycle of Xenopus laevis. Gen. Comp. Endocrinol. 39, 309 (1979).

32. Jokura, Y. and Urano, A. An immunohistochemical study of seasonal changes in luteinizing hormone-releasing hormone and vasotocin in the forebrain and the neurohypophysis of the toad, Bufo japonicus. Gen. Comp. Endocrinol. 59, 238 (1985).

33. Zoeller, R.T. and Moore, F.L. Seasonal changes in luteinizing hormone-releasing hormone concentrations in microdissected brain regions of male rough-skinned newts (Taricha granulosa). Gen. Comp. Endocrinol. 58, 222 (1985).

34. King, J.A. and Millar, R.P. TRH, GH-RIH and LH-RH in metamorphosing Xenopus laevis. Gen. Comp. Endocrinol. 44, 20 (1981).

35. Barnett, F.H., Sohn, J., Reichlin, S. and Jackson, I.M.D. Three

luteinizing hormone-releasing hormone-like substances in a teleost fish brain : none identical with the mammalian LH-RH decapeptide. Biochem. Biophys. Res. Commun. 105, 209 (1982).

36. King, J.A. and Millar, R.P. Multiple molecular forms of gonadotropin-releasing hormone in teleost fish brain. Peptides 6, 689 (1985).

37. Powell, R.C., Millar, R.P. and King, J.A. Diverse molecular forms of GnRH in an elasmobranch and a teleost fish. Gen. Comp. Endocrinol. 63, 77 (1986).

38. Jackson, I.M.D. and Pan, J.X. Evidence for five separate LH-RH-like substances but not LH-RH itself in the brain of the codfish. Program of the 65th Annual Meeting of The Endocrine Society, San Antonio, TX, 1983, p. 157 (abstract).

39. Sherwood, N.M., Harvey, B., Brownstein, M.J. and Eiden, L.E. Gonadotropin-releasing hormone (Gn-RH) in striped mullet (Mugil cephalus), milkfish (Chanos chanos), and rainbow trout (Salmo gairdneri) : comparison with salmon Gn-RH. Gen. Comp. Endocrinol. 55, 174 (1984).

40. Sherwood, N.M. Evolution of a neuropeptide family : gonadotropin-releasing hormone. Amer. Zool. (in press).

41. Breton, B., Motin, A., Kah, O., Lemenn, F., Geoffre, S., Precigoux, G. and Chambolle, P. Dosage radio-immunologique homologue d'un facteur hypothalamique de stimulation de la fonction gonadotrope hypophysaire de Saumon s-Gn-RH. C. R. Acad. Sci. Paris 299, 383 (1984).

42. Crim, J.W., Rajjo, I. and Vigna, S.R. Brain-gut peptides in holostean fish. Tenth International Symposium on Comparative Endocrinology, Colorado, USA, July 1985 (abstract).

43. Jackson, I.M.D. Distribution and evolutionary significance of the hypophysiotropic hormones of the hypothalamus. Front. Horm. Res. 6, 35 (1980).

44. Sherwood, N.M. and Sower, S.A. A new family member for gonadotropin-releasing hormone. Neuropeptides 6, 205 (1985).

45. Nozaki, M., Tsukahara, T. and Kobayashi, H. An immunocyto-chemical study on the distribution of neuropeptides in the brain of certain species of fish. Biomed. Res. 4, 135 (1984).

46. Demski, L.S. and Northcutt, R.G. The terminal nerve : a new chemosensory system in vertebrates? Science 220, 435 (1983).

47. Stell, W.K., Walker, S.E., Chohan, K.S. and Ball, A.K. The goldfish nervus terminalis : a luteinizing hormone-releasing hormone and molluscan cardioexcitatory peptide immunoreactive olfacto-retinal pathway. Proc. Natl. Acad. Sci. USA 81, 940 (1984).

48. Dufour, S., Pasqualini, C., Kerdelhue, B. and Fontaine, Y.A. Presence and distribution of radioimmunoassayable LHRH in the European eel, Anguilla anguilla. Neuropeptides 3, 159 (1982).

49. Crim, J.W., Urano, A. and Gorbman, A. Immunocytochemical studies of luteinizing hormone-releasing hormone in brains of agnathan fishes I. Comparisons of adult Pacific lamprey (Entosphenus tridentata) and the Pacific hagfish (Eptatretus stouti). Gen. Comp. Endocrinol. 37, 294 (1979).

50. Crim, J.W., Urano, A. and Gorbman, A. Immunocytochemical studies of luteinizing hormone-releasing hormone in brains of agnathan fishes II. Patterns of immunoreactivity in larval and

maturing Western brook lamprey (<u>Lampetra richardsoni</u>). Gen. Comp. Endocrinol. <u>38</u>, 290 (1979).

51. Nozaki, M. and Kobayashi, H. Distribution of LHRH-like substance in the vertebrate brain as revealed by immunohisto-chemistry. Arch. Histol. Japon. <u>42</u>, 201 (1979).

52. Georges, D. and Dubois, M.P. Mise en evidence par les techniques d'immunofluorescence d'un antigene de type LH-RH dans le systeme nerveux de <u>Ciona intestinalis</u> (Tunicier ascidiacae). C. R. Acad. Sci. Paris Serie D <u>290</u>, 29 (1980).

53. Loumaye, E., Thorner, J. and Catt, K.J. Yeast mating pheromone activates mammalian gonadotrophs : evolutionary conservation of a reproductive hormone? Science <u>218</u>, 1323 (1982).

54. Millar, R.P. and King, J.A. Synthesis, luteinizing hormone releasing activity, and receptor binding of chicken hypothalamic luteinizing hormone-releasing hormone. Endocrinology <u>113</u>, 1364 (1983).

55. Hasegawa, Y., Miyamoto, K., Igarashi, M., Chino, N. and Sakaki-bara, S. Biological properties of chicken luteinizing hormone-releasing hormone : gonadotropin release from rat and chicken cultured anterior pituitary cells and radioligand analysis. Endocrinology <u>114</u>, 1441 (1984).

56. Milton, R.C.deL., King, J.A., Badminton, M.N., Tobler, C.J., Lindsey, G.G., Fridkin, M. and Millar, R.P. Comparative structure-activity studies on mammalian [Arg^8]LH-RH and chicken [Gln^8]LH-RH by fluorimetric titration. Biochem. Biophys. Res. Commun. <u>111</u>, 1082 (1983).

57. Hattori, A., Ishii, S., Wada, M., Miyamoto, K., Hasegawa, Y., Igarashi, M. and Sakakibara, S. Effects of chicken (Gln^8)- and mammalian (Arg^8)-luteinizing hormone-releasing hormones on the release of gonadotrophins <u>in vitro</u> and <u>in vivo</u> from the adenohypophysis of Japanese quail. Gen. Comp. Endocrinol. <u>59</u>, 155 (1985).

58. Johnson, A.L., Johnson, P.A. and van Tienhoven, A. Ovulatory response, and plasma concentrations of luteinizing hormone and progesterone following administration of synthetic mammalian or chicken luteinizing hormone-releasing hormone relative to the first or second ovulation in the sequence of the domestic hen. Biol. Reprod. <u>31</u>, 646 (1984).

59. Sterling, R.J. and Sharp, P.J. A comparison of the luteinizing hormone-releasing activities of synthetic chicken LH-RH, synthetic porcine LH-RH and buserelin, an LH-RH analogue, in the domestic fowl. Gen. Comp. Endocrinol. <u>55</u>, 463 (1984).

60. Chan, S.T.H., Follett, B.K. and Millar, R.P. Comparison of synthetic ovine LHRH, avian LHRH, and their analogues by various biological and immunological assays. Gen. Comp. Endocrinol. <u>53</u>, 487 (1983) (abstract).

61. Chou, H.F., Johnson, A.L. and Williams, J.B. Luteinizing hormone releasing activity of [Gln^8]-LHRH and [His^5,Trp^7,Tyr^8]-LHRH in the cockerel, <u>in vivo</u> and <u>in vitro</u>. Life Sci. <u>37</u>, 2459 (1985).

62. Hattori, A. and Ishii, S. Stimulation of FSH and LH releases by two chicken LHRH's and mammalian LHRH <u>in vitro</u> and <u>in vivo</u>. J. Steroid Biochem. <u>20</u>(6B), 1548 (1984).

63. King, J.A., Davidson, J.S. and Millar, R.P. Desensitization to

gonadotropin-releasing hormone in perifused chicken anterior pituitary cells. Endocrinology 119 (in press, 1986).

64. Callard, I.P. and Lance, V. The control of reptilian follicular cycles. In "Reproduction and Evolution", J.H. Calaby and C.H. Tyndale-Biscoe (Eds.), Australian Acad. Sci., Canberra City, 1977, p. 199.

65. Licht, P., Owens, D.W., Cliffton, K. and Penaflores, C. Changes in LH and progesterone associated with the nesting cycle and ovulation in the olive ridley sea turtle, Lepidochelys olivacea. Gen. Comp. Endocrinol. 48, 247 (1982).

66. Licht, P., Millar, R., King, J.A., McCreery, B.R., Mendonca, M.T., Bona-Gallo, A. and Lofts, B. Effects of chicken and mammalian gonadotropin-releasing hormones (GnRH) on in vivo pituitary gonadotropin release in amphibians and reptiles. Gen. Comp. Endocrinol. 54, 89 (1984).

67. Licht, P. and Porter, D.A. In vivo and in vitro responses to gonadotropin releasing hormone in the turtle, Chrysemys picta, in relation to sex and reproductive stage. Gen. Comp. Endocrinol. 60, 75 (1985).

68. Licht, P. and Porter, D.A. LH secretion in response to gonadotropin releasing hormone (GnRH) by superfused pituitaries from two species of turtles. Gen. Comp. Endocrinol. 59, 442 (1985).

69. Phillips, J.A., Alexander, N., Karesh, W.B., Millar, R. and Lasley, B.L. Stimulating male sexual behaviour with repetitive pulses of GnRH in female green iguanas, Iguana iguana. J. Exp. Zool. 234, 481 (1985).

70. Ciarcia, G., Angelini, F. and Botte, V. Effects of a chronic treatment with the luteinizing hormone-releasing hormone agonist, buserelin, on the gonads of the lizard Podarcis s. sicula. Atti Acc. Lincei Rend. 74, 425 (1983).

71. McCreery, B.R. and Licht, P. The role of androgen in the development of sexual differences in pituitary responsiveness to gonadotropin releasing hormone (GnRH) agonist in the bullfrog, Rana catesbeiana. Gen. Comp. Endocrinol. 54, 350 (1984).

72. Mazzi, V., Vellano, C., Colucci, D. and Merlo, A. Gonadotropin stimulation by chronic administration of synthetic luteinizing hormone-releasing hormone in hypophysectomized pituitary grafted male newts. Gen. Comp. Endocrinol. 24, 1 (1974).

73. Vellano, C., Bona, A., Mazzi, V. and Colucci, D. The effect of synthetic luteinizing hormone releasing hormone on ovulation in the crested newt. Gen. Comp. Endocrinol. 24, 338 (1974).

74. Porter, D.A. and Licht, P. Pituitary responsiveness to super-fused GnRH in two species of ranid frogs. Gen. Comp. Endocrinol. 59, 308 (1985).

75. McCreery, B.R. and Licht, P. Pituitary and gonadal responses to continuous infusion of gonadotropin-releasing hormone in the male bullfrog, Rana catesbeiana. Biol. Reprod. 29, 129 (1983).

76. McCreery, B.R. and Licht, P. Induced ovulation and changes in pituitary responsiveness to continuous infusion of gonadotropin-releasing hormone during the ovarian cycle in the bullfrog, Rana catesbeiana. Biol. Reprod. 29, 863 (1983).

77. Ball, J.N. Hypothalamic control of the pars distalis in fishes, amphibians, and reptiles. Gen. Comp. Endocrinol. 44, 135

(1981).

78. Peter, R.E. Evolution of neurohormonal regulation of reproduction in lower vertebrates. Amer. Zool. 23, 685 (1983).

79. Crim, L.W., Evans, D.M., Coy, D.H. and Schally, A.V. Control of gonadotropin hormone release in trout : influence of synthetic LH-RH and LH-RH analogues in vivo and in vitro. Life Sci. 28, 129 (1981).

80. MacKenzie, D.S., Gould, D.R., Peter, R.E., Rivier, J. and Vale, W.W. Response of superfused goldfish pituitary fragments to mammalian and salmon gonadotropin-releasing hormones. Life Sci. 35, 2019 (1984).

81. Peter, R.E. Structure-activity studies on gonadotropin-releasing hormone in teleosts, amphibians, reptiles and mammals. In "Comparative Endocrinology : Developments and Directions", C.L. Ralph (Ed.), Alan R. Liss, Inc., New York, 1986, p. 75.

82. Peter, R.E., Chang, J.P., Nahorniak, C.S., Omeljaniuk, R.J., Sokolowska, M., Shih, S.H. and Billard, R. Interactions of catecholamines and GnRH in regulation of gonadotropin secretion in teleost fish. Rec. Prog. Horm. Res. 42 (in press).

83. King, J.A., Rivier, J.E., Vale, W.W. and Millar, R.P. Stimulation of testosterone and 17-β-estradiol secretion by synthetic salmon gonadotropin-releasing hormone in a teleost, Tilapia sparrmanii. S. Afr. J. Sci. 80, 430 (1984).

84. Peter, R.E., Nahorniak, C.S., Sokolowska, M., Chang, J.P., Rivier, J.E., Vale, W.W., King, J.A. and Millar, R.P. Structure-activity relationships of mammalian, chicken, and salmon gonadotropin releasing hormones in vivo in goldfish. Gen. Comp. Endocrinol. 58, 231 (1985).

85. Sower, S.A., Plisetskaya, E. and Gorbman, A. Steroid and thyroid hormone profiles following a single injection of partly purified salmon gonadotropin or GnRH analogues in male and female sea lamprey. J. Exp. Zool. 235, 403 (1985).

86. Pfaff, D.W. Luteinizing hormone-releasing factor potentiates lordosis behaviour in hypophysectomized ovariectomized female rats. Science 182, 1148 (1973).

87. Moss, R.L. and McCann, S.M. Induction of mating behaviour in rats by luteinizing hormone-releasing factor. Science 181, 177 (1973).

88. Witkin, J.W. and Silverman, A.J. Luteinizing hormone-releasing hormone (LHRH) in rat olfactory systems. J. Comp. Neurol. 218, 426 (1983).

89. Demski, L.S. The evolution of neuroanatomical substrates of reproductive behavior : sex steroid and LHRH-specific pathways including the terminal nerve. Amer. Zool. 24, 809 (1984).

90. Sharpe, R.M. Cellular aspects of the inhibitory actions of LH-RH on the ovary and testis. J. Reprod. Fert. 64, 517 (1982).

91. Millar, R.P., Garritsen, A. and Hazum, E. Characterization of Leydig cell gonadotropin-releasing hormone binding sites utilizing radiolabeled agonist and antagonist. Peptides 3, 789 (1982).

92. Dutlow, C.M. and Millar, R.P. Rat testis immunoreactive LH-RH differs structurally from hypothalamic LH-RH. Biochem. Biophys. Res. Commun. 101, 486 (1981).

93. Belisle, S., Guevin, J.F., Bellabarba, D. and Lehoux, J.G. Luteinizing hormone-releasing hormone binds to enriched human placental membranes and stimulates in vitro the synthesis of bioactive human chorionic gonadotropin. J. Clin. Endocrinol. Metab. 59, 119 (1984).

94. Eidne, K.A., Hendricks, D.T. and Millar, R.P. Demonstration of a 60K molecular weight luteinizing hormone-releasing hormone receptor in solubilized adrenal membranes by a ligand-immunoblotting technique. Endocrinology 116, 1792 (1985).

95. Eidne, K.A., Flanagan, C.A. and Millar, R.P. Gonadotropin-releasing hormone binding sites in human breast carcinoma. Science 229, 989 (1985).

96. Seppala, M. and Wahlstrom, T. Identification of luteinizing hormone-releasing factor and alpha-subunit of glycoprotein hormones in human pancreatic islets. Life Sci. 27, 395 (1980).

97. Hazum, E. Hormones and neutrotransmitters in milk. Trends in Pharmacological Sciences 4, 454 (1983).

98. Seppala, M. and Wahlstrom, T. Identification of luteinizing hormone-releasing factor and alpha-subunit of glycoprotein hormones in ductal carcinoma of the mammary gland. Int. J. Cancer 26, 267 (1980).

99. Hertelendy, F., Lintner, F., Asem, A.K. and Raab, B. Synergistic effect of gonadotropin releasing hormone on LH-stimulated progesterone production in granulosa cells of the domestic fowl (Gallus domesticus). Gen. Comp. Endocrinol. 48, 117 (1982).

100. Cheng, M.F. Role of gonadotropin releasing hormones in the reproductive behaviour of female ring doves (Streptopelia risoria). J. Endocr. 74, 37 (1977).

101. Jan, L.Y., Jan, Y.N. and Brownfield, M.S. Peptidergic transmitters in synaptic boutons of sympathetic ganglia. Nature 288, 380 (1980).

102. Jan, Y.N. and Jan, L.Y. A LHRH-like peptidergic neurotransmitter capable of 'action at a distance' in autonomic ganglia. Trends Neurosci. 6, 320 (1983).

103. Jones, S.W., Adams, P.R., Brownstein, M.J. and Rivier, J.E. Teleost luteinizing hormone-releasing hormone : action on bullfrog sympathetic ganglia is consistent with role as neurotransmitter. J. Neurosci. 4, 420 (1984).

104. Wilson, J.X. Conjugated catecholamines and pressor responses to angiotensin, luteinizing hormone-releasing hormone and prazosin in conscious toads. Br. J. Pharmac. 85, 647 (1985).

105. Sandow, J. Gonadotropic and antigonadotropic actions of LH-RH analogues. In "Neuroendocrine Perspectives, Volume 1", E.E. Muller and R.M. Macleod (Eds.), Elsevier Biomedical Press, Amsterdam, 1982, p. 339.

106. Gregory, H., Taylor, C.L. and Hopkins, C.R. Luteinizing hormone release from dissociated pituitary cells by dimerization of occupied LHRH receptors. Nature 300, 269 (1982).

SECTION 2

MECHANISMS OF ACTION OF HYPOTHALAMIC LHRH AND ANALOGS

6
Molecular Mechanism of LHRH Action in the Gonadotrope

C. A. McARDLE and P.M. CONN

Department of Pharmacology, The University of Iowa, College of Medicine, Iowa City, IA 52242, USA

INTRODUCTION

Luteinizing hormone-releasing hormone, (LHRH) is a hypothalamic decapeptide which stimulates the release of follicle stimulating hormone (FSH) and luteinizing hormone (LH) from pituitary gonadotropes. These glycoprotein hormones regulate steroidogenesis and gamete maturation in the gonadal tissue. LHRH and its analogs have great therapeutic potential as clinical and physiological studies indicate that the hormone can be used to regulate serum gonadotropin levels in vivo. Accordingly these compounds have been used successfully in the treatment of cryptorchidism, hypogonadotropic hypogonadism, endometriosis, steroid-dependent neoplasia and precocious puberty. Such clinical advances have occurred largely as a result of improved understanding of the molecular and cellular mechanism of action of LHRH at the gonadotrope.

LHRH RECEPTORS

Localization and characterization of LHRH receptors

The linear amino acid sequence of LHRH is pyro-Glu^1,His^2,Trp^3,- Ser^4,Tyr^5,Gly^6,Leu^7,Arg^8,Pro^9,Gly^{10}-NH$_2$. Structure-activity relationships have been examined in detail elsewhere [1] and in this volume. In early studies of the LHRH receptor the radioligands, [^{3}H]LHRH and [^{125}I]LHRH were used. These ligands were however, susceptible to proteolytic degradation, rapidly dissociated from the receptor and, in the case of [^{3}H]LHRH, of low specific activity [2]. These problems were overcome by the use of high affinity, metabolically stable agonists (such as buserelin and [D-Ala^6,Pro^9- NHEt]LHRH), which can be readily iodinated at Tyr^5. Studies with these ligands revealed a single class of highly specific, saturable LHRH binding sites in pituitary membranes [2,3]. Morphological studies and studies of radioligand binding to subcellular fractions indicate that the vast majority of LHRH receptors are located in the plasma membrane [4]. In order to estimate the size of the receptor Hazum et al. used a radiolabeled photoaffinity ligand to label LHRH binding sites of pituitary cell cultures [5]. Subsequent sodium dodecylsulphate-polyacrylamide gel electrophoresis (SDS-PAGE) separation revealed a binding protein with an apparent molecular weight of about 60,000. This estimate of the binding protein size was confirmed by SDS-PAGE separation followed by immunoblotting [6]. It is important to note that these estimates were obtained with denatured proteins extracted from the cellular membranes. A functional molecular weight can be obtained by target size analysis (radiation inactivation [7]), which is based upon the observation that the probability of inactivation of a protein by ionizing radiation is proportional to its size. This method provides an estimated molecular weight of the LHRH receptor of approximately 136,000 [8]. It is possible therefore, that the previously reported 60,000 protein is a subunit of the receptor which is associated with ligand binding.

Although the pituitary is clearly the target organ for hypo-thalamic LHRH, extrapituitary LHRH receptors have been demonstrated in gonadal tissue [9], adrenal cortex [6], and the central nervous system [10]. Evidence for the expression of the LHRH gene in brain tissue has also been presented [11]. Extrapituitary LHRH receptors and actions are reviewed in detail elsewhere [9].

Effects of endocrine status and development on LHRH receptors

Studies of LHRH receptors during development and in varied endo-crine states have revealed that receptor numbers change, whereas receptor affinity is relatively constant (typically $Ka = 1-3 \times 10^{10}$ M^{-1}, 3). Hence, the number of pituitary LHRH receptors is reduced in conditions such as aging and lactation, when serum gonadotropins are depressed, and receptor numbers are increased following ovari-ectomy (serum LH is elevated), and on the afternoon of proestrus (the time of the LH surge). As LHRH receptor numbers appear to be generally predictive of serum gonadotropin levels it seems likely that gonadotrope responsiveness is regulated, at least in part, by alteration of receptor numbers. The mechanisms by which LHRH receptor numbers and gonadotrope responsiveness to LHRH are regu-lated are discussed below.

LHRH receptor mobility and receptor-receptor interactions

The interaction of LHRH with its plasma membrane receptor is thought to be the first step in a series of events which lead to gonadotropin release. This interaction has been visualized direct-ly using fluorescent and radiolabeled derivatives of LHRH, and derivatives conjugated to ferritin or colloidal gold. When pitu-itary cells were lightly fixed prior to exposure to ferritin-conjugated LHRH, ferritin was seen evenly distributed over the cell surface [12]. In contrast, when cells were exposed to the ligand for 15 minutes prior to fixing, the ferritin granules (and presum-ably therefore the receptors) were aggregated and concentrated at one area of the cell surface. In subsequent studies the binding of a rhodamine derivative of [D-Lys⁶]LHRH, which binds to LHRH receptors with high affinity (Kd = 3 nM), was visualized by fluorescence microscopy coupled with image intensification [13]. Fluorescently labeled receptors were evenly distributed over the cell surface at 4°C, but at 37°C they rapidly aggregated into patches and became internalized into endocytic vesicles.

Studies of the fate of internalized receptors (using radio-labeled or colloidal gold conjugated ligands) have verified the previously described sequence of receptor binding, patching, and internalization and have identified the lysosomal and Golgi com-partments as major sites of accumulation of internalized receptors [14–16]. Receptor bound agonists are internalized more rapidly than receptor bound antagonists [17]. This observation is indica-tive of both continuous turnover of LHRH receptors and of agonist induced receptor internalization.

The demonstration of LHRH receptor mobility raises the ques-tions of the role of receptor and ligand internalization and move-ment in signal transduction at the gonadotrope. The possible role of internalized LHRH was investigated simply by removal of LHRH from the extracellular medium of dispersed pituitary cells after internalization had occurred. The prompt extinction of the secre-tory response on removal of LHRH indicated that the internalized ligand could not support LH release [18].

In order to test the possibility that receptor internalization might be involved in stimulus-release coupling, the effects of agonists were determined in conditions in which internalization was prevented. In the first experimental approach, the agonist [D-Lys^6]LHRH was coupled (via the ε amino group of Lys^6) to a N-hydroxysuccimide ester, and then via a 10 Å spacer arm, to a cross-linked agarose matrix [18]. The immobilized agonist caused LH release from pituitary cell cultures with the same efficacy as LHRH. Release of LH presumably occurred in the absence of receptor internalization because the agonist was attached to a support matrix which was larger than the cells, and because the agonist was resistant to liberation from the matrix. Although a ligand with high receptor affinity was used the possibility of receptor internalization after dissociation from the immobilized ligand could not be excluded. However fluorescence microscopy studies revealed that the microtubule disrupting agent vinblastine blocked both patching and internalization of LHRH receptors without affecting LHRH-stimulated LH release from pituitary cell cultures [19]. This indicates that receptor internalization and patching can be uncoupled from LHRH-evoked LH release.

Although the preceding experimental data indicate that large scale receptor patching and internalization are not prerequisites of agonist-stimulated LH release, it remains possible that these processes are involved in chronic regulation of gonadotrope respon-siveness. Moreover, as the fluorescence microscopy techniques used only enable visualization of aggregates of > 20-50 receptors, these data do not exclude the possibility that aggregation of small num-bers of receptors (microaggregation) may be involved in signal transduction. Indeed, several lines of evidence indicate that ligands with the ability to bring receptors together, are able to act as agonists. For example, autoantibodies to the insulin receptor which occur in some disease states, are able to mimic the biological effects of insulin [20]. Studies using monovalent and divalent F_{ab} fragments of these antibodies indicate that both fragments are able to bind to the receptor, but that the agonist activity is only observed with divalent antibodies. Accordingly, molecular probes were sought which might restrict the movement of LHRH receptors in the plane of the plasma membrane.

Since LHRH receptor antibodies were not available, LHRH receptors were cross-linked by means of antibody-conjugated ligands. In the first such study, the antagonist [p-Glu^1,D-Phe^2,D-Trp^3,D-Lys^6]-LHRH was dimerized using the bifunctional crosslinker, ethylene glycol bis-succinimidyl succinate (EGS, 21). This dimerized molecule, which was apparently too small to cross-link LHRH receptors, displayed comparable antagonist activity to the parent compound. The antagonist dimer was then incubated with cross reacting immunoglobulin. The resultant antibody-antigen conjugate, which consists of an immunoglobulin molecule with a LHRH antagonist dimer at the end of each F_{ab} arm, behaved as an agonist when added to pituitary cell cultures [21]. Stimulation of LH release by this molecule displayed characteristics of LHRH-stimulated LH release, in that it was Ca^{2+}-dependent and was blocked by calmodulin antagonists. These data demonstrate that a pure antagonist can be converted to an agonist when administered in a form which is able to cross-link receptors. Specifically, it appears that LH release occurs as a result of microaggregation of receptors, such that two receptors are brought within a critical distance of less than 150 Å (the maximum distance between the two F_{ab} associated ligands), and greater than 15 Å (the distance spanned by the antagonist dimer). Importantly, neither the bivalent antibody, nor the monovalent F_{ab} fragments (produced by papain digestion) exerted agonist activity [21]. Indeed, the monovalent antibody complex reverted to a pure antagonist as judged by inhibition of LHRH-stimulated release.

Further support for the contention that receptor microaggregation alone is sufficient to provoke LH release was obtained with the EGS dimer of the agonist [D-Lys^6]LHRH [22]. When pituitary cells were incubated with sufficient of the agonist dimer to produce an ED_{10} response, subsequent addition of antibody significantly enhanced LH secretion. Again this effect was not observed with monovalent immunoglobulin fragments and could be blocked by removal of extracellular Ca^{2+} or by addition of calmodulin inhibitors.

Although it is clear that receptor microaggregation results in Ca^{2+}-calmodulin dependent LH release, the mechanisms by which LHRH might produce such an effect remain a matter of speculation. Indeed, in the absence of specific means for inhibition of microaggregation it is not possible to test the necessity of microaggregation for receptor mediated stimulus-release coupling. Receptor occupancy by agonists (but not antagonists) may produce conformational changes, which expose complimentary binding sites, or may activate enzymes which catalyze the formation of receptor-receptor complexes. Alternatively, agonists may increase the mobility of receptors, and thereby increase the probability of receptor-receptor interactions, perhaps by interfering with the anchoring of receptors in the plasma membrane, or by producing localized changes in membrane fluidity. The means by which such receptor-receptor interactions provoke the secretory response are as yet unknown.

Introduction

As noted above, the number of pituitary LHRH receptors varies with age, sex and endocrine status [3]. Numerous groups have demonstrated the regulation of LHRH receptor number and pituitary responsiveness by LHRH (homologous regulation) as well as by other chemical messengers including steroids, opiates, catecholamines, and indoleamines (heterologous regulation, 23-25). The mechanisms by which gonadotrope responsiveness is regulated provide an important area of study, as it is the reduction in gonadotrope responsiveness produced on administration of stable agonist analogs of LHRH which provides the rationale for their use as contraceptives. Studies in our laboratory have focused on the relationship between LHRH-stimulated alteration of gonadotrope responsiveness and density of LHRH receptors, and on the role of signal transduction pathways in such alterations.

Desensitization

Several groups have demonstrated that LHRH receptor occupancy in gonadotropes produces homologous desensitization (refractoriness of the cells to LHRH as a result of prior exposure to the releasing hormone, 26-28). This effect, which has been observed both in vitro and in vivo, is markedly dependent on the concentration and duration of the LHRH challenge. In superfusion systems continuous exposure of dispersed pituitary cells to high doses of LHRH rapidly produces desensitization [27,29], whereas, pulsatile administration (e.g. brief pulses at hourly intervals) can prevent or delay desensitization [27] or even increase the sensitivity of gonadotropes to LHRH (the "self priming effect", 30).

Using a superfusion system, Conn et al. [31] demonstrated that exposure of cells to LHRH (10^{-8}-10^{-9} M for 20 minutes) reduced the response of the cells (LH release) to a subsequent dose. In contrast, when LH release was provoked first by the calcium ionophore A23187, and then by LHRH, no measurable desensitization was observed. These observations suggested that the desensitization observed could not be explained in terms of depletion of cellular LH_2 and provided the first indication that the process might be Ca^{2+}-independent. Further studies using static cultures of pituitary cells revealed that desensitization could be achieved by pretreating the cells with LHRH in the presence of the Ca^{2+} chelator EGTA [32]. Taken together, these experiments provide convincing evidence that homologous desensitization of gonadotropes differs fundamentally from the releasing process in that it is, at least in part, independent of Ca^{2+} mobilization from the extracellular space. However, although desensitization develops in the absence of extracellular Ca^{2+} the effect is less marked than that produced when cells are pretreated with LHRH in the presence of Ca^{2+} [33]. The possibility of a Ca^{2+}-dependent component of gonadotrope desensitization cannot therefore be excluded.

Interestingly, desensitization does not occur as a result of antagonist occupancy of LHRH receptors, but is produced when a dimerized antagonist with agonist activity is used [34].

Regulation of LHRH receptor number

In addition to effects on LH release and gonadotrope responsiveness, several groups have demonstrated that LHRH alters the number of LHRH receptors in pituitary tissue. Thus in superfused pituitary cells LHRH causesd both desensitization and a reduction in number of LHRH receptors [29]. In static cultures the effect of LHRH on the number of receptors is biphasic [26], the number of receptors being reduced (to approximately 60% of control) 1-3 hours after administration of 1 nM LHRH, and elevated (to approximately 140% of control) at 6-9 hours [26]. These effects occurred without a measurable change in receptor affinity and were not provoked by antagonist occupancy of the receptors. Chelation of extracellular Ca^{2+} with EGTA revealed the initial down-regulation to be Ca^{2+}-independent. In contrast, the up-regulation of receptors requires extracellular Ca^{2+} and is provoked by agents which elevate intracellular Ca^{2+} (A23187 and veratridine). The increase in receptor number was dependent on both protein and RNA synthesis (blocked by cycloheximide or actinomycin, 26).

It is tempting to speculate that gonadotrope responsiveness could be regulated by these alterations in LHRH receptor number. For example, the LHRH-provoked internalization of receptors could both reduce the number of cell surface receptors and target internalized receptors for metabolism (leading to a reduced receptor number). However, considerable evidence exists to suggest that such a relationship can not be absolute. First, the time course of development of desensitization (measurable 20 minutes after addition of LHRH and increasing for at least 6-12 hours, 33) differs from the time course of reduction in receptor number. Second, the time course of recovery from desensitization (gradual over 1-5 days, 35) differs from the time course of increase in receptor number [26]. Third, LHRH causes desensitization even when internalization of the receptor is blocked [36]. These observations suggest that factors other than altered receptor number may be important in regulation of gonadotrope responsiveness. The possibility that such factors might include altered coupling of the LHRH receptor to its effector molecules has not yet been tested.

STIMULUS-LH RELEASE COUPLING AT THE GONADOTROPE

Introduction

Studies of the mechanism by which LHRH provokes LH release have been facilitated by the availability of numerous specific agonist and antagonist probes for the LHRH receptor, and of compounds which can be used to manipulate signal transduction pathways. These studies have also been aided by the use of primary cell cultures.

Although early studies implicated cAMP as a potential second messenger for LHRH, subsequent investigations demonstrated that changes in cAMP levels could be uncoupled from LH release [37]. For example, elevation of intra- and extracellular levels of cAMP, inhibition of cyclic nucleotide phosphodiesterase, or administration of cAMP or dibutyryl cAMP, did not stimulate LH release or potentiate the ability of LHRH to do so. Similarly, although LHRH has been reported to elevate gonadotrope cGMP this effect has been uncoupled from LHRH-stimulated LH release with an inhibitor of cGMP formation [38]. Moreover, active analogs of cGMP do not provoke LH release from pituitary cell cultures [38]. The data dealing with the role of cyclic nucleotides in signal transduction at the gonadotrope has been reviewed elsewhere [39].

LHRH-stimulated LH release is dependent upon Ca^{2+} mobilization

Calcium is an important intracellular mediator involved in signal transduction in numerous tissues and cell types [for review see 40]. Several lines of evidence indicate that Ca^{2+} performs a second messenger function in LHRH-stimulated LH release.

First, Ca^{2+} is essential for LHRH-stimulated LH release. Early studies with hemi-pituitaries and pituitary slices demonstrated that the release of gonadotropins in response to crude hypothalamic extracts was abolished in Ca^{2+}-free medium [41,42]. Subsequent studies with the chemically pure releasing hormone revealed that LHRH-stimulated LH release was inhibited in Ca^{2+}-free medium or in medium to which EDTA or EGTA were added to chelate extracellular Ca^{2+} [32,43,44]. This inhibitory effect occured rapidly (< 2 minutes) and was reversed by addition of $CaCl_2$ to the incubation medium [45]. The binding of ligands to the LHRH receptor is not inhibited in the absence of Ca^{2+} or the presence of EGTA or EDTA. Calcium channel blockers (ruthenium red, verapamil, methoxyverapamil) provided a further means for demonstration of the role of Ca^{2+} in stimulated LH release. These compounds, and $LaCl_3$ (which inhibits the action of Ca^{2+} by displacing it from cellular binding sites) all inhibit LHRH-stimulated LH release [32,43,44].

Second, procedures which elevate intracellular Ca^{2+}, without LHRH receptor occupancy, also provoke LH release. These procedures include the application of Ca^{2+} selective ionophores (A23187 and ionomycin, 44,46,47) which allow Ca^{2+} to enter cells following its concentration gradient. The effects of these compounds are both time- and dose-dependent and are inhibited by chelation of extracellular calcium with EGTA [44,46,47]. LH release is also provoked by liposomes loaded with Ca^{2+}, but not by liposomes loaded with Mg^{2+} or with monovalent cations [46]. The vincal alkaloid veratridine is another secretagogue which is thought to provoke LH release by elevation of intracellular Ca^{2+} [44,48]. In neural tissue this compound opens Na^+ channels and this effect can be blocked with tetrodotoxin (TTX). The secretory response of gonadotropes to veratridine can be inhibited by removal of extracellular Na^+, by addition of TTX or by chelation of extracellular Ca^{2+} [48]. Thus LH release in response to veratridine is dependent on both extracellular Na^+ and Ca^{2+}, in contrast to

LHRH-stimulated LH release, which is Na^+-independent [48]. Presumably LHRH-stimulated LH release does not require the operation of Na^+ channels whereas the veratridine-induced operation of voltage sensitive Na^+ channels also causes the opening of Ca^{2+} channels [48].

A final line of evidence indicating that Ca^{2+} performs a second messenger function in this model is the demonstration that intracellular Ca^{2+} is elevated in response to LHRH. Early attempts to investigate this possibility using $^{45}Ca^{2+}$ were hampered by the fact that the mass of the calcium pool of interest (cytoplasmic ionized calcium) is extremly small compared to the mass of the other pools (intracellular sequestered calcium, and intra- and extracellular bound calcium). In spite of this problem, it was possible to show that stimulation with LHRH increases the rate of accumulation of $^{45}Ca^{2+}$ by pituitary tissue and the rate of efflux of $^{45}Ca^{2+}$ from prelabeled tissue [39,44]. This efflux was assumed to occur in response to elevation of intracellular Ca^{2+}. However, $^{45}Ca^{2+}$ flux provides only an indirect measure of cellular calcium metabolism which could conceivably be altered by changes in the influx, efflux or cellular distribution of Ca^{2+}. Moreover, the experimental manipulations required for accurate measurement of Ca^{2+} flux ($LaCl_3$ treatment to displace extracellular bound Ca^{2+}, preloading with $^{45}Ca^{2+}$ in low Ca^{2+} concentration medium) submit the cells to conditions known to inhibit LH release.

An alternative means of measuring intracellular Ca^{2+} involves the use of Ca^{2+} indicating compounds. Until recently this method was only applicable to large cells into which membrane impermeant Ca^{2+} indicators could be injected. However, a significant advance in the study of intracellular Ca^{2+} was achieved by the development of highly fluorescent Ca^{2+} indicators, such as Quin2, which could be loaded into cells without injection [49]. Quin2 is a fluorescent derivative of EGTA which can be loaded into cells as the lipophilic acetoxymethyl ester of Quin2. Once inside the cell this compound is hydrolyzed by non-specific esterases to free Quin2 which becomes sequestered within the cells because it is charged and does not readily cross lipid membranes. A shift in the wavelength of maximal fluorescence emission is seen when Quin2 binds Ca^{2+}. Using this method, Clapper and Conn [50], demonstrated a rise in intracellular Ca^{2+} concentration on addition of LHRH to suspensions of gonadotrope enriched pituitary cells. The average intracellular Ca^{2+} concentration in gonadotropes was estimated to be increased from approximately 100 to 130 nM on addition of LHRH. This effect was observed within 10 seconds of addition of LHRH and is thus the first measurable effect of the releasing hormone. No such effect was seen on addition of low affinity analogs or of LHRH antagonists. Interestingly, if intracellular levels of Quin2 are increased, the amount of intracellular Ca^{2+} chelated is also increased and a blunted secretory response to LHRH is observed.

The data outlined above demonstrate that a) Ca^{2+} is essential for LHRH-stimulated LH release, b) elevation of intracellular Ca^{2+} provokes LH release, and c) LHRH causes a measurable increase in intracellular Ca^{2+}. Taken together, these data provide convincing evidence that Ca^{2+} performs a second messenger function in this system.

In some systems in which Ca^{2+} performs a second messenger function, intracellular Ca^{2+} is thought to be elevated by mobilization of intracellular stores [for review see 51]. However, the evidence suggests that this is not the case for LHRH-stimulated LH release. For example, calcium antagonists such as methoxyverapamil prevent LH release by inhibiting the influx of extracellular Ca^{2+}, and addition of EGTA, or methoxyverapamil to superfused gonadotropes causes a prompt (< 2 minutes) extinction of LH release [56]. A further test of the relative roles of intra- and extracellular Ca^{2+} sources was achieved using dantrolene and 8-(N,N-diethylamino) octyl-3,4,5-trimethyloxybenzoate (TMB-8). These compounds which are thought to stabilize intracellular Ca^{2+} stores without inhibiting the mobilization of extracellular Ca^{2+} have no effect on LHRH-stimulated LH release [45]. Again, these observations indicate that extracellular Ca^{2+} is mobilized in response to LHRH, presumably by the opening of plasma membrane Ca^{2+} channels.

Recent electrophysiological studies in gonadotropes [52] have revealed that LHRH does not depolarize the plasma membrane, but causes a large increase in membrane voltage fluctuations (background noise). As this effect was Ca^{2+}-dependent and was inhibited by a calcium antagonist it was suggested that it was caused by conductance changes associated with the activation of Ca^{2+} channels (or Ca^{2+}-dependent channels). The depolarization independent effect of LHRH on LH release is inhibited by calcium antagonists with the same order of potency as that in which the depolarization evoked effect of veratridine is inhibited (methoxyverapamil > verapamil > diltiazem > nifedepine, 53). This order of potency is the reverse of that observed for inhibition of stimulus-contraction coupling in smooth muscle or cardiac tissue [54] where action potentials play a prominent role in Ca^{2+} entry. These observations provide evidence that the Ca^{2+} channels found in gonadotropes differ from those in non-secretory tissues, and that voltage-dependent and receptor-operated Ca^{2+} channels of gonadotropes are similar.

Calmodulin: an intracellular receptor for Ca^{2+}

Calmodulin is an ubiquitous intracellular Ca^{2+} receptor, which is known to regulate the activity of many Ca^{2+}-dependent enzymes. Such enzymes include adenylate cyclase, cyclic nucleotide phosphodiesterases, and several protein kinases, including myosin light chain kinase and phosphorylase kinase [55]. Since Ca^{2+} performs a second messenger role in LHRH-stimulated LH release, the possibility that calmodulin mediates this effect was investigated.

Using a sensitive and highly specific radioimmunoassay for calmodulin, Conn et al. [56] demonstrated that administration of LHRH to ovariectomized rats caused an increase in calmodulin associated with the plasma membrane, and a concomitant reduction in cytosolic calmodulin. These effects were dose- and time-dependent (maximal effect observed 15 minutes after LHRH administration) and were not observed with [des^1]LHRH which has a receptor affinity 1,000 fold less than that of LHRH. As no change in total cellular calmodulin was observed, these results are consistent with the translocation of calmodulin from the cytoplasm to the plasma membrane. Subsequent studies using the indirect immunofluorescence technique (fluorescein isothiocyanate and rhodamine labeled second antibodies) have provided morphological evidence for the association of calmodulin with LHRH receptor patches [57].

Although LHRH-stimulated redistribution of calmodulin and the association of calmodulin with the LHRH receptor patch may have functional significance, these observations do not necessarily indicate a role for calmodulin in LHRH-stimulation of LH release. Data indicating such a role has been obtained using drugs which bind to calmodulin and prevent the regulation of enzyme activity by the Ca^{2+}-calmodulin complex [58]. Calmodulin inhibitors of several chemical classes (penfluridol, pimozide, chlordiazepoxide, chlorpromazine and napthalene sulphonamides) all inhibit LHRH-stimulated LH release [59,60]. Moreover, the potency of these compounds at inhibition of LH release correlates well with their potency at inhibition of Ca^{2+}-calmodulin activation of cyclic nucleotide phosphodiesterase [59,61]. A further indication of the specificity of this effect is that pimozide inhibits LH release in response to LHRH and to the ionophore A23187 but does not alter the LH releasing effect of phorbol myristate acetate (PMA) or dioctanoylglycerol [62]. The latter compounds are thought to provoke LH release in a Ca^{2+}-calmodulin independent manner by direct activation of protein kinase C.

The above data indicate that calmodulin acts as an intracellular receptor, mediating the effects of Ca^{2+} mobilized in response to LHRH. The molecular mechanisms underlying these effects are not yet known. By analogy with other systems, it seems probable that the LHRH-provoked elevation of intracellular Ca^{2+} enables the production of a Ca^{2+}-calmodulin complex, which in turn regulates the activity of as yet undetermined enzymes.

LHRH alters phospholipid metabolism in gonadotropes

Recent evidence provides support for the role of various classes of lipids (arachidonic acid, prostaglandins, thromboxanes, leukotrienes, phospholipids and diacylglycerols) as informational molecules. Many hormones and neurotransmitters which act by mobilization of Ca^{2+} also alter inositol phospholipid metabolism [63], this is also the case for LHRH [64-68].

In cultures of anterior pituitary cells LHRH has been reported to cause a dose-dependent incorporation of [^{32}P] into phosphatidylinositol (PI) at doses which also stimulate LH release [66]. Incorporation of [^{32}P] into phosphatidic acid and into other lipids (phosphatidylcholine and lysophosphatidylcholine) was unaffected by LHRH. Subsequent studies with gonadotrope enriched cell cultures [65,67,68] have demonstrated LHRH-stimulated incorporation of [^{32}P] into both PI and phosphatidic acid. It seems likely that the latter effect was masked in the earlier studies by the large proportion of cells other than gonadotropes (estimated as approximately 85%).

Using gonadotrope enriched cell cultures, Andrews and Conn [65] have extended previous studies by the demonstration that LHRH provokes a rapid and specific incorporation of [^{32}P] into phosphatidic acid, PI_{b2}, PI-4-phosphate and PI-4,5-bisphosphate (figure 1a). In the [^{32}P] incorporation studies described above, cells were pretreated with [$^{32}PO_4$] for 10-60 minutes prior to challenge with LHRH. These protocols provide insufficient time for labeling of cellular phospholipid pools to isotopic equilibrium. Effects seen under these conditions are therefore likely to be indicative of altered rates of turnover of phospholipid pools and do not necessarily reflect changes in the mass of these pools. In order to investigate the possibility of mass changes in phospholipid pools, gonadotrope enriched pituitary cell cultures were labeled with [^{33}P] for 48 hours (to achieve isotopic equilibrium) and also with [^{32}P] for 1 hour [65]. Under these conditions LHRH provoked a rapid (45-60 seconds) reduction of the [^{33}P] content of the inositol phospholipid, indicating a reduction in the mass of this pool. A subsequent increase in the [^{32}P] content of the inositol phospholipid was also observed indicating an increase in the rate of turnover of this pool. These results are consistent with LHRH-stimulated hydrolysis of inositol phospholipids by a phospholipase C-type reaction, as has been suggested for several other systems.

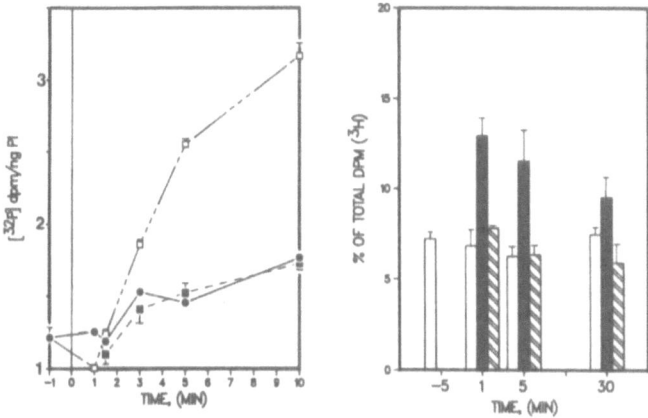

Figure 1.   LHRH-stimulated phospholipid and DAG turnover. Panel a: Cells were labeled for 1 hour with [$^{32}PO_4$] and then challenged with vehicle (●), PMA (3 ng.ml^{-1}, ■) or LHRH (10^{-8}M, □) for the indicated time. The [^{32}P] content of PI-4,5-bisphosphate pool was then determined. Qualitatively similar patterns of LHRH-stimulated turnover were seen for phosphatidic acid, PI and PI-4-phosphate. Panel b: Cells were labeled for 48 hours with [^{3}H]-arachidonic acid and then challenged for the indicated time with vehicle (open column), PMA (3 ng.ml^{-1}, shaded column) or LHRH (10^{-8}M, black column). The [^{3}H] content of the DAG pool was then determined. Andrews and Conn 1986, [65] with permission.

The products of inositol phospholipid hydrolysis by phospholipase C are inositol phosphates (IPs) and diacylglycerols (DAGs). Thus stimulation of phospholipase C by LHRH would be expected to increase the rate of turnover of IPs and DAGs. In order to measure the effect of LHRH on DAG production cells were labeled with [^{3}H]-arachidonic acid prior to determination of the amount of [^{3}H] in DAG. This protocol is dependent upon the observation that the sn-2 position of DAGs is rich in arachidonic acid so that the rate of incorporation of [^{3}H] into DAG is dependent on the rate of DAG turnover. LHRH provokes a rapid and transient (1-5 minutes) increase in the rate of DAG production (figure 1b).

The effect of LHRH on the rate of formation of IPs has also been determined. Using LiCl to block the recycling of IPs to inositol, Huckle and Conn [64] were able to demonstrate a LHRH-stimulated increase in IP accumulation. This effect was dose- and time-dependent, was blocked by LHRH antagonists, and was mimicked by an agent which provokes receptor aggregation (the antibody-conjugated agonist described above).

The demonstration of a LHRH-stimulated phospholipase C-type hydrolysis of inositol phospholipids raises the question of the means by which receptor occupancy by the releasing hormone is coupled to activation of the enzyme. Evidence obtained in several systems [69-71] indicates that hormone and neurotransmitter receptors may be functionally coupled to phospholipase C by regulatory guanine nucleotide-binding proteins (G-proteins). This relationship is analogous to that seen with adenylate cyclase which is thought to be coupled to numerous receptors by inhibitory or stimulatory G-proteins [72]. When GTP or a stable GTP analog (guanylyl-imidodiphosphate) were administered to permiabilized pituitary cells, both LH release and PI turnover were stimulated [73]. Pertussis toxin ("islet activating protein") and cholera toxin (which ADP ribosylate the inhibitory and stimulatory G-proteins regulating adenylate cyclase, respectively) both elevated cellular cAMP levels but were without effect on guanine nucleotide-stimulated LH release or PI turnover. These observations suggest that the G-protein involved in the regulation of gonadotrope phospholipase C differs from those known to regulate adenylate cyclase. Interestingly, the effects of GTP on LH release and PI turnover were inhibited by pretreatment with a LHRH receptor antagonist indicating the intimate association of a G-protein with LHRH recognition site of the receptor.

The data above indicate that LHRH increases the rate of inositol phospholipid turnover in gonadotropes. The enhanced rate of PI hydrolysis yields DAGs and IPs, both of which have been proposed as informational molecules, (DAGS as endogenous regulators of protein kinase C, PKC) and IPs (specifically inositol 1,4,5-trisphosphate) as regulators of the release of intracellular Ca^{2+}. An informational role for IPs in gonadotropes however, has not yet been established. Although IP$_3$ may mobilize intracellular Ca^{2+} in permeabilized cells [74], it appears that LHRH action requires mobilization of extracellular rather than intracellular Ca^{2+} [45].

Finally, it should be noted that the demonstration of LHRH-stimulated PI turnover and LH release does not necessarily indicate the former to be a prerequisite of the latter. Indeed, the Ca^{2+}-ionophore A23187 and a phorbol ester (PMA) provoke LH release without increasing the rate of PI turnover [65]. LHRH-stimulated inositol phospholipid turnover has also been uncoupled from LH release in the presence of the Ca^{2+} antagonist methoxyverapamil which was found to inhibit LH release, but not inositol phospholipid turnover [65] or IP production (at 1-10 μM methoxyverapamil, 64). These experiments indicate that unlike LHRH-stimulated LH release, LHRH-stimulated polyphosphoinositide turnover is not dependent on Ca^{2+} influx. The effects of the PKC activators PMA and dioctanoylglycerol, are particularly noteworthy. These compounds which provoke LH release both in the presence and absence of LHRH exert an inhibitory effect on LHRH-stimulated IP accumulation [64]. The inhibition of IP production indicates a possible mechanism for negative feedback of PKC on DAG production as has been suggested by groups studying other models [75].

Protein kinase C: an intracellular receptor for DAGs

PKC is the Ca^{2+} and phospholipid dependent kinase first described in brain tissue by Nishizuka [76]. This enzyme, has been demonstrated in both cytosolic and particulate fractions of numerous tissues [77,78]. The activity of PKC in vitro is dependent on the presence of Ca^{2+} and phospholipid. Phosphatidylserine supports PKC activity more effectively than other phospholipids. [77-79]. In the presence of phosphatidylserine, DAGs also stimulate PKC activity [80]. Kinetic analysis reveals that DAGs (but not monoacylglycerols or triacylglycerols) activate PKC by increasing the affinity of the enzyme for Ca^{2+} and phospholipid [77-81]. Thus in the presence of phosphatidylserine alone the enzyme requires high concentrations of Ca^{2+} (10-100 μM) for activity, whereas in the presence of DAG and phosphatidylserine activation requires lower Ca^{2+} concentrations (< 1-10 μM). The dependence of PKC on phosphatidylserine indicates that enzyme activation might involve association of the enzyme with cell membranes (the inner leaflet of plasma membranes is rich in phosphatidylserine). Subsequent production of DAG could then activate the enzyme.

The first indication of a possible role for PKC in LH release was the demonstration that the phorbol esters, phorbol dibutyrate (PDBu) and PMA stimulated LH release from pituitary cell cultures [34,62,82]. Phorbol esters are a class of tumor promoters which are thought to exert their biological effects, at least partly, by activation of PKC. Evidence in support of this includes the demonstration that a) cellular PKC activity co-purifies with the phorbol ester receptor [83,84], b) DAGs competetively inhibit the binding of PDBu to its cellular receptor [85,86], and c) phorbol esters can substitute for DAGs in activation of PKC in vitro [87,88]. Thus the ability of phorbol esters to stimulate LH release is attributed to the ability of these compounds to mimic the effects of endogenous DAG in activation of PKC. To test this possibility it was necessary to synthesize DAGs which could be readily administered to cells in culture (long chain DAGs are insoluble in aqueous media). Accordingly, a range of DAGs were synthesized with varying acyl chain length (4-10 carbons) in the sn-1 and 2 positions. These compounds stimulate both LH release from pituitary cells and PKC in tissue homogenates [89]. sn-1,2-Dioctanoylglycerol (DiC_8) proved to be the most potent of these compounds and analogs with hydrogen, chloride or sulfydryl groups substituted for the hydroxyl group were inactive in both assays. Importantly, structure-activity relationships revealed a good correlation between potency of the DAGs at stimulation of LH release and PKC activity [89].

As noted above, PKC activity is observed at low Ca^{2+} concentrations in the presence of DAG and phosphatidylserine. It has therefore been suggested that DAG production could lead to activation of PKC without elevation of intracellular Ca^{2+} [91]. In accord with this suggestion is the observation that phorbol ester-stimulated and DiC_8-stimulated LH release have been reported not to be inhibited in the absence of extracellular Ca^{2+} [34,89]. A further point of interest is that PKC activators, at doses which alone exert minimal effects on LH release (approximately ED_{10} doses) synergistically enhance A23187-stimulated LH release [62]. The implications of this observation are discussed further below.

LHRH or the superagonist buserelin cause the redistribution of PKC from the cytosolic to the particulate fraction of pituitary homogenates at doses which also provoke LH release. This effect, which is in many respects similar to the observed redistribution of calmodulin, occurs both in vivo and in vitro [90,91]. The effect observed in vitro was apparently gonadotrope-specific as it was most marked in gonadotrope-enriched populations. The effect observed in vivo was also gonadotrope-specific as it was inhibited by LHRH antagonists and was observed in ovariectomized rats (in which the proportion of gonadotropes in the pituitary is increased) but not in intact rats [91].

Agonist-evoked redistribution of PKC occurs in several systems [92-95] although the mechanism underlying this effect remains unclear. Interestingly, the effect of buserelin on PKC distribution was inhibited by pretreatment with the Ca^{2+} channel blocker methoxyverapamil [91]. This observation suggests that PKC redistribution occurs as a consequence of Ca^{2+}-mobilization. In support of this possibility it has been found that the inclusion of Ca^{2+} in homogenization solution increases the proportion of cellular PKC associated with the particulate fraction of rat brain [83], and GH_4C_1 cells [93]. Alternatively, since phorbol esters can provoke the redistribution of PKC to cell membranes [92], it is conceivable that endogenous DAGs produce similar effects. Finally, both Ca^{2+} mobilization and DAG production may be necessary to provoke the redistribution of PKC under physiological conditions. Using the binding of purified PKC to inside-out vesicles prepared from human erythrocytes as a model system, Wolf et al. [95] demonstrated that the Ca^{2+}-dependent association of PKC with plasma membranes is synergistically enhanced in the presence of PMA. Such an effect could clearly underly the synergistic activation of LH release by PMA and the Ca^{2+} ionophore A23187 [62].

Together, these data indicate that activation of PKC in vivo may require redistribution of the enzyme from the cytoplasm to cell membranes. The Ca^{2+}-dependent association of PKC with membranes rich in phosphatidylserine would favor the activation of the enzyme by endogenous DAGs (produced by LHRH-stimulated PI hydrolysis). Since both DAG production and PKC redistribution occur in response to LHRH it is likely that PKC mediates the effect of exogenous DAGs and the presumed effects of endogenous DAGs on LH release.

Modulation of Ca^{2+}-calmodulin action by PKC

In accord with the direct action of phorbol esters and DAGs on PKC, experiments in our laboratory have shown that the LH releasing effects of PMA and DiC_8 are not inhibited by the calcium-antagonist methoxyverapamil or by the calmodulin inhibitor pimozide [62]. In contrast, the effect of Ca^{2+} ionophores (A23187 and ionomycin) is markedly inhibited (at low doses) in the presence of pimozide [62]. Thus, it appears that DiC_8 and PMA can be used to selectively activate PKC mediated LH release and A23187 to selectively activate Ca^{2+}-calmodulin dependent release. It has been reported [62,96] that low concentrations of PMA or DiC_8 (approximately ED_{10}) can synergistically enhance the LH releasing effect of A23187 (1-15 μM). These observations raise the possibility that PKC, activated synergistically by DAG and elevated intracellular Ca^{2+}, could play a role in LHRH-stimulated LH release and that PKC activation may modulate or amplify Ca^{2+}-calmodulin dependent LH release. Although the mechanism underlying such modulation has not been investigated in gonadotropes, studies in other systems have revealed that PKC activation can alter the activity of ion channels [97] and can alter the rate or magnitude of secretagogue-induced changes in intracellular Ca^{2+} concentration [98]. Further modulatory effects of PKC activation could conceivably involve regulation of receptor-effector coupling, or negative feedback effects on IP turnover as noted above [64,75]. It should also be noted that the potential modulatory effects of PKC on established signal transduction pathways are reciprocated by the fact that activation of these pathways involves the production of second messengers (Ca^{2+} and DAGs) which regulate PKC activity.

Arachidonic acid and its metabolites

There is some evidence to indicate that arachidonic acid or its metabolites may play an informational role in gonadotropes. For example, it has been reported that arachidonic acid and leukotriene C_4 (LTC_4) provoke LH release and that lipoxygenase inhibitors can reduce LHRH-stimulated LH release [99-102]. However, it should be noted that the available data is somewhat sparce and often contradictory. Thus, the lipoxygenase inhibitor 5,8,11,14-eicosatetraynoic acid has been reported to inhibit [100], or when purified, to provoke [102], LH release. Moreover, LTC_4 and arachidonic acid have independently been reported to have no effect on LH release [100,102] or to provoke LH release [99,101]. A physiological role for arachidonic acid or its metabolites, in the action of LHRH, is therefore yet to be firmly established.

MULTIPLE SIGNAL TRANSDUCTION PATHWAYS AND POSSIBLE INTERACTIONS

In the preceding sections we have described the biological actions of LHRH, and reviewed the evidence indicating a role for several classes of informational molecules in signal transduction at the gonadotrope. A major question remaining to be answered concerns

91

the physiological relevance of the various putative second messengers. Investigations of this question are complicated by the fact that the relative importance of the various informational molecules is likely to be dependent upon the biological effect studied. For example, it is clear that LHRH-stimulated LH release and receptor up-regulation are Ca^{2+}-dependent whereas LHRH-stimulated receptor down-regulation and desensitization appear to be Ca^{2+}-independent.

The demonstration that LHRH-stimulated LH release is associated with [50,39], and is absolutely dependent upon [32,43,44], Ca^{2+} mobilization, indicates the central role of this cation in signal transduction at the gonadotrope. In contrast, although LHRH provokes the production of several other putative second messengers (DAGs, IPs, cyclic nucleotides, arachidonic acid and its metabolites) the absolute dependence of LHRH-stimulated LH release on production of these compounds has either not been demonstrated, or has been disproved. When considering the relative importance of the various informational molecules it should be noted that calmodulin inhibitors such as pimozide reduce LHRH-stimulated LH release (up to 80%) at concentrations which have no effect on PMA-stimulated LH release [62] or on lipid-stimulated PKC activity (unpublished observations).

In addition to the clear importance of the Ca^{2+}-calmodulin pathway, several lines of evidence indicate that other signal transduction pathways may be of physiological relevance. For example, although Ca^{2+}-ionophores and veratridine have been shown to provoke LH release with the same efficacy as LHRH, the doses used would be expected to produce a greater elevation of intracellular Ca^{2+} concentration than LHRH does. Thus although LHRH-stimulated LH release requires activation of a Ca^{2+}-calmodulin mediated signal transduction pathway, it is likely that this pathway is modulated or amplified by other effector systems.

The suggestion of multiple effector pathways has not been rigorously tested experimentally, but has been used successfully in construction of mathematical models of LHRH-stimulated LH release [103]. An unusual feature of LHRH-stimulated LH release in cultures of pituitary cells is that is that the dose-response curve spreads over a wide concentration range (10^{-11} - 10^{-6} M LHRH). This broad dose-response curve cannot be attributed to multiple classes of receptor as binding studies indicate a single class of LHRH receptor [3]. Mathematical models have been constructed based on the assumptions that the ligand-receptor complex, or a dimerized ligand-receptor complex, causes the secretory response by interaction with two effector systems [103]. Comparison of the predicted dose-response curves with experimental data revealed that the model provided an excellent fit for the dose-response curves obtained with LHRH and its agonist analogs.

In addition to recognizing the the possibility of multiple effector systems it is important to note that such systems may interact. For example, the demonstration that PKC activators can synergistically enhance the effects of low doses of a Ca^{2+} ionophore on LH release suggests the possibility that DAG production and consequent PKC activation may modulate the Ca^{2+}-calmodulin dependent signal-transduction pathway.

In figure 2 we have focused on LH release as the biological end-point about which most is known. We have stressed the clear importance of Ca^{2+}-calmodulin dependent cellular activity and have also indicated the means by which LHRH-stimulated PI turnover and PKC activation may provoke LH release or modulate Ca^{2+}-calmodulin dependent LH release. Finally, it should be noted that the mechanisms underlying other cellular effects, such as regulation of receptor number and cellular responsiveness are likely to differ from those underlying LH release.

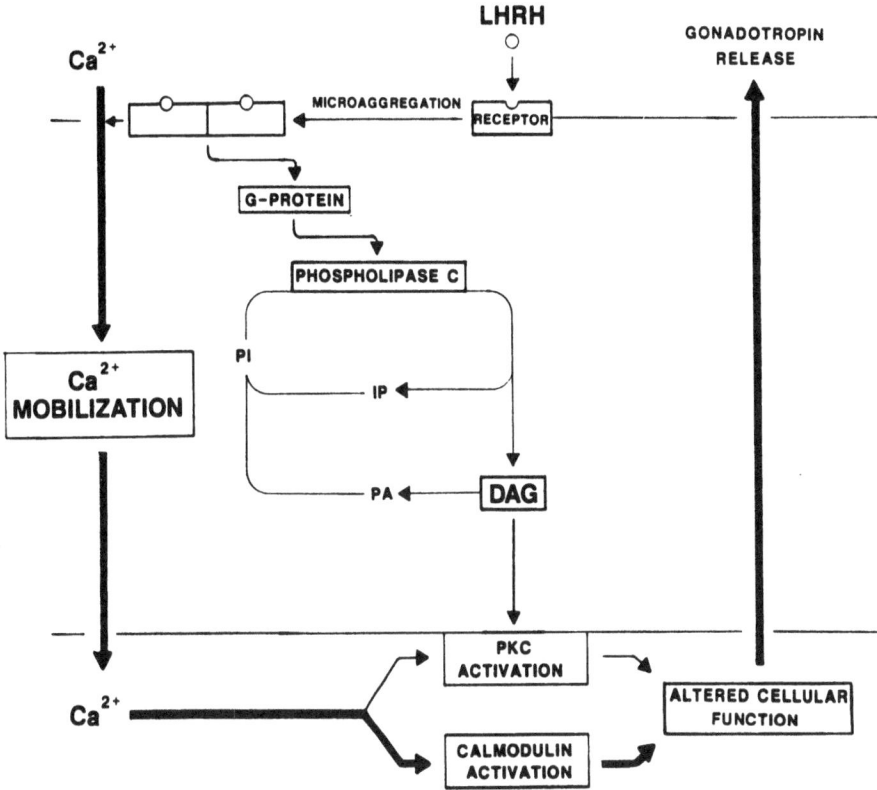

Figure 2. Schematic representation of the molecular events mediating LHRH-stimulated LH release. See text for details.

Acknowledgment. We thank Elizabeth McDonald for typing this manuscript and William Huckle and William Andrews for their helpful discussions. Work from our laboratory was supported by HD19899.

REFERENCES

1. Karten, M.J. and Rivier, J.E. Gonadotropin-releasing hormone analog design. Structure-function studies toward the development of agonists and antagonists: Rationale and perspectives. Endocr. Rev. **7**, 44 (1986).

2. Clayton, R.N. and Catt, K.J. Gonadotropin-releasing hormone receptors: Characterization, physiological regulation, and relationship to reproductive function. Endocr. Rev. 2, 186 (1981).

3. Marian, J., Cooper, R.L. and Conn, P.M. Regulation of the rat pituitary gonadotropin-releasing hormone receptor. Mol. Pharmacol. 19, 399 (1981).

4. Marian, J. and Conn, P.M. Subcellular localization of the receptor for gonadotropin-releasing hormone in pituitary and ovarian tissues. Endocrinology 112, 104 (1983).

5. Hazum, E. Photoaffinity labeling of luteinizing hormone releasing hormone receptor of rat pituitary membrane preparations. Endocrinology 109, 1281 (1981).

6. Eidne, K.A., Hendricks, D.T. and Millar, R.P. Demonstration of a 60K molecular weight luteinizing hormone-releasing hormone receptor in solubilized adrenal membranes by ligand-immunoblotting technique. Endocrinology 116, 1792 (1985).

7. Venter, J.C. Size of neurotransmitter receptors as determined by radiation inactivation/target size analysis. In "The Receptors", vol. II, P.M. Conn (ed.), Academic press, New York, p. 245, (1985).

8. Conn, P.M. and Venter, J.C. Radiation inactivation (target size analysis) of the gonadotropin releasing hormone receptor: Evidence for a high molecular weight complex. Endocrinology 116, 1324 (1985).

9. Hsueh, A.J.W. and Jones, P.B.C. Extrapituitary actions of gonadotropin releasing hormone. Endocr. Rev. 2, 437 (1981).

10. Reubi, J.C. and Maurer, R. Visualization of LHRH receptors in the rat brain. European J. Pharmacol. 106, 453 (1985).

11. Shivers, B.D., Harlan, R.E., Hejtmancik, J.F., Conn, P.M. and Pfaff, D.W. Localization of cells containing LHRH-like mRNA in rat forebrain using in situ hybridization. Endocrinology 118, 883 (1986).

12. Hopkins, C.R. and Gregory, H. Topographical localization of the receptors for luteinizing hormone-releasing hormone on the surface of dissociated pituitary cells. J. Cell Biol. 75, 528 (1977).

13. Hazum, E., Cuatrecasas, P., Marian, J. and Conn, P.M. Receptor mediated internalization of fluorescent gonadotropin releasing hormone by pituitary gonadotropes. Proc. Nat. Acad. Sci. U.S.A. 77, 6692 (1980).

14. Pelletier, G., Dube, D., Guy, J., Seguin, C. and Lefebvre, F.A. Binding and internalization of a luteinizing hormone-releasing hormone agonist by rat gonadotrophic cells. A radioautographic study. Endocrinology 111, 1068 (1982).

15. Duello, T.M., Nett, T.M. and Farquhar, M.G. Fate of a gonadotropin-releasing hormone agonist internalized by rat pituitary gonadotrophs. Endocrinology 112, 1 (1983).

16. Jennes, L., Stumpf, W.E. and Conn, P.M. Intracellular pathways of electronopaque gonadotropin-releasing hormone derivatives bound by cultured gonadotropes. Endocrinology 113, 1683 (1983).

17. Jennes, L., Coy, D. and Conn, P.M. Receptor-mediated uptake of GnRH agonist and antagonists by cultured gonadotropes:

Evidence for differential intracellular routing. "in press".

18. Conn, P.M., Smith, R.G. and Rogers, D.C. Stimulation of pituitary gonadotropin release does not require internalization of gonadotropin releasing hormone. J. Biol. Chem. **256**, 1098 (1981).

19. Conn, P.M. and Hazum, E. Luteinizing hormone release and gonadotropin-releasing hormone (GnRH) receptor internalization: Independant actions of GnRH. Endocrinology **109**, 2040 (1981).

20. Jacobs, S., Chang, K-J. and Cuatrecasas, P. Antibodies to purified insulin receptor have insulin-like activity. Science **200**, 1283 (1978).

21. Conn, P.M. Ligand dimerization: A technique for assessing receptor-receptor interactions. In "Methods in Enzymology", P.M. Conn (ed.), Academic press, New York, p. 49, (1983).

22. Conn, P.M., Rogers, D.C. and McNeil, R. Potency enhancement of a GnRH agonist: GnRH-receptor microaggregation stimulates gonadotropin release. Endocrinology **111**, 335 (1982).

23. Meites, J. and Sonntag, W.E. Hypothalamic hypophysiotropic hormones and neurotransmitter regulation: Current views. Ann. Rev. Pharmacol. Toxicol. **21**, 295 (1981).

24. Barraclough, C.A. and Wise, P.M. The role of catecholamines in the regulation of pituitary luteinizing hormone and follicle-stimulating hormone secretion. Endocr. Rev. **3**, 91 (1982).

25. Barkan, A., Regiani, S., Duncan, J., Papvasilion, S. and Marshall, J.C. Opioids modulate pituitary receptors for gonadotropin-releasing hormone. Endocrinology **112**, 387 (1983).

26. Conn, P.M., Rogers, D.C. and Seay, S.G. Biphasic regulation of the gonadotropin-releasing hormone receptor by receptor microaggregation and intracellular calcium levels. Mol. Pharmacol. **25**, 51 (1984).

27. Badger, T.M., Loughlin, J.S. and Naddaff, P.G. The luteinizing hormone-releasing hormone (LHRH)-desensitized rat pituitary: Luteinizing hormone responsiveness to LHRH in vitro. Endocrinology **112**, 793 (1983).

28. deKonig, J., van Dieten, J.A.M.J. and van Rees, G.P. Refractoriness of the pituitary gland after continuous exposure to luteinizing hormone releasing hormone. J. Endocrinol. **79**, 311 (1978).

29. Zilberstein, M., Zakut, H. and Naor, Z. Coincidence of downregulation and desensitization in pituitary gonadotrophs stimulated by gonadotropin releasing hormone. Life Sci. **32**, 663 (1983).

30. Evans, W.S., Uskavitch, D.R., Kaiser, D.L., Hellman, P., Borges, J.L.C. and Thorner, M.O. The self-priming effect of gonadotropin-releasing hormone on luteinizing hormone release: observations using rat anterior pituitary fragments and dispersed cells continuously perifused in parallel. Endocrinology **114**, 861 (1984).

31. Smith, W.A. and Conn, P.M. GnRH-mediated desensitization of the pituitary gonadotrope is not calcium dependent. Endocrinology **112**, 408 (1983).

32. Marian, J. and Conn, P.M. Gonadotropin releasing hormone stimulation of cultured pituitary cells requires calcium. Mol. Pharmacol. **16**, 196 (1979).

33. Jinnah, H.A. and Conn, P.M. Gonadotropin-releasing hormone-mediated desensitization of cultured rat anterior pituitary cells can be uncoupled from luteinizing hormone release. Endocrinology **118**, 2599 (1986).

34. Smith, W.A. and Conn, P.M. Microaggregation of the gonadotropin-releasing hormone-receptor: Relation to gonadotrope desensitization. Endocrinology **114**, 553 (1984).

35. Jinnah, H.A. and Conn, P.M. GnRH-stimulated LH release from pituitary cells in culture: Refractoriness and recovery. Am. J. Physiol. (Endocrinol. and Metab.) **249**, E619 (1985).

36. Gorospe, W.C. and Conn, P.M. Agents which decrease GnRH-receptor internalization do not inhibit GnRH-mediated gonadotrope desensitization. Endocrinology, "in press" (1986).

37. Conn, P.M., Morrell, D.V., Dufau, M.L. and Catt, K.J. Gonadotropin-releasing hormone action in cultured pituicytes: Independence of luteinizing hormone release and adenosine 3',5'-monophosphate production. Endocrinology **104**, 448 (1979).

38. Naor, Z. and Catt, K.J. Independent actions of GnRH upon cGMP production and LH release. J. Biol. Chem. **255**, 342 (1980).

39. Conn, P.M., Marian, J., McMillian, M., Stein, J., Rogers, D., Hamby, M., Penna, P. and Grant, E. Gonadotropin-releasing hormone action in the pituitary: A three step mechanism. Endocr. Rev. **2**, 174 (1981).

40. Rasmussen, H. and Barrett, P.Q. Calcium messenger system: An integrated view. Physiol. Rev. **64**, 938 (1984).

41. Wakabayashi, K., Kamberi, I.A. and McCann, S.M. _In vitro_ response of the rat pituitary to gonadotropin releasing factors and to ions. Endocrinology, **85**, 1046 (1969).

42. Samli, M.H. and Geshwind, I.I. Some effects of energy-transfer inhibitors and of Ca^{2+}-free and K^+-enhanced media on the release of LH from the rat pituitary gland _in vitro_. Endocrinology **82**, 225 (1968).

43. Stern, J.E. and Conn, P.M. Perifusion of rat pituitaries: Requirements for optimal GnRH-stimulated LH release. Am. J. Physiol. (Endocrinol. and Metab.) **240**, E504 (1981).

44. Hopkins, C.R. and Walker, A.M. Calcium as a second messenger in the stimulation of luteinizing hormone secretion. Mol. Cell. Endocrinol. **12**, 189 (1978).

45. Bates, M.D. and Conn, P.M. Calcium mobilization in the pituitary gonoadtrope: Relative roles of intra- and extracellular sources. Endocrinology **115**, 1380 (1984).

46. Conn, P.M., Rogers, D.C. and Sandhu, F.S. Alteration of the intracellular calcium level stimulates gonadotropin release from cultured rat anterior pituitary cells. Endocrinology **105**, 1122 (1979).

47. Conn, P.M., Kilpatrick, D. and Kirshner, N. Ionophoretic Ca^{2+} mobilization in rat gonadotropes and bovine adrenomedullary cells. Cell Calcium **1**, 129 (1980).

48. Conn, P.M. and Rogers, D.C. Gonadotropin release from pitu-

itary cultures following activation of endogenous ion channels. Endocrinology **107**, 2134 (1980).

49. Tsien, R.Y., Pozzan, T. and Rink, T.J. Calcium homeostasis in intact lymphocytes: Cytoplasmic free calcium monitored with a new, intracellularly trapped fluorescent indicator. J. Cell. Biol. **94**, 325 (1982).

50. Clapper, D.A. and Conn, P.M. GnRH stimulation of pituitary gonadotrope cells produces an increase in intracellular calcium. Biol. Reprod. **32**, 269 (1985).

51. Berridge, M.J. and Irvine, R.F. Inositol trisphosphate, a novel second messenger in cellular signal transduction. Nature **312**, 315 (1984).

52. Mason, W.T. and Waring, D.W. Electrophysiological recordings from gonadotrophs. Evidence for Ca^{2+} channels mediated by gonadotropin-releasing hormone. Neuroendocrinology **41**, 258 (1985).

53. Conn, P.M., Rogers, D.C. and Seay, S.G. Structure-function relationship of calcium ion channel antagonists at the pituitary gonadotrope. Endocrinology **113**, 1592 (1983).

54. Triggle, D.J. Calcium antagonists: Basic chemical and pharmacological aspects. In "New Perspectives in Calcium Antagonists," G.B. Weiss (ed.), Ann. Physiol. Soc., Bethesda, p. 1, (1981).

55. Means, A.R. and Dedman, J.R. Calmodulin, an intracellular calcium receptor. Nature **285**, 73 (1980).

56. Conn, P.M., Chafouleas, J.G., Rogers, D. and Means, A.R. Gonadotropin releasing hormone stimulates calmodulin redistribution in rat pituitary. Nature **292**, 264 (1981).

57. Jennes, L., Bronson, D., Stumpf, W.E. and Conn, P.M. Evidence for an association between calmodulin and membrane patches containing gonadotropin-releasing hormone-receptor complexes in cultured gonadotropes. Cell Tissue Res. **239**, 311 (1985).

58. Levin, R.M. and Weiss, B. Mechanism by which psychotropic drugs inhibit cyclic AMP phosphodiesterase. Mol. Pharmacol. **12**, 581 (1976).

59. Conn, P.M., Rogers, D.C. and Sheffield, T. Inhibition of gonadotropin-releasing hormone-stimulated luteinizing hormone release by pimozide: Evidence for a sight of action after calcium mobilization. Endocrinology **109**, 1122 (1981).

60. Conn, P.M., Bates, M.D., Rogers, D.C., Seay, S.G. and Smith, W.A. GnRH-receptor-effector-response coupling in the pituitary gonadotrope: A Ca^{2+} mediated system. In "The Role of Drugs and Electrolytes in Hormonogenesis," K. Fotherby and S.B. Pal (eds.), Walter de Gruyter and Co., Berlin, p. 85, (1984).

61. Levin, R.M. and Weiss, B. Selective binding of antipsychotics and other psychoactive agents to the calcium-dependent activator of cyclic nucleotide phosphodiesterase. J. Pharm. Exp. Ther. **208**, 454 (1979).

62. Harris, C.E., Staley, D. and Conn, P.M. Diacylglycerols and protein kinase C: Potential amplifying mechanism for Ca^{2+}-mediated GnRH stimulated LH release. Mol. Pharmacol. **27**, 532 (1985).

63. Berridge, M.J.   Inositol phosphate and diacylglycerol as second messengers. Biochem. J. **220**, 345 (1984).
64. Huckle, W.R. and Conn, P.M. The relationship between gonadotropin releasing hormone-stimulated luteinizing hormone release and inositol phosphate production: Studies with calcium antagonists and protein kinase C activators. Endocrinology "in press" (1987).
65. Andrews, W.V. and Conn, P.M. Gonadotropin-releasing hormone stimulates mass changes in phosphoinositides and diacylglycerol accumulation in purified gonadotrope cell cultures. Endocrinology **118**, 1148 (1986).
66. Snyder, G.D. and Bleasdale, J.E. Effect of LHRH on incorporation of [^{32}P]-orthophosphate into phosphatidylinositol by dispersed anterior pituitary cells. Mol. Cell. Endocrinol. **28**, 55 (1982).
67. Raymond, V., Leung, P.C.K., Veilleux, R., Lefevre, G. and Labrie, F.   LHRH rapidly stimulates phosphatidylinositol metabolism in enriched gonadotrophs. Mol. Cell. Endocrinol. **36**, 157 (1984).
68. Kiesel, L. and Catt, K.J. Phosphatidic acid and the calcium-dependent actions of gonadotropin-releasing hormone in pituitary gonadotropes. Arch. Biochem. Biophys. **231**, 202 (1984).
69. Litosch, I., Wallis, C. and Fain, J.N. 5-Hydroxytryptamine stimulates phosphate production in a cell-free system from blowfly salivary glands. J. Biol. Chem. **260**, 5464 (1985).
70. Wallace, M.A. and Fain, J.N. Guanosine 5'-o-thiotrisphosphate stimulates phospholipase C activity in plasma membranes of rat hepatocytes. J. Biol. Chem. **260**, 9527 (1985).
71. Haslam, R.J. and Davidson, M.M.L. Receptor-induced diacylglycerol formation in permeabilized platelets; possible role for GTP binding proteins. J. Receptor Res. **4**, 605 (1984).
72. Rodbell, M. The role of hormone receptors and GTP-regulatory proteins in membrane transduction. Nature **284**, 17 (1980).
73. Andrews, W.V., Staley, D.D., Huckle, W.R. and Conn, P.M. Stimulation of LH release and phospholipid breakdown by GTP in ATP-permeabilized pituitary cell cultures: Inhibition by GnRH antagonists suggests functional association of the G-protein and the GnRH receptor. Endocrinology "in press" (1986).
74. Streb, H., Irvine, R.F., Berridge, M.J. and Schulz, I. Release of calcium from a nonmitochondrial intracellular store in pancreatic acinar cells by inositol-1,4,5-triphosphate. Nature **306**, 67 (1983).
75. Watson, S.P. and Lapetina, E.G. 1,2-Diacylglycerol and phorbol ester inhibit agonist-induced formation of inositol phosphates in human platelets: Possible implications for negative feedback regulation of inositol phospholipid hydrolysis. Proc. Natl. Acad. Sci. U.S.A. **82**, 2623 (1985).
76. Takai, Y., Kishimoto, A., Iwasa, Y., Kawahara, Y., Mori, T. and Nishizuka, Y. Calcium-dependent activation of a multifunctional protein kinase by membrane phospholipids. J. Biol. Chem. **254**, 3692 (1979).
77. Kuo, J.F., Andersson, R.G.G., Wise, B.C., Mackerlova, L., Salmonsson, I., Brackett, N.L., Katoh, N., Shoji, M. and

Wrenn, R.W. Calcium-dependent protein kinase: Widespread occurance in various tissues and phyla of the animal kingdom and comparison of effects of phospholipid, calmodulin and trifluoperazine. Proc. Natl. Acad. Sci. U.S.A. **77**, 7093 (1980).

78. Takai, Y., Kikkawa, U., Kaibuchi, K. and Nishizuka, Y. Membrane phospholipid metabolism and signal transduction for protein phosphorylation. In "Advances in cyclic nucleotide and protein phosphorylation research," P. Greengard and G.A. Robinson (eds.), Raven, New York, p. 119, (1984).

79. Nishizuka, Y. The role of protein kinase C in cell surface signal transduction and tumour promotion. Nature **308**, 693 (1984).

80. Kishimoto, A., Takai, Y., Mori, T., Kikkawa, U. and Nishizuka, Y. Activation of calcium and phospholipid-dependent protein kinase by diacylglycerol, its possible relation to phosphatidylinositol turnover. J. Biol. Chem. **255**, 2273 (1980).

81. Nishizuka, Y. Turnover of inositol phospholipids and signal transduction. Science **225**, 1365 (1984).

82. Smith, M.A. and Vale, W.W. Superfusion of rat anterior pituitary cells attached to cytodex beads: Validation of a technique. Endocrinology **107**, 1425 (1980).

83. Niedel, J.E., Kuhn, L.J. and Vanderbark, G.R. Phorbol receptor copurifies with protein kinase C. Proc. Natl. Acad. Sci. U.S.A. **80**, 36 (1983).

84. Ashendel, C.L., Staller, J.M. and Boutwell, R.K. Protein kinase activity associated with a phorbol ester receptor purified from mouse brain. Cancer Res. **43**, 4333 (1983).

85. Sharkey, N.A., Leach, K.L. and Blumberg, P.M. Competitive inhibition by diacylgycerol of specific phorbol ester binding. Proc. Natl. Acad. Sci. U.S.A. **81**, 607 (1984).

86. Jaken, S. Increased diacylglycerol content with phospholipase C or hormone treatment: Inhibition of phorbol ester binding and induction of phorbol ester-like biological responses. Endocrinology **117**, 2301 (1985).

87. Castagna, M., Takai, Y., Kaibuchi, K., Sano, K., Kikkawa, U. and Nishizuka, Y. Direct activation of calcium-activated, phospholipid-dependant protein kinase by tumor-promoting phorbol esters. J. Biol. Chem. **257**, 7847 (1982).

88. Kikkawa, U., Takai, Y., Tanaka, Y., Miyake, R. and Nishizuka, Y. Protein kinase C as a possible receptor protein of tumor promoting phorbol esters. J. Biol. Chem. **258**, 11442 (1983).

89. Conn, P.M., Ganong, B.R., Ebeling, J., Staley, D., Neidel, J.E. and Bell, R.M. Diacylglycerols release LH: Structure-activity relations and protein kinase C. Biochem. Biophys. Res. Commun. **126**, 532 (1985).

90. Hirota, K., Hirota, T., Aguilera, G. and Catt, K.J. Hormone-induced redistribution of calcium-activated phospholipid-dependant protein kinase in pituitary gonadotrophs. J. Biol. Chem. **260**, 3243 (1985).

91. McArdle, C.A. and Conn, P.M. Hormone stimulated redistribution of gonadotrope protein kinase C *in vivo*: Dependence on calcium influx. Mol. Pharmacol. **29**, 570 (1986).

92. Kraft, A.S. and Anderson, W.B. Phorbol esters increase the amount of calcium phospholipid-dependant protein kinase associated with the plasma membrane. Nature **301**, 621 (1983).

93. Faeron, C.W. and Tashjian, A.H. Thyrotropin-releasing hormone induces redistribution of protein kinase C in GH_4C_1 rat pituitary cells. J. Biol. Chem. **260**, 8366 (1985).

94. Hannun, Y.A., Loomis, C.R. and Bell, R.M. Activation of protein kinase C by Triton X-100 mixed micelles containing diacylglycerol and phosphatidylserine. J. Biol. Chem. **260**, 10039 (1985).

95. Wolf, M., LeVine III, H., May Jr, S., Cuatrecacasas, P. and Sahyoun, N. A model for intracellular translocation of protein kinase C involving synergism between calcium and phorbol esters. Nature **317**, 546 (1985).

96. Naor, Z. and Eli, Y. Synergistic stimulation of leutenizing hormone (LH) release by protein kinase C activators and calcium ionophore. Biochem. Biophys. Res. Commun. **130**, 848 (1985).

97. Baraban, J.N., Snyder, S.H. and Alger, B.E. Protein Kinase C regulates ionic conductance in hippocampal pyramidal neurons: Electrophysiological effects of phorbol esters. Proc. Natl. Acad. Sci. U.S.A. **82**, 2538 (1985).

98. Drummond, A.H. Bidirectional control of cytosolic free calcium by thyrotropin-releasing hormone in pituitary cells. Nature **315**, 752 (1985).

99. Naor, Z. and Catt, K.J. Mechanism of action of gonadotropin-releasing hormone. Involvement of phospholipid turnover in luteinizing hormone release. J. Biol. Chem. **256**, 2226 (1981).

100. Naor, Z., Vanderhoek, J.Y., Lindner, H.R. and Catt, K.J. Arachidonic acid products as possible mediators of the action of gonadotropin-releasing hormone. In "Advances in Prostaglandin, Thromboxane, and Leukotriene Research, Vol. 12" B. Samuelsson, R. Paoletti and P. Ramwell (eds.), Raven Press, New York, (1983).

101. Hulting, A.L., Lindgren, J.A., Hokfelt, T., Eneroth, P., Werner, S., Patrono, C. and Samuelsson, B. Leukotriene C_4 as a mediator of luteinizing hormone release from rat anterior pituitary cells. Proc. Natl. Acad. Sci. U.S.A. **82**, 3834 (1985).

102. Conn, P.M., Whorton, R. and Lazar, J. An inhibitor of arachidonic acid metabolism stimulates luteinizing hormone (LH) release from cultured pituitary cells. Prostaglandins **19**, 873 (1980).

103. Leiser, J., Conn, P.M. and Blum, J.J. Interpretation of dose-response curves for luteinizing hormone release by GnRH, related peptides, and leukotriene C_4 according to a hormone/receptor/two effector model. Proc. Natl. Acad. Sci. U.S.A. **83**, 5963 (1986).

7
Mediation of the Preovulatory LH Surge: LHRH Pulsatility and Opioid Modulation

A. L. BARKAN amd J. C. MARSHALL

Division of Endocrinology and Metabolism, Department of Internal Medicine,
University of Michigan Hospital and VA Medical Center, University of Michigan,
Ann Arbor, MI 48109 - 0368, USA

INTRODUCTION

The development of specific radioimmunoassays for luteinizing hormone (LH) and follicle-stimulating hormone (FSH) allowed elucidation of the mechanisms of pituitary gonadotropin secretion and indicated the crucial role of hypothalamic LHRH in regulating gonadotropin release. Early studies of LH secretion showed marked variability of LH concentrations in peripheral blood. Serial measurements of plasma LH at 5-30 minute intervals demonstrated the periodic nature of LH secretion which is characterized by well-defined secretory pulses interspersed with periods of relative quiescence. Moreover, the patterns of LH secretion were altered in different physiological circumstances, and, for example, puberty was heralded by the appearance of a nocturnal, sleep-related augmentation in LH pulsatility. This suggested a central control of pulsatile gonadotropin secretion, and implied that hypothalamic LHRH secretion also occurred in a pulsatile manner. The proof of this hypothesis, however, was elusive. Measurement of LHRH in the peripheral blood was unhelpful, due to the limited sensitivity of LHRH radioimmunoassays and the dilution of hypothalamic-pituitary stalk blood into the systemic circulation. Other studies utilized collection of pituitary portal blood over 30 min periods in rats and showed that LHRH output was augmented on the afternoon of proestrus [1]. However, these experiments did not detect spontaneous LHRH pulses, as blood was collected over prolonged periods of time. Thus, the initial evidence of the pulsatile nature of hypothalamic LHRH secretion was only recently obtained [2] and has since been confirmed using various experimental paradigms.

LHRH SECRETION IN VITRO

McKibbin and Belchetz [3] showed that mediobasal guinea pig hypothalami secreted LHRH in a pulsatile manner for up to 72 h of incubation. However, they were unable to detect changes in pulse frequency or amplitude between ovariectomized animals and animals studied during the estrous cycle. On the other hand, a five to ten fold puberty-associated acceleration of pulsatile LHRH release from the hypothalami of male rats has been found in vitro [4].

LHRH SECRETION IN VIVO

Electrophysiological studies

Hypothalamic multiple unit activity (MUA) has been studied in ovariectomized animals to correlate electrical activity of hypothalamic neurons with pituitary LH release. Striking increases in MUA associated with the initiation of each LH pulse have been recorded in monkeys [5,6] and in rats [7]. Administration of the alpha$_1$-adrenoreceptor blocker phenoxybenzamine arrested the MUA and also terminated pulsatile LH release. Similarly, the dopaminergic receptor antagonist metoclopramide suppressed or abolished both MUA and LH pulsatility. These results agree with the known effects of norepinephrine and dopamine upon hypothalamic LHRH secretory neurons [8] and with the LH release-promoting effect of electrical stimulation of the hypothalamus [9]. These data suggest strongly that periodic excitation of LHRH-secreting hypothalamic neurons is responsible for pulsatile LHRH release and consequent pulsatile LH secretion.

Push-pull hypothalamic perfusion studies

This technique makes use of a stereotactically implanted cannula in the hypothalamus [10]. Subsequently, an inner cannula of smaller diameter is inserted into the outer cannula and serves as a route for continuous delivery of artificial CSF. Samples are drawn through the space between the inner and the outer cannulae for determination of LHRH, and LH is measured in simultaneous samples obtained from a peripheral vein. This technique has been successfully used in monkeys [11], sheep [12] and rats [13]. In all species studied, a clearly pulsatile LHRH secretory pattern was detected and each pulse of LH was coincident with a LHRH pulse.

Direct portal sampling

Although direct sampling of pituitary portal blood has been used by various groups in the past [1,2], the recently developed technique of Clarke and Cummins [14] has provided convincing evidence of the temporal relationships between LHRH and LH secretion. In this method, an artificial sinus is created in front of the anterior pituitary and two needles are inserted. At a later time, the upper needle is gently advanced to make a stab incision in the hypophysial portal vessels. This is followed by the continuous sampling of blood from the artificial sinus through the lower needle (portal blood for LHRH determination) and from the jugular vein for LH measurement. The nature of pituitary portal LHRH discharge was shown to be unequivocally pulsatile, and each pulse of LH was preceded by an LHRH pulse.

Thus, an impressive body of evidence has been collected to show that the pulsatile nature of LH secretion by the pituitary gland is the direct result of pulsatile secretion of LHRH from the hypothalamus via the hypothalamo-hypophysial portal vessels. Therefore, estimation of LH pulse frequency may provide valuable information about the frequency of endogenous hypothalamic LHRH pulsatile secretion. However, some caution

102

should be exercised in equating these phenomena. First, detection of LH pulses depends upon assay sensitivity and reproducibility, upon the frequency of sampling and upon the criteria used to define the amplitude of an LH pulse. High sampling frequencies are necessary to detect rapid LH pulsatile secretion and samples need to be obtained over prolonged periods of time to reliably show changes in LH pulse frequency. Second, gonadal steroids (and possibly other factors) can influence pituitary sensitivity to LHRH. Thus, in certain steroid milieu LH responses to LHRH may be attenuated and not detectable in the peripheral circulation.

NEURAL REGULATION OF LHRH SECRETION

Neurotransmitters

Multiple neurotransmitters have been shown to affect the activity of LHRH-secreting hypothalamic neurons, but the majority of data relate to the effects of norepinephrine (NE), epinephrine (E), dopamine (DA), and serotonin (5-HT).

Both inhibitory and excitatory components of NE have been recognized. Intra-cerebroventricular infusion of NE or administration of clonidine suppressed pulsatile LH discharge in ovariectomized rats [15,16]. However, acute suppression of hypothalamic NE or blockade of central adrenoreceptors in this model also caused a decline in LH pulsatility [17] which could be restored after administration of clonidine [18]. These opposing effects of NE in ovariectomized rats may reflect the existence of alpha$_1$ (stimulating) and alpha$_2$ (inhibiting) receptors, but the mechanisms remain unclear. In contrast, in cycling and castrate steroid-primed rats, alpha-adrenergic agonists increased LH release [19,20] and antagonists suppressed pulsatile LH release and blocked the gonadotropin surge [21,22].

Epinephrine does not alter LH pulse frequency in ovariectomized rats, but it is more potent than NE or dopamine in eliciting an LH rise in proestrous or estrogen-primed rats [23]. Also, inhibition of the conversion of NE to E blocks the gonadotropin surge in both models [24,25]. E pinephrine turnover in the mediobasal hypothalamus is increased at the time of the LH surge [26] and thus, the function of E may be limited to the promotion of LHRH discharge during the surge.

Activation of DA receptors in ovariectomized rats slows LH pulses [17], but some [27], though not all [19], studies have shown that DA may stimulate LH release in steroid-primed rats. In vitro, DA stimulated LHRH release from the mediobasal hypothalamus [28] whereas metoclopramide arrested the electrophysiological activity of the hypothalamic LHRH pulse generator in vivo [5]. The reasons for the variable results in different studies are not certain and the precise role of DA in regulation of LHRH secretion awaits clarification.

There is considerable, though controversial evidence to support a regulatory role of 5-HT in the stimulation of both tonic and phasic LHRH secretion. Suppression of hypothalamic 5-HT by neurotoxin suppressed LH pulsatility [29] and 5-HT receptor blockers attenuated LH pulse amplitude [30]. Also, manipulation of brain 5-HT levels can block estradiol (E$_2$)-induced LH surges [31], and hypothalamic 5-HT levels fall on the afternoon of proestrus, coincident with the increased LH secretion [32].

Endogenous Opioid Peptides

As discussed above, pulsatile LHRH release may be stimulated or inhibited by several neurotransmitters and their effects may be modified by the prevailing steroid milieu. It is unlikely that each neurotransmitter affects LHRH secretion in an independent fashion, and the effects of each neurotransmitter system are probably coordinated. In recent years, evidence has accumulated that the endogenous opioid peptide (EOP) system acts as a neuromodulator of other neurotransmitter systems involved in the regulation of pulsatile LHRH discharge.

Endogenous opioid peptides belong to the proopiomelanocortin family of peptides and are widely distributed throughout various body systems. Different EOP, such as beta-endorphin, met-enkephalin, leu-enkephalin and dynorphin may elicit variable physiological responses, depending on the properties of the affected system and the type of tissue receptor (mu, delta, kappa, sigma, etc). In general, opioid agonists suppress and opioid antagonists increase gonadotropin secretion, and these actions are exerted predominantly on the central nervous system.

The amygdala and the periaqueductal central gray are the highest centers known to be involved in opioid inhibition of LH secretion. Microinjections of beta-endorphin [33] or morphine [34] into these areas suppress pituitary LH secretion and injections of naloxone increase plasma LH. Thus, these neural tissues may initiate opioid effects and transmit the signal to the hypothalamus [35]. Considerable evidence indicates that opioids regulate LHRH secretion, acting directly at the level of hypothalamus. Morphine suppresses the proestrous surge of LHRH in pituitary portal plasma of rats [36], and opioids inhibit and naloxone augments LHRH secretion from isolated hypothalami [37-39]. Several studies also suggest that opioids may modulate LH secretion directly at the pituitary level. Leu-enkephalin potentiated the LH response to LHRH [40]. In contrast, beta-endorphin and met-enkephalin suppressed LH release in vitro, and naloxone blocked the inhibitory action of beta-endorphin and itself elicited LH release [41,42]. Interestingly, both beta and gamma-endorphin stimulated LH release from ovine pituitaries [43] suggesting that species differences may exist in the pituitary actions of opioid compounds. Opioid peptides did not alter LHRH binding to pituitary LHRH receptors [44] and the direct pituitary effects of opioids may be due to paracrine influences of opioid peptides upon LH secretion.

Opioid-neurotransmitter interrelations

The question whether opioid peptides act directly on LHRH neurons or alter the activity of other neurotransmitter systems, which in turn influence LHRH secretion, has been addressed in a series of studies. In ovariectomized, E_2 and progesterone (P) pretreated rats, the LH-releasing effect of naloxone was blocked by phenoxybenzamine and by dopamine beta-hydroxylase inhibitors [45]. Clonidine, but not naloxone, was able to elicit LH release in animals whose catecholamine synthesis was abolished by dopamine beta-hydroxylase blockers. These and other data suggested that the opiate-induced modulation of LH (and by inference LHRH) release required NE participation. Beta-endorphin reduced hypothalamic dopamine secretion [46], but no effect of dopaminergic drugs was observed in naloxone-treated rats [45], suggesting that dopamine may not be important in opioid regulation of LHRH secretion. Opioids may also modify serotoninergic systems and hypothalamic serotonin turnover was altered in rats given morphine and naloxone [47]. Pretreatment with 5-hydroxytryptophan to increase hypothalamic serotonin content prevented naloxone-induced LH secretion, while depletion of hypothalamic tryptophan potentiated naloxone-induced LH release [48].

Opioid–steroid interactions

The activity of the endogenous opioid system is influenced by gonadal steroids and this interaction may play a significant role in opioid regulation of reproductive cyclicity. Mediobasal hypothalamic beta-endorphin and dynorphin neurons possess nuclear estrogen receptors [49] and castration decreases and estradiol increases hypothalamic beta-endorphin content in rats [50]. Pituitary portal beta-endorphin levels are low in castrate monkeys and during the early follicular phase, but are increased during the late follicular and especially during the luteal phases of the cycle [51]. The augmented beta-endorphin secretion during the luteal phase appears to be due to the additional effects of P in the pre-existing high E_2 milieu [52]. The low activity of the EOP system in castrated animals or during low E_2 states (i.e. early follicular phase) is associated with the inability of opiate blockade by naloxone to elicit increased LH secretion. This effect is manifest when E_2 levels are increased during the late follicular or luteal phases of the cycle [53-55].

PULSATILE LHRH SECRETION

Gonadotrope Function

Several studies have documented the requirement for a pulsatile LHRH stimulus to maintain LH secretion in several species. Continuous infusions of LHRH or administration of long acting LHRH agonists desensitize LH secretion, whereas the intermittent pulsatile delivery of LHRH maintains LH secretion in monkeys and humans [56,57]. An LHRH pulse frequency of 1 pulse/hour maintains release of LH and FSH in sheep, monkeys and humans. Faster frequencies of 3/hour reduce both LH and FSH in plasma, whereas slower frequencies of 1 pulse every 3-4 hours results in a decline in LH but a rise in plasma FSH [58-60]. The frequency of LHRH pulses may also modulate the amount of LH released. LH pulse amplitude is low after fast LHRH frequencies but increases when a slower LHRH frequency is used [59].

The initial event in LHRH action is binding to specific receptors in the gonadotrope cell membrane [61] and LHRH is known to increase LH and FSH synthesis. LHRH pulse frequency and amplitude also appear to regulate the concentration of both LHRH receptors (LHRH-R) and steady state levels of mRNAs for the alpha and LH beta subunits. In LHRH deficient animals exogenous LHRH increases LHRH-R [62] and this effect is dependent upon the dose of LHRH per pulse. In castrate testosterone-replaced male rats, a dose of 25 ng results in a maximum increase in LHRH-R, but at higher physiologic levels of testosterone (5ng/ml), five fold lower doses of LHRH produce maximal LHRH-R responses [63]. In the same model, using a constant dose of LHRH/pulse, the frequency of the LHRH signal regulates

LHRH-R and LH release [64]. An LHRH pulse given every 30 min produced a maximum rise in LHRH-R whereas faster or slower frequencies resulted in smaller responses. LHRH pulses also increased steady state concentrations of both alpha and LH beta mRNAs. In castrate male rats, testosterone replacement reduced mRNA levels to lower values than were observed in intact animals. LHRH pulses given every 30 min increased alpha and LH beta mRNAs in castrate testosterone-replaced rats. The increase in LH beta mRNA was dose dependent however, and 25 ng LHRH/pulse produced a maximal increase with smaller responses being seen after larger or smaller LHRH doses. Thus, in male rats an LHRH stimulus of 25 ng/pulse given every 30 min produces the maximal responses in LHRH-R, LH beta subunit mRNA and maintains LH release over a period of 1-2 days [65].

These data suggest that the gonadotrope appears to be able to recognize changes in the pattern of LHRH stimulation. Alterations in the frequency or amplitude of the LHRH signal can produce changes in LHRH-R, LH subunit mRNA concentrations and can also modify the amount of LH released.

Regulation of reproductive cyclicity

Cyclic changes in the function of the reproductive system is a feature present in females of all species. Ovarian function is characterized by the sequential secretion of estradiol and progesterone that is required for preparation of the endometrium to accept and to retain a fertilized ovum. Additionally, changes in ovarian steroids can regulate pituitary gonadotropin output, which in turn controls ovarian follicular growth and probably determines the number of follicles which mature during a particular cycle. A marked increase in gonadotropin secretion is needed to induce ovulation. These finely tuned alterations in gonadotropin secretion and in ovarian function are regulated by the central nervous system. For example, in cattle and sheep, the timing of ovulation is dictated by day length ("seasonal breeders"). Cats and rabbits, the so-called "reflex ovulators", manifest gonadotropin surges only after coitus. In primates (including humans) and in some rodents such as rats, reproductive cycles seem to be spontaneous and follow one another in an uninterrupted fashion (monthly in women, or every 4-5 days in rats). However, even in these species, reproductive cyclicity can be disrupted by external stimuli, such as stress of various types. Thus, even in "spontaneous ovulators", reproductive function is governed by the central nervous system, and the hypothalamic LHRH neuronal activity seems to be the final common pathway by which this influence is exerted. Such changes in hypothalamic LHRH neuronal activity may be translated into a form "readable" by the pituitary gonadotropes in one of two ways: changes in the frequency of the LHRH signal, changes in the amplitude of the LHRH signal, or by a combination of both.

Pulsatile LH secretion during rat estrous cycles

Relatively little is known about the patterns of pulsatile LH (and by inference LHRH) secretion in rats and some existing data are conflicting. The technical difficulties of conducting such studies are considerable in that the amount of blood which can be drawn is limited and the stress of sampling may disrupt LHRH pulsatility. A summary of existing information in rats is given in Table 1.

Table 1: Pulsatile LH Secretion During the Rat Estrous Cycle

Author	Sampling Interval (minutes)	LH Interpulse Interval (minutes)			
		Metestrus	Diestrus	Proestrus	Estrus
Higuchi et al (66)	5	40	43	35	ND
Fox et al (67)	6-10	46	49	60	ND
Levine et al (13)*	12			48	
Gallo et al (68)	6-8	62			106
Leipheimer et al (69)	6		78	90	
Leipheimer et al (70)	6	69			

* Hypothalamic LHRH output as measured by the push-pull cannula technique. ND - not detected

Although data from different groups are somewhat heterogenous, the general concensus is that the frequency of LH secretion shows little or no change during the rat estrous cycle, with the exception of the day of estrus, which is characterized by a significant slowing or absence of LH (and by inference LHRH) pulses. Thus, the transition from estrus to metestrus is accompanied by the acceleration of LHRH pulse frequency.

Pulsatile LH secretion during menstrual cycles

Although the central mechanisms governing reproductive cyclicity may not be identical in humans and rats, the fact that both species exhibit spontaneous regular ovulation, suggests that they may be similar. Studies in humans and primates are easier to perform, as frequent blood samples can be obtained over a prolonged period of time. Present data in humans are summarized in Table 2 together with data from studies in Rhesus monkeys.

Table 2: Pulsatile LH Secretion During Menstrual Cycles

Author	Sampling Interval (minutes)	LH Pulses per 12 Hours					
		EF	MF	LF	EL	ML	LL
Yen et al (71)	15	7.5		8.0	3.1		3.0
Santen & Bardin (72)	20	6.6		-	3.2		-
Backstrom et al (73)	15	6.6	8.2	8.8	3.2		6.8
Reame et al (74)	20	7.7		7.4	5.6		5.3
Soules et al (75)	20	7.2		8.5	2.2		-
Reame et al (74)	10	11.8		14.3	8.0		7.8
Filicori et al (76)	10	-		-	7.6	4.4	4.2
Filicori et al (77)	10	7.7	10.7	10.1	7.0	3.5	3.3
Djahanbakhch et al (78)	5	-		16.4	-	-	
Veldhuis et al (79)	10-15	9.7		13.6	4.4		-
Veldhuis et al (80)	5	10.3		-	-		-
Steele et al (81)	5	6.0	11.7	11.1	-	-	
Norman et al (82)*	10-15	9.6	12.5	10.0	3.7	3.7	2.3
Van Vugt et al (83)*	15	6.0		-	1.7		-

Data have been recalculated and normalized to a 12 hour observation period. (*) indicate studies performed in Rhesus monkeys. EF, MF, LF, EL, ML, LL indicate early, mid, and late follicular or luteal phases of the cycle respectively.

These results demonstrate clearly that the frequency of LH pulses increases gradually from the early to the late follicular phase and then slows during the luteal phase of the cycle. An example of changing LH pulsatility during the human menstrual cycle is shown in Figure 1.

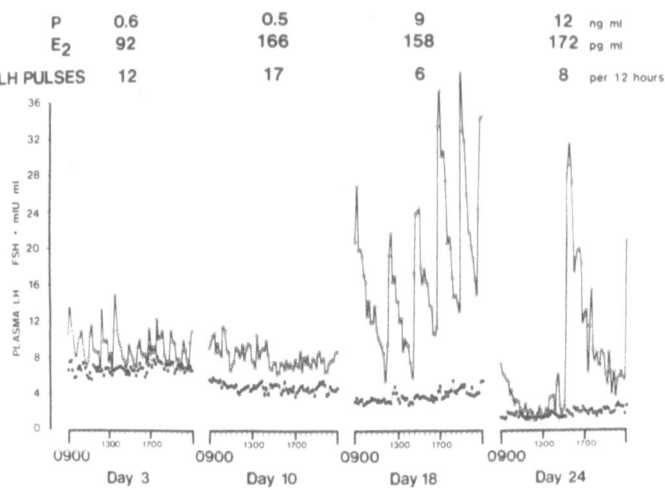

Figure 1

Plasma LH, FSH, estradiol (E_2) and progesterone (P) during an ovulatory menstrual cycle. Samples were drawn at 10 min intervals for 12 hours on Days 3, 10, 18 and 24 of the cycle. Reproduced from Marshall, J.C. et.al. Pulsatile gonadotropin-releasing hormone (GnRH) - studies of puberty and the menstrual cycle. In: Labrie, F. and Proulx, L. (eds). Endocrinology. Elsevier Sci. Publishers 1984, pp. 25-32 (with permission).

Pulsatile LH secretion during the preovulatory gonadotropin surge

In both rats and humans the preovulatory gonadotropin surge is preceded by a significant elevation in plasma estradiol (E_2) and by the initial rise in plasma progesterone (P). The exact mechanisms involved in the genesis of the preovulatory surge remain uncertain. Increased LHRH secretion appears to play a role, as increased hypothalamic LHRH secretion has been observed during surges in different species, including rats [84], rabbits [85] and monkeys [86]. The increase in LHRH secretion is mediated by the changing levels of gonadal steroids, and the interplay between the effects of E_2 and P upon LHRH release and upon pituitary sensitivity to LHRH are both crucial aspects in the generation of the surge. This ability of gonadal steroids to elicit LH surges has been used to establish a model of ovariectomized E_2-replaced (or E_2+P-replaced) females. In this model, regular gonadotropin surges occur daily (in rats), or 48 hours after administration of E_2 in higher species. The resultant gonadotropin surges are similar to the spontaneous surges in cycling animals both in timing, magnitude, duration, and existence of critical period, as well as in responsiveness to pharmacological stimuli (blockade by barbiturates or morphine). Thus, the ovariectomized E_2-replaced ($\pm$ P) model has been used to study the mechanisms involved in the generation of the preovulatory gonadotropin surges.

E_2 acts at both the pituitary and hypothalamic levels to promote the LH surge. At the pituitary, elevation of plasma E_2 concentrations initially decreases LH secretion (negative feedback), but after a period of time which varies in different species, pituitary sensitivity to LHRH increases - the so-called positive feedback effect [87]. The appearance of positive feedback phase requires the presence of higher circulating E_2 concentrations. The second effect of an elevation in plasma E_2 is to increase hypothalamic LHRH secretion [87]. This combination of increased hypothalamic LHRH output and heightened pituitary sensitivity to LHRH promotes marked gonadotropin secretion - the gonadotropin surge. Thus, an increase in estradiol is important in producing the LH surge but the magnitude of the E_2-induced surge can be augmented by P. Although P augments pituitary sensitivity to LHRH in vitro [88], the effect of P in vivo appears to be at the hypothalamic level, where it augments hypothalamic LHRH secretion [89,90]. This action probably requires previous hypothalamic exposure to E_2 and in cycling animals is manifest only on the afternoon of proestrus [90].

The preovulatory elevations of estradiol and progesterone also affect pulsatile LHRH secretion. In rats, Gallo [91] has reported increased LH pulse frequency during the ascending part of the surge. LH pulse frequency was unchanged in other studies [67], but LH pulse amplitude was increased during the surge. It is uncertain whether the increase in LH amplitude results from increased LHRH pulse amplitude or from enhanced pituitary sensitivity to LHRH. In primates, high-frequency, high-amplitude LH pulses were observed during the preovulatory gonadotropin surge [82]. In women, LH pulse amplitude was significantly increased [74,81], but LH pulse frequency was similar to that observed during the late follicular phase. Considerable clarification of events at the time of the surge has been obtained from measurements of portal LHRH and peripheral LH in ovariectomized ewes [92]. Injection of E_2 resulted in a bi-phasic LH response (negative and positive feedback), and the LH surge was accompanied by increased LHRH output. During the negative feedback phase, LHRH pulse frequency was similar to that observed in castrated controls (interpulse interval of 50 min), but the LH pulses, present in castrates, were obliterated. During the positive feedback phase, LHRH pulse frequency increased (interpulse interval of 27min) and pulsatile LH secretion, concordant with the LHRH pulses, was restored. These data indicate that the initial negative effects of E_2 are due to reduced pituitary sensitivity to LHRH whereas the positive effects of E_2 are exerted at both the hypothalamic and pituitary levels.

LHRH receptors and LH mRNA during estrous cycles

LHRH receptor concentrations (LHRH-R) vary during the estrous cycle and studies have shown that LHRH-R is low on metestrus, increases two to three fold on diestrus through the afternoon of proestrus, and then declines rapidly toward estrus [93]. These dynamics are similar to the changes in pituitary sensitivity to LHRH during the estrous cycle and suggests that LHRH-R may constitute an important part of the mechanisms regulating responses to LHRH.

Recent studies from our laboratory have shown that LH subunit mRNA concentrations also change during the estrous cycle in rats. Both alpha and LH beta mRNA levels are low on metestrus and both increase 2 fold during diestrus before falling during the night of diestrus/proestrus. On proestrus, alpha mRNA is unchanged, but concentrations of LH beta mRNA increase a few hours prior to the LH surge and remain elevated (3 fold) for 6-8 hours. Both alpha and LH beta mRNAs are low during estrus [94].

The mechanisms regulating LHRH-R and LH subunit mRNA concentrations during the estrus cycle remain uncertain. The increase in LHRH-R and subunit mRNAs occurs after the appearance of pulsatile LH secretion on metestrus. As LHRH pulses can increase LHRH-R and subunit mRNA concentrations in males, this suggests that an increase in LHRH pulsatile secretion may be the underlying mechanism. The increase in plasma E_2 which also begins on diestrus may also play a role and could augment the effects of LHRH on receptors and LH subunit gene expression. Similarly, the changing ovarian steroid milieu on diestrus-proestrus may differentially modify receptor and mRNA responses to pulsatile LHRH. Progesterone has been shown to reduce the frequency of LHRH pulses [95] and this may account for the decline in LHRH-R after the gonadotropin surge. The mechanisms of the changes in LHRH-R and subunit mRNA concentrations at the time of the LH surge are also unclear. Immediately prior to the LH surge, LHRH-R transiently falls by 50% [96]. This change in LHRH-R is independent of the changing plasma concentrations of E_2 and P as it also occurs prior to the afternoon LH surge in ovariectomized E_2-treated rats [97]. The acute reduction in LHRH-R also appears to be independent of changes in gonadotropins or prolactin as it could not be reproduced by administration of LH, FSH or prolactin to ovariectomized E_2-rats [97,98]. However, suppression of hypothalamic LHRH release by pentobarbital abolished both the fall in LHRH-R and the LH surge [96,97]. This suggested that an increase in LHRH secretion may be the mechanism involved in acutely reducing LHRH-R and increasing LH release. Administration of exogenous LHRH (225 ng every 10 or 30 min) did not acutely reduce LHRH-R, however, and the changes in receptors may reflect a specific pattern (amplitude or frequency) of the LHRH signal. This currently remains unproven, but as LH beta mRNA is increased prior to the LH surge and specific LHRH dose/frequency combinations can selectively increase LH beta mRNA in males [65] such a mechanism may explain the observed events at the level of the gonadotrope during the LH surge (see below).

Endogenous opiates and the preovulatory gonadotropin surge

Administration of morphine or opioid peptides abolishes the afternoon gonadotropin surge in both cycling and ovariectomized E_2-treated rats [99-101]. The specific opioid nature of this phenomenon is confirmed by the ability of naloxone to prevent this effect of opiate agonists. Subsequent studies have shown that hypothalamic beta-endorphin content declines rapidly and transiently prior to, or concomitant with, the preovulatory LH surge [102-104]. Naloxone did not elicit LH secretion at this time [105,106], supporting the view that opioid inhibition of LHRH secretion was diminished prior to or during the LH surge. These data suggested that the central signal leading to the generation of the gonadotropin surge may involve a sudden fall in hypothalamic opioid inhibition of LHRH secretion. Indeed, prevention of opioid inhibition by naloxone was followed by the premature appearance of an LH surge of similar pattern and magnitude to the spontaneous preovulatory surge [107]. To examine this issue, we have studied the effects of opioid-active drugs in ovariectomized E_2 treated--rats. In this model, as

110

in its proestrous counterpart, the gonadotropin surge is preceded by a transient fall in the number of pituitary LHRH receptors [93,96,97]. Both the LHRH-R fall and the LH surge were blocked by pentobarbital and morphine [96,97]. This suggested that the LHRH-R fall may serve as a marker of the action of the presumed central "ovulatory" signal - increased LHRH secretion. Between 0900 h and 1400 h both LHRH-R and LH are stable in ovariectomized-E_2 treated rats, but administration of naloxone (mimicking the presumed fall in opioid influence) was immediately followed by a transient fall in LHRH-R and a rise in plasma LH. Conversely, morphine elicited a prompt rise in LHRH-R and a fall in plasma LH concentrations [44]. In animals with radiofrequency-induced mediobasal hypothalamic lesions, and in those pretreated with LHRH-antiserum, both morphine and naloxone were ineffective [98]. These data strongly suggested that the opioid-induced changes in LHRH-R and LH were mediated through altered function of LHRH neurons. Indeed, stimulation of LHRH neurons with the alpha-adrenoreceptor agonist clonidine reproduced the changes seen after administration of naloxone, a fall in LHRH-R and a rise in LH, whereas blockade by phenoxybenzamine had opposite, morphine-like effects. Inhibition of LHRH secretion by the dopamine agonists L-DOPA and bromocriptine, was followed by a rise in LHRH-R and a fall in plasma LH [98]. Thus, modulation of endogenous opioid tone may elicit changes in hypothalamic neurotransmitter activity, resulting in increased LHRH secretion, which in turn produces a transient fall in LHRH-R and the increase in LH secretion - the gonadotropin surge.

These effects of opioids may be mediated through alterations of both the frequency of LHRH secretion as well as the amplitude of LHRH pulses [108] and both factors may be involved in regulating LHRH-R and LH release. Acute exposure of dispersed pituitary cells to LHRH was followed by a transient fall in LHRH-R which occurred prior to maximal LH secretion [109]. Also an increase in frequency of LHRH pulses may play a role in the fall in LHRH-R. Frequent LHRH injections (every 8-15min) were less effective in increasing LHRH-R and in promoting LH release in male rats [64]. Thus, a change in the pattern of LHRH delivery to the gonadotrope may reduce LHRH-R and augment LH secretion. This remains to be demonstrated in vivo but the requirement for a specific LHRH frequency or amplitude may explain why exogenous LHRH did not reduce LHRH-R in ovariectomized E_2-treated rats [97].

CONCLUDING REMARKS

The information summarized above indicates that alterations in the patterns of LHRH secretion play an important role in the regulation in reproductive cyclicity in mammals. While evidence for changes in LHRH pulse frequency in rodents is not compelling, marked changes in LHRH pulse frequency during the menstrual cycle have been well documented in primates and humans. The exact roles of alterations in the LHRH signal remain to be clarified, however, and it is important to note that LH surges and ovulation can be induced in LHRH deficient women and primates by LHRH pulses given at a constant frequency [110]. The effects of altered LHRH pulse frequency may be subtle and possibly related to the maintenance of continuing cyclicity. Some patients treated with constant frequency LHRH regimens exhibit deficient luteal phase function, and a recent study has suggested that an increase in LHRH frequency produces optimal follicular development and luteal phase function [111]. In that study, a majority of women treated with a constant LHRH frequency had rapid luteolysis and this did not occur when the initial LHRH frequency of 1 pulse every 4 hours was progressively increased to 1 pulse every 90 min during the earlier part of the follicular phase. The role of changing LHRH pulse frequency as a determining factor in the generation of reproductive cyclicity in women is shown schematically in Figure 2.

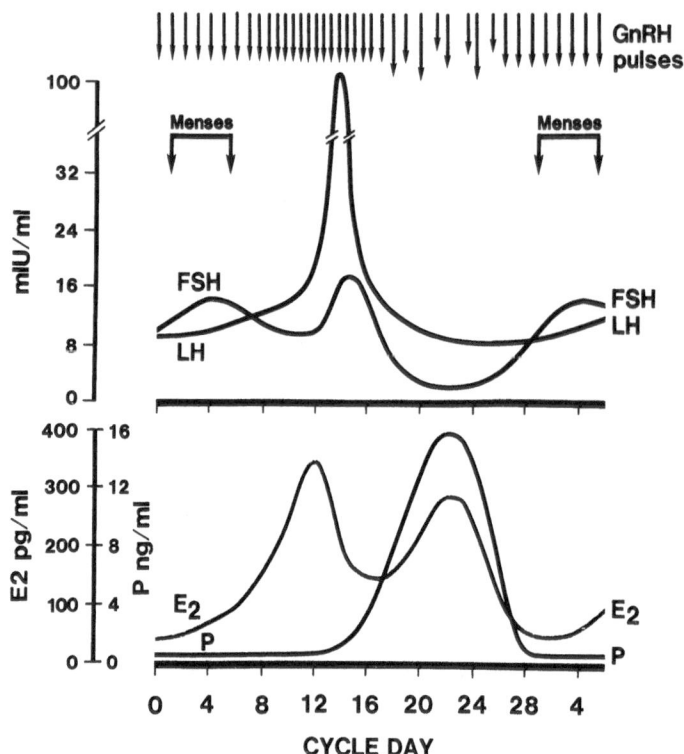

<u>Figure 2</u>

Suggested role of altered LHRH pulse frequency in the regulation of the menstrual cycle. The length of the arrow indicates LHRH pulse amplitude and the interval between the arrows indicates LHRH pulse frequency. Reproduced from Marshall, J.C., et.al. Pulsatile gonadotropin-releasing hormone (GnRH) - studies of puberty and the menstrual cycle. In Labrie, F. and Proulx, L. (eds.) Endocrinology. Elsevier Sci. Publishers 1984, pp. 25-32.

The gradual acceleration of LHRH pulse frequency between the early and the late follicular stages increases LH synthesis and secretion, and the combination of high E_2 (positive feedback) and a fast LHRH pulse frequency results in the generation of the preovulatory gonadotropin surge. High P and E_2 levels during the luteal stage increase endogenous opioid peptides in the hypothalamus and this results in a slow frequency and irregular amplitude LHRH secretion. The slow LHRH stimulus may not be optimal for LH synthesis but, as FSH release is inhibited by the elevated E_2 [112], pituitary

112

stores of FSH are maintained. When P and E_2 levels fall as a result of luteolysis, LHRH pulse frequency increases, and this results in preferential secretion of FSH, induction of ovarian LH receptors and aromatase enzymes, and follicular maturation. This sequence of events allows continuation of sequential reproductive cyclicity.

Overall, present data suggest that changes in the patterns of LHRH secretion can regulate pituitary and ovarian function in mammals. Alterations in the activity of central neurotransmitter systems regulate LHRH secretion and these changes are in part dependent upon the prevailing ovarian steroid milieu. In turn, the gonadotrope recognizes the alterations in LHRH signal patterns and this, together with the direct effects of ovarian hormones on the gonadotrope, results in changes in gonadotropin synthesis and secretion during the estrous and menstrual cycles.

REFERENCES

1.	Sarkar, D.K., Chiappa, S.A., Fink, G., and Sherwood, N.M. Gonadotropin-releasing hormone surge in proestrous rats. Nature 264,461 (1976)
2.	Carmel, P.W., Araki, S. and Ferin, M. Pituitary stalk portal blood collection in rhesus monkeys: evidence for pulsatile release of gonadotropin-releasing hormone. Endocrinology 99,243 (1976)
3.	McKibbin, P.E. and Belchetz, P.E. Prolonged pulsatile release of gonadotropin-releasing hormone from the guinea pig hypothalamus in vitro. Life Sci 38,2145 (1986)
4.	Bourguignon, J.P. and Franchimont, P. Puberty-related increase in episodic LHRH release from rat hypothalami in vitro. Endocrinology 114,1941 (1984)
5.	Kaufman, J.M., Kesner, J.S., Wilson, R.C. and Knobil, E. Electrophysiological manifestation of LHRH pulse generator activity in the rhesus monkey: influence of alpha-adrenergic and dopaminergic blocking agents. Endocrinology 116,1327 (1985)
6.	Kesner, J.S., Kaufman, J.M., Wilson, R.C., Kuroda, G. and Knobil, E. On the short-loop feedback regulation of the hypothalamic luteinizing hormone-releasing hormone "pulse generator" in the rhesus monkey. Neuroendocrinology 42,109 (1986)
7.	Kawakami, M., Uemura, T. and Hayashi, R. Electrophysiological correlates of pulsatile gonadotropin release in rat. Neuroendocrinology 35,63 (1982)
8.	Kalra, S.P. and Kalra, P.S. Neural regulation of luteinizing hormone secretion in the rat. Endocrine Rev 4,311 (1983)
9.	Sirett, N.E., Hyland, B.I., Hubbard, J.I., Lapwood, K.R. and Elgar, H.J. Luteininzing hormone release in the anesthetized cat following electrical stimulation of limbic structures. Neuroendocrinology 42,128 (1986)
10.	Levine, J.E. and Ramirez, V.D. In vivo release of luteinizing hormone-releasing hormone estimated with push-pull cannulae from the mediobasal hypothalami of ovariectomized, steroid-primed rats. Endocrinology 107,1782 (1980)
11.	Levine, J.E., Norman, R.L., Gliessman, P.M., Oyama, T.T., Bansberg, D.R. and Spies, H.G. In vivo gonadotropin-releasing hormone release of serum luteinizing hormone measurements in ovariectomized, estrogen-treated rhesus macaques. Endocrinology 117,711 (1985)

12. Levine, J.E., Pau, K.Y.F., Ramirez, V.D. and Jackson, G.L. Simultaneous measurement of luteinizing hormone-releasing hormone and luteinizing hormone release in unanesthetized, ovariectomized sheep. Endocrinology 111,1449 (1982)

13. Levine, J.E. and Ramirez, V.D. Luteinizing hormone-releasing hormone release during the rat estrous cycle and after ovariectomy, as estimated with push-pull cannulae. Endocrinology 111,1439 (1982)

14. Clarke, I.J. and Cummins, J.T. The temporal relationship between gonadotropin releasing hormone (GnRH) and luteinizing hormone (LH) secretion in ovariectomized ewes. Endocrinology 111,1737 (1982)

15. Gallo, R.V. Neuroendocrine regulation of pulsatile luteinizing hormone release in the rat. Neuroendocrinology 30,122 (1980)

16. Leung, P.C.K., Adrendash, G.W., Whitmayer, D.I., Gorski, R.A. and Sawyer, C.H. Differential effects of central adrenoreceptor agonists on luteinizing hormone release. Neuroendocrinology 34,207 (1982)

17. Weick, R.F. Acute effects of adrenergic receptor blocking drugs and neuroleptic agents on pulsatile discharges of luteinizing hormone in ovariectomized rats. Neuroendocrinology 26,108 (1978)

18. Estes, K.S., Simpkins, J.W. and Kalra, S.P. Resumption with clonidine of pulsatile LH release following acute norepinephrine depletion in ovariectomized rats. Neuroendocrinology 35,56 (1982)

19. Kreig, R.J. and Sawyer, C.H. Effects of intraventricular catecholamines on luteinizing hormone release in ovariectomized steroid-primed rats. Endocrinology 99,411 (1976)

20. Rubinstein, L. and Sawyer, C.H. Role of catecholamines in the release of pituitary ovulating hormone(s) in rat. Endocrinology 86,988 (1970)

21. Kalra, P.S., Kalra, S.P., Krulich, L., Fawcett, C.P. and McCann, S.M. Involvement of norepinephrine in transmission of the stimulatory influence of progesterone on gonadotropin release. Endocrinology 90,1168 (1972)

22. Kalra, S.P. and McCann, S.M. Effects of drugs modifying catecholamine synthesis on plasma LH and ovulation in the rat. Neuroendocrinology 15,79 (1974)

23. Kalra, S.P. Catecholamine involvement in preovulatory LH release: reassessment of the role of epinephrine. Neuroendocrinology 40,139 (1985)

24. Crowley, W.R., Terry, L.C. and Johnson, M.D. Evidence for the involvement of central epinephrine systems in the regulation of luteinizing hormone, prolactin and growth hormone release in female rats. Endocrinology 110,1102 (1982)

25. Crowley, W.R. and Terry, L.C. Effects of an epinephrine synthesis inhibitor, SKF 64139, on the secretion of luteinizing hormone in ovariectomized rats. Brain Res 204,231 (1981)

26. Adler, B.A., Johnson, M.D., Lynch, C.O. and Crowley, W.R. Evidence that norepinephrine and epinephrine systems mediate the stimulatory effects of ovarian hormones on luteinizing hormone and luteinizing hormone-releasing hormone. Endocrinology 113,1431 (1983)

27. Vijayan, E. and McCann, S.M. Re-evaluation of the role of catecholamines in control of gonadotropin and prolactin release. Neuroendocrinology 25,150 (1978)

28. Rasmussen, D.D., Liu, J.H., Wolf, P.L. and Yen, S.S.C. Gonadotropin-releasing hormone neurosecretion in the human hypothalamus: in vitro regulation by dopamine. J Clin Endocrinol Metab 62,479 (1986)

29. Wuttke, W., Hancke, J.L, Hohn, K.G. and Baumergarten, H.G. Effect of intraventricular injection of 5,7-dihydroxytryptamine on serum gonadotropins and prolactin. Ann NY Acad Sci 305,423 (1978)

30. Rasmussen, D.D., Jacobs, W., Kissinger, P.T. and Malven, P.V. Plasma luteinizing hormone in ovariectomized rats following pharmacologic manipulation of endogenous brain serotonin. Brain Res 229,230 (1981)

31. Walker, R.F. Quantitative and temporal aspects of serotonin's facilitatory action on phasic secretion of luteinizing hormone in female rats. Neuroendocrinology 36,468 (1983)

32. Quay, W.B. Differences in circadian rhythms in 5-hydroxytryptamine according to brain region. Am J Physiol 214,1448 (1968)

33. Parvizi, N. and Ellendorf, F. Beta-endorphin alters luteinizing hormone secretion via the amygdala but not the hypothalamus. Nature 286,812 (1980)

34. Lakoski, J.M. and Gebhart, G.F. Morphine administration in the amygdala or periaqueductal central gray depress serum levels of luteinizing hormone. Brain Res 232,231 (1982)

35. Krettek, J.E. and Price, J.L. Amygdaloid projections to subcortical structures within the basal forebrain and brainstem in the rat and cat. J Compar Neurol 178,225 (1978)

36. Ching, M. Morphine suppresses the proestrous surge of GnRH in pituitary portal plasma of rat. Endocrinology 112,2209 (1983)

37. Rotsztejn, W.H., Drouva, S.V., Patlou, E. and Kordon, C. Met-enkephalin inhibits in vitro dopamine-induced LHRH release from mediobasal hypothalamus of male rats. Nature 274,281 (1978)

38. Wilkes, M.M. and Yen, S.S.C. Augmentation by naloxone of efflux of LRF from superfused medial basal hypothalamus. Life Sci 28,2355 (1981)

39. Leadem, C.A., Crowley, W.R., Simpkins, J.W. and Kalra, S.P. Effects of naloxone or catecholamine on LHRH release from the perifused hypothalamus of the steroid-primed rat. Neuroendocrinology 40,497 (1985)

40. May, P.B., Mittler, J.C. and Ertel, N.H. Enkephalins and pituitary hormone release. Modification of responsiveness to LHRH. Hormone Res 10,57 (1979)

41. Cacicedo, L. and Sanchez Franco, F. Direct action of opioid peptides and naloxone on gonadotropin secretion by cultured rat anterior pituitary cells. Life Sci 38,617 (1986)

42. Blank, M.S., Fabbri, A., Catt, K.J. and Dufau, M.L. Inhibition of luteinizing hormone release by morphine and endogenous opiates in cultured pituitary cells. Endocrinology 118,2098 (1986)

43. Matleri, R.L. and Moberg, G.P. The effect of opioid peptides on ovine pituitary gonadotropin secretion in vitro. Peptides 6,957 (1985)

44. Barkan, A., Regiani, S., Duncan, J., Papavasiliou, S. and Marshall, J.C. Opioids modulate pituitary receptors for gonadotropin-releasing hormone. Endocrinology 112,387 (1983)

45. Kalra, S.P. and Simpkins, J.W. Evidence for noradrenergic mediation of opioid effects on luteinizing hormone secretion. Endocrinology 109,776 (1981)

46. Wilkes, M.M. and Yen, S.S.C. Reduction by beta-endorphin of efflux of dopamine and DOPAC from superfused medial basal hypothalamus. Life Sci 27,1387 (1980)

47. Johnson, M.D. and Crowley, W.R. Effects of opiate antagonists on serotonin turnover and on luteinizing hormone and prolactin secretion in estrogen- or morphine-treated rats. Neuroendocrinology 38,322 (1984)

48. Ieiri, T., Chen, H.T. and Meites, J. Naloxone stimulation of luteinizing hormone release in prepubertal female rats: role of serotonergic system. Life Sci 26:1269 (1980)

49. Morrell, J.I., McGinty, J.W. and Pfaff, D.W. A subset of beta-endorphin or dynorphin-containing neurons in the medial basal hypothalamus accumulates estradiol. Neuroendocrinology 41,417 (1985)

50. Forman, L.J., Sonntag, W.E, Hylka, V.W. and Meites, J. Mediation by gonadal steroids of plasma beta-endorphin and LH in castrate female and male rats. Peptides 6,835 (1985)

51. Wehrenberg, W.B., Wardlow, S.L., Frantz, A.G. and Ferin, M. Beta-endorphin in hypophysial portal blood: variations throughout the menstrual cycle. Endocrinology 111,879 (1982)

52. Wardlaw, S.L., Wehrenberg, W.B., Ferin, M., Antunes, J.L. and Frantz, A.G. Effect of sex steroids on beta-endorphin in hypophysial portal blood. J Clin Endocrinol Metab 55,877 (1982)

53. Petraglia, F., Locatelli, V., Penalva, A., Cocchi, D., Genazzani, A.R. and Muller, E.E. Gonadal steroid modulation of naloxone-induced LH secretion in the rat. J Endocrinol 101,33 (1984)

54. Quigley, M.E. and Yen, S.S.C. The role of endogenous opiates on LH secretion during the menstrual cycle. J Clin Endocrinol Metab 51,179 (1980)

55. Blankstein, J., Reyes, F.I., Winter, J.S.D. and Faiman, C. Endorphins and the regulation of the human menstrual cycle. Clin Endocrinol 14,287 (1981)

56. Belchetz, P.E., Plant, T.M., Nakai, Y., Keogh, E.G. and Knobil, E. Hypophysial responses to continuous and intermittent delivery of hypothalamic gonadotropin-releasing hormone. Science 202,631 (1978)

57. Marshall, J.C. and Kelch, R.P. Low dose pulsatile gonadotropin-releasing hormone in anorexia nervosa - a model of human pubertal development. J Clin Endocrinol Metab 51,730 (1979)

58. Wildt, L., Hausler, A., Marshall, G., Hutchison, J.S., Plant, T.M., Belchetz, P.E. and Knobil, E. Frequency and amplitude of gonadotropin-releasing hormone stimulation and gonadotropin secretion in the rhesus monkey. Endocrinology 109,376 (1981)

59. Clarke, I.J., Cummins, J.T., Findlay, J.K., Burman, K.J. and Daughton, B.W. Effects on plasma LH and FSH of varying frequency and amplitude of gonadotropin-releasing hormone pulses in ovariectomized ewes with hypothalamic-pituitary disconnection. Neuroendocrinology 39,214 (1984)

60. Pohl, C.R., Richardson, D.W., Hutchinson, J.S., Germak, J.A. and Knobil, E. Hypophysiotropic signal frequency and the functioning of the pituitary - ovarian system in the rhesus monkey. Endocrinology 112,2076 (1983)

61. Clayton, R.N., Shakespear, R.A., Duncan, J.A. and Marshall, J.C. Radioiodinated nondegradeable gonadotropin-releasing hormone analogues - New probes for the investigation of pituitary GnRH receptors. Endocrinology 60,1369 (1979)

116

62. Frager, M.S., Pieper, D.R., Tonetta, S.A., Duncan, J.A. and Marshall, J.C. Pituitary gonadotropin-releasing hormone (GnRH) receptors - effects of castration, steroid replacement and the role of GnRH in modulating receptors in the rat. J Clin Invest 67,615 (1981)

63. Garcia, A., Schiff, M. and Marshall, J.C. Regulation of pituitary gonadotropin-releasing hormone receptors by pulsatile gonadotropin releasing hormone - modulation by testosterone. J Clin Invest 74:920 (1984)

64. Katt, J.A., Duncan, J.A., Herbon, L., Barkan, A. and Marshall, J.C. The frequency of gonadotropin-releasing hormone stimulation determines the number of pituitary gonadotropin-releasing hormone receptors. Endocrinology 116,2113 (1985)

65. Papavasiliou, S.S., Zmeili, S., Khoury, S., Landefeld, T.D., Chin, W.W. and Marshall, J.C. Gonadotropin-releasing hormone differentially regulates expression of the alpha and luteinizing hormone beta subunit genes in male rats. Proc Natl Acad Sci USA 83,4026 (1986)

66. Higuchi, T. and Kawakami, M. Changes in the characteristics of pulsatile luteinizing hormone secretion during the estrous cycle and after ovariectomy and estradiol treatment in female rats. J Endocrinol 94,77 (1982)

67. Fox, S.R. and Smith, M.S. Changes in the pulsatile pattern of luteinizing hormone secretion during the rat estrous cycle. Endocrinology 116,1485 (1985)

68. Gallo, R.V. and Bona-Gallo, A. Lack of ovarian steroid negative feedback on pulsatile luteinizing hormone release between estrus and diestrous day 1 in the rat estrous cycle. Endocrinology 116,1525 (1985)

69. Leipheimer, R.E., Bona-Gallo, A. and Gallo, R.V. Ovarian steroid regulation of pulsatile luteinizing hormone release during the interval between the morning of Diestrus 2 and Proestrus in the rat. Neuroendocrinology 41,252 (1985)

70. Leipheimer, R.E., Bona-Gallo, A. and Gallo, R.V. The influence of progesterone and estradiol on the acute changes in pulsatile luteinizing hormone release induced by ovariectomy on Diestrus day 1 in the rat. Endocrinology 114,1605 (1984)

71. Yen, S.S, Tsai, C.C., Naftolin, F., Vandenberg, G. and Ajabor, L. Pulsatile patterns of gonadotropin release in subjects with and without ovarian function. J Clin Endocrinol Metabol 34,671 (1972)

72. Santen, R.J. and Bardin, C.W. Episodic luteinizing hormone secretion in man. J Clin Invest 52,2617 (1973)

73. Backstrom, C.T., McNeilly, A.S., Leask, R.M. and Baird, D.T. Pulsatile secretion of LH, FSH, prolactin, estradiol and progesterone during the human menstrual cycle. Clin Endocrinol (Oxf) 17,29 (1982)

74. Reame, N., Sauder, S.E., Kelch, R.P. and Marshall, J.C. Pulsatile gonadotropin secretion during the human menstrual cycle - evidence for altered frequency of gonadotropin-releasing hormone secretion. J Clin Endocrinol Metab 59,:328 (1984)

75. Soules, M.R., Steiner, R.A., Clifton, D.K., Cohen, N.L., Aksel, S. and Bremner, W.J. Progesterone modulation of pulsatile luteinizing secretion in normal women. J Clin Endocrinol Metab 58,378 (1984)

76. Filicori, M., Butler, J.P. and Crowley, W.F. Neuroendocrine regulation of the corpus luteum in the human - evidence for pulsatile progesterone secretion. J Clin Invest 73,1638 (1984)

77. Filicori, M., Santoro, N., Merriam, G.R. and Crowley, W.F. Characterization of the physiological pattern of gonadotropin secretion throughout the human menstrual cycle. J Clin Endocrinol Metab 62,1136 (1986)

78. Djahanbakhch, O., Warner, P., McNeilly, A.S. and Baird, D.T. Pulsatile release of LH and estradiol during the periovulatory period in normal women. Clin Endocrinol (Oxf) 20,579 (1984)

79. Veldhuis, J.D., Beitins, I.Z., Johnson, M.L., Serabian, M.A. and Dufau, M.L. Biologically active luteinizing hormone is secreted in episodic pulsations that vary in relation to the stage of the menstrual cycle. J Clin Endocrinol Metab 58,1050 (1984)

80. Veldhuis, J.D., Evans, W.S., Johnson, M.L., Willis, M.R. and Rogol, A.D. Physiological properties of the luteinizing hormone pulse signal: impact of intensive and extended venous sampling paradigms on its characterization in healthy men and women. J Clin Endocrinol Metab 62,881 (1986)

81. Steele, P.A., McDonnell, L.F. and Judd, S.J. Activity of gonadotropin-releasing hormone neurons during the preovulatory gonadotropin surge. Fertil Steril 45,179 (1986)

82. Norman, R.L., Linstrom, S.A., Bansberg, D., Ellinwood, W.E., Gliessman, P. and Spies, H.G. Pulsatile secretion of luteinizing hormone during the menstrual cycle of rhesus macaques. Endocrinology 115,261 (1984)

83. VanVugt, D.A., Lam, N.Y. and Ferin, M. Reduced frequency of pulsatile luteinizing hormone secretion in the luteal phase of the rhesus monkey. Involvement of endogenous opioids. Endocrinology 115,1095 (1984)

84. Ching, M. Correlative surges of LHRH, LH and FSH in pituitary staln plasma and systemic plasma of rat during proesturs. Neuroendocrinology 34,279 (1985)

85. Tsou, R.C., Dailey, R.A., McLanahon, C.S., Parent, A.D., Tindall, G.T. and Neill, J.D. Luteinizing hormone-releasing hormone (LHRH) in pituitary stalk plasma during the preovulatory gonadotropin surge of rabbits. Endocrinology 101,534 (1977)

86. Neill, J.D., Patton, J.M., Dailey, R.A., Tsou, R.C. and Tindall, G.T. Luteinizing hormone-releasing hormone (LHRH) in pituitary stalk blood of rhesus monkeys: relationship to levels of LH release. Endocrinology 101,430 (1977)

87. Kesner, J.S., Convey, E.M. and Anderson, C.R. Evidence that estradiol induces the preovulatory LH surge in cattle by increasing pituitary sensitivity to LHRH and then increasing LHRH release. Endocrinology 108,1386 (1981)

88. Turgeon, J.L. and Waring, D.W. Acute progesterone and 17-beta-estradiol modulation of luteinizing hormone secretion by pituitaries of cycling rats superfused in vitro. Endocrinology 108:413 (1981)

89. Kim, K. and Ramirez, V.D. In vitro luteinizing hormone-releasing hormone release from superfused rat hypothalami: site of action of progesterone and effect of estrogen priming. Endocrinology 116,252 (1985)

90. Kim, K. and Ramirez, V.D. In vitro LHRH release from hypothalamus as a function of the rat estrous cycle: effects of progesterone. Neuroendocrinology 42,392 (1986)

91. Gallo, R.V. Pulsatile LH release during the ovulatory LH surge on proestrus in the rat. Biol Reprod 24,100 (1981)

92. Clarke, I.J. and Cummins, J.T. Increased gonadotropin-releasing hormone pulse frequency associated with estrogen-induced luteinizing hormone surges in ovariectomized ewes. Endocrinology 116,2376 (1985)

93. Savoy-Moore, R.T., Schwartz, N.B., Duncan, J.A. and Marshall, J.C. Pituitary gonadotropin-releasing hormone receptors during the rat estrous cycle. Science 209,942 (1980)

94. Zmeili, S., Papavasiliou, S.S., Marshall, K.C. and Landefeld, T.D. Alpha and LH beta mRNAs are differentially regulated during the proestrus LH surge of the rat estrous cycle. Proc 68th Meeting Endocrine Soc Abstract 35,39 (1986)

95. Goodman, R.L. and Karsch, F.J. Pulsatile secretion of luteinizing hormone: differential suppression by ovarian steroids. Endocrinology 107,1286 (1980)

96. Savoy-Moore, R.T., Schwartz, N.B., Duncan, J.A. and Marshall, J.C. Pituitary gonadotropin-releasing hormone receptors on proestrus: effects of pentobarbital blockade of ovulation in the rat. Endocrinology 109,1360 (1981)

97. Barkan, A.L., Regiani, R.A., Duncan, J.A. and Marshall, J.C. Pituitary gonadotropin-releasing hormone receptors during gonadotropin surges in ovariectomized estradiol-treated rats. 112,1042 (1983)

98. Barkan, A.L., Duncan, J.A., Schiff, M., Papavasiliou, S., Garcia-Rodriguez, A., Kelch, R.P. and Marshall, J.C. Opioid and neurotransmitter regulation of pituitary gonadotropin-releasing hormone (GnRH) receptors in the ovariectomized estradiol-treated rat: role of altered GnRH secretion. Endocrinology 116,1003 (1984)

99. Pang, C.N., Zimmermann, E. and Sawyer, C.H. Morphine inhibition of the preovulatory surge of plasma luteininzing hormone and follicle stimulating hormone in the rat. Endocrinology 101,1726 (1977)

100. Koves, K., Marton, J., Molnar, J. and Halasz, B. (D-Met$_2$, Pro$_5$) enkephalinamide-induced blockade of ovulation and its reversal by naloxone in the rat. Neuroendocrinology 32,82 (1981)

101. Sylvester, P.W., Chen, H.T. and Meites, J. Effects of morphine and naloxone on phasic release of luteinizing hormone and follicle-stimulating hormone. Proc Soc Exp Biol and Med. 164,207 (1980)

102. Barden, N., Merand, Y., Rouleau, D., Garon, M. and Dupont, A. Changes in the beta-endorphin content of discrete hypothalamic nuclei during the estrous cycle in the rat. Brain Res 204,441 (1981)

103. Knuth, U.A., Sikand, G.S., Casanueva, F.F., Havlicek, V. and Friesen, H.G. Changes in beta-endorphin content in discrete areas of the hypothalamus throughout proestrus and diestrus of the rat. Life Sci 33,1443 (1983)

104. Hulse, G.K., Coleman, G.J., Copolov, D.L. and Clements, J.A. Relationship between endogenous opioids and the oestrous cycle in the rat. J Endocrinol 100,271 (1984)

105. Piva, F., Maggi, R., Limonta, P., Motta, M. and Martini, L. Effect of naloxone on luteinizing hormone, follicle-stimulating hormone and prolactin secretion in the different phases of the estrous cycle. Endocrinology 117,766 (1985)

106. Gabriel, S.M., Berglund, L.A. and Simpkins, J.W. A decline in endogenous opioid influence during the steroid-induced hypersecretion of luteinizing hormone in the rat. Endocrinology 118,558 (1986)

119

107. Allen, L.G. and Kalra, S.P. Evidence that a decrease in opioid tone may evoke preovulatory luteinizing hormone release in the rat. Endocrinology 118,2375 (1986)

108. Leadem, C.A. and Kalra, S.P. Effects of endogenous opioid peptides and opiates on luteinizing hormone and prolactin secretion in ovariectomized rats. Neuroendocrinology 41,342 (1985)

109. Loumaye, E. and Catt, C.J. Agonist-induced regulation of pituitary receptors for gonadotropin-releasing hormone. Dissociation of receptor recruitment from hormone release in cultured gonadotrophs. J Biol Chem 258,12002 (1983)

110. Knobil, E., Plant, T.M., Wildt, L., Belchetz, P.E. and Marshall, G. Control of the rhesus monkey menstrual cycle: permissive role of hypothalamic gonadotropin-releasing hormone. Science 207,1371 (1980)

111. Hanker, J.P., Nieschlag, E. and Schneider, H.P.G. Frequency-varied versus unvaried pulsatile LHRH substitution in hypothalamic amenorrhea. Europ J Obstet Gynecol Reprod Biol 17,103 (1984)

112. Marshall, J.C., Case, G.D., Valk, T.W., Corley, K.P., Sauder, S.E. and Kelch, R.P. Selective inhibition of follicle-stimulating hormone secretion by estradiol. Mechanism for modulation of gonadotropin responses to low dose pulses of gonadotropin-releasing hormone. J Clin Invest 73,248 (1983)

SECTION 3

EXTRA-HYPOTHALAMIC
LHRH-LIKE MATERIALS

8
LHRH Binding Sites in Human Tissues

T. A. BRAMLEY

Department of Obstetrics and Gynaecology, University of Edinburgh, Centre for
Reproductive Biology, 37 Chalmers Street, Edinburgh, Scotland

INTRODUCTION

Paracrine regulation, (secretion of a factor or hormone by one
cell type which acts locally to modify the function of a
different cell type) requires the satisfaction of the
following criteria:
1. The factor must be produced locally, in close proximity to
    its target tissue.
2. Target tissue must possess specific receptors for the
    hormone.
3. Termination of hormone action demands rapid local hormone
    inactivation.
4. The factor must achieve a biological response.
5. Changes in hormone production/action and/or changes in
    receptor concentrations must correlate with changes in
    physiological status.
    There is evidence that LHRH-like peptides fully satisfy
these conditions in the rat ovary [1-3] and testis [4,5], and
LHRH-like peptides (along with a range of other factors) are
now well established as intragonadal paracrine hormones [6,7].
However, the reported absence of specific LHRH receptors in
the ovary of the mouse, cow, pig, sheep, monkey and human,
coupled with the frequent failure to demonstrate effects of
LHRH and its analogues on steroid secretion (particularly in
the primate and human ovary) suggested that LHRH-like peptides
were of little importance in species other than the rat (see
[5] for refs).
    Recently, specific LHRH-binding sites have been described
in a number of extrapituitary human tissues, and other
evidence has been presented which meets many of the five
criteria outlined, inferring a possible paracrine role for
LHRH-like factors in a number of human tissues, particularly
placenta, gonads and breast cancer cells. These findings are
reviewed below.

1. LOCAL PRODUCTION OF AN LHRH-LIKE FACTOR

Placenta   Immunohistochemical   localization   of LHRH
demonstrated activity in the cytotrophoblast, villous stroma
[8,9] and on the outer surface of the syncytiotrophoblast
[8,10].   Since hCG is produced and released from the
syncytiotrophoblast, the hypothesis was advanced that LHRH
produced by the cytotrophoblast acted on receptors on the
syncytiotrophoblast membrane to stimulate hCG secretion, in an
analogous fashion to the stimulation of pituitary LH release
by hypothalamic LHRH.   Certainly, material which is
immunologically, chromatographically and chemically identical
to the hypothalamic decapeptide can be extracted from human
placentae [11-14] and placental tissue can synthesize LHRH de
novo [14-16].   However, placental extracts contained much
greater amounts of higher molecular weight LHRH-like
molecules, which were considered to be more important than the
decapeptide [14,17 - see chapter 10].
        Isolation of the cDNA for LHRH precursor from human
placenta showed a C-terminal extension of 56 aminoacid [18]:
this LHRH-associated peptide displayed gonadotrophin-releasing
activity and suppressed prolactin release by pituitary tissue
in vitro [19].   The actions of this peptide on placental
function, and its relationship, if any, to the high-MW
LHRH-like molecules synthesised by the placenta are awaited
with great interest.
        Gonads   LHRH-like peptides were isolated from ovarian
extracts of rat [20,21] and pig [22,23] and rat testis (see
Chapter 9   ).   Moreover, LHRH bioactivity may be present in
peritoneal fluid of women [24].   These peptides differed
immunologically from, and were larger than LHRH. However,
efforts to demonstrate similar factors in human follicular
fluid and ovarian extracts have been inconsistent, and
confounded by occasional activity in control tissues.
        Breast   LHRH-like factors have been detected in human
breast milk [25] and localized immunohistochemically in some
ductal breast carcinomas [26]. Moreover, there is presumptive
evidence that certain breast tumour cell lines may produce an
LHRH-like substance (K. Eidne, personal communication).

2.   PERIPHERAL LHRH RECEPTORS

        Placenta   Radioiodinated LHRH agonists bind specifically
to human placental membranes [27-29].   Binding was
displaceable by LHRH and its analogues, but not by a wide
range of other peptides and hormones. Placental binding could
not discriminate between LHRH and its agonist analogues, in
marked contrast to rat pituitary and gonadal receptors, where
the affinity for the LHRH agonist buserelin was 10-500 fold
higher than for LHRH (Table 1). However, since the endogenous
ligand acting on placental LHRH receptors appears to differ
from LHRH (see above), receptor affinity for this factor may
be much higher than for the hypothalamic decapeptide.
Notwithstanding their apparently low affinity, sufficiently

TABLE 1. COMPARISON OF HUMAN AND RAT LHRH BINDING SITES

| Species | Tissue | AFFINITY (k_d/K_a^{-1};M) | | MW (kDa) | Reference |
		LHRH	LHRH Agonist		
HUMAN	Placenta	$5\text{-}10\times10^{-7}$	$3\text{-}5\times10^{-7}$		27
		$2\text{-}4\times10^{-7}$	$2\text{-}3\times10^{-7}$		28
		9×10^{-7}	$2\text{-}5\times10^{-7}$	53.7	29
		$3\text{-}10\times10^{-7}$	$1\text{-}2\times10^{-7}$		33,36
	Corpus Luteum	10×10^{-7}	$2\text{-}5\times10^{-7}$		30
		20×10^{-7}	$3\text{-}8\times10^{-7}$		31
		$10\text{-}20\times10^{-7}$	$3\text{-}4\times10^{-7}$		36
	Breast Cancer	0.2×10^{-7}		64.0	37
	MCF-7 Cells		10^{-5}		38
	Testis		10^{-4}		36
	Pituitary	4.8×10^{-9}	0.3×10^{-9}	64.0	39
RAT	Pituitary	4.7×10^{-9}	0.3×10^{-9}	60.0	39
		1.4×10^{-9}	0.2×10^{-9}		40
		20.0×10^{-9}	0.2×10^{-9}	60.0	41
		48.0×10^{-9}	0.1×10^{-9}		33
	Ovary	5×10^{-9}	0.5×10^{-9}		40
		10×10^{-9}	$0.2\text{-}0.8\times10^{-9}$	60.0+54.0	42
		$30\text{-}100\times10^{-9}$	$0.1\text{-}0.3\times10^{-9}$		33,36
	Testis	3×10^{-9}	0.3×10^{-9}		40
		100×10^{-9}	0.5×10^{-9}		43
		50×10^{-9}	0.3×10^{-9}		33

high concentrations may be achieved locally within the placenta to activate these receptors.

Ovary The presence of specific binding sites for LHRH and its analogues in the human corpus luteum is now well established [30,31]. Previous reports which failed to measure binding can be attributed largely to a number of crucial differences in receptor assay methodology (for detailed discussion, see [32]). Human luteal (and placental) binding sites and rat pituitary and gonadal receptors required both N- and C- terminal regions of the molecule for binding [33]. However, whereas amino acid substitutions at position 6 enhanced, and at position 8 decreased, potency for rat gonadal and pituitary receptors, these modifications had only minor effects on binding to human luteal sites, suggesting differences in the receptor and/or endogenous LHRH-like factors related to the mid-chain region of the molecule [33].

Because of their low affinity, luteal LHRH binding sites were thought by some to represent binding to peptide-degrading enzymes. However, this is unlikely, for the following reasons:

(a) Human luteal (and placental) binding sites have an impressive specificity for LHRH and its analogues [32]: a range of proteins, protein hormones, peptides, peptide hormones, steroids and general reagents failed to displace LHRH agonist binding to these tissues [33].

(b) Substances with N-terminal pGlu or C-terminal glycinamide residues failed to compete for binding, indicating that ligand was not binding to the active sites of pyroglutamyl amino-peptidase, carboxy-peptidase C or post-proline cleaving enzymes [33].

125

(c) Both (^{125}I) labelled LHRH and agonist were bound specifically by human luteal tissue, and displaced by similar concentrations of unlabelled LHRH or agonist. Thus, binding was unrelated to amino-acid substitutions conferring resistance to peptide degradation [31].

(d) Inhibitors of the different classes of tissue proteases failed to block binding to luteal (and placental) tissue [33], though these inhibitors block the various LHRH-degrading activities of the hypothalamus and pituitary [34].

(e) Sub-cellular fractionation of human luteal tissue showed that specific LHRH binding activity was enriched in cell-surface (and endoplasmic reticulum) membrane fractions, but not in lysosomes [35].

Other tissues Specific binding of LHRH agonist has been demonstrated in human Leydig cells [36], ductal breast carcinomas [37] and MCF-7 breast tumour cells [38]. Binding to all human extra-pituitary tissues tested was of low affinity (Table 1), suggesting a possible species difference between rat and human LHRH receptors. However, human pituitary LHRH receptors had affinities for LHRH and LHRH agonist [39] which were similar to those of the rat pituitary (Table 1).

3. RAPID LOCAL INACTIVATION OF LHRH

Placenta Partially-purified placental membranes rapidly decrease LHRH agonist immunoactivity in a time- and temperature-dependent manner, (Fig 1). Heating of placental membranes (95°C; 10min) prevented LHRH agonist inactivation. Furthermore, the ability of [^{125}I]-labelled LHRH and buserelin to rebind to fresh placental membranes was also decreased rapidly following preincubation with placental membranes (Fig. 2A). [^{125}I]-LHRH was degraded more rapidly than the superagonist, buserelin. Loss of intact LHRH and agonist was accompanied by the appearance of degradation products on TLC-autoradiography.

Ovary Preincubation of [^{125}I]-labelled buserelin or LHRH with human CL tissue also showed a rapid time- and temperature-dependent inactivation (Fig 2B). As with placenta, LHRH was inactivated more rapidly than buserelin.

4. BIOLOGICAL EFFECTS ON PERIPHERAL TISSUE

Placenta Most studies showed no response of a range of placental functions to LHRH or its agonist analogues in vivo [10,44-46], though several studies were conducted at early gestational ages, at which time placental tissue may be unresponsive to exogenous LHRH (see below). However, stimulatory responses have been reported in normal pregnancy

126

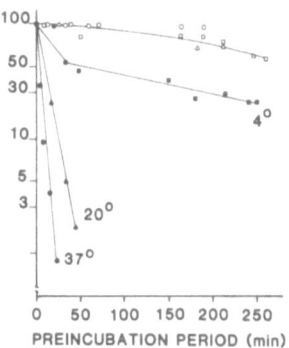

IMMUNOACTIVE BUSERELIN REMAINING
(% CONTROL)

FIGURE 1   LHRH agonist inactivation by placental membranes.
100µg Buserelin was preincubated with partially purified
placental membranes at 4°C, 20°C or 37°C for the periods
shown.   After acidification ten-fold dilution and boiling (10
min) to stop the reaction, LHRH agonist remaining was
immunoassayed using a specific anti-buserelin antibody (R103).
Note that heat pretreatment of placental membranes (open
symbols) prevented degradation at all temperatures (A. Currie
& H.M. Fraser; unpublished data with permission).

[47] and in certain patients with trophoblastic tumours.   LHRH
can also suppress placental progesterone secretion in women at
mid-gestation   [48]   and   acutely   stimulate   chorionic
gonadotrophin (CG)   secretion in the pregnant macaque [48].
Furthermore,   administration of an LHRH antagonist to pregnant
baboons suppressed both CG and steroid secretion [49].
     In vitro, LHRH stimulated the release of hCG by static
cultures of placental villous explants [50] and by perfused
trophoblast cells [51].   hCG secretion was stimulated via
specific   LHRH receptors,   as LHRH antagonists suppressed
hormone   release   [52].   However,   human   chorionic
somatomammotrophin (HCS), which like hCG, is synthesized and
secreted by syncytiotrophoblast, showed little or no response
to LHRH [50,53]. LHRH effects on placental steroid secretion
were   inconsistent, with stimulation [54], no effect [55] or
inhibition [56] reported.   Steroids and lipoproteins could
modulate the hCG response to LHRH in vitro [55,56].
     Ovary   Conflicting effects of LHRH and its agonist
analogues in vivo on luteal function in humans and primates

127

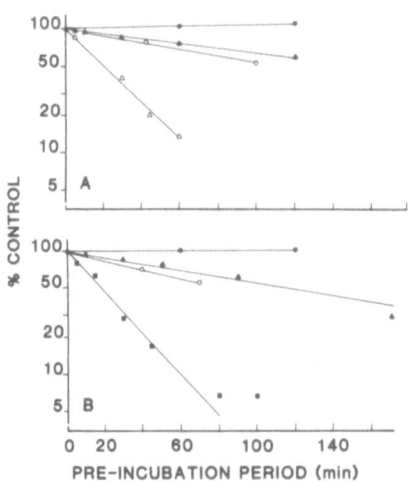

LHRH—RECEPTOR BINDING

PRE-INCUBATION PERIOD (min)

FIGURE 2 LHRH and LHRH agonist inactivation. 100pg [^{125}I]-labelled LHRH (open symbols) or buserelin (solid symbols) was preincubated with partially-purified membranes of placenta (A) or corpus luteum (B) for the periods shown at 0°C (●,○); 20°C (▲,△) or 37°C (■). After rapid filtration (Whatman GF/C filters), ability of tracers to rebind to fresh placental (A) or CL (B) membranes was measured.

have been reported. In women, administration of LHRH or LHRH agonist in the early luteal phase (days 1-5 after ovulation) suppressed progesterone secretion somewhat, but with little or no change in luteal phase length [57-60], whereas treatment in the mid-luteal phase (days 4-9) resulted in major suppression of progesterone and significant shortening of the luteal phase [57,59]. However, similar doses administered to early pregnant women [61,62] or to women treated with exogenous hCG [61,63] were not luteolytic, indicating that high hCG levels could overide LHRH effects.

In baboons, agonist treatment in the early luteal phase had little or no effect on progesterone secretion [64,65]. However, LHRH agonist given at the time of CL rescue by CG markedly reduced progesterone levels and terminated pregnancy [65, 66]. Furthermore, these agonist effects disappeared after the luteo-placental shift had occurred [66], showing that (unlike the human) LHRH agonists blocked the effects of CG on the corpus luteum.

Studies in the Rhesus monkey have shown a narrow luteolytic window for agonist administration in the early luteal phase (day 3, 5 but not 7): however, inhibitory effects were lost following hypophysectomy, implying that luteolysis required the presence of the pituitary gland in this species

[67]. As in the baboon, LHRH agonist implants blocked the stimulation of the Rhesus monkey CL by CG [68]. Finally, LHRH agonists reduced luteal progesterone levels but not luteal phase length in M. Fascicularis [69].

In vitro, nanomolar concentrations of [D-Trp^6,Nα MeLeu^7,Pro^{9}NHEt]LHRH markedly reduced progestin secretion by human granulosa cells, but only after 96h in culture [70]. Inhibition was reversed by an LHRH antagonist, which had no effect alone. Moreover, testosterone secretion by cells derived from a virilizing ovarian tumour was inhibited by low concentrations (10^{-8} to 10^{-6}M) of [D-Ser(tBu)^6, AzaGly^{10}]LHRH [71]. In contrast, steroidogenesis by cultured human granulosa cells was unaffected by 10^{-10} to 10^{-7}M [D-Trp^6,Pro^{9}NHEt]LHRH ethylamide [72]. Moreover, collagenase-dispersed human luteal cells [73-75] failed to respond to LHRH and LHRH agonist analogues whereas, under the same conditions, rat luteal cells showed a clear response [75].

Breast tumour cells. The growth of the breast is clearly under endocrine control, and roughly one-third of breast tumours require hormones for their continued growth. LHRH agonists suppress ovarian steroid secretion and can be used therapeutically in premenopausal women to bring about "chemical gonadectomy" and tumour regression [76]. However, agonist treatment of post-menopausal women with breast cancer also produced objective responses in some women [77], suggesting direct anti-tumour effects.

The growth of MCF-7 human breast cancer cells in culture was inhibited by low concentrations of LHRH agonist (buserelin, 10^{-10} to 10^{-9}M) or LHRH (10^{-7} to 10^{-5}M) [38]. Levels of agonist in excess of 10^{-7}M resulted in a progressive decrease in cell numbers. These effects were reversed by removal of agonist from the culture medium, or by inclusion of a specific LHRH antagonist [38]. These findings have been essentially confirmed by others, though higher agonist levels were required for an effect to be shown [78]. In contrast, T-47D and MDA-MB-231 cells were unaffected by LHRH agonist concentrations which inhibited MCF-7 cell growth [38].

5. CHANGES IN LEVELS OF LHRH-LIKE PEPTIDES AND/OR RECEPTORS WITH PHYSIOLOGICAL STATUS

Placenta Immunoreactive LHRH content varied, rising to mid-gestation and falling at term [11]. Furthermore, "endogenous releasable" hCG (hormone release during the first 24h of culture of placental explants; ref [48,51]) and in vitro responsiveness to LHRH (measured on day 4 of culture when responsiveness had returned to maximum) varied markedly depending on the stage of gestation (Fig 3). "Releasable" hCG increased to a maximum at 9-10 weeks gestation, (reflecting peak maternal hCG levels in vivo), but responsiveness to exogenous LHRH was minimal (Fig 3). However, after 10 weeks

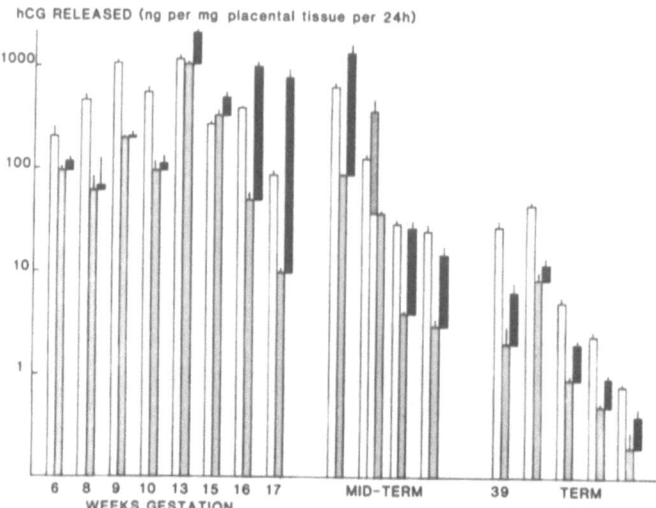

hCG RELEASED (ng per mg placental tissue per 24h)

WEEKS GESTATION

FIGURE 3   Changes in hCG secretion and LHRH response of
placental explants in vitro with gestational age. (□),
release of hCG during 0-24h in culture ("endogenous
releasable" hCG);
(▨), release of hCG during 96-120h in culture (baseline
production);
(■), stimulation of hCG secretion above baseline by 10μg/ml
LHRH (96-120h in culture);
(▧), LHRH- antagonist sensitive hCG secretion (96-120h).
Note logarithmic scale. [Data compiled from refs: 17, 48, 49,
52].

gestation, hCG levels in vivo fell and "endogenous" hCG
content declined progressively.   At the same time,
responsiveness to LHRH in vitro rose progressively, so that by
13-17 weeks gestation LHRH-stimulated hCG secretion exceeded
initial "endogenous" levels. In term placenta, endogenous hCG
content fell to very low levels, although stimulation by LHRH
was still demonstrable (Fig 3).
      Ovary   Our recent studies have shown a high correlation
between LHRH agonist binding levels in human CL tissue
throughout the luteal phase, and a number of important indices
of luteal function.   Agonist binding levels were highly
correlated with unoccupied (p<0.001;n=49) and occupied
(p<0.001; n=49) LH receptors, and with LDL (p<0.01;n=25) and
PRL receptors (p<0.05; n=21), but not with FSH binding (p=0.4;
n=25).   There was also a significant correlation with luteal
content of progesterone (p <0.05; n=27), but not oestradiol,
androstenedione, testosterone or DHT. LHRH binding was low
in stromal, thecal and granulosa cell homogenates, but rose

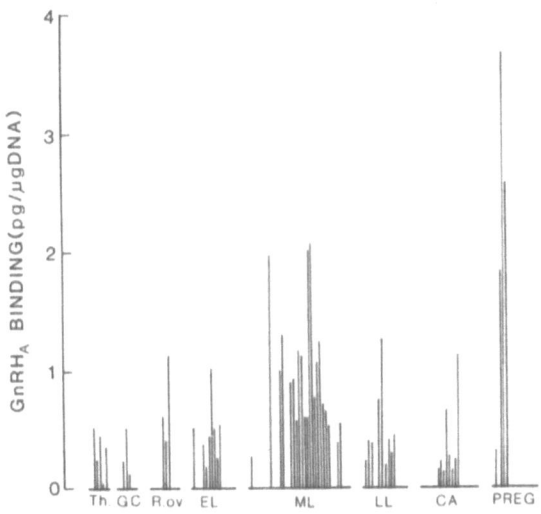

FIGURE 4 [125]-LHRH agonist binding to human ovarian tissue. Th, Theca; GC, Granulosa cell; R.OV, recent ovulation; EL, early-luteal; ML, mid-luteal; LL, late-luteal; CA, corpus albicans; PREG, CL of pregnancy.

with luteinization, reaching highest levels in the mid-luteal phase, then fell with luteolysis (Fig 4). Binding was also high in three of four CL of pregnancy tested.

These findings suggest that human luteal LHRH binding may be of physiological relevance.

CONCLUSIONS

Evidence for the involvement of LHRH-like factors in human placental regulation is now quite convincing (see also Chapter 10) and studies in breast cancers suggest important regulatory effects (inhibition of growth in vivo and in vitro - criterion 4; specific binding of LHRH; criterion 2) though these are demonstrable in some cell lines only, and there is a major discrepancy between the 50% inhibitory dose for cell growth $(10^{-10}M)$ and for LHRH agonist binding (5×10^{-5}M;38).

In the human corpus luteum, specific binding sites are present (criterion 2), though of low affinity, binding site concentrations correlate with other important indices of luteal function (criterion 5), and there is rapid hormone inactivation (criterion 3). However, local production of LHRH-like factors by the human ovary (criterion 1) has not yet been demonstrated, and there are major inconsistencies in LHRH effects on ovarian function (criterion 4). However, a number

131

of different factors can confound the demonstration of LHRH effects.

FACTORS CONFOUNDING DEMONSTRATION OF LHRH EFFECTS IN HUMAN EXTRA-PITUITARY TISSUES

Tissue response may vary:
(a) Between species (e.g. LHRH antagonised CL stimulation by CG in baboons [65,66] and macaque [68], but not woman [61-63]):
(b) Between individuals (e.g. marked differences in luteal LHRH binding in mid-luteal CL [Fig. 4]):
(c) With stage of development (e.g. the markedly different responses of placental explants to LHRH throughout gestation [Fig. 3]; the narrow luteolytic window for LHRH in the human [57-60] and primate [67] in vivo; the inhibition of steroidogenesis by LHRH agonist following culture of granulosa cells with LH for 96h [70], suggesting a requirement for luteinization):
(d) With the action of other hormones (e.g. possible effects of insulin and oestradiol on LHRH responsiveness of MCF-7 cells [38]; LHRH effects on rat gonads are influenced by gonadotrophin environment [1-5]):
(c) With receptor occupancy by endogenous ligand (e.g. lack of LHRH effect in early gestation [Fig. 3]).
Methodology may be inappropriate:
(a) Use of isolated cells (e.g. collagenase - dispersion of human CL [73-75] destroys luteal LHRH binding sites [31]; cell-cell interactions may be important for LHRH effects [6,7]):
(b) Inappropriate incubation conditions. Incubation for 2-4h [72-75] may be too short to demonstrate LHRH effects as longer periods (>4h) are usually required for clear-cut effects on rat gonadal steroid secretion [1-4]. Conversely, long-term cultures may also be inappropriate, since added LHRH and buserelin are degraded very rapidly by CL and placenta at 37°C (T_{50}, 5-20 min; Figs. 1,2). If the continuous presence of moderate hormone concentrations is necessary, changes will be seen only with analogues which are resistant to degradation. Interestingly, the only study to demonstrate LHRH effects on human ovarian steroidogenesis in vitro [70] used an analogue with an [Nα MeLeu]' substitution, which reportedly confers greater resistance to degradation. LHRH degradation may also contribute to differences between LHRH-responsive breast tumour cell lines (e.g. MCF-7; low degradation?) and unresponsive (high degradation?) T-47D and MDA-MD-231 cells:
(c) Inappropriate end-point. LHRH effects may be quite specific (e.g. LHRH stimulates release of hCG, but not hCS from syncytiotrophoblast cells [50,53]). Thus, LHRH changes in steroid secretion may be small/transient,

whereas larger changes may occur with other end-points [see 1-3].

Use of inappropriate hormone. LHRH analogues with superagonist activity in the rat pituitary and gonad may not necessarily have enhanced activity in the human [32,33]. Moreover, the endogenous ligands for human extra-pituitary receptors are not yet known (though GAP and endogenous LHRH-like factors are prime candidates). LHRH and its analogues may be induced to fit the receptor site, but with much lower affinity than the endogenous ligand. Thus, chorionic LHRH-like factor is much more potent than LHRH in stimulating CG release from placental explants [48]. The resolution of these discrepancies should clarify whether LHRH-like factors are, indeed, involved as paracrine regulatory factors in the human ovary.

The corpus luteum is essential for the establishment and maintainance of early pregnancy in the human [79]. Better understanding of the factors regulating its formation, maintenance and regression may enable the design of agents which specifically interrupt its normal function. A great many analogues of LHRH have been synthesized, and much is now known of their actions, dynamics and pharmacology. If it is confirmed that LHRH-like peptides do, indeed, play a role in the regulation of the human ovary and placenta, the synthesis of LHRH analogues which can interact selectively with these receptors may produce specific, effective and safe agents for the control of human fertility.

REFERENCES

1. Hsueh, A.J.W. & Jones, P.B.C. Extrapituitary actions of gonadotropin-releasing hormone. Endocr. Rev., 2, 437 (1981).
2. Labrie, F., Seguin, C., Lefebvre, F-A., Massicotte, J., Pelletier, G., Borgus, J-P., Kelly, P-A., Reeves, J.J. & Belanger, A. Intraovarian actions of GnRH. In "Intraovarian Control Mechanisms", C.P. Channing & S.J. Segal (Eds). Plenum Press, New York, 1982, p 211.
3. Knecht, M., Ranta, T., Naor, Z. & Catt, K.J. Direct effects of GnRH on the ovary. In "Factors Regulating Ovarian Function", G.S. Greenwald & P.F. Terranova, (Eds). Raven Press. New York, p 225, 1983.
4. Sharpe, R.M. Intratesticular factors controlling testicular function. Biol. Reprod., 30, 29 (1984).
5. Sharpe, R.M. Intragonadal hormones. Biblio. Reprod., 44, C1 (1984).
6. Hsueh, A.J.W. Paracrine mechanisms involved in granulosa cell differentiation. Clinics in Endocrinol. & Metab., 15, 117 (1986).
7. Sharpe, R.M. Paracrine control of the testis. Clinics in Endocrinol. Metab., 15, 185 (1986).
8. Khodr, G.S. & Siler-Khodr, T. Localization of luteinizing hormone-releasing factor in the human placenta. Fertil.

Steril., 29, 523. (1978).

9. Miyake, A., Sakumoto, T., Aono, T., Kawamura, Y., Maeda, T. & Kurachi, K. Changes in luteinizing hormone-releasing hormone in human placenta throughout pregnancy. Obstet. & Gynecol., 60, 444 (1982).

10. Seppala, M., Wahlstrom, T., Lehtovirta, P., Lee, J.N. & Leppalouto, J. Immunohistochemical demonstration of luteinizing hormone-releasing factor-like material in human syncytiotrophoblast and trophoblastic tumours. Clinical Endocr., 12, 441. (1980).

11. Siler-Khodr, T.M. & Khodr, G.S. Content of luteinizing hormone - releasing factor in the human placenta. Am. J. Obstet. Gynecol., 130, 216 (1978).

12. Lee, J.N., Seppala, M. & Chard, T. Characterization of placental luteinizing hormone - releasing factor-like material. Acta Endocr., 96, 394 (1981).

13. Osathanondh, R. & Elkind-Hirsch, K.E. Presence of immunoreactive luteinizing hormone - releasing hormone factor in hydatidiform mole as compared with normal trophoblastic tissue. Placenta (suppl 3), 257 (1981).

14. Tan, L. & Rousseau, P. The chemical identity of the immunoreactive LHRH-like peptide biosynthesized in the human placenta. Biochem. Biophys. Res. Comm., 109, 1061. (1982).

15. Gibbons, J.M., Mitnick, M. & Chieffo, V. In vitro biosynthesis of TSH- and LH-releasing factors by the human placenta. Am. J. Obstet. Gynecol., 121, 127 (1975).

16. Khodr, G.S. & Siler-Khodr, T. Placental luteinizing hormone-releasing factor and its synthesis. Science, 207, 315. (1980).

17. Siler-Khodr, T.M. Hypothalamic-like peptides of the placenta. Sem. Reprod. Endocr., 1, 321 (1983).

18. Seeburg, P.H. & Adelman, J.R. Characterization of cDNA for precursor of human luteinizing hormone releasing hormone. Nature (London), 311, 666 (1984).

19. Nikolics, K., Mason, A.J., Szonyi, E., Ramachandran, J. & Seeburg, P.H. A prolactin inhibiting factor within the precursor for human gonadotropin - releasing hormone. Nature (London), 316, 511 (1985).

20. Ying, S.Y, Ling, N., Bohlen, P. & Guillemin, R. Gonadocrinins: peptides in ovarian follicular fluid stimulating the secretion of pituitary gonadotropins. Endocrinology, 108, 1206 (1981).

21. Aten, R.F., Williams, T., Behrman, H.R. & Wolin, D.L. Ovarian gonadotropin - releasing hormone-like protein(s): demonstration and characterisation. Endocrinology, 118, 961 (1986)

22. Williams, A.T. & Ulmanis, M.A. "Macromolecular-bound antigonadotrophin in porcine follicular fluid with LHRH immunoactivity. Biol. Reprod., 28 (Suppl 1) 161, Ab 258 (1983).

23. Minaguchi, H., Mori, J. & Vemura, T. Partial isolation of gonadotrophin releasing hormone (GnRH) like substance from the porcine ovary. In 7th Int. Congress Endocrinol., Abstr

No. 1560. Exerpta Medica. Amsterdam (1984).

24. Demoulin, A. Donnez, J., Volders-Keuliens, L., Thomas, K., Lambotte, R. & Franchimont, P. Activite de type gonadocrinine dans le liquide peritoneal pendant le cycle menstruel chez la femme normale. C. R. Soc. Biol. (Paris), 175, 377 (1981).

25. Amarant, T., Fridkin, M. & Koch, Y. Luteinizing hormone - releasing hormone and thyrotropin - releasing hormone in human and bovine milk. Eur. J. Biochem., 127, 647 (1982).

26. Seppala, M. & Wahlstrom, T. Identification of luteinizing hormone - releasing factor and alpha subunit of glycoprotein hormones in ductal carcinoma of the mammary gland. Int. J. Cancer., 26, 267 (1980).

27. Currie, A.J., Fraser, H.M. & Sharpe, R.M. Human placental receptors for luteinizing hormone releasing hormone. Biochem. Biophys. Res. Comm., 99, 332 (1981).

28. Belisle, S., Guevin, J-F., Bellabarba, D & Lehoux, J-G. Luteinizing hormone-releasing hormone binds to enriched human placental membranes and stimulates in vitro the synthesis of bioactive human chorionic gonadotropin. J. Clin. Endocrinol. Metab., 59, 119 (1984).

29. Iwashita, M., Evans, M.I. & Catt, K.J. Characterization of a gonadotropin - releasing hormone receptor site in term placenta and chorionic villi. J. Clin. Endocrinol. Metab., 52, 127 (1986).

30. Popkin, R., Bramley, T.A., Currie, A., Shaw, R.W. Baird, D.T. & Fraser, H.M. Specific binding of luteinizing hormone releasing hormone to human luteal tissue. Biochem. Biophys. Res. Comm., 114, 750 (1983).

31. Bramley, T.A., Menzies, G.S. & Baird, D.T. Specific binding of gonadotrophin - releasing hormone and an agonist to human corpus luteum homogenates: characterization, properties and luteal phase levels. J. Clin. Endocrinol. Metab., 61, 834 (1985).

32 Fraser, H.M., Bramley, T.A., Miller, W.R. & Sharpe, R.M. Extrapituitary actions of LHRH analogues in tissues of the human female and investigation of the existence and function of LHRH-like peptides. In "Gonadotropin Down-Regulation in Gynaecological Practice" D.R. Chadha, & R. Rolland. (eds). Alan R. Liss Inc., New York (in press).

33. Bramley, T.A., Menzies, G.S. & Baird, D.T. Specificity of gonadotrophin - releasing hormone binding sites of the human corpus luteum: comparison with receptors of rat pituitary gland. J. Endocrinol., 108, 323 (1986).

34. Griffiths, E.C. & McDermott, J.R. Enzymic inactivation of hypothalamic regulatory hormones. Molec. Cell. Endocr. 33, 1 (1983).

35. Bramley, T.A. & Menzies, G.S. Subcellular fractionation of the human corpus luteum: distribution of GnRH agonist binding sites. Molec. Cell. Endocr., 45, 27 (1986).

36. Popkin, R.M., Bramley, T.A., Currie, A., Sharpe, R.M. & Fraser, H.M. Binding sites for LH-RH in the human - does LH-RH exert extrapituitary actions in man?: In "LHRH and its Analogues. Fertility & Antifertility Aspects". (M.

Schmidt-Gollwitzer, & R. Schley eds) Walter de Gruyter, Berlin. p 61 (1985).

37. Eidne, K.A., Flanagan, C.A. & Millar, R.P. Gonadotropin - releasing hormone binding sites in human breast carcinoma. Science, 229, 989 (1985).

38. Miller, W.R., Scott, W.N., Morris, R., Fraser, H.M. & Sharpe, R.M. Growth of human breast cancer cells inhibited by a luteinizing hormone - releasing hormone agonist. Nature (London), 313, 231 (1985).

39. Wormald, P.J., Eidne, K.A. & Millar, R.P. Gonadotropin - releasing hormone receptors in human pituitary: ligand structural requirements, molecular size and cationic effects. J. Clin. Endocrinol. Metab., 61, 1190 (1985).

40. Clayton, R.N. & Catt, K.J. Gonadotropin - releasing hormone receptors: characterization, physiological regulation and relationship to reproductive function. Endocr. Rev., 2, 186 (1981).

41. Hazum, E. Photoaffinity labeling of luteinizing hormone releasing hormone receptor of rat pituitary membrane preparations. Endocrinology, 109, 1281 (1981).

42. Hazum, E. & Nimrod, A. Photoaffinity-labeling and fluorescence-distribution studies of gonadotropin - releasing hormone receptors in ovarian granulosa cells. Proc. Nat. Acad. Sci. (USA), 79, 1747 (1982).

43. Sharpe, R.M. & Fraser, H.M. Leydig cell receptors for luteinizing hormone - releasing hormone and their modulation by administration or deprivation of the releasing hormone. Biochem. Biophys. Res. Communs., 95, 256 (1980).

44. Tolis, G., Comaru-Schally, A.M., Mehta, A.E. & Schally, A.V. Failure to interrupt established pregnancy in humans by D-tryptophan-6-luteinizing hormone - releasing hormone. Fertil. Steril., 36, 241 (1981).

45. Tsai, C.C., Mathur, R.S., Baker, E.R. & Nair, R.M.G. Lack of hormonal changes in response to 1mg luteinizing hormone - releasing hormone injection during early human gestation. Neuroendocrinol. Lett., 44, 51 (1982).

46. Rubinstein, L.M., Parlow, A.F., Derzko, C. & Hershman, J. Pituitary gonadotropin response to LHRH in human pregnancy. Obstet. Gynecol., 52, 172 (1978).

47. Egyed, J. & Gati, I. Elevated serum HCG level after intravenous LH-RH administration in human pregnancies. Endocrinologica Experimentalis, 19, 11 (1983).

48. Siler-Khodr, T.M. & Khodr, G.S. Production and activity of placental releasing hormones. In "Fetal Endocrinology". M.J. Novy & J.A. Resko (Eds) Acad. Press. London (1981) p 183.

49. Siler-Khodr, T.M., Kuehl, T.J. & Vickery, B.H. Effects of a gonadotropin - releasing hormone antagonist on hormonal levels in the pregnant baboon and on fetal outcome. Fertil. Steril., 41, 448 (1984).

50. Siler-Khodr, T.M., Khodr, G.S., Valenzuela, G. & Rhode, J. Gonadotropin - releasing hormone effects on placental hormones during gestation: I Alpha-human chorionic

gonadotropin, human chorionic gonadotropin and human chorionic somatomammotropin. Biol. Reprod., <u>34</u>, 245 (1986).

51. Butzow, R. Luteinizing hormone - releasing factor increases release of human chorionic gonadotrophin in isolated cell columns of normal and malignant trophoblasts. Int. J. Cancer, <u>29</u>, 9 (1982).

52. Siler-Khodr, T.M., Khodr, G.S., Vickery, B.H. & Nestor, J.J.Jr. Inhibition of hCG, αhCG and progesterone release from human placental tissue in vitro by a GnRH antagonist. Life Science., <u>32</u>, 2741 (1983).

53. Golander, A., Barrett, J.R., Tyrey, L., Fletcher, W.H. and Handwerger, S. Differential synthesis of human placental lactogen and human chorionic gonadotropin in vitro. Endocrinology, <u>102</u>, 597 (1978).

54. Siler-Khodr, T.M., Khodr, G.S., Valenzuela, G. & Rhode, J. Gonadotropin-releasing hormone effects on placental hormones during gestation: II. Progesterone, Estrone, Estradiol & Estriol. Biol. Reprod., <u>34</u>, 255 (1986).

55. Haning R.V.Jr., Choi, L., Kiggens, A.J., Kuzma, D.L. & Summerville, J.W. Effects of dibutyryl adenosine 3', 5'-Monophosphate, luteinizing hormone-releasing hormone, and aromatase inhibitor on simultaneous outputs of progesterone, 17β-estradiol, and human chorionic gonadotropin by term placental explants. J. Clin. Endocrinol. Metab., <u>55</u>, 213 (1982).

56. Wilson, E.A., Jawad, M.J. & Dickson, L.R. Suppression of human chorionic gonadotropin by progestational steroids. Am. J. Obstet. Gynecol., <u>138</u>, 708 (1980).

57. Lemay, A., Faure, N. & Labrie, F. Induction of luteolysis by postovulatory intranasal administration of [D-Ser (TBU)^6-des-Gly-NH$_2$ ^{10}]-LHRH ethylamide (Buserelin): A postcoital contraceptive approach. In "LHRH peptides as Female and Male Contraceptives". G. I. Zatuchni, J.D. Shelton & J. J. Sciarra (Eds.), Harper & Row, Philadelphia, (1982) p 184.

58. Koyama, T., Ohkura, T., Kumasaka, T. & Saito, M. Effect of postovulatory treatment with a luteinizing hormone - releasing hormone analog on the plasma level of progesterone in women. Fertil. Steril., <u>30</u>, 549 (1978).

59. Sheehan, K.L., Casper, R.F. & Yen, S.S.C. Induction of luteolysis by luteinizing hormone - releasing factor (LRF) agonist: sensitivity, reproducibility and reversibility. Fertil. Steril., <u>37</u>, 209 (1982).

60. Lemay, A., Faure, N. & Labrie, F. Sensitivity of pituitary and corpus luteum responses to single intranasal administration of (D-Ser[TBU]^6-des-Gly-NH$_2$ ^{10})luteinizing hormone - releasing hormone ethylamide (Buserelin) in normal women. Fertil. Steril., <u>37</u>, 193 (1982).

61. Casper, R.F., Sheehan, K.L. & Yen, S.S.C. Chorionic gonadotropin prevents LRF-agonist-induced luteolysis in the human. Contraception, <u>21</u>, 471 (1980).

62. Skarin, G., Nillius, S.J. & Wide, L. Failure to induce early abortion by huge doses of a superactive LRH agonist

in women. Contraception. 26, 457 (1982).

63. Bergquist, C., Nillius, S.J. & Wide, L. Luteolysis induced by a luteinizing hormone - releasing hormone agonist is prevented by human chorionic gonadotropin. Contraception., 22, 341 (1980).

64. Hagino, N., Nakamoto, O., Kunz, Y., Arimura, A., Coy, D.H. & Schally, A.V. Effect of D-Trp 6-LH-RH on the pituitary - gonadal axis during the luteal phase in the baboon. Acta. Endocr. (Kbh), 91, 217 (1979).

65. Das, C. & Talwar, G.P. Pregnancy-terminating action of a luteinizing hormone - releasing hormone agonist D-Ser(Bu^t)^6 des Gly^{10} Pro EA in baboons. Fertil. Steril., 39, 218 (1983).

66. Vickery, B.H., McRae, G.I. & Stevens, V.C. Suppression of luteal and placental function in pregnant baboons with agonist analogs of luteinizing hormone - releasing hormones. Fertil. Steril., 36, 664 (1981).

67. Balmaceda, J.P. & Asch, R.H. The effects of LHRH agonistic analogs during the luteal phase of the Rhesus monkey. In "LHRH Peptides as Female and Male Contraceptives" G.I. Zatuchni, J.D. Shelton & J.J. Sciarra (Eds.), Harper and Row, Philadelphia, p 85 (1984).

68. Vickery, B.H. & McRae, G.I. Antagonism by an LHRH agonist of the steroidogenic effects of exogenous human chorionic gonadotrophin in the rhesus monkey. Life Sciences, 27, 1409 (1980).

69. Raynaud, J-P., Mary, I., Moguilewsky, M., Mouren, M. & Labrie, F. Inhibition of progesterone secretion during the luteal phase by two luteinizing hormone - releasing hormone agonists in Macaca Fascicularis. Fertil. Steril., 34, 593 (1980).

70. Tureck, R.W., Mastroianni, L.Jr., Blasco, L. & Strauss, J.F. III. Inhibition of human granulosa cell progesterone secretion by a gonadotropin - releasing hormone agonist. J. Clin. Endocrinol. Metab., 54, 1078 (1982).

71. Lamberts, S.W.J., Timmers, J.M., Oosterom, R., Verleun, T., Rommerts, F.G. & de Jong, F.H. Testosterone secretion by cultured arrhenoblastoma cells: suppression by a luteinizing hormone - releasing hormone agonist. J. Clin. Endocrinol. Metab., 54, 450 (1982).

72. Casper, R.F., Erickson, G.F., Rebar, R.W. & Yen, S.S.C. The effect of luteinizing hormone - releasing factor and its agonist on cultured human granulosa cells. Fertil. Steril., 37, 406 (1982).

73. Tan, G.J.S. & Biggs, J.S.G. Absence of effect of LH-RH on progesterone production by human luteal cells in vitro. J. Reprod. Fert., 67, 411 (1983).

74. Casper, R.F., Erickson, G.F. & Yen, S.S.C. Studies on the effect of gonadotropin-releasing hormone and its agonist on human luteal steroidogenesis in vitro. Fertil. Steril., 42, 39 (1984).

75. Richardson, M.C., Hirji, M.R., Thompson, A.D. & Masson, G.M. Effects of a long - acting analogue of LH-releasing hormone on human and rat corpora lutea. J. Endocrinol.,

101, 163 (1984).
76. Schally, A.V., Comaru-Schally, A.M. & Redding, T.W. Antitumour effects of analogues of hypothalamic hormones in endocrine-dependent cancers. Proc. Soc. Exptl. Biol. Med., 175, 259 (1984).
77. Harvey, H.A., Lipton, A. & Max, D.T. LHRH analogues for human mammary carcinoma: In "LHRH and Its Analogues: Contraceptive and Clinical Applications", B.H. Vickery, J.J. Nestor, Jr. & E.S.E. Hafez (Eds.), MTP Press, Lancaster, (1984) p 329.
78. Blankenstein, M.A., Henkelman, M.S. & Klijn, J.G.M. Direct inhibitory effect of a luteinizing hormone - releasing hormone agonist on MCF-7 human breast cancer cells. Eur. J. Cancer Clin. Oncol., 21, 1493 (1985).
79. Csapo, A.I., Pulkkinen, M.O., Ruttner, B., Sauvage, J.P. & Wiest, W.G. The significance of the human corpus luteum in pregnancy maintenance. Am. J. Obstet. Gynecol., 112: 1061 (1972).

9
LHRH and "LHRH-Like" Factors in the Male Reproductive Tract

M.P. HEDGER*, D.M. ROBERTSON and D.M. de KRETSER

Department of Anatomy, Monash University, Melbourne, Victoria 3168, Australia. *Gamete Biology Section, Laboratory of Reproductive and Developmental Toxicology, National Institute of Environmental Health Sciences, Research Triangle Park, NC 27709, USA

INTRODUCTION

A testicular site of action for LHRH was first indicated by observations that LHRH agonists bound to high-affinity receptors in the interstitial tissue of the adult rat testis[1-5] and inhibited Leydig cell function in hypophysectomized rats *in vivo*[6-8]. Although there have been several reports since of proteins or peptides in testicular tissue and seminal plasma that have "LHRH-like" properties[9-24], the biochemical characteristics of most of these molecules, their relationships to the mammalian hypothalamic LHRH decapeptide and to one another, and their physiological significance remain poorly understood.

DIRECT ACTIONS OF LHRH AND LHRH AGONISTS ON THE MALE REPRODUCTIVE TRACT

Numerous *in vivo* and *in vitro* studies in the immature and adult rat have clearly established the ability of LHRH and LHRH agonists to modulate testicular function by a direct mechanism in this species [see review 25]. During short-term (less than 24h) treatment in the hypophysectomized rat and in testicular cells or Leydig cell cultures, these peptides stimulate basal and hCG-stimulated steroidogenesis, while longer periods of exposure lead to an inhibition of steroidogenesis in the same experimental models[8,26-32]. The direct actions on Leydig cell steroidogenesis are blocked by concomitant treatment with LHRH antagonists, confirming that they are receptor mediated[31,33] and high-affinity receptors for LHRH agonists are located on the rat Leydig cell[34,35]. These receptors are almost identical in their specificity for different analogues of LHRH to the anterior pituitary LHRH-receptor[2,3,34,36] and appear to have the same subunit structure[34,36].

In addition to direct effects on Leydig cell function, there is evidence to suggest that LHRH and LHRH agonists influence the function of other testicular cells directly. In the hypophysectomized rat, LHRH agonists induce an increase in testicular blood flow[37] and when injected directly into one testis of the intact rat, LHRH agonists cause a unilateral decrease in interstitial fluid volume[33], suggesting an effect on the permeability characteristics of the vascular endothelial cells. Although it is possible that this action is mediated by the Leydig cell, there is autoradiographical evidence for LHRH receptors on intertubular cells other than Leydig cells in dispersed testicular cells fractionated on Percoll density gradients[35].

LHRH and its agonists also have direct actions on accessory reproductive organs in the male rat. They have been shown to inhibit androgen stimulated growth of the ventral prostate and seminal vesicles of castrated and hypophysectomized castrate rats[38] and RNA and protein synthesis and ornithine decarboxylase activity in the ventral prostate of castrate rats[39]. The significance of these observations is unclear as LHRH receptors have not been detected in these tissues of the normal rat, although there are binding sites for LHRH agonists in rat prostatic tumour cell lines[40].

It should be noted that most studies on the direct actions of LHRH agonists at the testicular level have been performed in the rat. Evidence for direct actions of these peptides or the presence of LHRH-receptors in the testes of other species, including the human, is limited [see review 41].

THE TESTIS: A SOURCE OF "LHRH-LIKE" PEPTIDES?

The levels of hypothalamic LHRH in peripheral blood are not sufficient to activate the testicular receptor, due to the large dilution of portal blood in the peripheral circulation and rapid degradation of LHRH by peripheral tissues[42,43]. This indicates that either (a) the testicular LHRH receptors and attendant biochemical machinery have no physiological role; (b) there are peripheral sources for LHRH; or (c) the receptors mediate the action of a molecule other than LHRH. Early impetus for the last two proposals was provided by reports that LHRH was produced by another reproductive tissue, the human placenta[44], and that the ovarian follicular fluid of several species contained an "LHRH-like" peptide that stimulated the release of LH and FSH from the pituitary *in vitro*, but which was chromatographically and immunologically distinct from LHRH[45].

In the testis, Sharpe and colleagues demonstrated that interstitial fluid from hCG-treated rats, and acetic acid or acidified ethanol extracts of stump-tailed Macaque testes, collagenase-dispersed rat seminiferous tubules or spent medium from immature rat Sertoli cell cultures displaced a radiolabelled LHRH agonist (LHRH-A = [D-Ser(tBu)^6,Pro^9-NHEt]LHRH) from the testicular LHRH receptor[9,11,12]. The acidified ethanol extracts of the rat seminiferous tubules and Macaque testes and interstitial fluid also stimulated the release of LH from rat hemi-pituitaries *in vitro*. However, the rat tissue extracts did not cross-react in an LHRH radioimmunoassay employing antiserum R42, which requires both terminals of the LHRH decapeptide for activity[46], indicating the absence of significant amounts of LHRH from the extracts. Consequently, it was suggested that the extracts contained an

"LHRH-like" peptide which bound to the LHRH-receptor and stimulated the release of LH at the pituitary level, but which was immunologically, and therefore chemically, distinct from LHRH. Surprisingly, the same extracts did cross-react in a radioimmunoassay that was specific for LHRH-A but which did not recognize LHRH[47]. Stimulation of both LH and FSH by organic solvent extracts of the spent media from immature rat Sertoli cells in culture has been confirmed by others[14].

PEPTIDASES IN TESTICULAR EXTRACTS

In this laboratory, initial studies were directed towards isolating the testicular factor(s) responsible for these "LHRH-like" activities[20].

The LHRH-A antiserum was generously provided by Drs Richard Sharpe and Hamish Fraser. It was confirmed that both high-speed supernatant and acetic acid extracts of adult rat testes suppressed [^{125}I]-LHRH-A binding to the anterior pituitary and testicular LHRH-receptors and LHRH-A antiserum, but following further extraction in acidified ethanol, there was a 98-99% loss of these activities. The apparent immuno- and receptor-activities were located exclusively in the seminiferous tubule compartment of the rat testis, were heat sensitive and appeared to be 40-fold larger than LHRH following gel filtration. The extracts did not stimulate LH or FSH release in an *in vitro* LHRH bioassay employing anterior pituitary cells in monolayer culture, but were actually found to antagonize the ability of LHRH or LHRH-A to stimulate gonadotrophin release.

Co-incubation of unlabelled or [^{125}I]-labelled LHRH and LHRH-A with the testicular supernatants or acetic acid extracts resulted in rapid degradation of the peptides, as assessed by radioimmunoassay and reversed-phase (RP)-HPLC (Fig. 1), establishing the presence of substantial peptidase activity in the extracts. It was concluded that this peptidase activity was responsible for both the displacement of ^{125}I-LHRH-A in the radioreceptor and radioimmunoassays and the antagonism of LHRH and LHRA-A activity *in vitro*.

The peptidase which degrades both LHRH and LHRH-A in testicular extracts has been partially characterized[48]. It has an apparent molecular weight (MW) of 43,000 following gel filtration, is principally produced by the Sertoli cell and is present in interstitial fluid (Fig. 2).

As the possibility of peptidase contamination had not been excluded in earlier studies, the displacement of radiolabelled LHRH-A from either antiserum or receptor cannot be considered as sufficient evidence for the presence of "LHRH-like" activity in testicular tissue[9,11,12]. The observation of such high levels of protease in our extracts also raised the possibility that many peptides, including LHRH, in these preparations had been modified or destroyed during extraction, fractionation or assay. When the testicular extracts were boiled to inactivate the peptidase, concentrated, and de-salted on octadecylsilyl (ODS)-silica

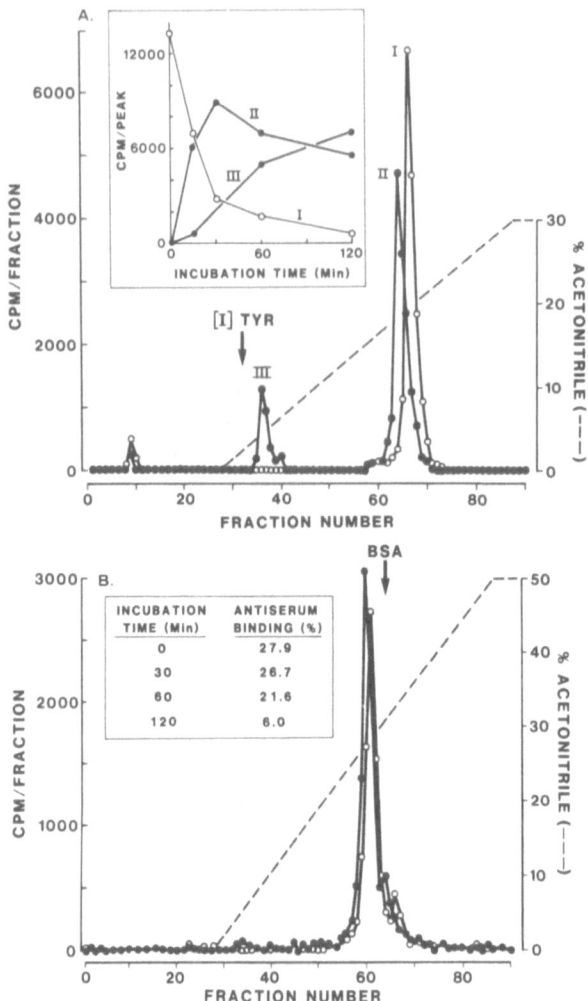

FIGURE 1 Reversed-phase HPLC radioactivity profiles of (A) [^{125}I]-
LHRH and (B) [^{125}I]-LHRH-A before (o–o) and after (o–o)
incubation with rat testicular supernatant at 25°C, pH
7.4 A: [^{125}I]-LHRH incubated with supernatant for 40
min. B: [^{125}I]-LHRH-A incubated with supernatant for 120
min. Inset A: radioactivity in peaks I to III during
degradation of [^{125}I]-LHRH. Elution positions of iodo-
tyrosine ([I]-Tyr) and bovine serum albumin (BSA) are
indicated. Reproduced from Hedger MP et al., Mol.
Cell. Endocrinol., 46, 59 (1986) by permission.

cartridges, we were unable to detect LHRH-receptor binding activity
or gonadotrophin-releasing activity, although, using a very similar
procedure, Sharpe and colleagues were able to detect greatly
reduced levels of both activities in their testicular extracts[15).

144

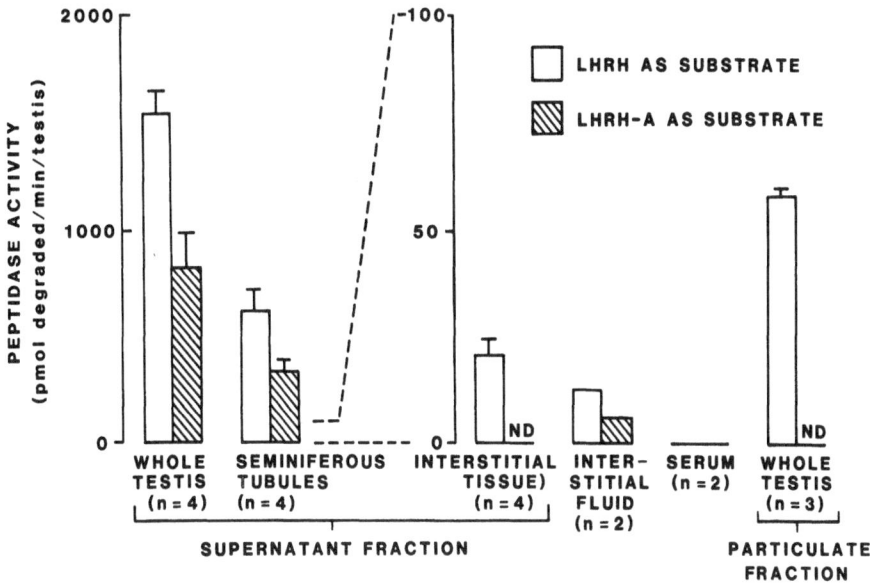

FIGURE 2 Compartmentalization of testicular peptidases using LHRH
(□) and LHRH-A (▨) as substrate at 25°C, pH 7.4.
Values are mean ± SEM, n = number of preparations
assayed.   ND: not detectable (< 3.0) pmol
degraded/min/testis).

LARGER MOLECULAR WEIGHT LHRH-IMMUNOREACTIVE FACTORS

On the assumption that a testicular "LHRH-like" factor might
possess immunological similarities with LHRH, some groups have
employed LHRH antisera to extract and identify molecules of
interest in testicular extracts.   Studies have established the
presence of multiple LHRH-immunoreactive species in immunoaffinity-
purified rat testicular extracts, ranging in size from >100,000 to
1000 Da following gel filtration under non-reducing, non-
dissociating conditions[10,13].   In both studies, the affinity
purified molecules was found to cross-react with LHRH antisera
directed against the C-terminal sequence of LHRH (-Leu[7]-Arg[8]-
Pro[9]Gly[10]-NH$_2$), but to a much lesser or negligible degree with
antiserum R42.   In another series of studies, Arimura and
Turkelson[17] reported that the major LHRH-immunoreactive species
in acid extracts of rat testes eluted just after the void volume on
a Sephadex G-50 gel filtration column (exclusion limit 30,000 Da),
but dissociated into a lower weight form eluting just prior to the
salt peak following boiling with 8M guanidine hydrochloride and 5%
dithiothreitol.   It was suggested that the large MW form was due to
either aggregation of the smaller MW factor or binding to a larger
MW protein.   This small MW factor was found to be distinct from
LHRH following further purification by RP-HPLC and the significant
cross-reactivity of this partially purified factor with several

LHRH antisera of differing specificities suggested that the testicular molecule differed only slightly from LHRH, but chromatographically and immunologically distinct from LHRH, was also reported by Dutlow and Millar[10].

As was reported by Sharpe et al.[11], detectable levels of a molecule with properties identical to LHRH itself were not demonstrated in any of these extracts, although Bhasin and colleagues treated their extracts with charcoal to remove steroids which would also have removed any endogenous free LHRH or smaller MW LHRH-immunoreactive peptide, if present[13]. This latter group has also provided indirect evidence that at least some of the LHRH-immunoreactive factors are synthesized in the testis. Incubation of rat testis slices with $[3_H]$-tyrosine resulted in the incorporation of radioactivity into three immunoprecipitable peaks by gel filtration, the two larger ones corresponding to the large MW (>15,000 Da) and 6000 Da molecules also found in testicular extracts, and one unidentified peak eluting somewhat later[18], possibly the small MW LHRH-immunoreactive species[10,17].

Bhasin and colleagues indicated that at least two of the LHRH-immunoreactive species, with apparent molecular weights of >15,000 and 6000 Da following gel filtration, displaced LHRH agonists from the LHRH-receptor[13]. It was confirmed that this activity was not due to peptidase contamination. Treatment of the unfractionated affinity-purified extract with a peptidase led to a loss of receptor assay activity, indicating the proteinaceous nature of these factors[18]. The unfractionated extract also inhibited oLH-stimulated testosterone production by mixed testicular cell monolayers during incubation for 48h, and this activity was prevented by pre-treatment of the cultures for 24h with an LHRH antagonist, indicating that the effect was LHRH-receptor mediated[19]. Unfortunately, the testicular factor(s) mediating this bio-activity was not identified. It was also reported that the small MW LHRH-immunoreactive factor weakly stimulated LH and FSH release from pituitary fragments and weakly antagonized the action of added LHRH[17].

FURTHER STUDIES IN THIS LABORATORY

As none of these groups had excluded the presence of testicular peptidase activity during extraction and fractionation, the possibility that proteins and peptides in their extracts may have been destroyed or modified had to be considered. In this laboratory, a preparative method, involving extraction in strong acid in the presence of a high ionic strength, absorption onto ODS-silica, extraction in acidified ethanol/chloroform and ether-extraction, was designed. This method provided an optimized recovery of LHRH, eliminated peptidase activity and produced a substantial reduction in protein, salt and steroid loads, which might interfere in the assays[20,21]. Recoveries were monitored by addition of $[^{125}I]$-LHRH or unlabelled LHRH to tissue prior to extraction, and the integrity of the added peptide at the end of extraction was confirmed by RP-HPLC. LHRH-immunoreactive species in the resulting highly purified testicular extracts were investigated with antisera directed against the LHRH C-terminal (T2

146

and Caraty antisera) and antisera which required both ends of the LHRH decapeptide for activity (R42 and Rice No. 5 antisera). The antisera were generously provided by Drs Ron Swerdloff, Iain Clarke and Greg Rice. Biological activity in the testicular extracts was assessed using the *in vitro* LHRH bioassay.

As has been reported by others[10,13], LHRH-immunoreactivity in extracts prepared by this method was detected with antisera directed against the LHRH C-terminal sequence (Table 1), including the T2 antiserum used by Bhasin and colleagues[13].

TABLE 1 Levels of immunoreactivity in a highly purified testicular extract as assessed by LHRH and LHRH-A radioimmunoassays.

Radioimmunoassay	Activity	
	pg/mg extract	pg/testis
LHRH antiserum (T2)	126	138
LHRH antiserum (Caraty)	91*	100
LHRH antiserum (R42)	<15	<16
LHRH antiserum (Rice No. 5)	< 3.3	< 3.6
LHRH-A antiserum (R102)**	480	520

* Preparation gave non-parallel dose-response curves when compared with the standard.

** Values are pg LHRH-A.

Immunoreactivity was not detectable in the extracts using antisera which recognize the native molecule only indicating that the levels of LHRH in the extracts were considerably less than the levels of LHRH-immunoreactivity indicated by the antisera directed against the C-terminal sequence. The profiles of activity following fractionation on a Sephadex G-15 column (exclusion limit 1500 Da) indicated multiple overlapping peaks of activity eluting in the void volume and just after, but earlier than exogenous LHRH fractionated under the same conditions (Fig. 3).

The highly purified extracts in our hands still cross-reacted in the LHRH-A radioimmunoassay as originally reported by Sharpe et al.[11]. The significance of this is unclear, as the antiserum apparently requires the presence of the synthetic residue, Proline-ethylamide, for recognition [47].

Both the unfractionated extracts and void volume gel-filtration fractions stimulated the release of LH and FSH in anterior pituitary cell cultures (Fig.3). However, TSH and prolactin were also released by these fractions and co-incubation with a potent LHRH antagonist did not block release of any of these hormones, indicating non-specific stimulation of anterior pituitary hormone release by a factor (or factors) in the testis extract which was excluded from the Sephadex G-15 column. There was no detectable gonadotrophin-releasing activity in the remainder of the gel filtration profile corresponding either to later eluting peaks of LHRH-immunoreactivity or the elution position of exogenous

LHRH. These observations also demonstrate that the stimulation of

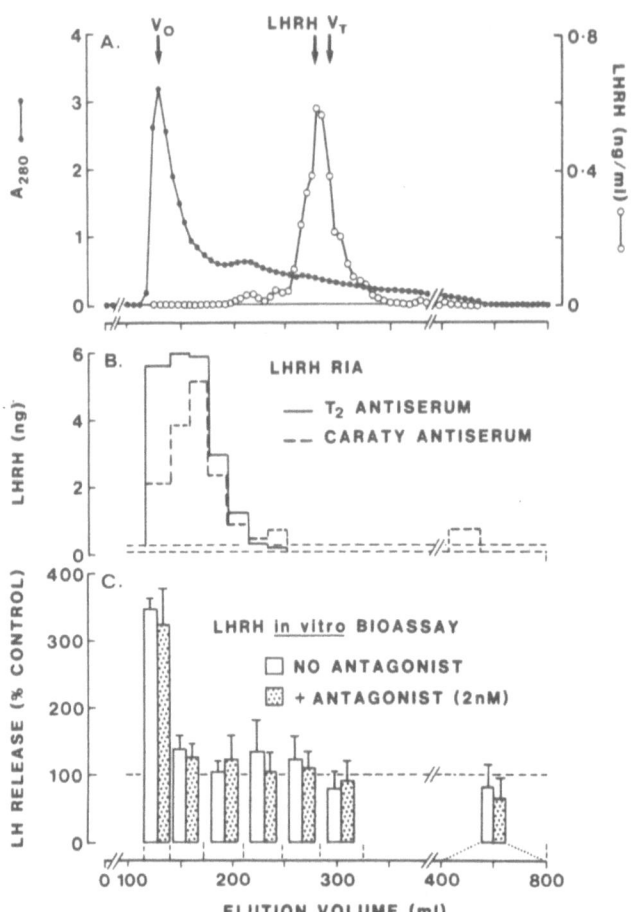

FIGURE 3 Profiles of LHRH-immunoreactivity and *in vitro* LHRH
bioactivity following gel filtration fractionation of
highly purified testicular extract on a Sephadex G-15
column with 0.1M acetic acid as elution buffer at 4°C.
SA: immunoreactivity in testicular extract containing
added LHRH; B: immunoreactivity in pooled gel filtration
fractions using the T2 and Caraty antisera;   C:
stimulation of LH release by pooled gel filtration
fractions in the presence and absence of the potent LHRH
antagonist, [AC-Ala^1,pCl-D-Phe^2,D-Trp^{3,6}]LHRH, Bars are
mean ± SD; n = 3 determinations;   -----, limit of assay
sensitivity; Vo, void volume; LHRH, elution position of
unextracted LHRH fractionated in the presence of
testicular extract; Vt, total volume.

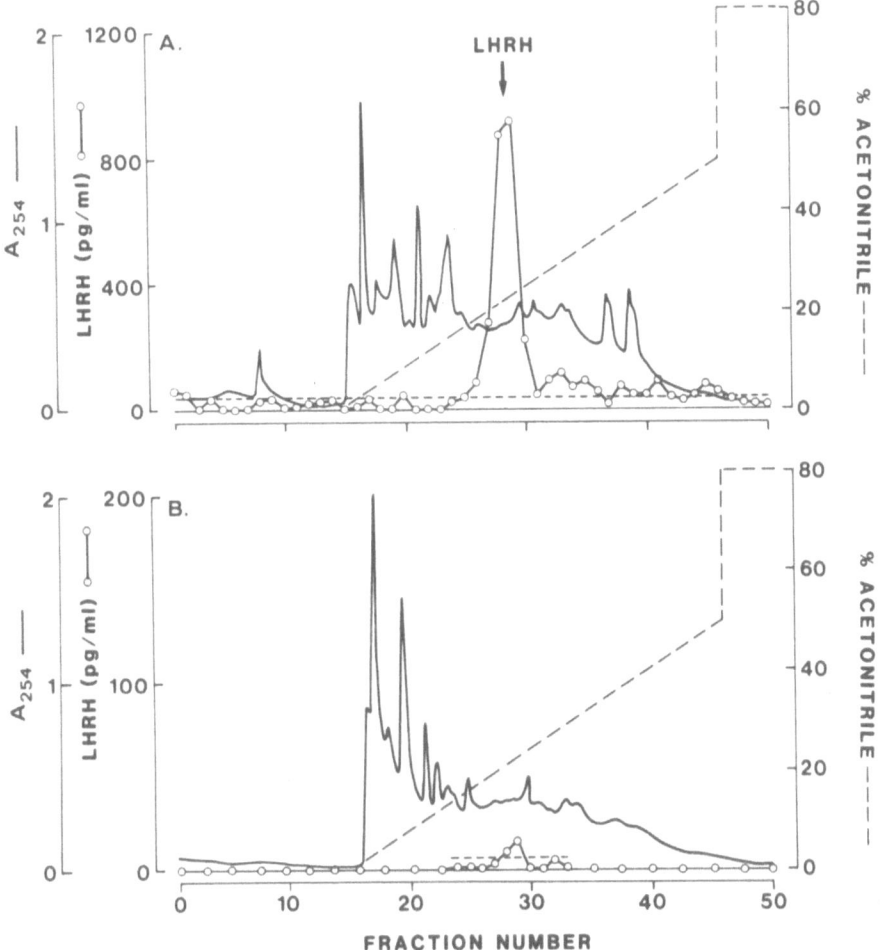

FIGURE 4 Reversed-phase HPLC absorbance and LHRH-immunoreactivity profiles of Sephadex G-15 gel filtration fractions corresponding to the elution position of LHRH as described in figure 3. A: highly purified extract with added LHRH; B: extract without added LHRH. ----, limit of assay sensitivity; -O-LHRH, elution position of LHRH fractionated alone.

LH or FSH release alone, as has been reported for extracts of
Sertoli cell medium, interstitial fluid or testis
extracts[9,11,12,14,17] is insufficient evidence for the presence
of a bioactive "LHRH-like" peptide. Gonadotrophin release should
be prevented by administration of an LHRH antagonist, to confirm
activity is mediated via the LHRH-receptor.

MEASUREMENT OF LHRH IN TESTICULAR TISSUE

Using the optimized extraction procedure in conjunction with gel
filtration, RP-HPLC and a highly sensitive LHRH radioimmunoassay,
endogenous LHRH-immunoreactivity which corresponded
chromatographically to authentic LHRG extracted under the same
conditions was detected in rat testicular extracts (Fig. 4). Using
the estimate of recovery derived from the addition of exogenous
LHRH to some samples extracted in parallel, a concentration of 1.0
pg free LHRH per testis was estimated to be present in the rat
testis prior to extraction[35].
    This level of activity was too small to confirm the
bioactivity of the peptide, although the peptide was (a)
chromatographically identical to LHRH by both gel filtration and
RP-HPLC; and (b) gave dose-response curves that were parallel to
the LHRH standard in a radioimmunoassay which was highly specific
for LHRH (using Rice No. 5 antiserum).

IMMUNOCYTOCHEMICAL STUDIES

By immunohistochemistry, employing an antiserum directed against
the middle of the LHRH sequence, one group demonstrated reactivity
over the interstitial cell cytoplasm and nuclei of spermatogonia in
rat testis paraffin sections[49]. A similar distribution of
immunoreactivity was observed by Bhasin and Swerdloff[18], although
this group reported that immunoreactivity was not removed by pre-
absorbing the antiserum with LHRH indicating this activity was most
likely the result of non-specific binding or antiserum cross-
reactivity with molecules unrelated to LHRH.

LHRH-IMMUNOREACTIVE FACTORS IN HUMAN SEMINAL PLASMA

Radioimmunoassayable "LHRH-like" activity has also been found in
organic solvent extracts of human seminal plasma[16,22-24]. This
immunoreactivity was detectable with antisera directed against the
C-terminal of LHRH, but not with antiserum R42, indicating that
this activity is not due to the presence of LHRH[23,24].
Incubation of [^{125}I]-LHRH with extracted seminal plasma did not
affect the immunological or chromatographic properties of the

150

peptide, indicating that peptidases were not interfering in the assays[24]. Employing the same antisera used to detect "LHRH-like" peptides in rat testicular extracts, Swerdloff et al.[22] has reported that there are two LHRH-immunoreactive species (2600 and 5000 Da), following gel filtration. Extracted seminal plasma also displaced the binding of a radiolabelled LHRH agonist to the pituitary receptor[24]. Seminal plasma from normal, oligospermic and vasectomized men contain the same levels of this radioimmunoassayable activity, indicating that the primary source of this activity is unlikely to be the testis[16,24]. Bioactivity has not been assessed in any of these studies.

SIGNIFICANCE AND BIOCHEMICAL NATURE OF "LHRH-LIKE" PEPTIDES

In the absence of detectable amounts of LHRH in their testicular tissue extracts, several groups have suggested that one or more of the LHRH-immunoreactive species in these extracts may be biologically active at the testicular receptor. There is evidence from the chicken that multiple forms of gonadotrophin-releasing peptides with very similar sequences can exist in the hypothalamus of a single species[50]. In those extrahypothalamic mammalian tissues where an LHRH-immunoreactive peptide has been both reported and characterized, which includes the rat brain, ovine pineal gland, human placenta, and human milk, the peptide has been found to be identical in characteristics to hypothalamic LHRH [51-53]. The same now appears to be true of the rat testis. Although there is limited evidence for a peptide similar in size to LHRH with immunological similarities, but chromatographically distinct from LHRH, in testicular extracts[10,17], receptor-mediated biological activity of this factor has not been demonstrated.

There is evidence that some of the factors in testicular and seminal plasma extracts and immunoaffinity-purified fractions displace the binding of radiolabelled LHRH agonists from the LHRH-receptor once peptidase contamination has been excluded, indicating affinity for the receptor binding site[13,15,24]. However, it should be pointed out that similar results may be attributable to factors which displace ligand from the LHRH-receptor but which are otherwise unrelated to LHRH. For example, inhibition of the binding of LH and FSH to their respective receptors by several factors present in testicular and seminal plasma extracts which are chemically unrelated to either gonadotrophin has been well characterized[54-56]. In only one study has LHRH-receptor mediated bioactivity of a testicular extract at the pituitary or testicular level been demonstrated[19]. However, the factor(s) responsible remain to be identified. Moreover, as a mixed testicular cell preparation was used, it cannot be ruled out that the action of the extract on Leydig cell function was exerted indirectly through another testicular cell type. In our laboratory, evidence for a factor capable of selectively stimulating gonadotrophin-release via the LHRH-receptor *in vitro* was not detected in a highly purified testicular extract optimized for recovery of LHRH, although it should be pointed out that the rigorous extraction method employed may have excluded larger proteins or peptides with different chemical characteristics to LHRH.

Identification of the mRNA coding for LHRH in the human placenta and rat and human hypothalamus has confirmed that LHRH in these tissues is synthesized as a larger MW precursor which possesses a signal peptide sequence of 23 amino acids, followed by the LHRH decapeptide sequence and a terminal sequence of 59 amino acids[57]. Presumably, the signal peptide is cleaved off in the endoplasmic reticulum leaving a 69 amino acid precursor intermediate (approximate MW 8000 Da) which is subsequently processed enzymatically to native LHRH in the secretory granule[58]. It is yet to be determined where and in what sequence the precursor peptide is cleaved during processing, although the precursor possesses several protease-sensitive regions[57]. Most studies of LHRH-immunoreactive species in the hypothalamus, placenta and testis have demonstrated molecules with molecular weights which are intermediate between the precursor and LHRH [10,13,59,60]. These data suggest that LHRH-immunoreactive peptides in the hypothalamus ranging in size from 5000 Da to 2000 Da may be precursor-LHRH intermediates[59,61]. The possibility that the testicular LHRH-immunoreactive species ranging in apparent MW from 6000 Da to around 1000 Da on gel filtration[10,13,17] are either precursor-LHRH intermediates or degradation products of the precursor produced by the action of testicular proteases during extraction also needs exploration. The cross-reactivity of testicular extracts with various LHRH antisera would suggest that at least part of the C-terminal sequence of the LHRH decapeptide is exposed in the intermediates and the inability to detect these peptides with more discriminating antisera, such as R42, may be due to the fact that the LHRH conformation and/or N- and C-terminal modifications are absent. The cross-reactivity pattern of this antiserum is similar to that described for LHRH-immunoreactive species in the hypothalamus[61]. Moreover, if the testicular molecules are LHRH precursors, the ratio of this larger MW LHRH-immunoreactivity in the testis to free LHRH indicates that the bulk of LHRH in the testis is incompletely processed.

Although this may explain the presence of intermediate size LHRH-immunoreactive species in testicular extracts, some of the testicular LHRH-immunoreactive species appear to be considerably larger than the LHRH precursor on gel filtration[10,13,17]. As these larger MW species were observed following gel filtration under non-reducing, non-dissociating conditions, it is possible that these are aggregates of LHRH or LHRH binding to larger proteins as suggested by Arimura and Turkelson[17]. Another possibility that has not been excluded in any study, including our own, is that cross-reactivity with at least some of the testicular or seminal plasma LHRH-immunoreactive species is due to antibodies in the antiserum which recognize an epitope found not only on the LHRH peptide but which is shared by several other, potentially unrelated, proteins or peptides[62]. The cross-reactivity of testicular extracts with the LHRH-A antiserum (R103) is probably due to this kind of interaction. Such proteins or peptides are unlikely to be able to bind to the LHRH-receptor to elicit a biological response.

The amount of LHRH found in extracts of adult rat testes is too large to be attributable to simple contamination by hypothalamic LHRH in the testicular vasculature at the time of death[21]. It is conceivable that the testicular levels of LHRH are derived from the plasma by accumulation or active uptake, although this is difficult to reconcile with the extremely active degrading activity of the rat testis, and interstitial fluid. A second possible source of testicular LHRH might be from peripheral LHRH-containing neurones terminating within the testis. Neurones containing LHRH are widely distributed throughout the central nervous system, where LHRH has been implicated as a neurotransmitter involved in the regulation of reproductive behaviour[63]. In the testis, nerves terminate in the interstitial tissue where the LHRH receptors are located and some of these neurones may utilize LHRH as the neurotransmitter. Evidence for a third possibility, that LHRH may be synthesized in the testis, has been discussed in the previous section.

On first glance, the considerably lower level of LHRH present in the testis, when compared with the concentration of the hormone in the hypothalamus (approximately 0.02%), suggests that testicular LHRH may not be physiologically significant. However, in a recent study using both immature and adult rats, it was demonstrated that continuous infusion of an LHRH antagonist into one testis produced greater than 90% occupancy of the LHRH receptors in the infused testis, but only a 50% reduction in LHRH-receptor numbers in the contralateral testis[64]. At the dose of antagonist employed, serum LH, FSH, prolactin and testosterone were not affected, but the infused testis displayed a significant reduction in testosterone content and LH-, FSH- and prolactin-receptor numbers compared with the contralateral testis. These data indicate that the antagonist interferes with the action of a locally produced ligand for the testicular LHRH-receptor and that the ligand has a supportive role in maintaining Leydig cell function. Studies in this and other laboratories have provided evidence that the seminiferous tubules, specifically the Sertoli cell, exert regulatory influences on the Leydig cell, mediated by one or more unidentified factors[65-68] and testicular LHRH is one potential candidate for mediating this influence. The low testicular concentration of LHRH may be indicative of a highly localized role for LHRH in the testis.

In contrast to the hypothalamus, where a ready store of LHRH needs to be held for rapid release due to the fact that LHRH is synthesized in the neuronal cell body some distance from its site of release, synthesis of LHRH by seminiferous tubule cells can occur very near to its site of release. The levels of large MW LHRH-immunoreactivity in testicular extracts suggest that LHRH in the testis may exist chiefly as the larger MW prohormone, as appears to be the case in the perikarya of the preoptic and arcuate nuclei where hypothalamic LHRH is synthesized [61]. Moreover, the events of spermatogenic development are comparatively slow compared to the rapid events that occur during the pulsatile release of gonadotrophins. These factors could contribute to a reduced requirement to store free LHRH prior to release, which might in part explain the low testicular content of the decapeptide hormone.

Furthermore, if most of the free LHRH in the testis was present in the interstitial fluid, allowing for an interstitial fluid volume of 76 ul/testis in the adult rat[69], a testicular level of 1 pg could represent an interstitial fluid concentration as high as 14 pg/ml, approaching mean portal plasma levels [70,71]. As LHRH release from the tubules at certain stages of the cycle of the seminiferous epithelium might vary, local concentrations of LHRH surrounding individual Leydig cell clusters could be expected to be even higher. The failure of secreted LHRH to accumulate in the interstitial fluid, which would result in a greater overall testicular concentration and diffusion to more distant Leydig cells, may be attributable to its rapid degradation by interstitial fluid peptidases secreted by adjacent Sertoli cells[48]. It is therefore possible that, given a very rapid sequence of LHRH precursor processing, release and degradation within highly localized regions of the testis, the concentration of LHRH in certain areas of the intertubular space could be more than adequate for LHRH to have a significant biological effect even though the overall concentration in the testis is low. In fact, such a mechanism may be essential to support paracrine interaction within any system as completely open as the testicular interstitial fluid.

The significance of LHRH-immunoreactive species in the seminal plasma is unclear. There are no reports of receptors for LHRH in the male reproductive tract, although androgen-stimulated growth of both the prostate and seminal vesicles is inhibited by LHRH agonists[38]. This raises the possibility that locally produced LHRH has direct actions in these tissues. Alternatively, seminal plasma peptides may have a site of action in the female tract, which is also responsive to the direct effects of LHRH agonists[39]

CONCLUSIONS

In summary, although there is considerable evidence for a role of LHRH in regulating testicular function, our own studies have indicated that the levels of LHRH in the rat testis are extremely small compared with the levels of LHRH found in the rat hypothalamus. Whether the extremely low levels of LHRH in the rat testis are indicative of residual levels of hypothalamic LHRH, or the consequence of a highly localized mode of action and rapid turnover of the peptide, consistent with the proposed physiological role of LHRH as a local regulator of Leydig cell function, remains to be established.

Studies in our laboratory, and in others, have confirmed the presence in testicular extracts of considerably larger amounts of factors which cross-react with antisera directed against the C-terminus of LHRH, but not with antisera directed against the entire molecule or both termini. Similar LHRH-immunoreactive factors are present in seminal plasma, but these do not appear to originate from the testis. Earlier evidence that any of these factors bind to the LHRH-receptor and either stimulate gonadotrophin release or modulate Leydig cell functions has yet to be confirmed. The physiological significance of these "LHRH-like" factors is at

154

present unknown, but they may represent peptides related to or homologous with LHRH, LHRH precursors or intermediate LHRH bound to larger MW proteins or merely molecules that non-specifically interfere with radioimmunoassay or radio receptor assay procedures.

REFERENCES

1.   Bourne, G.A., Regiani, S., Payne, A.H. and Marshall, J.C.: Testicular GnRH receptors - characterization and localization on interstitial tissue. J. Clin. Endocrinol. Metab., 51, 407 (1980).
2.   Clayton, R.N., Katikineni, M., Chan, V., Dufau, M.L. and Catt, K.J.: Direct inhibition of testicular function by gonadotropin-releasing hormone: mediation by specific gonadotropin-releasing hormone receptors in interstitial cells. Proc. Nat. Acad. Sci. (USA), 77, 4459 (1980).
3.   Lefebvre, F., Reeves, J.J., Seguin, C., Massicotte, J. and Labrie, F.: Specific binding of a potent LHRH agonist in rat testis. Molec. Cell. Endocrinol., 20, 127 (1980).
4.   Perrin, M.H., Vaughan, J.M., Rivier, J.E. and Vale, W.W.: High affinity GnRH binding to testicular membrane homogenates. Life Sci., 26, 2251 (1980).
5.   Sharpe, R.M. and Fraser, H.M.: Leydig cell receptors for luteinizing hormone releasing hormone and its agonists and their modulation by administration or deprivation of the releasing hormone. Biochem. Biophys. Res. Comm., 95, 256 (1980).
6.   Arimura, A., Serafini, P., Talbot, S. and Schally, A.V.: Reduction of testicular luteinizing hormone/human chorionic gonadotropin receptors by [D-Trp^6]-luteinizing hormone releasing hormone in hypophysectomized rats. Biochem. Biophys. Res. Comm., 90, 687 (1979).
7.   Hsueh, A.J.W and Erickson, G.F.: Extra-pituitary inhibition of testicular function by luteinizing hormone releasing hormone. Nature, 281, 66 (1979).
8.   Bambino, T.H., Schreiber, J.R. and Hsueh, A.J.W.: Gonadotropin-releasing hormone and its agonist inhibit testicular luteinizing hormone receptor and steroidogenesis in immature and adult hypophysectomized rats. Endocrinology, 107, 908 (1980).
9.   Sharpe, R.M. and Fraser, H.M.: hCG stimulation of testicular LHRH-like activity. Nature, 287, 642 (1980).
10. Dutlow, C.M. and Millar, R.P.: Rat testis immunoreactive LH-RH differs structurally from hypothalamic LH-RH. Biochem. Biophys. Res. Comm., 101, 486 (1981).
11. Sharpe, R.M., Fraser, H.M., Cooper, I. and Rommerts, F.F.G.: Sertoli-Leydig cell communication via an LHRH-like factor. Nature, 290, 785 (1981).
12. Sharpe, R.M., Fraser, H.M., Cooper, I. and Rommerts, F.F.G.: The secretion, measurement, and function of a testicular LHRH-like factor. Ann. N.Y. Acad. Sci., 383, 272 (1982).
13. Bhasin, S., Heber, D., Peterson, M. and Swerdloff, R.: Partial isolation and characterization of testicular GnRH-like factors. Endocrinology, 112, 1114 (1983).

14. Nagendranath, N., Jose, T.M. and Juneja, H.S.: Bioassayable gonadotropin releasing hormone-like activity in the spent nutrient medium of rat Sertoli cells in primary cultures. Horm. Metab. Res., 15, 99 (1983).

15. Sharpe, R.M. and Harmer, T.J.: The nature and biological actions of testicular LHRH. In: "Hormones and Cell Regulation." Vol. 7. J.E. Dumont, J. Nunez and R.M. Denton (Eds). Elsevier Biomedical Press, Amsterdam. p. 217 (1983).

16. Chan, S.Y.W. and Tang, L.C.H.: Immunoreactive LHRH-like factor in human seminal plasma. Arch. Androl., 10, 29 (1983).

17. Arimura, A. and Turkelson, C.M.: LHRH-like substance in the rat testis. Ann. N.Y. Acad. Sci., 438, 390 (1984).

18. Bhasin, S. and Swerdloff, R.S.: Rat testicular GnRH-like factors. In "Gonadal Proteins and Peptides and their Biological Significance." M.R. Sairam and L.E. Atkinson (Eds). World Scientific Publishing Company, Singapore, 1984, p. 327.

19. Bhasin, S. and Swerdloff, R.S.: Testicular GnRH-like factors: characterization of biologic activity. Biochem. Biophys. Res. Comm., 122, 1071 (1984).

20. Hedger, M.P., Robertson, D.M., Browne, C.A. and de Kretser, D.M.: Studies on the identification of a LHRH-like peptide in the rat testis. Ann. N.Y. Acad. Sci., 438, 371 (1984).

21. Hedger, M.P., Robertson, D.M., Browne, C.A. and de Kretser, D.M.: The isolation and measurement of luteinizing hormone-releasing hormone (LHRH) from the rat testis. Molec. Cell. Endocrinol., 42, 163 (1985).

22. Swerdloff, R.S., Bhasin, S. and Sokol, R.Z.: GnRH-like factors in the rat testis and human seminal plasma. Ann. N.Y. Acad. Sci., 438, 382 (1984).

23. Izumi, S-I., Makino, T. and Iizuka, R.: Immunoreactive luteinizing hormone-releasing hormone in the seminal plasma and human semen parameters. Fertil. Steril., 43, 617, (1985).

24. Sokol, R.Z., Peterson, M., Heber, D. and Swerdloff, R.S.: Identification and partial characterization of gonadotropin-releasing hormone-like factors in human seminal plasma. Biol. Reprod., 33, 370 (1985).

25. Cooke, B.A. and Sullivan, M.H.F.: The mechanisms of LHRH agonist action in gonadal tissues. Molec. Cell. Endocrinol., 41, 115 (1985).

26. Hsueh, A.J.W., Schreiber, J.R. and Erickson, G.F.: Inhibitory effect of gonadotropin releasing hormone upon cultured testicular cells. Molec. Cell. Endocrinol., 21, 43 (1981).

27. Cao Y-Q., Sundaram, K., Bardin, C.W., Rivier, J. and Vale, W.: Direct inhibition of testicular steroidogenesis and gonadotrophin receptor levels by [(imBzl)-D-His^6,Pro^9-NEt]GnRH and [D-Trp^6,Pro^9-NEt]GnRH, potent agonists of GnRH. Int. J. Androl., 5, 158 (1982).

28. Hunter, M.G., Sullivan, M.H.F., Dix, C.J., Aldred, L.F. and Cooke, B.A.: Stimulation and inhibition by LHRH analogues of cultured rat Leydig cell function and lack of effect on mouse Leydig cells. Molec. Cell. Endocrinol., 27, 31 (1982).

29. Sharpe, R.M. and Cooper, I.: Stimulatory effect of LHRH and its agonists on Leydig cell steroidogenesis *in vitro*. Molec. Cell. Endocrinol., 26, 141 (1982).

30. Browning, J.Y., D'Agata, R., Steinberger, A., Grotjan, H.E., Jr. and Steinberger, E.: Biphasic effect of gonadotropin-releasing hormone and its agonist analog (HOE766) on *in vitro* testosterone production by purified rat Leydig cells. Endocrinology, 113, 985 (1983).

31. Hsueh, A.J.W., Bambino, T.H., Zhuang, L-Z, Welsh, T.H., Jr. and Ling, N.C.: Mechanism of the direct action of gonadotropin-releasing hormone and its antagonist on androgen biosynthesis by cultured rat testicular cells. Endocrinology, 112, 1653 (1983).

32. Sharpe, R.M., Doogan, D.G. and Cooper, I.: Factors determining whether the direct effects of an LHRH agonist on Leydig cell function *in vivo* are stimulatory or inhibitory. Molec. Cell. Endocrinol., 32, 57 (1983).

33. Sharpe, R.M., Doogan, D.G. and Cooper, I.: Direct effects of a luteinizing hormone-releasing hormone agonist on intratesticular levels of testosterone and interstitial fluid formation in intact male rats. Endocrinology, 113, 1306 (1983).

34. Hazum, E. and Keinan, D.: Testicular GnRH receptors: photoaffinity labelling and fluorescence distribution studies. Peptides, 5, 119 (1984).

35. Hedger, M.P., Risbridger, G.P. and de Kretser, D.M.: Autoradiographical localization of luteinizing hormone releasing hormone (LHRH) receptors on rat testicular intertubular cells fractionated on Percoll density gradients. Aust. J. Biol. Sci., 38, 435 (1985).

36. Iwashita, M. and Catt, K.J.: Photoaffinity labeling of pituitary and gonadal receptors for gonadotropin-releasing hormone. Endocrinology, 117, 738 (1985).

37. Damber, J-E., Bergh, A. and Daehlin, L.: Stimulatory effect of an LHRH-agonist on testicular blood flow in hypophysectomized rats. Int. J. Androl., 7, 236 (1984).

38. Sundaram, K., Cao, Y-Q., Wang, N-G., Bardin, C.W., Rivier, J. and Vale, W.: Inhibition of the action of sex steroids by gonadotropin-releasing hormone (GnRH) agonists: a new biological effect. Life Sci., 28, 83 (1981).

39. Reddy, P.R.K., Rao, I.M., Raju, V.S., Rukmini, V. and Reddy,R.L.: Direct inhibitory actions of GnRH on accessory reproductive organs of rat. J. Steroid Biochem., 23, 819 (1985).

40. Hierowski, M.T., Altamirano, P., Redding, T.W. and Schally, A.V.: The presence of LHRH-like receptors in Dunning R3327H prostate tumors. FEBS Lett., 154, 92 (1983).

41. Hsueh, A.J.W. and Schaeffer, J.M.: Gonadotropin-releasing hormone as a paracrine hormone and neurotransmitter in extra-pituitary sites. J. Steroid Biochem., 23, 757 (1985).

42. Redding, T.W. and Schally, A.V.: The distribution, half-life, and excretion of tritiated luteinizing hormone-releasing hormone (LH-RH) in rats. Life Sci., 12, 23 (1973).

43. Nett, T.M., Akbar, A.M. and Niswender, G.D.: Serum levels of luteinizing hormone and gonadotropin-releasing hormone in cycling, castrated and anestrous ewes. Endocrinology, 94, 713 (1974).

44. Khodr, G.S. and Siler-Khodr, T.M.: Placental luteinizing hormone-releasing factor and its synthesis. Science, 207, 315 (1980).

45. Ying, S-Y., Ling, N., Bohlen, P. and Guillemin, R.: Gonadocrinins: peptides in ovarian follicular fluid stimulating the secretion of pituitary gonadotropins. Endocrinology, 108, 1206 (1981).

46. Nett, T.M., Akbar, A.M., Niswender, G.D., Hedlund, M.T. and White, W.F.: A radioimmunoassay for gonadotropin-releasing hormone (Gn-RH) in serum. J. Clin. Endocrinol. Metab., 36, 880 (1973).

47. Fraser, H.M., Sandow, J. and Krauss, B.: Antibody production against an agonist analogue of luteinizing hormone-releasing hormone: evaluation of immunochemical and physiological consequences. Acta Endocrinol., 103, 151 (1983).

48. Hedger, M.P., Robertson, D.M., Tepe, S.J., Browne, C.A. and de Kretser, D.M.: Degradation of luteinizing hormone-releasing hormone (LHRH) and an LHRH agonist by the rat testis. Molec. Cell. Endocrinol., 46, 59 (1986).

49. Paull, W.K., Turkelson, C.M., Thomas, C.R. and Arimura, A.: Immunohistochemical demonstration of a testicular substance related to luteinizing hormone-releasing hormone. Science, 213, 1263 (1981).

50. Miyamoto, K., Hasegawa, Y., Nomura, M., Igarashi, M., Kangawa, K. and Matsuo, H.: Identification of the second gonadotropin-releasing hormone in chicken hypothalamus: evidence that gonadotropin secretion is probably controlled by two distinct gonadotropin-releasing hormones in avian species. Proc. Nat. Acad. Sci. (USA), 81, 3874, (1984).

51. King, J.A. and Millar, R.P.: Decapeptide luteinizing hormone releasing hormone in ovine pineal gland. J. Endocrinol., 91, 405 (1981).

52. Amarant, T., Fridkin, M. and Koch, Y.: Luteinizing hormone-releasing hormone and thyrotropin-releasing hormone in human and bovine milk. Eur. J. Biochem., 127, 647 (1982).

53. Tan, L. and Rousseau, P.: The chemical identity of the immunoreactive LHRH-like peptide biosynthesized in the human placenta. Biochem. Biophys. Res. Comm., 109, 1061 (1982).

54. Reichert, L.E., Jr. and Abou-Issa, H.: Studies on a low molecular weight testicular factor which inhibits binding of FSH to receptor. Biol. Reprod., 17, 614 (1977).

55. Reichert, L.E., Jr., Sanzo, M.A. and Dias, J.A.: Studies on purification and characterization of gonadotropin binding inhibitors and stimulators from human serum and seminal plasma. In: "Intragonadal Regulation of Reproduction." P. Franchimont and C.P. Channing (Eds). Academic Press, New York, p. 61 (1981).

56. Dias, J.A., Treble, D.H. and Reichert, L.E., Jr.: Effect of bacitracin and polyamines on follicle-stimulating hormone binding to membrane-bound and detergent-solubilized bovine calf testis receptor. Endocrinology, 113, 2029 (1983).

57. Adelman, J.P., Mason, A.J., Hayflick, J.S. and Seeburg, P.H.: Isolation of the gene and hypothalamic cDNA for the common precursor of gonadotropin-releasing hormone and prolactin release-inhibiting factor in human and rat.   Proc. Nat. Acad. Sci. (USA), 83, 179 (1986).

58. Gainer, H., Russell, J.T. and Loh, Y.P.: The enzymology and intracellular organization of peptide precursor processing: the secretory vesicle hypothesis. Neuroendocrinol., 40, 171 (1985).

59. Millar, R.P., Aehnelt, C. and Rossier, G.: Higher molecular weight immunoreactive species of luteinizing hormone releasing hormone: possible precursors of the hormone. Biochem. Biophys. Res. Comm., 74, 720 (1977).

60. Gautron, J.P., Pattou, E. and Kordon, C.: Occurrence of higher molecular forms of LHRH in fractionated extracts from rat hypothalamus, cortex and placenta.   Molec. Cell. Endocrinol., 24, 1 (1981).

61. Millar, R.P., Wegener, I. and Schally, A.V.   Putative prohormonal luteinizing hormone-releasing hormone.   In: "Neuropeptides. Biochemical and Physiolgical Studies." R.P. Millar (Ed).   Churchill Livingstone, Edinburgh. pp. 111 (1981).

62. Berzofsky, J.A. and Schechter, A.N.:   The concepts of crossreactivity and specificity in immunology.   Molec. Immunol., 18, 751 (1981).

63. Witter, A. and de Wied, D.:   Hypothalamic-pituitary oligopeptides and behaviour.   In: "Physiology of the Hypothalamus." Handbook of the Hypothalamus, Vol. 2. P.J. Morgane and J. Panksepp (Eds). Marcel Dekker, New York. pp. 307 (1980).

64. Clayton, R.N., Detta, A., Nikula, H. and Huhtaniemi, I.T.: Physiological role of putative testicular gonadotrophin releasing hormone (GnRH). Med. Biol., 63, 201 (1985).

65. Aoki, A. and Fawcett, D.W.: Is there a local feedback from the seminiferous tubules affecting activity of the Leydig cells? Biol. Reprod., 19, 144 (1978).

66. Risbridger, G.P., Kerr, J.B. and de Kretser, D.M.: Evaluation of Leydig cell function and gonadotropin binding in unilateral and bilateral cryptorchidism: evidence for local control of Leydig cell function by the seminiferous tubule. Biol. Reprod., 24, 534 (1981).

67. Bergh, A.:   Local differences in Leydig cell morphology in the adult rat testis: evidence for a local control of Leydig cells by adjacent seminiferous tubules. Int. J. Androl., 5, 325 (1982).

68. Parvinen, M., Nikula, H. and Huhtaniemi, I.: Influence of rat seminiferous tubules on Leydig cell testosterone production in vitro. Molec. Cell Endocrinol., 37, 331 (1984).

69. Sharpe, R.M. and Cooper, I.: Testicular interstitial fluid as a monitor for changes in the intratesticular environment in the rat. J. Reprod. Fert., 69, 125 (1983).

70. Fink, G. and Jamieson, M.G.: Immunoreactive luteinizing hormone releasing factor in rat pituitary stalk blood: effects of electrical stimulation of the medial preoptic area. J. Endocrinol., 68, 71 (1976).

71. Eskay, R.L., Mical, R.S. and Porter, J.C.: Relationship between luteinizing hormone releasing hormone concentration in the hypophysial portal blood and luteinizing hormone release in intact, castrated and electrochemically-stimulated rats. Endocrinology, 100, 263 (1977).

10
Placental LHRH-Like Activity

T.M. SILER-KHODR
Department of Obstetrics and Gynecology, The University of Texas
Health Science Center at San Antonio, San Antonio, TX 78284, USA

INTRODUCTION

Multiple endocrine functions of the placenta have long been recognized. However, only recently has the presence of hypothalamic-like release and inhibiting activities in the placenta been realized. One of these activities is similar to LH-RH and recent studies indicate that chorionic LH-RH-like activity interacts within a paracrine system involving chorionic gonadotropin, steroid and prostaglandin (PG) releases. The delineation of this paracrine system within the placenta has led us to reassess and broaden our understanding of the control of placental endocrine function.

This chapter will review what is currently known about LH-RH-like activity in the placenta, its receptor interaction and its effect on release of other placental hormones. In addition, effects of LH-RH analogues on placental function, their significance and possible applications will be discussed.

PRESENCE OF LH-RH-LIKE ACTIVITY

The presence of an LH-RH-like bio-activity in the human placenta was first reported by Gibbons et al. [1], who observed that placental extracts stimulated rat LH release in vivo. They also showed that placental explant culture incorporated ^{3}H-amino acids into a substance which eluted from CM-cellulose as did LH-RH. Subsequently, we demonstrated the presence of apparent LH-RH immunoactivity in placental extracts and quantitated the apparent LH-RH immunoactivity in the human placenta throughout gestation [2]. We found that the highest concentration occurred in early pregnancy and demonstrated a similar pattern of apparent LH-RH immunoreactivity in maternal circulation (Fig. 1). Localization of this LH-RH-like activity in the placental villus has been done by ourselves [3] using immuno-fluorescence and by Miyaki et al. [4] using immuno-enzymatic localization. LH-RH was predominantly localized in the cytotrophoblast and absent from the syncytium (Fig. 2). There was also specific uptake along the outer cell membrane of the syncytiotrophoblast. Placental production of LH-RH-like immunoactivity was indicated, since the release of apparent LH-RH immunoactivity increased after

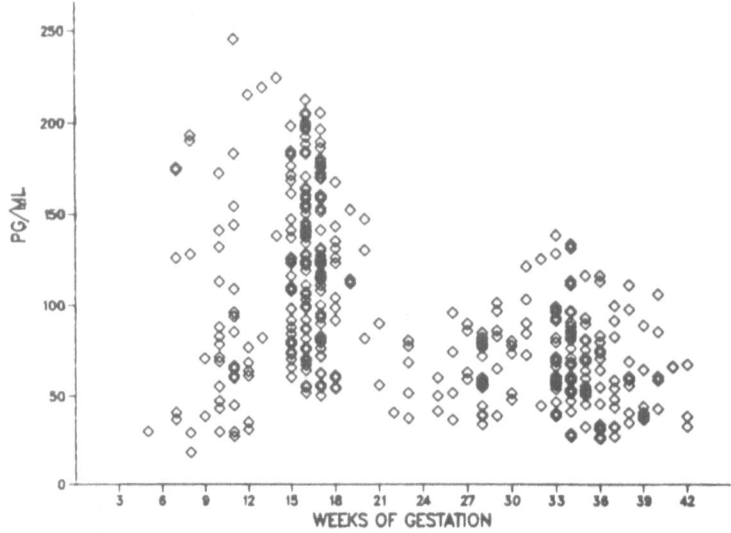

FIGURE 1 Apparent LH-RH immunoactivity in maternal circulation throughout gestation. Reproduced from Siler-Khodr et al., Am. J. Obstet. Gynecol., 150, 376 (1984) with permission.

4 days of culture and total release exceeded the original tissue content [5]. We directly studied the synthesis of LH-RH-like immunoactivity by the human placenta using ^{3}H-amino acids. ^{3}H-peptide was recovered in the area that synthetic LH-RH eluted. Analysis of concentrates of this eluate showed that they contained equipotent immuno- and bio-assayable LH-RH-like activity [6]. Thus, the placental and hypothalamic LH-RH were very similar. Subsequently, Lee et al. [7], using acid extracts of human placenta, confirmed the presence of immunoreactive LH-RH-like material which eluted as

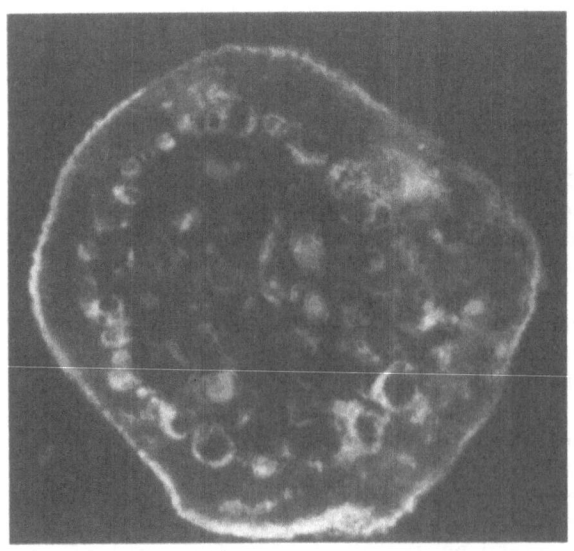

FIGURE 2
Immunofluorescent localization of GnRH-like material in a human placental villus using anti-GnRH. Reproduced from Siler-Khodr, Clin. Perinatol. 10, 553 (1983) with permission.

162

did synthetic LH-RH on HPLC. Tan and Rosseau [8] have also isolated
a peptide, having the identical decapeptide sequence of synthetic
LH-RH, from acid extracts of human placenta. More recently, Seeburg
and Adelman [9] have isolated from human placenta, an mRNA which
codes for a 92 amino acid peptide containing the decapeptide
sequence of LH-RH. These data clearly establish the presence and
expression of LH-RH in the human placenta.

LH-RH-like activity in the placenta of other species has also
been demonstrated [10,11]. However, the apparent LH-RH immunoactivity found in the rat placenta was largely due to a high
molecular weight material [10]. Nowak et al. [11] have also
observed LH-RH-like bioactivity in the rabbit placenta [11].
However, only a portion of this activity could be inhibited with an
antagonist of LH-RH. Thus, the presence of another molecule with
LH-RH-like activity was postulated. Recently, Millar et al. [12]
have reported a 13-amino acid sequence different from LH-RH, yet
having LH-RH-like bioactivity. Interestingly, this sequence is
contained in the 92-amino acid peptide described by Seeburg et al.
[8], which also contains the decapeptide LH-RH. Thus, there is
evidence supporting the hypothesis that the placenta may contain
more than one LH-RH-like activity.

We have noted that the apparent immunoactive LH-RH in the human
placenta is far greater than the LH-RH-decapeptide content [13-15].
Isolation procedures known to result in high recoveries of LH-RH
(acid, methanol or ethanol extractions), yielded only 10 ng LH-RH-
like activity/term placenta. However, extraction procedures using
neutral pH buffers resulted in 5-10 µg of apparent LH-RH immunoactivity per term placenta. We have isolated the substance effecting
this apparent LH-RH immunoactivity, and have found it to be a glycoprotein of ~60,000 mol wt. It is biologically active in stimulating
LH release from rat pituitary cell cultures, but with only about
1/1000 the potency of LH-RH. It stimulates hCG, αhCG, prostaglandin
E (PGE) and 13,14-dihydro-15-keto-prostaglandin F (MPF) release from
placental explants with 200 to 600 times, respectively, the molar
potency than does LH-RH (Fig. 3). We have therefore named it human
chorionic gonadotropin releasing factor (hCG-RF). Further studies
have demonstrated that this substance inactivates LH-RH. The precise
mechanism of this inactivation is under investigation. Inhibition of
this activity, i.e. hCG-RF inactivation of LH-RH, can be effected by
heating hCG-RF or exposure to acid or certain peptidase inhibitors,
but the ability of hCG-RF to stimulate placental prostaglandins and
hCG release remains. We have postulated that this hCG-RF has enzymatic activity to degrade LH-RH as well as capability to stimulate
prostaglandin synthesis which, in turn, stimulates hCG. This
hypothesis is compatible with the findings of Nowak et al. [11], who
reported that rabbit placenta extracts contain LH-stimulating
activity that could be antagonized only partially by an LH-RH
antagonist. Further studies, separating the prostaglandin stimulation and LH-RH-related stimulation of hCG from the human placenta,
may better define these activities and their interrelations.

There is increasing evidence for a physiologic role for LH-RH-
like activity in the placenta. The presence of LH-RH receptors in
the human placenta has been demonstrated [16-18]. Belisle et al.
[17] have reported that the number of these receptors is higher at

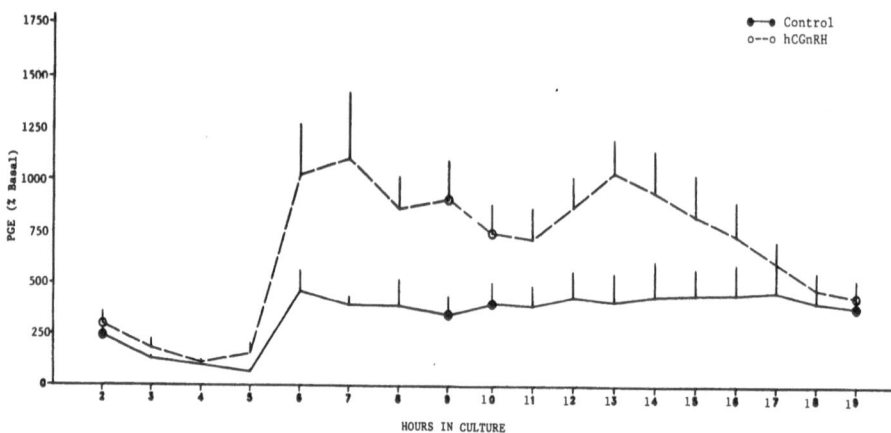

FIGURE 3 The release over control (mean ± SEM) of PGE from placental explants perifused with control medium (•——•) or
starting at the fifth hour with hCG-RH (208 nM, o---o).

midgestation than at term. However, the affinity of the receptor is
only 10^{-7} for LH-RH and no greater for superagonists of LH-RH, compared to 10^{-10} in the pituitary [16,18]. These findings have led to
the hypothesis that there may be yet another more active LH-RH-like
activity in the placenta that binds to this receptor and/or, since
LH-RH acts via a paracrine system in the placenta, higher concentrations of LH-RH may exist at the receptor and thus, this low affinity
constant may be physiological. Other studies [19-22] have shown that
cAMP or dibutyryl cAMP stimulates hCG, steroid and PG releases,
supporting the theory that their release may be receptor-mediated.

IN VITRO STUDIES

Numerous studies exist studying the biological action of LH-RH and
its analogs. LH-RH stimulates the release of hCG and αhCG from
early [23] and term [21,22,24,25] placentas _in vitro_ in a dose-
related fashion. HCS was not affected, indicating the action to be
specific. Also, we have shown that the basal hormonal release and
response to LH-RH varied with gestational stages of the placenta
[26]. Using placental explant cultures, we found that basal release
of αhCG and hCG was greatest at 9-13 weeks of gestation (Fig. 6) and
lowest at term. These basal hormonal releases declined with extended
culture, except from 13- and 15-week placental cultures, where the
initially high release continued throughout the eight days of
culture. Initial release of hCS was low at six weeks and increased
to maximum rates by 15 weeks, retaining this high level to term.
    Stimulation of hCG in response to LH-RH was observed from
placental explants of 13, 15, 16, 17, 39 and 40 weeks of gestation
[26] (Fig. 4). However, in early placentas, when basal hCG release
was highest, no further stimulation of hCG by LH-RH was effected.
LH-RH stimulated the release of αhCG and hCG most dramatically in

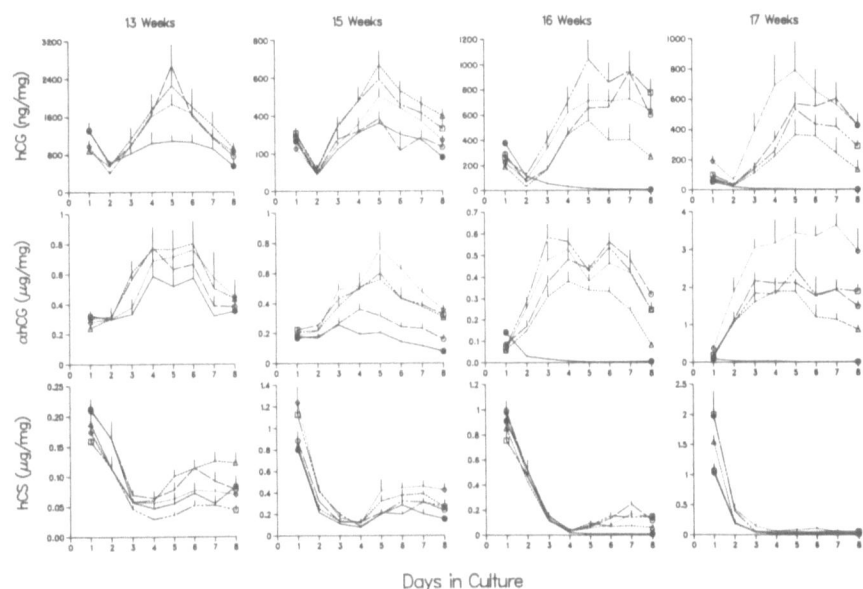

Days in Culture

FIGURE 4 Mean (±SEM) release of hCG, αhCG and hCS from human placental explants of varying gestational ages over 8 days of culture when incubated with LH-RH (control ●——●, 0.2 μg/ml o---o, 1.0 μg/ml Δ---Δ, 10.0 μg/ml □-----□, 50 μg/ml ◇···◇). Reproduced from Siler-Khodr et al., Biol. Reprod., 34, 245 (1986) with permission.

cultures of 16- and 17-week placentas, where increases of as much as 400- and 250-fold, respectively, were observed on day 6 of culture. In term placental cultures after 6 days in vitro, a 20-fold stimulation of αhCG and a 10-fold increase of hCG were caused by LH-RH. The largest responses of αhCG and hCG to LH-RH were observed when estrogen levels were low. Dose-related responses were observed in some placentas, yet in some instances, maximal effects were attained with all doses utilized (0.2 to 50 μg/ml). LH-RH did not stimulate a significant increase of hCS release at any gestational stage.

Steroid release was also determined [27], although it should be noted the estrogen precursors, DHEA-S or 16-OH-DHEA-S, were not present in the media, thus accounting for the rapid decline in estrogen production over the culture period. However, the initial basal release of the steroids was related to the gestational age of the placenta. Basal release of P, E_1 and E_2 on day 1 of culture was highest from placentas of early gestation (9-13 weeks). Release of P then declined, reaching a nadir by 15 weeks, and continuing at that level, whereas the release of E_1 and E_2, which reached a nadir at 17 weeks, again increased by term. In contrast, the basal release of E_3 increased with increasing gestational age of the placenta.

Stimulation of P by LH-RH was greatest in placentas of 16 and 17 weeks' gestation after extended culture when the basal release of P had declined [27] (Fig. 5). As much as a 240-fold increase was observed on the eighth day of culture. A large stimulation of P

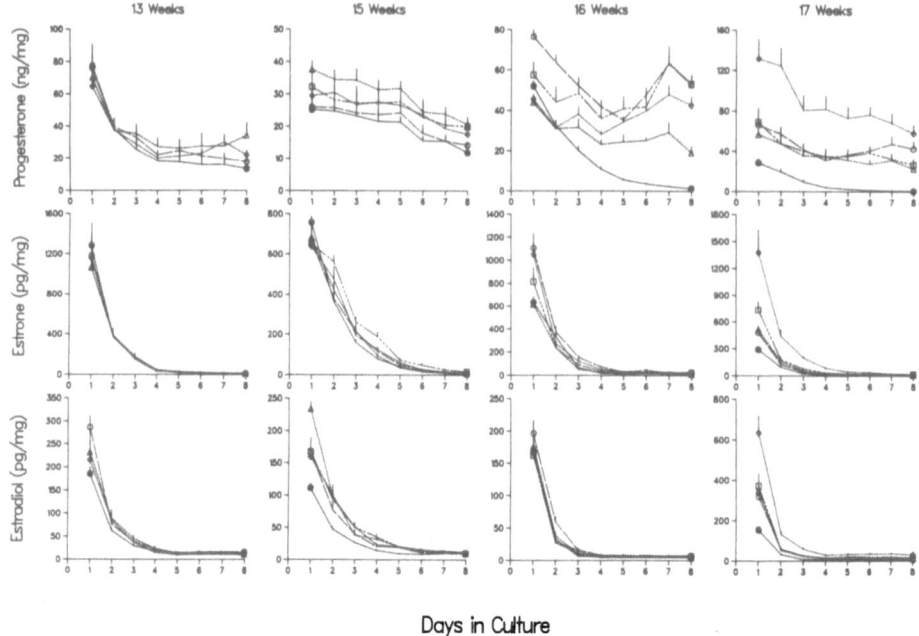

Days in Culture

FIGURE 5 Mean (±SEM) release of progesterone, estrone and estradiol from human placental explants of varying gestational ages over 8 days of culture when incubated with LH-RH. Symbols as in Fig. 4. Reproduced from Siler-Khodr et al., Biol. Reprod., 34, 255 (1986) with permission.

(32-fold) was also observed in term placental cultures. A stimulation of E_1 and E_2 by LH-RH was observed during the initial days of culture and in mid-gestational cultures (16-17 weeks). Stimulation of E_2 only was also observed at 13-15 weeks and at term. A stimulation of E_3 was observed in certain individual placentas. A correlation of the P and hCG response to LH-RH stimulation was noted, as was an inverse relation of estrogens and hCG stimulation by LH-RH.

These data demonstrate that human placentas of different gestational ages have varying hormonogenic capabilities in vitro and establish that synthetic LH-RH is capable of stimulating αhCG, hCG and steroid production, although the degree and pattern of response to LH-RH stimulation are related to the gestational age of the placental tissue and its time in culture. The most responsive period to exogenous LH-RH stimulation of αhCG, hCG and P release was on days 5 and 6 of culture, when basal estrogen release was very low. These data support the hypothesis that hCG release might be controlled by a chorionic LH-RH stimulation and suggest that local steroid levels may modulate the hCG response to LH-RH stimulation. Supporting the steroid feedback action are our studies and those of Branchaud et al. [28], showing that addition of DHEA-S to the media resulted in increased E_2 release and blocked hCG response to LH-RH stimulation.

LH-RH also affects prostaglandin release [20,21,29]. As for the other hormones, we found very significant effects, but only at cer-

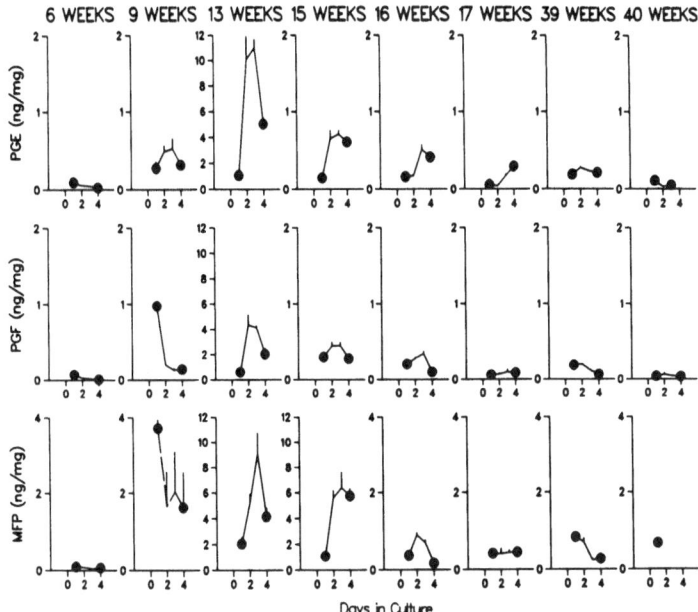

6 WEEKS 9 WEEKS 13 WEEKS 15 WEEKS 16 WEEKS 17 WEEKS 39 WEEKS 40 WEEKS

FIGURE 6 Basal release (mean ± SEM) of PGE, PGF and MPF from human
placental explants of varying gestational ages over 4 days
of culture. Reproduced from Siler-Khodr et al., Biol.
Reprod., in press, with permission.

tain gestational stages [29]. The greatest basal release of PGE,
PGF and MPF was from the 9 to 13-week placental cultures, with the
release on the second and third days increasing 4 to 10-fold from
that of the first day of culture (Fig. 6). From 15 weeks to term,
the initial basal release (day 1) of these prostaglandins was only
slightly higher than at 6 weeks and, by term, the later increase
with extended culture was absent or very small. Addition of synthetic LH-RH to cultures of 6- or 9-week placentas effected no
significant change in any of these prostaglandins (Fig. 7). However,
LH-RH added to the 13-week placental cultures gave a dose-related
inhibition of these prostaglandins, especially on days 2 and 3 of
culture, when the basal release normally increased 10-fold. However,
after 15 weeks, a stimulation of these prostaglandins by LH-RH was
observed and was as much as 50-fold in the cultures of 16 and 17-
week placentas, as well as the term placental cultures. The LH-RH
effect on prostaglandins occurred from the first days of culture as
did the estrogen response. In some placentas, the lower doses were
more effective than higher ones.
　　　Studies using an LH-RH antagonist (Syntex, RS-29226), in an
attempt to interfere with endogenous LH-RH-like activity have also
been performed [30-32]. Placentas of 6, 9, 12 and 15 weeks were
cultured with only Medium 199, or Medium 199 with RS-29226,
(1 μg/ml) or this LH-RH antagonist (1 μg/ml) together with synthetic
LH-RH (10 μg/ml) and release of αnCG, hCG, hCS, P, E_1, E_2, PGE, PGF
and PFM was determined. In very early gestation (6 and 9 weeks),
none of these hormonal releases were affected by this dose of this

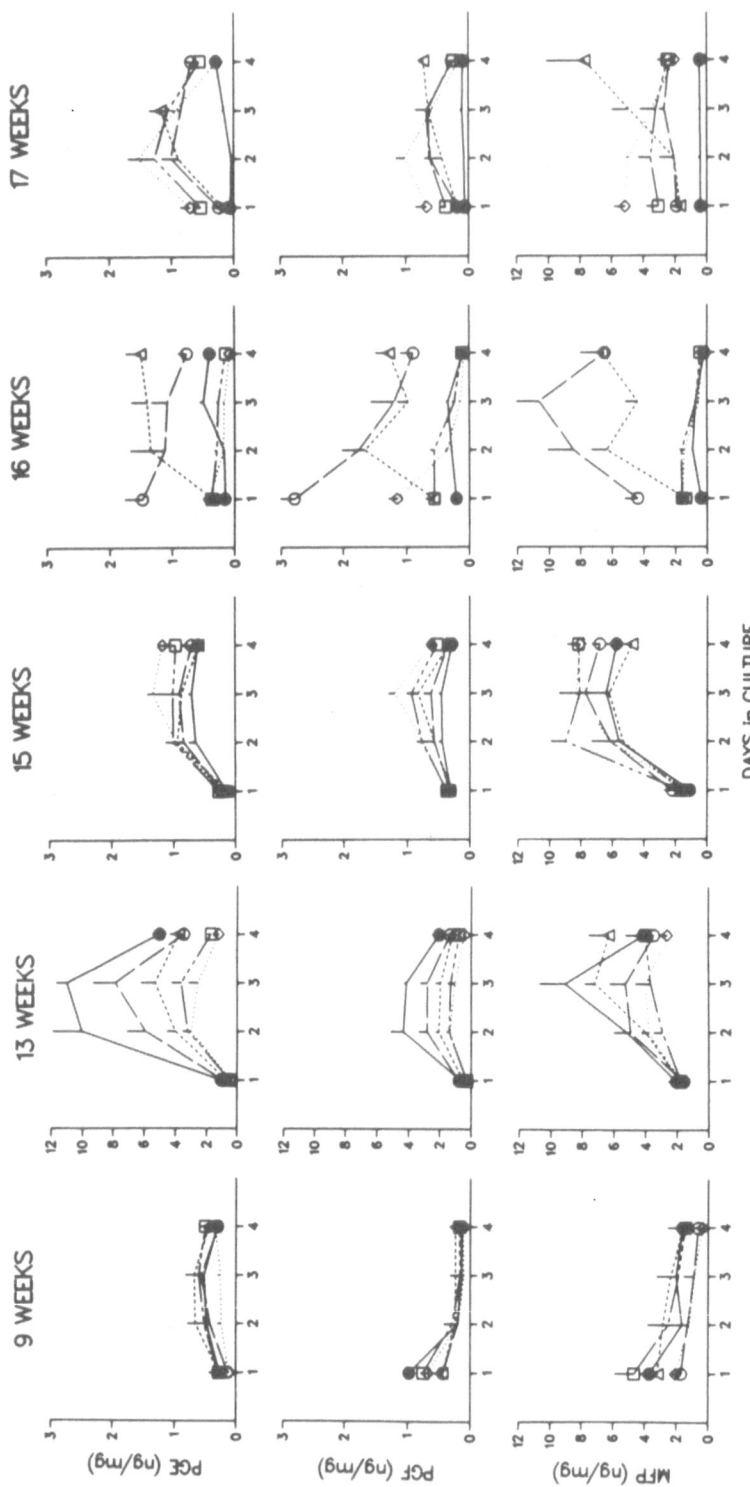

FIGURE 7 Mean (±SEM) PGE, PGF and MPF from human placental explants of varying gestational ages over 8 days of culture when incubated with LH-RH. Symbols as in Fig. 4. Reproduced from Siler-Khodr et al., in press, with permission.

168

LH-RH antagonist. However, by 13 weeks of gestation, a potent inhibition of αhCG, hCG, P, E_1, E_2, PGE, PGF and PFM release was observed (Fig. 8). Also, in the 15-week cultures, where basal hormonal releases had already declined, this antagonist again inhibited release of αhCG, hCG, P, E_1, PGE, PGF, PFM, but not E_2. Concomitant addition of synthetic LH-RH at 10 times the concentration of the antagonist did not override the effects of the antagonist at 13 weeks. However, at 15 weeks, this dose of synthetic LH-RH partially reversed the antagonist's inhibition of P and totally reversed the suppression of E_1, PGE, PGF and PFM. PG releases were even stimulated above the controls. These data demonstrated that an LH-RH antagonist can compete with endogenous placental LH-RH-like activity and that LH-RH can reverse its effects. Thus, it appears that endogenous placental LH-RH-like activity influences these hormonal releases and that the endogenous LH-RH-like receptors can be positively and negatively competed for using LH-RH or its antagonist.

These data on placental hormonal release in vitro have led to the following theory about placental endocrine function throughout gestation: The human placenta synthesizes a molecule or molecules which have LH-RH activity similar to that of the hypothalamic factor. One of these placental factors is chemically similar to LH-RH. Highest concentrations of placental LH-RH-like activity occur around the time of peak hCG production. Placental receptors for LH-RH-like activity are present by this stage of gestation. The basal release of αhCG, hCG, P, E_1, E_2, PGE, PGF and PFM can be inhibited by an LH-RH antagonist, indicating that their production is dependent on the endogenous LH-RH-like activity. The possibility exists that there is more than one endogenous placental LH-RH-like activity with one being more potent than LH-RH in effecting prostaglandin release, since LH-RH inhibits prostaglandin production at the gestational stage when endogenous LH-RH activity is highest and prostaglandin release per mg placental tissue is highest. As the placenta matures, the cytotrophoblasts, the source of LH-RH-like activity, decline, leaving free receptors which exogenous LH-RH can stimulate to increase hormonal production. With the progress of gestation and a further decline of endogenous LH-RH-like activity, the greatest percent response to LH-RH is observed. By term, although LH-RH still stimulated sizable releases of αhCG, hCG and P, it is attenuated when compared to that at 16 and 17 weeks, suggesting either a decline in receptors and/or a modulation of their response by higher steroid levels. Steroid modulation of αhCG and hCG stimulation by LH-RH was also indicated, since its maximal responses occurred in the absence of estrogens. Release of P appears to be tied to that of hCG, but estrogen and prostaglandin response to LH-RH appeared independent of hCG, since their increase to LH-RH occurred prior to that of hCG, and, in many instances, without any concomitant effect on hCG.

IN VIVO STUDIES

Several in vivo studies have also been completed. Concentrations of circulating immunoreactive LH-RH in maternal blood throughout pregnancy were highest in early pregnancy [33], as were placental LH-RH-like concentrations [2]. Additionally, throughout all of pregnancy,

169

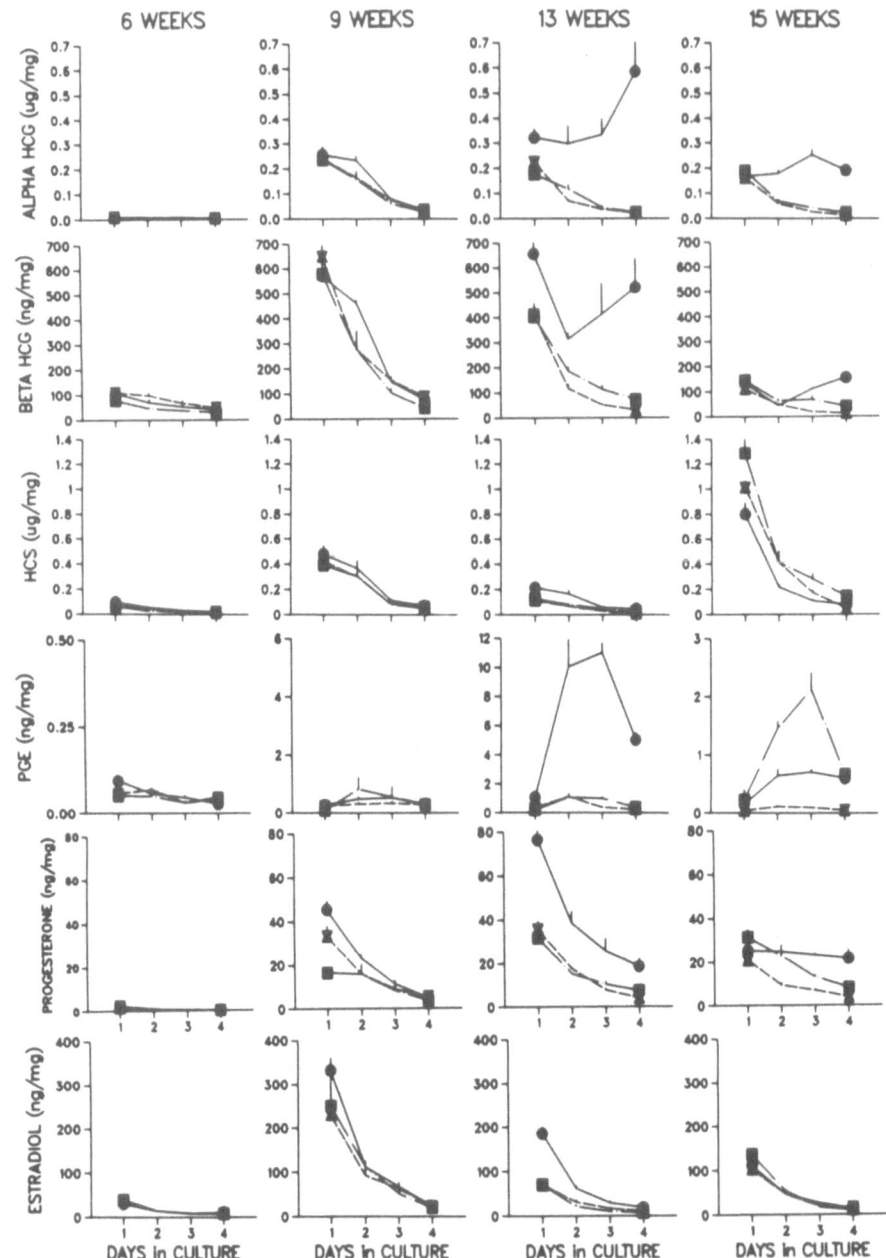

FIGURE 8 Release of αhCG, hCG, hCS, P, E₂ and PGE (mean ± SEM) from
human placental explants of varying gestational ages over
4 days of culture when incubated with 1 μg/ml LH-RH
antagonist (xx--xx), 1 μg/ml LH-RH antagonist and 10 μg/ml
LH-RH (■—·—■ or control (●——●). Reproduced from Siler-
Khodr et al., Placenta, in press and Siler-Khodr et al.,
Prostaglandins, 31, 1003 (1986), with permission.

circulating levels were increased above that in non-pregnant women, suggesting the apparent placental LH-RH immunoactivity may enter the maternal circulation. These levels may have predictive value as, in four cases with very low concentrations of apparent LH-RH immunoactivity in the maternal circulation, premature labor occurred.

In other studies, exogenous LH-RH was administered as an intravenous bolus to the mother. These studies were performed in pregnant women of 8-13 and 16-19 weeks gestation. A decrease of circulating αhCG and hCG was observed which was dose-related. Estrogens were increased, while progesterone was increased only at the lower doses and decreased at the higher doses. At midgestation, the only significant change which occurred following LH-RH administration of 0.2 or 0.5 µg/ml was a suppression of hCG. These findings indicate that the very high doses of LH-RH administered to women in early pregnancy can alter circulating αhCG, hCG, estrogens and P. Although the mechanisms of these effects cannot be delineated from these studies, it is of interest that, as in the placental culture studies, estrogens were increased by LH-RH without a concomitant increase in hCG.

In similar studies performed in pregnant monkeys at 22-30 days, 90-106 days and 155-162 days of gestation, circulating levels of monkey CG (mCG), and P were determined. At all stages of pregnancy, LH-RH caused a stimulation of P which was dose-related at mid and late gestation. MCG had a small increase, only in early pregnancy. Once again, an effect of an LH-RH-like activity on circulating hormone levels during pregnancy was indicated from these data and, since effects were also observed in mid and term pregnancies when ovarian steroidogenesis is no longer significant, it appears these progesterone changes should reflect a placental action of the LH-RH.

Other investigators [34] have actively immunized marmoset monkeys to LH-RH. One of these monkeys was two weeks pregnant at the time of primary injection. Maximum titres were reached by eight weeks, then circulating P concentrations declined and, by 12 weeks, the pregnancy was aborted. In two other studies [35,36], baboons received agonists of LH-RH during early pregnancy and abortion resulted in many of the animals. In one of these studies [35], bCG was shown to decrease following administration of the agonist. Other investigators [37-39] have shown that either LH-RH, LH-RH agonist or LH-RH antagonist administered to rats in early and late pregnancy resulted in pregnancy failure. Further studies showed a similar action of LH-RH in hypophysectomized rats in late pregnancy, demonstrating an extra-pituitary action of the LH-RH-like interactions.

The action of two different antagonists given to baboons during early pregnancy has also been studied [40,41]. In these studies, 6 animals were administered two different antagonists via a mini pump for 7 days at 35-45 days of pregnancy (well past the time of the ovarian-placental shift in this species [42]). One pregnancy ended in spontaneous abortion, two in stillbirths and one in neonatal death. Of the two animals delivering well live-borns, one developed antibodies to the antagonist which may have protected it from its deleterious action. Circulating baboon CG, P, E_1 and E_2 levels were determined before, during, and after antagonist administration and a transient suppression of progesterone during drug exposure was observed. Effects on bCG were difficult to assess, since it normally declines rapidly at this time of gestation. However, later in gestation, estrogens were lower in the animals that delivered stillborns, and labor was prolonged. We speculate that the early insult with this dose of antagonist may have been insufficient to abort the pregnancy, but damaged the placenta and its later ability to produce adequate estrogens and PGs for the normal progress of labor.

These studies in vivo indicate that LH-RH-like activity influences the level of maternal circulating hormones during pregnancy. One site of the LH-RH actions should be the placenta, since in each (the human, monkey, and baboon), when studies were done even after the time of the ovarian-placental shift, LH-RH altered hormonal releases and/or resulted in a deleterious outcome of pregnancy. These data also indicate that administration of LH-RH analogues to the mother may be effective in influencing placental endocrine function and thus the progress of pregnancy. Since, in some pregnancies, low LH-RH-like activity has been associated with abnormal outcome, possibly maternal circulating LH-RH-like activity could have predictive value and/or placental stimulation with LH-RH analogues be effective therapeutically. In addition, placental hormonal function is unquestionably affected by LH-RH and its response to LH-RH varies dramatically during gestation. It is indicated that the variations may be related to the concentration of endogenous placental LH-RH-like activity, the receptor number and/or the steroid milieu. Studies utilizing an antagonist of LH-RH demonstrate the specificity of this system and the importance of endogenous LH-RH-like activity in maintaining placental αhCG, hCG, PGs and steroids release.

CONCLUSIONS

In summary, the presence of LH-RH-like activities in the human placenta is well established. One of these activities is similar to the decapeptide LH-RH and specific receptors for this peptide are present in the placenta. In addition, yet another activity exists that is a potent stimulator of prostaglandin and placental hCG release. LH-RH like activity of the placenta affects CG, steroid and prostaglandin release, thus, in the placenta, there is a complete paracrine system involving these hormones. Delineation of this system needs further study. However, studies to date indicate that human placental endocrine function is responsive to exogenous GnRH or its antagonist by at least 9-13 weeks of gestation. The dynamic nature of placenal endocrine function and the presence of multiple feedback interaction has been demonstrated. These conclusions are supported by the finding that, around 13-15 weeks of gestation, high basal hCG release in vitro continues without further GnRH stimulation, yet by 16-17 weeks, exogenous GnRH and removal of estrogen precursors are needed to allow for continued hCG release. Even greater modulation of endocrine release to GnRH is observed at term. In addition, in vivo studies demonstrating the action of GnRH analogues on endocrine parameters in pregnant baboons support the hypothesis that GnRH-like activities play a physiologic role in pregnancy. Definition of the multiple factors that influence GnRH-like activities throughout gestation needs to be investigated. However, studies to date support the proposal that LH-RH or LH-RH analogue may be useful to affect placental function during pregnancy.

REFERENCES

1. Gibbons, J.M., Jr., Mitnick, M. and Chieffo, V. In vitro biosynthesis of TSH- and LH-releasing factors by the human placenta. Am. J. Obstet. Gynecol., 121, 127 (1975).
2. Siler-Khodr, T.M. and Khodr, G.S. Content of luteinizing hormone releasing factor in the human placenta. Am. J. Obstet. Gynecol., 130, 216, (1978).
3. Khodr, G.S. and Siler-Khodr, T.M. Localization of luteinizing hormone-releasing factor (LRF) in the human placenta. Fertil. Steril., 29, 523 (1978).
4. Miyake, A., Sakumoto, T., Aono, T., Kawamura, Y., Maeda, T. and Kurachi, K. Changes in luteinizing hormone-releasing hormone in human placenta throughout pregnancy. Obstet. Gynecol., 60, 444 (1982).
5. Siler-Khodr, T.M. and Khodr, G.S. Extrahypothalamic luteinizing hormone releasing factor (LRF): Release of immunoreactive LRF by the human placenta in vitro. Fertil. Steril., 32, 294 (1979).
6. Khodr, G.S. and Siler-Khodr, T.M. Placental LRF and its synthesis. Science, 207, 315 (1980).
7. Lee, J.N., Seppälä, M. and Chard, T. Characterization of placental luteinizing hormone-releasing factor-like material. Acta Endocrinol. (Copenh.), 96, 394 (1981).
8. Tan, L. and Rousseau, P. The chemical identity of the immunoreactive LHRH-like peptide biosynthesized in the human placenta. Biochem. Biophys. Res. Commun., 109, 1061 (1982).
9. Seeburg, P.H. and Adelman, J.P. Characterization of cDNA for precursor of human luteinizing hormone releasing hormone. Nature, 311, 666 (1984).
10. Gautron, J.P., Pattou, E. and Kordon, C. Occurrence of higher molecular forms of LHRH in fractionated extracts from rat hypothalamus, cortex and placenta. Mol. Cell. Endocrinol., 24, 1 (1981).
11. Nowak, R., Wiseman, B.S., Bahr, J.M. Identification of a GnRH-like factor in the rabbit fetal placenta. Biol. Reprod., 31, 67 (1984).
12. Millar, R.P., Wormald, P.J. and Milton, R.C. Stimulation of gonadotropin release by a non-GnRH peptide sequence of the GnRH precursor. Science, 232, 68 (1986).
13. Siler-Khodr, T.M. Hypothalamic-like peptides of the placenta. In "Seminars in reproductive endocrinology", G. Weiss (Ed.), Thieme-Stratton, New York, 1983, p. 321.
14. Siler-Khodr, T.M. Hypothalamic-like releasing hormones of the placenta. In "Clinics in perinatology", S.S.C. Yen (Ed.), W.B. Saunders, Philadelphia, 1983, p 553.
15. Siler-Khodr, T.M. Human chorionic gonadotropin releasing hormone. In "Gynecology and obstetrics. Proceedings of the XIth World Congress", K. Thomsen, H. Ludwig (Eds.), Springer Verlag, Heidelberg, in press.
16. Currie, A.J., Fraser, H.M. and Sharpe, R.M. Human placental receptors for luteinizing hormone releasing hormone. Biochem. Biophys. Res. Commun., 99, 332 (1981).

17. Belisle, S., Guevin, J.-F., Bellabarba, D. and Lehoux, J.-G. Luteinizing hormone-releasing hormone binds to enriched human placental membranes and stimulates in vitro the synthesis of bioactive human chorionic gonadotropin. J. Clin. Endocrinol. Metab., 59, 119 (1984).

18. Iwashita, M., Evans, M.I. and Catt, K.J. Characterization of a gonadotropin-releasing hormone receptor site in term placenta and chorionic villi. J. Clin. Endocrinol. Metab., 62, 127 (1986).

19. Miura, S., Osathanondh, R., Makris, A., Todd, R.B., Levesque, L.A. and Ryan, K.J. Effect of luteinizing hormone-releasing factor (LRF) on the concentrations of 3', 5'-cyclic adenosine monophosphate (cAMP) and human chorionic gonadotropin (hCG) in trophoblastic tissue in vitro. The 26th Annual Meeting of the Society for Gynecologic Investigation, San Diego, Abstract #168, p 102, 1979

20. Haning, R.V., Choi, L., Kiggens, A.J., Kuzma, D.L. and Summerville, J.W. Effects of dibutyl cAMP, LHRH, and aromatase inhibitor on simultaneous outputs of prostaglandin $F_{2\alpha}$ and 13,14-dihydro-15-keto prostaglandin $F_{2\alpha}$ by term placental explants. Prostaglandins, 23, 29 (1982).

21. Haning, R.V., Choi, L., Kiggens, A.J. and Kuzma, D.L. Effects of prostaglandins, dibutyryl cAMP, LHRH, estrogens, progesterone, and potassium on output of prostaglandin $F_{2\alpha}$, 13,14-dihydro-15-keto-prostaglandin $F_{2\alpha}$, hCG, estradiol, and progesterone by placental minces. Prostaglandins, 24, 495 (1982).

22. Haning, R.V., Jr., Chot, L., Kiggens, A.J., Kuzma, D.L. and Summerville, J.W. Effects of dibutyryl adenosine e', 5'-monophosphate, luteinizing hormone-releasing hormone, and aromatase inhibitor on simultaneous outputs of progesterone, 17 beta-estradiol, and human chorionic gonadotropin by term placental explants. J. Clin. Endocrinol. Metab., 55, 212 (1982).

23. Khodr, G.S. and Siler-Khodr, T.M. The effect of luteinizing hormone releasing factor (LRF) on hCG secretion. Fertil. Steril., 30, 301 (1978).

24. Siler-Khodr, T.M. and Khodr, G.S. Dose response analysis of GnRH stimulation of hCG release from human term placenta. Biol. Reprod., 25, 353 (1981).

25. Butzow, R. Luteinizing hormone-releasing factor increases release of human chorionic gonadotrophin in isolated cell columns of normal and malignant trophoblasts. Int. J. Cancer, 29, 9 (1982).

26. Siler-Khodr, T.M., Khodr, G.S., Valenzuela, G. and Rhode, J. GnRH effects on placental hormones during gestation. I. αhCG, hCG and hCS. Biol. Reprod., 34, 245 (1986).

27. Siler-Khodr, T.M., Khodr, G.S., Valenzuela, G. and Rhode, J. GnRH effects on placental hormones during gestation. II. Progesterone, estrone, estradiol and estriol. Biol. Reprod., 34, 255 (1986).

28. Branchaud, C.L., Goodyer, C.G. and Lipowski, L.S. Progesterone and estrogen production by placental monolayer cultures: Effects of dehydroepiandrosterone and luteinizing hormone-

releasing hormone. J. Clin. Endocrinol. Metab., **56**, 761 (1983).

29. Siler-Khodr, T.M. GnRH effects on placental hormones during gestation. III. Prostaglandin E, prostaglandin F and 13,14-dihydro-15-keto-prostaglandin F. Biol. Reprod., **34**, 312 (1986).

30. Siler-Khodr, T.M., Khodr, G.S., Vickery, B.H. and Nestor, J.J. Inhibition of hCG, αhCG and progesterone release from human placental tissue in vitro by a GnRH antagonist. Life Sci., **32**, 2741 (1983).

31. Siler-Khodr, T.M., Khodr, G.S., Harper, M.J.K., Rhode, J., Vickery, B.H. and Nestor, J.J., Jr. Differential inhibition of human placental prostaglandin release in vitro by a GnRH antagonist. Prostaglandins, **31**, 1003 (1986).

32. Siler-Khodr, T.M., Khodr, G.S., Rhode, J., Vickery, B.H. and Nestor, J.J., Jr. Gestational age related inhibition of placental hCG, αhCG and steroid hormone release in vitro by a GnRH antagonist. Placenta (1986) in press.

33. Siler-Khodr, T.M., Khodr, G.S. and Valenzuela, G. Immunoreactive GnRH level in maternal circulation throughout pregnancy. Am. J. Obstet. Gynecol., **150**, 376 (1984).

34. Hodges, J.K. and Hearn, J.P. Effects of immunisation against luteinising hormone releasing hormone on reproduction of the marmoset monkey. Callithrix jacchus. Nature, **265**, 746 (1977).

35. Vickery, B.H., McRae, G.I. and Stevens, V.C. Suppression of luteal and placental function in pregnant baboons with agonist analogs of luteinizing hormone-releasing hormones. Fertil. Steril., **36**, 664 (1981)

36. Das, C. and Talwar, G.P. Pregnancy-terminating action of a luteinizing hormone-releasing hormone agonist D-Ser (Bu^t)^{6}des Gly^{10}ProEA in baboons. Fertil. Steril., **39**, 218 (1983).

37. Macdonald, G.J. and Beattie, C.W. Pregnancy failure in hypophysectomized rats following LH-RH administration. Life Sci., **24**, 1103 (1979).

38. Bex, F.H. and Corbin, A. Luteinizing hormone-releasing hormone (LHRH) and LHRH agonist termination of pregnancy in hypophysectomized rats: Extrapituitary site of action. Endocrinology, **108**, 273 (1981).

39. Rivier, C. and Vale, W. Interaction of gonadotropin-releasing hormone agonist and antagonist with progesterone, prolactin, or human chorionic gonadotropin during pregnancy in the rat. Endocrinology, **110**, 347 (1982).

40. Siler-Khodr, T.M., Kuehl, T. and Vickery, B.H. Effects of a gonadotropin releasing hormone antagonist on hormonal levels in the pregnant baboon and on fetal outcome. Fertil. Steril., **41**, 448 (1980).

41. Siler-Khodr, T.M., Kuehl, T. and Vickery, B. Action of a GnRH antagonist on the pregnant baboon. The 32nd Annual Meeting of the Society for Gynecologic Investigation (Phoenix), Abstract #249:142, 1985

42. Castracane, V.D. and Goldzieher, J.W. Timing of the luteal-placental shift in the baboon (Papio cynocephalus). Endocrinology, **118**, 506 (1986).

SECTION 4

PHARMACOLOGY OF LHRH ANTAGONISTS

11

In Vitro Histamine Release with LHRH Analogs

M.J. KARTEN[1], W.A. HOOK[2], R.P. SIRAGANIAN[2], D.H. COY[3], K FOLKERS[4] J.E. RIVER[5] and R.W. ROESKE[6]

[1]Contraceptive Development Branch, Center for Population Research, NICHHD, NIH, Bethesda, MD 20892; [2]Clinical Immunology Section, Lab. Microbiol. Immunol., NIDR, NIH, Bethesda, MD 20892; [3]Tulane University, New Orleans, LA 70112; [4]University of Texas, Austin, TX 78712; [5]The Salk Institute, La Jolla, CA 92037; [6]Indiana University School of Medicine, Indianapolis, IN 46223, USA

INTRODUCTION

A variety of peptides such as substance P, somatostatin, vasoactive intestinal peptide, gastrin, etc., have been reported to trigger the release of histamine from mast cells [1-5]. These cells are found in many tissues, notably skin, gingiva, lung and mesentery. They have prominent granules which contain histamine and other mediators of inflammation which can be released causing dilation of capillaries and increased vascular permeability. However, the finding by Schmidt et al. that a potent LHRH antagonist, [N-Ac-D-Nal(2)^1,D-pF-Phe^2,D-Trp^3,D-Arg^6]LHRH, produced transient edema of the face and extremities when administered subcutaneously to rats at 1.25 mg/kg, or 50-100 times the effective antiovulatory dose [6], had a significant impact on the development of LHRH antago-nists as potential contraceptive agents. This observation suggest-ed that LHRH analogs might release histamine and other inflammatory mediators from cells. Subsequently, accounts of in vitro histamine release by LHRH analogs were reported by Nekola et al. [7], Hook et al. [8], and by Karten and Rivier [9]. Morgan et al. have compared several LHRH antagonists for histamine release in vivo and in vitro [10]. Roeske et al. [11], Rivier et al. [12], and Folkers et al. [13] have described some efforts to reduce the histamine releasing potential of LHRH antagonists through struct-ural modification.

Histamine release can also be triggered by antigen reacting with the antibody of allergy (IgE) attached to a histamine-con-taining cell. When two adjacent IgE molecules are bridged by a specific antigen, the cell is triggered to release histamine. In IgE-mediated, as well as some other mechanisms of release, fusion of the granule membrane with the cell membrane occurs causing the secretion of histamine and other mediators out of the cell in a non-cytotoxic manner [14]. We have seen no evidence that histamine release by LHRH is IgE-mediated.

The other histamine-containing leukocyte is the basophil, which can be triggered to release histamine by some of the same agents and by pathways similar to those found in mast cells. Baso-phils circulate in the blood of humans, rats and guinea pigs where they constitute less than 1% of the leukocytes. Like mast cells,

179

normal basophils do not replicate in culture. However, a histamine-containing cultured rat basophilic leukemia cell line (RBL-2H3) has been developed and used frequently for studies of the biochemical pathways involved in histamine release [15]. We have seen no evidence of histamine release from human basophils or cultured RBL-2H3 cells by LHRH or its analogs. Basophils differ from mast cells in several important ways [15] and these differences may account for the histamine release response to LHRH by one cell type and not the other.

The discovery of the edematogenic and anaphylactoid properties of the D-Arg[6]-related LHRH antagonist modifications necessitated further structural changes if these LHRH antagonists were to receive serious consideration as potential contraceptive agents. The release of histamine by LHRH agonists and antagonists, as well as by other peptides, appears to be a function of specific structural parameters which are independent of other inherent biological activities. It should therefore be possible to incorporate structural elements which would retain the gonadotropin-suppressive properties of the most potent LHRH antagonists and yet would greatly reduce the histamine releasing potency of these analogs. This chapter describes the methods used to measure peptide-induced histamine release from mast cells, the characteristics of the reaction, the reproducibility of the assay, structure-activity relationships of LHRH analogs with respect to histamine release, and observations on the separation of antiovulatory activity from histamine releasing activity for the LHRH antagonists.

METHODS FOR HISTAMINE RELEASE

The in vitro histamine release reaction is simple. A suspension of rat mast cells is added to increasing concentrations of peptide and the mixture is incubated for a few minutes followed by centrifugation to collect the histamine in the supernatant. A PIPES (piperazine-N,N'-bis[2-ethanesulfonic acid]) medium buffered at pH 7.4 containing NaCl 119 mM, KCl 5 mM, PIPES 25mM, NaOH 40 mM, glucose 5.6 mM, $CaCl_2$ 1 mM, and 0.1% bovine serum albumin was used. This was designated as PIPES AC. Peptides were dissolved in double distilled H_2O at a concentration of 2 mg/ml and stored at -20°C. They were thawed just prior to testing, diluted in PIPES AC and prewarmed for 5 min at 37°C. Peptides studied were stable to heating at 56°C for 2 hr, and to freezing and thawing.

Peritoneal cells were collected from male Sprague-Dawley rats weighing 200 to 250 gm and purchased from Harlan (Madison, WI). After euthanasia by CO_2, the peritoneal cavity was washed with 50 ml PIPES AC medium containing 20 units of heparin. Following centrifugation at 200 x g for 8 min at 4°C, cells were washed again and finally resuspended to a concentration of 8 to 24 x 10^5 total leukocytes/ml in PIPES AC. This suspension contained approximately 5-10% mast cells. Washed cells were used immediately after collection and were prewarmed for 5 min at 37°C prior to pipetting 0.25 ml aliquots into 12 x 75 mm polystyrene tubes containing 0.25 ml of diluted peptide. Mixtures were incubated for 15 min at 37°C and the reaction stopped by centrifugation at 400 x g for 15 min at 4°C. The cell supernatants were assayed for histamine content by the automated fluorometric assay procedure [16,17]. Alternatively, a more laborious manual fluorometric assay method may be employed which gives similar results [17]. The LHRH analog 4 (Table 1) was tested with the mast cells of each rat as a standard in each experiment.

CHARACTERISTICS OF THE HISTAMINE RELEASE REACTION

Figure 1 gives typical dose response curves and demonstrates how ED_{50} values, expressed in µg/ml, were determined. The most potent histamine releasing compounds were the LHRH antagonists such as compounds 1, 4 and 7, while the LHRH superagonists such as compounds 41 and 42 were markedly less potent as histamine releasers (Table 1). Dose response curves are typically steep across the 50% endpoint; the peptides usually achieved 100% histamine release at higher concentrations (Figure 1). In this experiment mast cells were purified to greater than 90% by centrifugation through

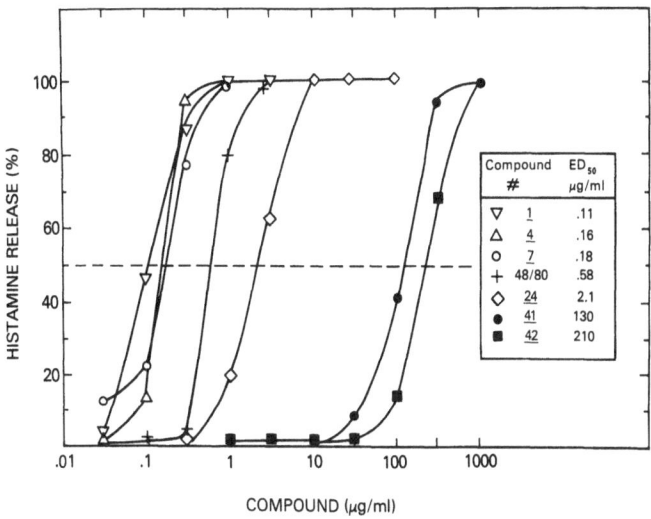

FIGURE 1 Typical dose response curves of six LHRH analogs and compound 48/80 demonstrating how ED_{50} values are graphically determined.

Percoll and incubated for 15 min with the histamine releasing compound. The response curves and ED_{50} values were similar to those obtained with unpurified cell suspensions, suggesting that other cell types are not required for histamine release. For routine testing, mast cells were not purified. In other experiments, where mast cell supernatants were concommitantly assayed for release of lactic dehydrogenase, there was no evidence seen of cell toxicity induced by LHRH or any analog tested (1, 4, 5, 7, 24, 38, 42). There was no enhancement of histamine release by

181

phosphatidyl serine with LHRH and the analogs listed above. This is in contrast to the IgE-triggered release reaction from rat mast cells which is highly dependent on the addition of phosphatidyl serine to reaction mixtures.

Other differences from allergic-type release include the short incubation time required and the lack of a calcium requirement. The time needed for maximal histamine release was less than 1 min, even at less than optimal peptide concentrations. Neither added calcium nor magnesium ions were essential for histamine release by LHRH, its analog 4, or compound 48/80. However, with these agents, greater release occurred when 1 mM Ca++ was included in the medium. Less release was seen when 1 mM Mg++ was substituted for 1 mM Ca++. Histamine release was greater at 25°C and 27°C than at 17°C, and no release occurred when cells were incubated with peptide at 1°C. This is further suggestive evidence that the histamine release is due to a secretory rather than a cytolytic effect of the peptides.

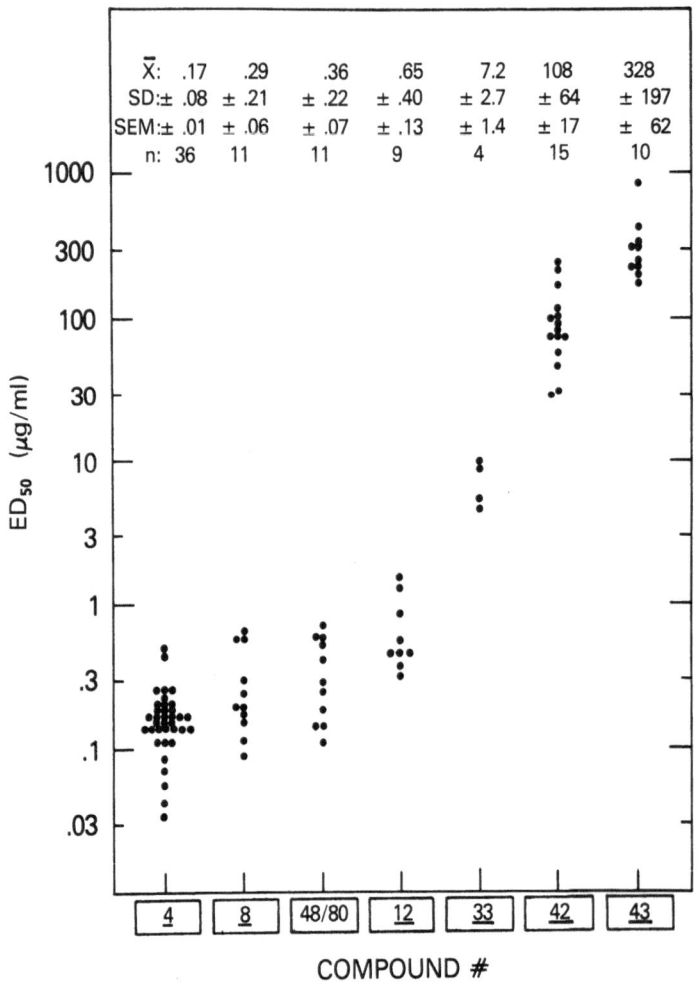

FIGURE 2   Reproducibility of histamine release results over a 20-month period.

Reproducibility of the histamine release reaction in multiple experiments is demonstrated in Figure 2 which gives results obtained over a 20-month period. The overall range seen for each compound is approximately 10-fold and this variation may be due to individual differences in sensitivity among rats. Each point represents the mean of duplicate or triplicate determinations. Figure 2 also shows that a similar variation in ED_{50} was encountered with compound 48/80 which differs in its basic structure from the LHRH analogs.

Certain peptides are not completely soluble in H_2O and this may affect the reproducibility of the assay. In these cases a suitable solvent such as DMSO or ethanol may be used to prepare the stock solution if suitable controls are included to assure that there is no effect of the solvent on the release reaction. All peptides were tested in duplicate or triplicate with mast cells from a minimum of 3 different rats. In general, variations in ED_{50} values obtained in day-to-day assays may be minimized by multiple tests using consistent technique, solubilizing the peptides and using a homogeneous source of rats.

STRUCTURE-ACTIVITY RELATIONSHIPS (SAR)

The SAR data in Table 1 are presented in order of decreasing histamine releasing potency of the LHRH analogs. The standard reference LHRH antagonist is [N-Ac-D-Nal(2)[1],D-pF-Phe[2],D-Trp[3],D-Arg[6]]LHRH, 4, which has an $ED_{50} = 0.17 + .01$ µg/ml. Comparisons of potency will refer to this standard unless otherwise indicated (e.g., comparisons with a parent analog). The relative potencies reported herein will differ slightly from some previously reported potencies [8,9] due to the inclusion of additional assay data.

Structural Characteristics for Potent Histamine Releasers

The structural characteristics of the most potent LHRH analogs in triggering histamine release in vitro involve a combination of a strongly basic D-amino acid side chain (Arg or Lys) at position 6 (in close proximity to Arg[8]) and a cluster of hydrophobic aromatic amino acids at the N-terminus (e.g., analogs 1-10). Thus, the standard, 4, is approximately 2000x more potent than LHRH, 43. The replacement of the aliphatic side chain in position 7 by an aromatic one (compare 3 with 4 and compare 6 and 9 with 1) has a slight, if any, modulating effect on in vitro histamine releasing potency. Although the basic guanidino function on the D-hArg(Et$_2$)[6] modification (8) is partially shielded, it still retains high histamine releasing potency - albeit approximately one-third that of its closely related parent (1). The Bal[3] (Bal = benzothienyl-alanine, the sulfur isostere of tryptophan) analog, 10, was only half as active as its parent, 7 in releasing histamine. The effect of D-Ala[10] in enhancing histamine releasing potency is unclear due to the unavailability of an adequate number of appropriate

Table 1. LHRH Analogs[a]: histamine releasing potency and antiovulatory potency

Analog	In Vitro Histamine Release[b] (μg/ml) $ED_{50} \pm$ SEM	Ovulation Inhibition[c] (μg/rat) Corn Oil ED_{100}
1. [N-Ac-D-Nal(2)[1], D-pCl-Phe[2], D-Trp[3], D-Arg[6], D-Ala[10]]LHRH	$0.10 \pm .02$	1.0
2. [N-Ac-D-Nal(2)[1], D-Phe[2,3], D-Arg[6], Phe[7], D-Ala[10]]LHRH	$0.11 \pm .04$	2.5
3. [N-Ac-D-Nal(2)[1], D-pF-Phe[2], D-Trp[3], D-Arg[6], Phe[7]]LHRH	$0.16 \pm .01$	-
4. [N-Ac-D-Nal(2)[1], D-pF-Phe[2], D-Trp[3], D-Arg[6]]LHRH	$0.17 \pm .01$	2.5
5. [N-Ac-D-pCl-Phe[1], D-pCl-Phe[2], D-Trp[3], D-Lys[6], D-Ala[10]]LHRH	$0.19 \pm .06$	>7.5[d]
6. [N-Ac-D-Nal(2)[1], D-pCl-Phe[2], D-Trp[3], D-Arg[6], Phe[7], D-Ala[10]]LHRH	$0.20 \pm .03$	>>0.5[e]
7. [N-Ac-D-pCl-Phe[1], D-pCl-Phe[2], D-Trp[3], D-Arg[6], D-Ala[10]]LHRH	$0.26 \pm .07$	3.0
8. [N-Ac-D-Nal(2)[1], D-pF-Phe[2], D-Trp[3], D-hArg(Et$_2$)[6], D-Ala[10]]LHRH	$0.29 \pm .06$	>1.5
9. [N-Ac-D-Nal(2)[1], D-pCl-Phe[2], D-Trp[3], D-Arg[6], pF-Phe[7], D-Ala[10]]LHRH	$0.32 \pm .13$	2.5
10. [N-Ac-D-pCl-Phe[1], D-pCl-Phe[2], D-Trp[3], D-Bal[3], D-Arg[6], D-Ala[10]]LHRH	$0.52 \pm .03$	>2.0
11. [N-Ac-D-pCl-Phe[1], D-pF-Phe[2], D-Trp[3], D-Arg[5]]LHRH	$0.60 \pm .01$	-
12. [N-Ac-D-Nal(2)[1], D-C$^\alpha$-Me-pCl-Phe[2], D-Pal[3], D-Arg[6], 4-Thia-Lys[8], D-Ala[10]]LHRH	$0.65 \pm .13$	1.0
13. [N-Ac-D-Nal(2)[1], D-pF-Phe[2], D-Trp[3], Arg[6]]LHRH	$0.83 \pm .12$	>>5.0
14. [N-Ac-D-Nal(2)[1], D-pCl-Phe[2], D-Pal[3], Arg[5], D-Glu(AA)[6], D-Ala[10]]LHRH[f]	$1.6 \pm .66$	1.5(s)[g]
15. [N-Ac-D-Nal(2)[1], D-pCl-Phe[2], D-Pal[3], Arg[5], D-Nal(2)[6], D-Ala[10]]LHRH	$1.9 \pm .10$	>>1.0
16. [N-Ac-D-Nal(2)[1], D-pCl-Phe[2], D-Pal[3], Arg[5], D-Trp[6], D-Ala[10]]LHRH	$2.1 \pm .23$	>>5.0
17. [N-Ac-D-pCl-Phe[1], D-pCl-Phe[2], D-Trp[3], D-Ala[10]]LHRH	$2.2 \pm .34$	-
18. [N-Ac-D-Nal(2)[1], D-pF-Phe[2], D-Trp[3], Arg[5]]LHRH	$2.2 \pm .05$	-
19. [N-Ac-D-Nal(2)[1], D-pF-Phe[2], D-Trp[3,6]]LHRH	$2.3 \pm .21$	-
20. [N-Ac-D-Nal(2)[1], D-pCl-Phe[2], D-Pal[3,6], Trp[7], D-Ala[10]]LHRH	$2.6 \pm .56$	(>>0.5)[h]
21. [N-Ac-D-Nal(2)[1], D-pCl-Phe[2], D-Pal[3,6], Arg[5], D-Ala[10]]LHRH	$2.9 \pm .33$	1.0
22. [N-Ac-D-Nal(2)[1], D-C$^\alpha$-Me-pCl-Phe[2], D-Pal[3], Lys(iPr)[5,8], D-Tyr[6], D-Ala[10]]LHRH	$3.2 \pm .41$	1.0
23. [N-Ac-D-Nal(2)[1], D-C$^\alpha$-Me-pCl-Phe[2], D-Trp[3], Aopmp[6-7], D-Ala[10]]LHRH[i]	$3.2 \pm .60$	10.0
24. [N-Ac-D-Nal(2)[1], D-C$^\alpha$-Me-pCl-Phe[2], D-Trp[3], Arg[5], D-Tyr[6], D-Ala[10]]LHRH	$3.7 \pm .80$	2.5
25. [N-Ac-D-Nal(2)[1], D-pCl-Phe[2], D-Pal[3], Arg[5], D-Tyr[6], D-Ala[10]]LHRH	$3.7 \pm .51$	>>0.5(s)

184

#	Analog[a]	Histamine release[b]	Antiovulatory[c]
26.	[N-Ac-D-Nal(2)^1,D-Cα-Me-pCl-Phe^2,D-Pal^3,D-Arg^6,Lys(iPr)^8,D-Ala^{10}]LHRH	$4.0 + .40$	1.0
27.	[N-Ac-D-Nal(2)^1,D-Cα-Me-pCl-Phe^2,D-Trp^3,D-Arg^6,His8,D-Ala^{10}]LHRH	$4.5 + .72$	>>5.0
28.	[N-Ac-D-Nal(2)^1,D-Cα-Me-pCl-Phe^2,D-Pal^3,D-Arg^6,hArg(Et$_2$)^8,D-Ala^{10}]LHRH	$4.9 + .33$	1.0
29.	[N-Ac-D-Nal(2)^1,D-pCl-Phe^2,D-Pal^{3,6},Pal^5,D-Ala^{10}]LHRH	$5.1 + 1.0$	(>1.0)
30.	[N-Ac-D-Nal(2)^1,D-Cα-Me-pCl-Phe^2,D-Trp^3,N-Me-Tyr^5,D-Arg^6]LHRH (1-6)	$5.7 + .19$	>>1000
31.	[N-Ac-D-Nal(2)^1,D-pCl-Phe^2,D-Pal^3,Arg^5,D-Trp^6,Tyr^8,D-Ala^{10}]LHRH	$5.8 + .17$	10.0
32.	[N-Ac-D-Nal(2)^1,D-pCl-Phe^2,D-Trp^3,D-Lys(iPr)^6,Lys(iPr)^8,D-Ala^{10}]LHRH	$6.6 + .32$	1.0
33.	[N-Ac-D-pCl-Phe^1,D-pCl-Phe^2,D-Trp^{3,6}]LHRH	$7.2 + 1.4$	—
34.	[N-Ac-D-Nal(2)^1,D-pCl-Phe^2,D-Pal^{3,6},D-Ala^{10}]LHRH	$9.8 + 1.5$	3.0
35.	[N-Ac-D-Nal(2)^1,D-pCl-Phe^2,D-Pal^3,Arg^5,D-Glu^6,D-Ala^{10}]LHRH	$17 + 3.7$	>>10.0(S)
36.	[N-Ac-D-Nal(2)^1,D-pF-Phe^2,D-Trp^3]LHRH	$18 + 3.0$	—
37.	[D-Arg^6]LHRH	$25 + 3.2$	—
38.	[N-Ac-$\triangle^3$-Pro^1,D-pF-Phe^2,D-Trp^{3,6}]LHRH	$39 + 5.6$	10.0
39.	[D-Trp^6]LHRH	$46 + 7.0$	—
40.	[Arg^6]LHRH	$46 + 4.6$	—
41.	[D-Lys^6,Pro^9-NHEt]LHRH	$59 + 24$	—
42.	[D-Trp^6,Pro^9-NHEt]LHRH	$108 + 17$	—
43.	LHRH	$328 + 62$	—

a The LHRH analogs were synthesized in the laboratories of the investigators as follows: 1, 2, 5-7, 10, 17, 33, 39 (D. Coy); 20, 21, 29, 33 (K. Folkers); 4, 9, 13-16, 25, 31, 34, 35, 38, 42 (J. Rivier); 12, 22-24, 26-28, 30, 32 (R. Roeske). Analogs 3, 8, 11, 18, 19, 36, 37, 40, 41 and 43 were synthesized under NIH contract NO1-HD-2-2824 with the Salk Institute.

b Histamine release determinations were performed in duplicate or triplicate using mast cells from a minimum of three individual rats. Results are given as the mean + standard error of the mean (SEM).

c Antiovulatory assays were conducted as described in [20] by Drs. Rehan Naqvi and Marjorie Lindberg of EG&G Mason Research Institute.

d The symbol (>) denotes the fact that there was a statistically significant reduction in the number of rats ovulating compared to the control although an ED$_{100}$ value was not achieved at the dose indicated.

e The symbol (>>) indicates that, at the dose tested, the analog was inactive.

f D-Glu(AA) = D-4-p-(methoxy)-benzoyl-2-aminobutyric acid; AA = anisole adduct.

g (S) denotes the use of saline as the vehicle.

h Assay conducted by Dr. C.Y. Bowers, Tulane University School of Medicine.

i Aopmp = 2-(3'-amino-2'-oxo-1'-pyrrolidino)-4-methyl-pentanoic acid.

pairs of analogs for comparison: one closely related pair (1 and 4) would suggest slight enhancement of potency due to D-Ala[10]. At the N-terminus, however, the enhancement of histamine releasing potency by the more hydrophobic Ac-D-Nal(2)[1] vis-à-vis Ac-D-pCl-Phe[1] can be seen by comparing 1 with 7 and comparing 19 with the closely related 33.

By themselves, two basic side chains, in close proximity, are insufficient to impart high histamine-releasing potency to LHRH analogs. Thus [D-Arg[6]]LHRH, 37, and [Arg[6]]LHRH, 40, are 147x and 271x, respectively, less potent than the standard and 13x and 7x, respectively, more potent than LHRH. Similarly, the cluster of hydrophobic amino acids at the N-terminus (in the absence of D-Arg[6]) is insufficient for high histamine releasing potency as demonstrated by the fact that [N-Ac-D-Nal(2)[1],D-pF-Phe[2],D-Trp[3]]LHRH, 36, and [N-Ac-D-pCl-Phe[1],D-pCl-Phe[2],D-Trp[3,6]]LHRH 33, are 106x and 42x, respectively, less potent than the standard.

It is important to note that even the hexapeptide fragment, 30, which contains the hydrophobic N-terminus but only a single positively charged residue (D-Arg), now at the C-terminus, possesses moderate histamine releasing potency of approximately 60x that of LHRH. This fragment is approximately 35x less potent than the standard in releasing histamine although it is at least 400x less potent than the standard with respect to its antiovulatory potency.

In general there is not necessarily a correlation between anti-ovulatory potency and in vitro histamine releasing potency of the LHRH antagonists. Examination of the tabulated data will reveal many examples in support of this conclusion.

The least potent LHRH analogs, in vitro, with respect to histamine release, are the superagonists (37 and 39-42), or, generally, those with the fewest structural modifications relative to LHRH (43).

In our experiments LHRH (43) and analogs 4, 5, 7 and 38 failed to release histamine from human basophils and RBL-2H3 cells. Other LHRH analogs have not yet been tested. The biological significance of histamine release by LHRH analogs from mast cells but not from basophils is unclear. Nevertheless, it is likely that the inflammatory effects seen in vivo with some of these peptides is related to the release of mediators from histamine-containing cells.

Apparent Topological Effects at Positions 5 and 6

Decreasing the spatial proximity of the arginine groups, for example, by introducing D-Arg at position 5 ([N-Ac-D-Nal(2)[1], D-pF-Phe[2],D-Trp[3],D-Arg[5]]LHRH, 11), rather than position 6, decreases histamine releasing potency three-fold relative to the standard. A subtle topological effect is revealed by inversion of configuration at position 6 with the replacement of D-Arg[6] by L-Arg[6] resulting in [N-Ac-D-Nal(2)[1],D-pF-Phe[2],D-Trp[3],Arg[6]]LHRH, 13, which is four-fold less potent than the standard in releasing histamine and at least two-fold less potent with respect to its antiovulatory properties. Further reduction in histamine releasing potency is observed by introducing L-Arg at position 5 (analogs 15, 16 and 18) with various non-basic groups at position 6. Comparison of 11 and 18 reveals a similar topological effect occurring with inversion of configuration at position 5 (D-Arg[5] versus L-Arg[5]). Apparently, the most potent analogs, with respect to histamine releasing activity, require a particular topological alignment of the basic amino acid at position 6 (or 5) with the hydrophobic N-terminus (all D-aromatic amino acids) for optimal binding to the histamine receptor. Deviations from this alignment appear to lower potency.

Elimination of D-Arg[6] and/or Arg[8]

The absence of D-Arg[6] (analogs 17 and 19) results in a level of histamine releasing potency 10% of that of the standard and approximately 150x that of LHRH. The replacement of D-Arg in position 6 with D-Pal [Pal = 3-(3-pyridyl)-alanine] in conjunction with D-Pal substitution at position 3 (to introduce some hydrophilicity at the N-terminus) results in reduced histamine releasing potency (see 20 and 21) approximately 15-fold with respect to the standard and 30-fold with respect to the parent, 1. The analog containing an Arg in position 5 retained high antiovulatory potency (21). The introduction of D-Pal in position 3 and 6 markedly decreases histamine releasing potency depending upon other positional variants but, taking their antiovulatory potencies into account, analogs 21, 29 and 34 appear to offer equivalent opportunities for further development (Folkers et al. [13]).

The elimination of both D-Arg[6] and L-Arg[8], with the simultaneous incorporation of the somewhat shielded and less basic L-Lys(iPr) residues at positions 5 and 8, resulted in [N-Ac-D-Nal(2)[1],D-C$^\alpha$-Me-pCl-Phe[2],D-Pal[3],Lys(iPr)[5,8],D-Tyr[6],D-Ala[10]]LHRH, 22, an analog with a 19-fold reduction in histamine releasing potency with respect to the standard while retaining high anti-ovulatory potency. Introduction of a lactam constraint at positions 6-7 results in 23, an analog with markedly reduced histamine releasing potency (approximately 20-fold with respect to the standard) as well as reduced antiovulatory potency (approximately four-fold). Interchanging Arg and Tyr provides the interesting analog, [N-Ac-D-Nal(2)[1],D-C$^\alpha$-Me-pCl-Phe[2],D-Trp[3],Arg[5],D-Tyr[6],D-Ala[10]]LHRH, 24, with 37x reduced histamine releasing potency compared with the closely related D-Arg[6] analog, 1, while its antiovulatory potency is decreased only slightly.

A comparison of the potencies of 26 and 28 shows that even in the presence of D-Arg[6], replacement of Arg[8] by Lys(iPr) or hArg(Et$_2$) results in analogs (26 and 28, respectively) with markedly reduced histamine releasing potency (24 to 29-fold with respect to the standard) and retention of high antiovulatory potency. The implication is that side chains with only slightly lower basicity than Arg and/or with hydrophobic N$^\omega$-alkyl groups shielding the charged group in position 8 reduce such potency. This effect is observed also at position 6 in conjunction with the naturally occurring Arg[8] (compare analogs 8 with 1 or 2) but to a much lesser extent. Incorporation of changes at both positions 6 and 8 with Lys(iPr) results in an important substitution model, [N-Ac-D-Nal(2)[1],D-pCl-Phe[2],D-Trp[3],D-Lys(iPr)[6], Lys-

(iPr)^8,D-Ala^{10}]LHRH, 32, which is 66x less potent than its parent, 1, for histamine release while retaining equal anti-ovulatory potency.

Introduction of an acidic function, e.g., D-Glu, into position 6 results in 35, with markedly reduced histamine releasing and anti-ovulatory potency. However, the neutral but hydrophobic D-Glu(AA)^6 modification (AA = anisole adduct) yields [N-Ac-D-Nal(2)^1, D-pCl-Phe^2,D-Pal^3,Arg^5,D-Glu(AA)^6,D-Ala^{10}]LHRH (14), which is ten-fold less potent than the standard but equipotent with the corresponding D-Nal(2)^6 analog, 15, with respect to histamine release.

Reduction of Hydrophobicity at Position 6 and at the N-Terminus

Even the presence of a hydrophobic side chain (D-Trp^6) combined with a hydrophobic N-terminus and Arg^8 is sufficient to impart fairly high (140x LHRH) histamine releasing potency to the analog, [N-Ac-D-Nal(2)^1,D-pF-Phe^2,D-Trp^{3,6}]LHRH, 19. Removal of only the hydrophobic side chain at position 6 (from 19), while leaving the hydrophobic N-terminus intact, results in [N-Ac-D-Nal(2)^1, D-pF-Phe^2,D-Trp^3]LHRH, 36, with an 8-fold reduction in histamine releasing potency. However, reducing the hydrophobic character of the N-terminus by replacing N-Ac-D-Nal(2)^1 with N-Ac-Δ^3-Pro^1 results in [N-Ac-Δ^3-Pro^1,D-pF-Phe^2,D-Trp^{3,6}]LHRH, 38, with a decrease in histamine releasing potency of approximately 17-fold with respect to the parent, 19. Thus 38 is approximately 229x less potent than the standard with respect to histamine release and 4x less potent with respect to inhibition of ovulation.

Correlation of In Vitro and In Vivo Activity

There appears to be a correlation between in vitro histamine release and in vivo activity. The most potent histamine releasers in vitro produce an edematogenic effect in rats at the doses tested while the less potent (e.g., analog 38 and some super-agonists) do not exhibit this edema effect at the doses tested [6,9]. Anaphylactoid-like reactions in rats have also been reported for LHRH antagonists which are potent in vitro releasers of histamine [10,18]. Clinically, mild local reactions have been reported when a LHRH superagonist (e.g., 42) has been injected subcutaneously [19]. In the case of the standard antagonist, 4, there appears to be a dose-response relationship in terms of local erythema and induration with scratch-testing and intradermal testing, but this has not been studied in the absence of benadryl for subcutaneous injection (W.F. Crowley, private communication). [N-Ac-D-Nal(2)^1,D-pCl-Phe^2,D-Trp^3,D-hArg(Et$_2$)^6,D-Ala^{10}]LHRH (closely related to analog 8) has produced a dose-related wheal and flare at the site of injection [M. Henzl, private communication].

DECREASED HISTAMINE RELEASE BY LHRH ANALOGS: PROGNOSIS

We believe that the prognosis for considerably reducing the histamine releasing potential of the LHRH antagonists, to at least that of the superagonists (while maintaining high gonadotropin inhibition), is good. Several analogs have already been cited above which possess 20-40x less histamine releasing potency than the standard while retaining equal or higher antiovulatory potency. Another ten-fold decrease will reduce the histamine releasing potency of these antagonists to the level of the superagonists. It is unlikely that the histamine releasing activity can be entirely eliminated from the LHRH antagonists. However, the mild reaction which has been seen at the site of injection with some superagonists has not limited their clinical potential. We believe that if the histamine releasing potency of the LHRH antagonists can be reduced to the level of the superagonists, then the clinical potential of the LHRH antagonists will not be limited by such a side effect.

ACKNOWLEDGEMENTS

Peptides were synthesized under the aegis of NIH contracts NO1-HD-4-2832 (DHC), NO1-HD-4-2831 (KF), NO1-HD-4-2833 (JER), NO1-HD-4-2834 (RWR). D.H. Coy acknowledges the assistance of Dr. Simon Hocart for the preparation of the peptides. K. Folkers acknowledges and expresses appreciation to the following coworkers for the peptides: Dr. Phi-Fun Louisa Tang, Dr. Minoru Kubota, and Xiao Shao-bo. J.E. Rivier acknowledges the assistance of John Porter and John Dykert for the preparation and characterization of the peptides. R.W. Roeske acknowledges the assistance of Dr. Nishith Chaturvedi, Dr. Tanya Hrinyo, and Maria Kowalizuk for the synthesis of the peptides. We express our appreciation to Dr. Rehan Naqvi and Dr. Marjorie Lindberg for the antiovulatory testing of the peptides.

REFERENCES

1. Theoharides, T.C. and Douglas, W.W. Mast cell histamine secretion in response to somatostatin analogues: structural considerations. Eur. J. Pharmacol., 73, 131 (1981).
2. Foreman, J. and Jordon, C. Histamine release and vascular changes induced by neuropeptides. Agents Actions, 13, 105 (1983).
3. Irman-Florjanc, T. and Erjavec, F. Compound 48/80 and substance P induced release of histamine and serotonin from rat peritoneal mast cells. Agents Actions, 13, 138 (1983).
4. Foreman, J.C. and Piotrowski, W. Peptides and histamine release. J. Allergy Clin. Immunol., 74, 127 (1984).
5. Tharp, M.D., Thirlby, R. and Sullivan, T.J. Gastrin induces histamine release from human cutaneous mast cells. J. Allergy Clin. Immunol., 74, 159 (1984).
6. Schmidt, F., Sundaram, K., Thau, R.B. and Bardin, C.W. [Ac-D-Nal(2)^1,4FD-Phe^2,D-Trp^3,D-Arg^6]-LHRH, a potent antagonist of LHRH produces transient edema and behavioral changes in rats. Contraception, 29, 283 (1984).

7. Nekola, M.V., O'Neil, C., Morgan, J. and Coy D.H. Antagonists of luteinizing hormone releasing hormone (LHRH): potent releasers of histamine in rats. Clin. Res., 32, 865A (1984)(Abstract).

8. Hook, W.A., Karten, M. and Siraganian, R.P. Histamine release by structural analogs of LHRH. Fed. Proc., 44, 1323 (1985).

9. Karten, M.J. and Rivier, J.E. Gonadotropin-releasing hormone analog design. Structure-function studies toward the development of agonists and antagonists: rationale and perspective. Endocr. Rev., 7, 44 (1986).

10. Morgan, J.E., O'Neil, C.E., Coy, D.H., Hocart, S.J. and Nekola, M.V. Antagonistic analogs of luteinizing hormone-releasing hormone are mast cell secretagogues. Int. Archs Allergy Appl. Immun., 80, 70 (1986).

11. Roeske, R.W., Chaturvedi, N.C., Rivier, J., Vale, W., Porter, J. and Perrin, M. Substitution of Arg[5] for Tyr[5] in GnRH antagonists. In "Peptides: Structure and Function." Proceedings of the Ninth American Peptide Symposium. C.M. Deber, V.J. Hruby, and K.D. Kopple (Eds.), Pierce Chemical Co., Rockford, IL, p. 561.

12. Rivier, J.E., Porter, J., Rivier, C.L., Perrin, M., Corrigan, A., Hook, W.A., Siraganian, R.P. and Vale, W.W. New effective gonadotropin releasing hormone antagonists with minimal potency for histamine release in vitro. J. Med. Chem. (In press).

13. Folkers, K., Bowers, C., Xiao, S., Tang, P.L. and Kubota, M. Increased potency of antagonists of the luteinizing hormone releasing hormone which have D-3-Pal in position 6. Biochem. Biophys. Res. Commun., 137, 709 (1986).

14. Ishizaka, T. and Ishizaka K. Activation of mast cells for mediator release through IgE receptors. Prog. Allergy, 34, 188 (1984).

15. Siraganian, R.P. Histamine secretion from mast cells and basophils. Trends in Pharmacologic Sciences, 4, 432 (1983).

16. Siraganian, R.P. An automated continuous flow system for the extraction and fluorometric analysis of histamine. Anal. Biochem., 57, 383 (1974).

17. Siraganian, R.P. and Hook, W.A. Histamine release and assay methods for the study of human allergy. In "Manual of Clinical Immunology" 3rd ed., N.R. Rose, H. Friedman, and J.L. Fahey (Eds.) Amer. Soc. for Microbiology, Washington, 1986, p. 808.

18. Hahn, D.W., McGuire, J.L., Vale, W.W. and Rivier, J. Reproductive/endocrine and anaphylactoid properties of an LHRH antagonist, ORF 19260 [Ac-D-Nal(2)[1],4FDPhe[2],D-Trp[3],D-Arg[6]]-GnRH. Life Sci., 37, 505 (1985).

19. Mansfield, M.J., Beardsworth, D.E., Loughlin, J.S., Crawford, J.D., Bode, H.H., Rivier, J., Vale, W., Kushner, D.C., Crigler, J.F. and Crowley, W.F. Long-term treatment of central precocious puberty with a long-acting analogue of luteinizing hormone-releasing hormone. N. Engl. J. Med., 309, 1386 (1983).

20. Corbin, A. and Beattie, C.W. Inhibition of the pre-ovulatory proestrous gonadotropin surge, ovulation and pregnancy with a peptide analogue of luteinizing hormone releasing hormone. Endocr. Res. Commun., 2, 1 (1975).

12
Anaphylactoid Properties of LHRH Analogs

A. PHILLIPS, D. W. HAHN, C. BISHOP,
R. J. CAPETOLA and J. L. McGUIRE

Research Laboratories, Ortho Pharmaceutical Corporation, Raritan,
NJ 08869, USA

INTRODUCTION

The isolation and structural elucidation of LHRH by Schally [1] and Guillemin [2] in 1971 led to the synthesis of analogs which have been proposed for use in a variety of clinical disorders such as endometriosis, precocious puberty and prostatic carcinoma. These analogs have included both agonists, many of which are currently being studied clinically, and more recently, competitive antagonists. The first LHRH antagonists which were synthesized in 1972 [3] were not very potent, but did support the feasibility of synthesizing competitive antagonists. This led to research in many laboratories to improve the potency of antagonists. As reviewed by Karten [4], a large number of chemical modifications of LHRH have been attempted. Substitutions at positions 2, 3 and 6 have been among the most effective, although the structure activity relationships in this work appear to be very complex. One series of analogs with an arginine substituted at position 6 appears to be most potent [5,6]. One of these, [N-Ac-D-Nal(2)^1, D-pF-Phe^2,D-Trp^3, D-Arg^6]LHRH has been proposed for clinical studies.

During drug toxicity studies with this peptide, Schmidt, et al. [7] observed vascular permeability changes in rodents treated with the compound. Studies in our laboratories to further characterize these changes led us to conclude that these changes were identical to cutaneous anaphylaxis reactions possibly as a result of a direct action of the drug on mast cell mediator release. A program in our laboratory [8,9] screening a full series of LHRH antagonists demonstrated that the potencies of these peptides, in assays measuring LHRH antagonist activity, do not correlate with their ability to cause cutaneous anaphylaxis. These data suggested that the LHRH inhibiting and anaphylactoid activities were not linked, and a potent LHRH antagonist with a minimal potential to cause an allergic reaction could be identified. Before describing the data of these peptides on histamine release, we will briefly outline some of the pertinent biochemical events that occur during mast cell/basophil secretion.

191

MAST CELL/BASOPHIL MEDIATORS

Mast cells and basophils secrete substances that mediate immedi-
ate-type hypersensitivity reactions when an appropriate stimulus
binds to cell surface IgE receptors and subsequently cross-link
these receptors. These mediators can be either pre-formed or
stored in secretory granules or are newly generated. In human
mast cells the pre-formed mediators include histamine, heparin,
and tryptase along with acid hydrolases, oxidative enzymes, and
chemotactic substances, whereas the newly formed mediators include
arachidonate-derived substances such as the slow-reacting substances (SRSs) and prostaglandin D_2 (PGD$_2$), in addition to
platelet activating factor (PAF). Because mast cells occupy
strategic positions in and around venules and in connective tissues of cutaneous, mucosal, and serosal surfaces, the mediators
exert their activity at these locations.

Activation of Mediator Secretion. Multiple mechanisms cause degranulation and mediator release from mast cells and basophils
(Fig. 1). Cross-linkage by specific antigen of IgE that is bound
to mast cell and basophil plasma membranes via receptors specific
for the Fc region of IgE is the mechanism most relevant to human
disease, such as asthma and allergic rhinitis.

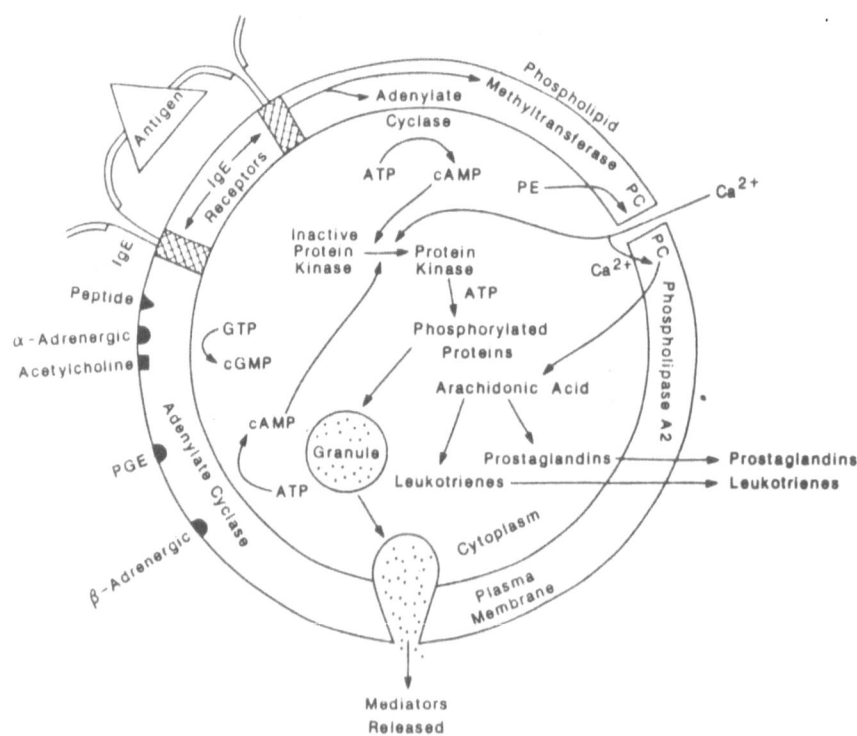

FIGURE 1   The mast cell

Agents that activate mast cells by nonimmunologic mechanisms may be relevant to iatrogenically induced anaphylaxis in patients [10]. These would include calcium ionophores (which translocate extracellular or membrane-associated calcium into cells), compound 48/80, hyperosmolar mannitol and mellitin from bee venom. The complement-derived anaphylatoxins C3a and C5a and peptides with basic amino acid sequences such as in Substance P [10] and some LHRH antagonists cause degranulation of mast cells and basophils.

Following activation of mast cells and basophils, both energy and calcium influx are essential for degranulation to occur. In addition, cyclic nucleotides appear to modulate the secretion of mediators from mast cells or basophils [11]. The intracellular levels of cAMP can be elevated by the addition of exogenous cAMP or its dibutyryl derivative and by the addition of inhibitors of the phosphodiesterase enzyme (e.g. theophylline) which is involved in the breakdown of cAMP. All of these agents have been reported to inhibit mediator release in a number of systems, including both human and rat basophils as well as mast cells.

Response to Histamine. Histamine secreted from mast cells stimulates a biologic response by binding to and activating the cell surface histamine receptors, designated H_1 and H_2. Contraction of bronchial and gastrointestinal smooth muscle occurs via H_1 receptors, whereas stimulation of gastric acid secretion by parietal cells is H_2-receptor mediated. The triple response elicited by intradermal injection of histamine consists of initial local erythema due to histamine-directed vasodilation, erythema due to vasodilation from an axon reflex, and finally a central edematous wheal due to a histamine-directed increase in vasopermeability representing combined H_1 and H_2 response. Enhancement of local vasopermeability by released histamine also facilitates the tissue deposition of pathobiologic serum components such as immune complexes and permits the interaction of serum and cellular components not normally in residence in connective tissue with the insoluble macromolecular complex of neutral proteases and heparin proteoglycan that is also released from rodent and human mast cells. These actions suggest a multifaceted role for histamine in acute allergic inflammation.

Lipoxygenase and Cyclooxygenase Products. Arachidonic acid can be metabolized by either the cyclooxygenase or the lipoxygenase pathway. The products of the lipoxygenase pathway are leukotrienes. There is some suggestive evidence for a role of a product from the lipoxygenase pathway in cell secretion. Among the lipoxygenase products, several compounds (e.g., 5-HPETE, 5-HETE, and 12-HETE) enhance IgE-mediated release, and 5-HPETE can release histamine in the presence of cytochalasin B, an agent which disrupts microfilaments. Thus, a role for a lipoxygenase product in the release process is suggested but has not been confirmed [10].

In mast cells/basophils the cyclooxygenase pathway leads predominantly to the formation of prostaglandin D_2. Inhibitors of the cyclooxygenase pathway (e.g., aspirin, indomethacin) have little or no effect on histamine release from cells. Therefore

193

products of this pathway appear not to be involved in the secretory process [10].

ANAPHYLACTOID ACTIVITY OF LHRH ANTAGONISTS

Cutaneous Anaphylactoid Activity in Rats and Monkeys. Anaphylactoid activity in female Wistar rats was measured by injecting Evan's blue dye intravenously into the tail vein. Immediately following, 0.05 ml of an LHRH analog dissolved in saline was injected intradermally into the shaved mid-dorsal area. Approximately twenty minutes after the injection, the rats were sacrificed. The dimensions of the blue wheal responses were recorded and the wheal areas (mm^2) calculated. Similar methods were used to measure the wheal response in rhesus monkeys.

The amino acid sequences of the peptides tested are presented in Table 1 in order of potency in the assay measuring anaphylactoid activity in rats. Some trends in a structure activity relationship were seen. Peptides which did not contain arginine in position 5 or 6 tended to be less potent. Other investigators conducting studies with other classes of peptides have also demonstrated that basic amino acid sequences impart increased anaphylactoid activity [12]. In our studies, Arg^5 or Arg^6 substitutions were equipotent, in contrast to other reports [13]. Peptide 12, which contains Arg^6 was the most potent anaphylactoid agent in the rat (Table 1). This LHRH antagonist has been reported previously to be a potent histamine-releasing agent [14] and to induce cutaneous anaphylaxis in rats [7].

Nine of the peptides were tested for anaphylactoid activity in the monkey. Seven of the 9 peptides were within a relatively narrow range of potency whereas peptides 7 and 10 were considerably less potent (Table 2).

Pulmonary Mechanics in the Guinea Pig. Male Hartley guinea pigs were anesthetized with urethane and placed in a whole body plethysmograph with a jugular vein cannulated for i.v. administration of test compounds, a carotid artery cannulated for monitoring blood pressure, and a tracheal cannulation was performed to maintain respiration at a constant volume via a miniature Starling pump. Transpleural pressure was obtained via insertion of a needle into the pleural cavity and a sidearm from the tracheal cannula in conjunction with a differential pressure transducer. Pressure changes within the plethysmograph were sensed via another differential pressure transducer and air flow, tidal volume, dynamic lung compliance (C_{dyn}), and lung resistance (R_L) were calculated. Arterial blood pressure and heart rate were also measured.

The animals were administered succinyl choline to arrest spontaneous respiration and allowed to stabilize. An intravenous infusion (1 ml/min, 20 min) of the test compound was then performed. Percent changes were calculated from the baseline values prior to i.v. drug administration. Maximum changes occurred during the infusion, and were recorded.

No significant alterations of pulmonary function were observed

Table 1. Anaphylactoid and antiovulatory activity of LHRH analogs

Peptide No.[a]	Anaphylactoid Activity Rat ED (8.75x8.75 mm wheal) μg/wheal	Antiovulatory Activity Rat ED$_{50}$ (μg/kg)	Therapeutic Index[b]
1 LHRH	NA	NA	—
2[c] [N-Ac-Δ^3-Pro^1,D-pF-Phe^2,D-Trp^{3,6}]LHRH	11.29	19.72	0.572
3[c] [N-Ac-D-Nal(2)^1,D-pCl-Phe^2,D-Trp^3,D-Arg^6]LHRH	9.54	7.20	1.325
4[d] [D-Trp^6,Pro^9-NHEt]LHRH	2.97	NA	—
5[d] [N-Ac-D-Nal(2)^1,D-αMe,pCl-Phe^2,D-Pal(3)^3,D-Arg^6,D-hArg(Et^2)8,D-Ala^{10})LHRH	0.81	2.00	0.405
6[c] [N-Ac-D-Nal(2)^1,D-pCl-Phe^2,D-Pal(3)^3,Arg^5,D-Glu(AA)^6,D-Ala^{10})LHRH	0.48	1.54	0.312
7[c] [N-Ac-Δ^3-Pro^1,D-Cl-Phe^2,D-Pal(3)^3,D-Nal(2)^6,D-Ala^{10})LHRH	0.21	3.59	0.058
8[c] [N-Ac-D-Nal(2)^1,D-pCl-Phe^2,DPal(3)^3,Arg^5,D-Nal(2)^6,D-Ala^{10}]LHRH	0.20	2.77	0.072
9[c] [N-Ac-D-Nal(2)^1,D-pCl-Phe^2,D-Pal(3)^3,Arg^5,D-Tyr^5,D-Ala^{10}]LHRH	0.15	2.77	0.054
10[d] [N-Ac-D-Nal(2)^1,D-αMe$_1$pCl-Phe^2,D-Pal(3)^3,D-Arg^6,Lys(iPr)^8]LHRH	0.12	1.00	0.120
11[d] [N-Ac-D-Nal(2)^1,D-pCl-Phe^2,D-Pal(3)^3,Arg-D-Pal(3)^6,D-Ala^{10}]LHRH	0.09	3.38	0.027
12[c] [N-Ac-D-Nal(2)^1,D-pF-Phe^2,D-Trp^3,D-Arg^6]LHRH	0.01	2.56	0.004

a Peptides numbered in order of potency in assay measuring rat anaphylactoid activity
b Therapeutic index = Anaphylactoid ED/Antiovulatory ED
c These peptides were obtained from Jean Rivier of the Salk Institute
d These peptides were obtained from Marvin Karten of the NIH
NA = not active

Table 2: Comparison of anaphylactoid activity of LHRH analogs in rats and monkeys

Peptide No.	Monkey ED (5.0x5.0 mm wheal) μg/wheal	Rat ED (5.0x5.0 mm wheal)[a] μg/wheal
3	0.028	0.04184
5	0.022	0.00347
6	0.058	0.00003
7	0.875	0.00199
8	0.021	0.00002
9	0.039	0.00416
10	0.223	0.00049
11	0.029	0.00067
12	0.027	0.00175

a For comparative purposes, rat ED (5.0 x 5.0 mm) values were extrapolated from same linear regression used for ED (8.75 x 8.75 mm) values presented in Table 1.

for any of the compounds studied at doses much higher than those required to inhibit ovulation (Table 3). Thus, although peptide 12 stimulates histamine-release in vitro [14] and causes a wheal response (Table 2), the potential for bronchospasm and cardiovascular appears to be small.

Table 3: Pulmonary effects[a] of 10 mg/kg i.v. infusions of LHRH and two analogs in the anesthetized guinea pig

Treatment	I.V. Dose (mg/kg)	Number of Guinea Pigs	CDYN[b]	RL[c]
Saline	20 ml	3	-11.7±1.2	4.3±4.8
Peptide 1	10	3	-31.3±14.0	41.0±36.5
Peptide 2	10	3	-13.7±2.7	14.0±5.0
Peptide 12	10	2	-21.0	21.0

a Data are expressed as % change from control baseline values for all parameters monitored
b CDYN – dynamic compliance
c RL   – lung resistance

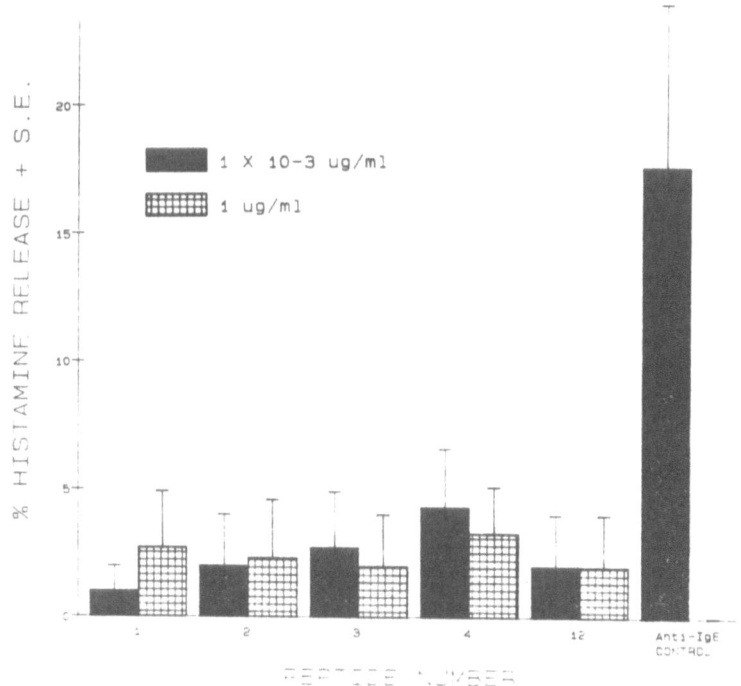

FIGURE 2 Spontaneous histamine release from human mast cells induced by several LHRH analogs. n=3 for each bar.

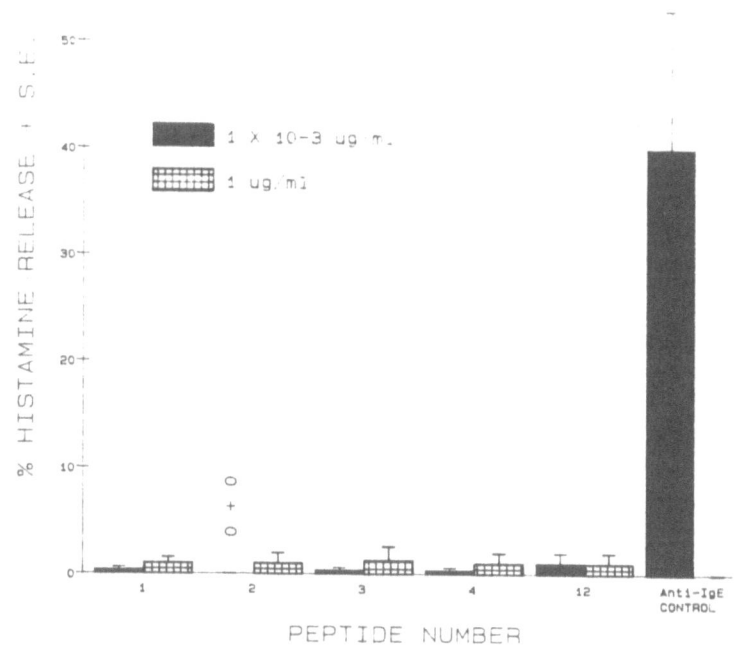

FIGURE 3 Spontaneous histamine release from human basophils induced by several LHRH analogs. n=3 for each bar.

197

Histamine Release from Human Basophils and Mast Cells. Histamine release from human mast cells and basophils are assayed according to Lichtenstein (personal communication). Briefly, basophils and mast cells were obtained from volunteers and placed in suspension. Aliquots of the cell pool were incubated at 37°C. Peptides were added to the cells. After a short incubation (~5 min) the cells were removed to a 4°C waterbath. The cells were separated from the supernatant buffer by centrifugation. Histamine was assayed in the supernatant. An equivalent aliquot of cells was challenged with anti-human IgE to provide a physiological control and showed that the cells are responsive in the assay. Another equivalent aliquot of the cell pool was lysed and centrifuged as described above to determine the total cellular histamine. Percent histamine release was calculated as (histamine in drug treated aliquot/histamine in lysed, treated aliquot) x 100.

An insignificant amount of histamine was released by either cell type after incubation with the peptides (Figs. 2 & 3). The physiological control (anti-human IgE) proved that the cells were capable of responding to a stimulus by releasing histamine and gives some indication of the quantity of histamine released in normal physiological responses.

Ovulation Inhibition in Rats. Rats were injected subcutaneously with an LHRH antagonist dissolved in saline at 1 to 2 pm on the day of proestrus. The doses tested were 0.3125, 0.625, 1.25, 2.5, 5.0 or 10.0 µg/kg. Each antagonist was tested at three or four of these doses and ten rats were tested per dose group. Control rats received saline only. The following morning, the animals were sacrificed and the oviducts examined microscopically for the presence of ova. A rat with one or more ova present in the oviducts was considered to have ovulated.

The antiovulatory potencies of the LHRH antagonists did not correlate to their ability to cause a wheal response (Table 1), suggesting that the LHRH antagonist properties are independent of their anaphylactoid activity. Peptides 2, 3, 5 and 6 have the best therapeutic indices. In addition to their better therapeutic index, the enhanced antiovulatory potencies of peptides 5 and 6 indicate that these peptides provide potent inhibition of LHRH with a minimal potential to cause an allergic response. Peptide 12, the most potent peptide in causing a wheal response in rats, also had the worst therapeutic index (Table 1).

CONCLUDING REMARKS

The structural identity of native LHRH gave impetus to the synthesis of both agonists and antagonists of this gonadotropin releasing-hormone. Compounds with basic amino acids at position 6 first emerged as the most potent antagonists. Initial toxicity studies with one of these compounds revealed that upon local injection, vascular permeability changes reminiscent of histamine release occurred that might preclude widespread clinical utility of this drug. Thus began the search for new potent antiovulatory analogs devoid of this liability.

As a primary screen for histamine releasibility we chose as our model the skin of rats or monkeys. This _in vivo_ model was selected primarily because certain agents can increase vascular permeability by means other than histamine release, e.g. by activation of H_1 receptors. Therapeutic indices were calculated from the potencies in these assays and the assay measuring the ability to inhibit ovulation. With the data from the compounds evaluated, no discernible relationship emerged between their anaphylactoid and antiovulatory activities indicating that the two events are not positively correlated, and potent LHRH antagonists without the potential to cause an allergic reaction exist. The safety of some LHRH antagonists is also indicated in studies in guinea pigs in which these compounds caused no significant changes in pulmonary resistance or compliance after intravenous infusion at large multiples of their antiovulatory dose.

Thus, it appears that although some LHRH antagonists may possess the potential for anaphylactoid activity, others represent significant advances in the development of relatively safe drugs with the potential to be used for the treatment of a variety of clinical disorders as well as contraceptives.

REFERENCES

1. Matsuo, H., Balea, Y., Nair, R.M., Arimura, A. and Schally, A.V. Structure of the porcine LH- and FSH-releasing hormone. I. The proposed amino acid sequence. Biochem. Biophys. Res. Commun., 43, 1334 (1971).
2. Burgus, R., Butcher, M., Amoss, M., Ling, N., Monahan, M.W., Rivier, J., Fellows, R., Blackwell, R., Vale, W., and Guillemin, R. Primary structure of the ovine hypothalamic luteinizing hormone releasing factor (LRF). Proc. Natl. Acad. Sci., 69, 278 (1972).
3. Vale, W., Grant, G., Rivier, J., Monahan, M., Amoss, M., Blackwell, R., Burgus, R. and Guillemin, R. Synthetic polypeptide antagonists of the hypothalamic luteinizing hormone releasing hormone factor. Science, 176, 933 (1972).
4. Karten, M.J. and Rivier, J.E. Gonadotropin-releasing hormone analog design, rationale and perspective. Endocr. Rev. 7(1), 44 (1986).
5. Rivier, J., Rivier,C., Perrin, M., Porter, J. and Vale, W. LHRH analogs as antiovulatory agents. In "LHRH and its Analogs", B.H. Vickery, J.J. Nestor, Jr. and E.S.E. Hafez (Eds.), MTP Press, Boston, 1984, p. 11.
6. Nekola, M.V. and Coy, D.H. LHRH antagonists in females. In "LHRH and its Analogs", B.H. Vickery, J.J. Nestor, Jr. and E.S.E. Hafez (Eds.), MTP Press, Boston, 1984, p. 125.
7. Schmidt, F., Sundaram, K., Thau, R.B. and Bardin, C.W. [Ac-D-Nal(2)^1,4FD-Phe^2,D-Trp^3,D-Arg^6]-LHRH, a potent antagonist of LHRH, produces transient edema and behavioral changes in rats. Contraception 29, 283 (1984).
8. Phillips, A., Hahn, D.W., Capetola, R.J., and McGuire, J.L. The antiovulatory and anaphylactoid activities of two potent LHRH antagonists. The Pharmacologist 28, Abs. #689 (1986).

9. Hahn, D.W., McGuire, J.L., Vale, W.W. and Rivier, J. Reproductive/endocrine and anaphylactoid properties of an LHRH antagonist, ORF 18260 [Ac-DNAL[1](2),4FDPhe[2],D-Trp[3], D-Arg[6]]-GnRH. Life Sci., $\underline{37}$, 505 (1985).
10. Schwartz, L. The Mast Cell. In "Allergy", A.P. Kaplan (Ed.), Churchill Livingston, New York, 1985, p. 53.
11. Bourne, H.R., Lichtenstein, L.M. and Melmon, K.L., Modulation of inflammation and immunity by cyclic AMP. Science, 184 (1974).
12. Stanworth, D.R., Kings, M., Roy, P.D., Moran, J.M. and Moran, D.M. Synthetic peptides comprising sequences of the human immunoglobulin E heavy chain capable of releasing histamine. Biochemical J., $\underline{180}$, 665 (1979).
13. Rivier, J.E., Porter, J., Rivier, C.L., Perrin, M., Corrigan, A., Hook, W.A., Siraganian, R.P. and Vale, W.W. New effective gonadotropin releasing hormone antagonists with minimal potency for histamine release in vitro. J. Med. Chem. $\underline{29}$, 1846 (1986).
14. Hook, W.A., Karten, M. and Siraganian, R.P. Histamine release by structural analogs of LHRH. Fed. Proc., $\underline{44}$, 1323 (1985).

13
Reproductive Physiology and General Pharmacology of LHRH Antagonists

B.H. VICKERY

Department of Physiology, Institute of Biological Sciences, Syntex
Research, Palo Alto, CA 94304, USA

INTRODUCTION

Competitive antagonism of LHRH at its pituitary receptors by a
peptide administered systemically would be expected, because of
the hemodilution involved, to require a dauntingly large dose to
be effective. Nonetheless, chemical manipulation and substitution
in the LHRH molecule [1-3] have now resulted in agents whose
potency is sufficient to permit clinical evaluation in humans
[4,5]. Pharmacological evaluation of these peptides has
demonstrated them to be powerful tools for dissecting reproductive
physiology and suggests that they may find contraceptive and
therapeutic niches as drugs which do not duplicate the utilities
of the LHRH agonist analogs. However, these studies have also
sounded a cautionary note since many degranulate mast cells with
consequent release of mediators including histamine and
serotonin. Available analogs differ in their histamine-releasing
potency relative to their LHRH antagonizing potency in vitro [6]
and in vivo [7], leading to the expectation that further chemical
manipulation of the LHRH molecule may be able to separate these
two activities [8-10].

REPRODUCTIVE PHYSIOLOGY

LHRH antagonists compete with endogenous LHRH for its receptor
binding sites [11]. These receptors are present on the
gonadotropes in the pituitary but are also reported with similar
affinity in rat gonads [12,13] or as lower affinity sites in human
corpora lutea [14,15], breast [16] and placenta [17]. Interaction
with the pituitary sites results acutely in abolition of a
preovulatory LH surge. Chronic administration, at higher dose
levels, suppresses basal gonadotropin levels, resulting in the
equivalent of a chemical castration. Although LH and FSH are
equally affected by the LHRH antagonists in vitro from pituitary
cells, LH levels decline more rapidly in vivo and to a greater
degree than do FSH levels. These in vivo effects probably reflect
interaction of other factors including the gonadal steroids,

inhibin, and differences in the circulatory half lives of LH and FSH. Chronic administration of LHRH antagonist will equally suppress both gonadotropins, particularly when bioactivity rather than immunoactivity is assessed.

LHRH agonists can interact with the extrapituitary receptor sites to cause a variety of direct suppressive effects on the respective tissue functions [18]. This has led to speculation on paracrine roles for LHRH or LHRH-like materials. However, while LHRH antagonists will block the effects of exogenous LHRH agonists working through these receptors [19-22], there are few reports of LHRH antagonists exerting direct extrapituitary effects in normal animals [23].

Effects in females

Administration of an LHRH antagonist at noon of proestrus in rats can successfully compete with the endogenous preovulatory LHRH rise, preventing the LH surge and ovulation [24]. In fact this has been adopted as a sensitive standard assay to gauge potencies of LHRH antagonists. This assay was modified to give an indirect measure of duration of action of LHRH antagonists either by monitoring days elapsing after proestrous dosing until ovulation occurs or by progressively increasing the gap between time of dosing and noon of proestrus while still successfully blocking ovulation at the normal time of estrus [25]. In primates LHRH antagonists can prevent the occurrence of both the spontaneous and the estrogen-induced preovulatory LH surge [26,27]. Administration during proestrus in the dog can suppress vaginal discharge, abrogate the progressive development in vaginal cytology and sexual behavior and prevent ovulation [28].

The ovariectomized animal or the postmenopausal woman provides a more precise as well as more sensitive model in which to assess effects on circulating levels of LH; effects on FSH are of lesser magnitude and are slower to develop [29,30].

Suppression of ovarian steroidogenic function (induction of medical castration) requires a much higher daily dose of LHRH antagonist than is required to lower gonadotropins for 24 hours in the castrate animal or to block ovulation when administered 24 hours before the anticipated LH surge [29]. This may be illustrated by the study showing that once weekly administration of an LHRH antagonist to female cynomolgus monkeys was capable of indefinitely postponing ovulation while leaving E_2 levels in the early follicular range [26]. It was concluded (from a different dosing regimen) that the mechanism was due to blockade of estrogen positive feedback, suggesting that atresia of dominant follicles was also involved. In light of other results demonstrating some LHRH antagonists to have very long circulating $T_{1/2}$ values and in the absence of measurements of blood levels of the antagonist in this study, it cannot be ruled out that the effects were due to continued presence of the analog. It is possible that this dosing regimen could form the basis of a contraceptive method, however the concern over unopposed estrogen stimulation and endometrial carcinoma would dictate the use of periodic progestational supplements to cause sloughing of the endometrium in a similar manner to that proposed for LHRH agonists [31,32].

Administration of LHRH antagonist to pregnant rats up to day 12 of gestation will terminate pregnancy [34-35] as will hypophysectomy or immuno-neutralization of circulating gonadotropins [36]. LHRH antagonist also will terminate pregnancy in dogs through suppression of luteal progesterone output [28]. However in this species the corpus luteum appears not to require pituitary gonadotropins until about the third week of gestation and the LHRH antagonist is ineffective until that time. Hypophysectomy in the dog does terminate luteal function if performed on or after day 18 of the luteal phase; the effect is precipitous at later stages but only a transient fall in progesterone levels follows early performance of the procedure [37,38]. Surprisingly, the pregnant cat at about 20 days of gestation shows no change in progesterone levels in response to LHRH antagonist suggesting total autonomy of the corpus luteum from pituitary control. The responses in both dog and cat are very similar to those noted for the luteolytic prostaglandin analogs [39, G. Stabenfeld, personal communication] which however are thought to act directly on the corpus luteum.

In nonpregnant primates, luteal function is rapidly and markedly suppressed by LHRH antagonist treatment [29,40,41]. Spontaneous recovery of luteal function will occur unless suppression is maintained for more than 3 days [40,42], which accords well with immunoneutralization studies and findings in hypothalamically lesioned animals [43-45]. Studies in women, while confirming the luteal suppression, showed however that exogenous hCG would override the effect [4]. This would suggest that the antagonists like the agonists [46,47], would be ineffective for terminating human pregnancy. More recently, detailed replacement studies in stumptailed macaques have suggested that a small window of a few days may exist when the luteal suppression resulting from antagonist may not be reversed by CG [42].

In vitro studies with human placental tissue explants showed LHRH antagonist to suppress placental production of both progesterone and CG [48,49]. This indicates that an antagonist, by blocking both pituitary and placental gonadotropin release, might be able to terminate pregnancy. Studies in pregnant baboons have so far been equivocal [50,51], perhaps indicating poor penetration to the syncytiocytotrophoblast and/or insufficient dosage. The production rate of the placental LHRH-like material is very high [52] and the placental binding sites, while of high specificity, are of low affinity [53]. Both of these findings would elevate the required circulating levels of antagonists for effective competition with endogenous ligand.

Effects in males

The castrate male rat is very sensitive to the effects of LHRH antagonists and the normally very elevated levels of LH can be decreased by 70% or more within 2 hours of injection [29]. The preparation has also been used to assess the durations of action of different analogs [29,54]. An 8-10 fold higher dose is required to suppress gonadotropin secretion for an equivalent period of time in the intact animal [29]; however, suppression is more complete and is reflected by shutdown of testicular function-lowering of circulating testosterone to castrate levels and cessation of spermatogenesis. The first effect of the antagonist appears to be to decrease frequency and amplitude of gonadotropin release [54]. This is followed by a decline in the basal levels.

Chronic treatment of male rats with LHRH antagonists causes infertility in breeding trials, initially due to inhibition of mating behavior [55]. Replacement of low levels of testosterone restores mating behavior but not fertility, while higher levels restore fertility also [56]. The latter effect was believed to be due to direct support of spermatogenesis by testosterone at the testicular level. However normal intratesticular levels of testosterone are certainly not achieved by such supplementation and much higher levels of testosterone are required in the hypophysectomized rat. Testosterone supplementation can re-elevate circulating levels of FSH in the face of LHRH antagonist treatment in rats [57,58]; it may be that the combined effect of testosterone and FSH is responsible for reinitiation or maintained support of spermatogenesis.

LHRH antagonists very effectively suppress gonadotropin secretion in dogs [59]. Interestingly, the pharmacokinetics are very different in dogs, at least for detirelix ([N-Ac-D-Nal(2)^1, D-pCl-Phe^2,DTrp^3,D-hArg(Et$_2$)^6,D-Ala^{10}]LHRH), and the plasma T$_{1/2}$ for this compound is about 15 times greater than that in rats. This is reflected by a lesser dosage requirement for gonadotropin and gonadal steroid suppression (Table 1). Chronic treatment suppresses spermatogenesis [59]. The effect is rapidly reversible with sperm reappearing in the ejaculate just over one spermatogenic cycle after stopping treatment. Supplementation of testosterone to the low normal range restores accessory organ secretion but does not prevent the achievement of azoospermia, merely extending from 6 to 18 weeks the time to expression.

There are now several reports of the efficacy of LHRH antagonist in male macaques [60-65]. Although azoospermia is induced routinely by LHRH antagonist alone, there is some controversy over the effect of testosterone supplementation. Because of differences in mode of administration of antagonist (daily versus continuous) and dose levels further studies on the interaction between testosterone and LHRH antagonists in monkeys will be required. However, it seems clear that azoospermia can be achieved in the face of testosterone supplementation if a high enough dose of LHRH antagonist is used. Two groups find a depression in body weight by LHRH antagonists, however, in one center (Chapter 15), this is stopped by testosterone replacement suggesting that it is due to loss of the anabolic effect of androgens. At the other center body weight declines even in the face of testosterone replacement [63].

Reversal of the suppressive effect on reproductive parameters is clear. In fact, a rebound elevation has been noted in

Table 1. Correlation between minimal effective dose of detirelix and plasma half life in various species.

Species	MED for 24 Hours Suppression of Testosterone	Plasma T½
rat	1600 µg/kg	96 min
dog	100 µg/kg	22 hrs
cynomolgus	250 µg/kg	19 hrs
man	14-70 µg/kg	48 hrs

gonadotropin levels, testosterone levels, testicular dimensions and sperm count [63]. This could be due to a temporary resetting of the feedback loops of gonadotropins and steroids at the hypothalamic level. This effect might form the basis of a temporary relief from oligospermia, as previously suggested for high dose testosterone therapy [66].

Single dose studies [67,68] suggest that these agents will also be effective suppressants of the pituitary gonadal axis in men. Again, for detirelix, the increased potency relative to that in other species correlates with a further extension in plasma T½ [68]. Theoretically, it should take about 9 days for a compound with such a long half life to reach steady state circulating levels from daily dosing (Fig. 1). During this time the minimal circulating levels should increase. Therefore the daily dose requirement for gonadal suppression after 1 week of dosing with such a long lived analog may be considerably less than the single dose required to suppress for 24 hours.

Antitumor effects

The blockade of gonadal steroidogenesis rapidly achieved with the LHRH antagonists suggests they may be better candidates for treatment of the classical gonadal steroid dependent neoplasias than the LHRH agonists. In addition, their reported efficacy against some other tumor models suggests a previously nonsuspected role for gonadal steroids in other tumors.

Two female rat tumors (MXT 3.2 and MT/W9A) were retarded in growth rate by daily administration of LHRH antagonists [69]. While the effects are no doubt mainly due to the ablation of circulating sex steroids, direct inhibitory effects cannot be ruled out [70].

Similarly LHRH antagonists retard growth (weight gain and volume) of the Segaloff 11095 squamous cell carcinoma and the Dunning prostate tumor in male rats [71,72]. The lack of the "flare" associated with LHRH agonist therapy of prostatic tumors [73-77] makes the LHRH antagonist analogs particularly attractive in this area.

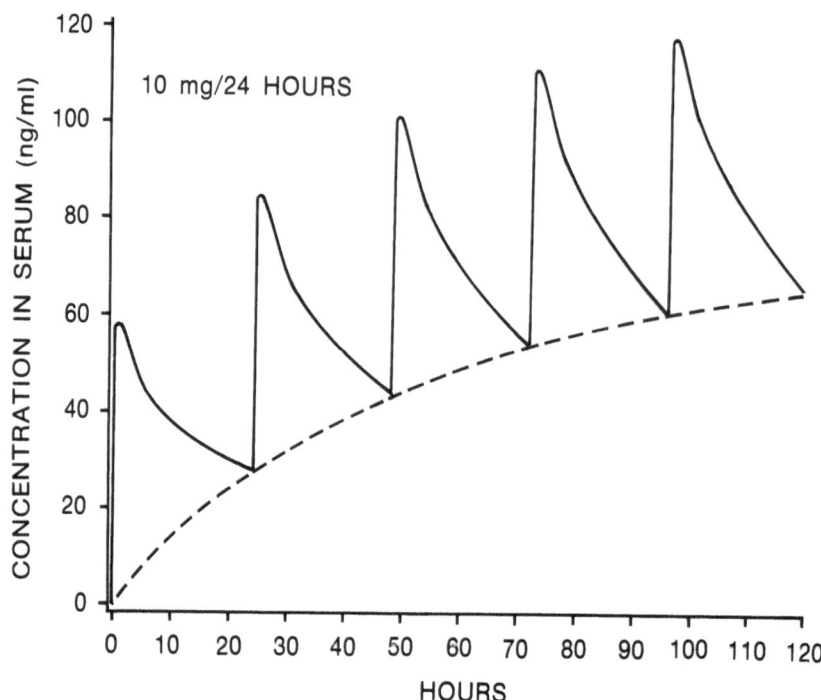

FIGURE 1. Computer simulation of circulating levels of detirelix
resulting from daily s.c. injection of 10 mg to man,
based upon levels measured following a single dose of
10 mg to man.

LHRH antagonists also retard the growth of a number of other
tumors in animal models. These include a prolactin and
ACTH-secreting pituitary tumor [78], osteo- and chondro-sarcomas
[79,80] and pancreatic tumors [81]. By inference, gonadal
steroids must play some part in the growth of these tumors in the
animal. Whether this will hold true for the human disease remains
to be determined.

GENERAL PHARMACOLOGY

Although there was an isolated report of elevated blood pressure
and decreased heart rate leading to death in rats following
intraperitoneal injection of some early LHRH antagonists [82], it
was generally believed that the effects of these agents were
specific to the reproductive system. Evaluation of a representative analog (detirelix) by injection in a wide range of standard
pharmacological tests, was without effect [31]. In 1984, however,
it was reported that another analog ([N-Ac-D-Nal(2)^1,D-pF-
Phe^2,D-Trp^3,D-Arg^6]LHRH), administered i.m. or s.c. at or below the
dose required for reproductive effects, caused a 6 hour edematous
swelling of the face and paws and cyanosis of the tails of rats
[83]. Intravenous administration to rats caused vasodilation of
peripheral vessels, respiratory depression, lethargy and cyanosis

206

followed by death in some cases. Administration of this analog to rhesus monkeys caused facial and scrotal flushing and profound, although transient, behavioral depression.

It was subsequently shown that detirelix was in fact a potent mast cell degranulator in vitro or by intravenous administration to rats. Subcutaneous administration of very high doses (many fold the dose affecting reproductive function) failed to cause symptoms consistent with histamine release in either rats or monkeys (Table 2). The reasons for this discrepancy are not established but may be connected with the fact that the low solubility of the compound in body fluids results in precipitation at the site of injection, with formation of a slowly releasing depot of peptide so that acutely high blood levels are not reached. These differences between compounds have carried forward into man: anaphylactoid responses (urticaria, wheals) have been noted following single injection of [D-Nal(2)^1,D-pF-Phe^2, D-Trp^3,D-Arg^6]LHRH in spite of predosing with Benadryl® (J. Hall and W. Crowley Jr., personal communication). However, no reactions were observed in 6 men and mild transient upper body flushing in only 1 of 6 women receiving 20 mg s.c. of detirelix (P. Hoffman and S.E. Monroe, personal communication). In this single responder much higher blood levels of detirelix were measured than in the other subjects suggesting a much more rapid absorption in this case. In all subjects studied, this dose caused a rapid fall in blood levels of the gonadotropins which were then maintained low for up to 48 hours [5]. In fact, maintained suppression of gonadotropins and gonadal function in men may be achieved with a daily dose of 1 mg. It does appear

Table 2. Comparison of the minimal dose (MED) requirement for effects of detirelix upon reproductive function and histamine release.

MED (S.C.)	Species	
	Rat	Monkey
suppression of gonadotropins	5 µg/kg	5–20 µg/kg
suppression of cycling	240 µg/kg	100 µg/kg
suppression of spermatogenesis	100 µg/kg	250 µg/kg
causing edema	>4 mg/kg (300 µg/kg)*	–
causing flushing	–	>20 mg/kg (500 µg/kg)*

*i.v. dose

therefore that separation of reproductive and adverse effects is possible for these compounds.

CONCLUDING REMARKS

LHRH antagonists are agents whose advantages of rapidity of action and lack of initial stimulatory action at the pituitary compared to the agonists has been tempered by their single adverse pharmacological effect mediated through degranulation of mast cells. The strong possibility that this latter activity will be minimized if not abolished leaves the way clear for LHRH antagonists as clinically useful agents. However the relative cost and dosage of these analogs versus the agonists still dictates that they be used either for very short term therapy or in situations where the agonists are not useful or are contraindicated. Such possibilities include once weekly administration (with a periodic progestogen supplement) for female contraception, luteal phase administration for progesterone mediated disorders, perhaps including premenstrual syndrome, and fertility control in pets. The LHRH agonists are clearly not going to be useful male contraceptives, except by heroic treatment regimens [84]. The LHRH antagonists may be effective for this purpose [85] but it is unlikely that this use will be economically viable unless analogs with at least a 10-fold increase in potency become available. Finally there are patients with gonadal hormone dependent cancers who are at risk during the early stimulation caused by LHRH agonist. Such patients may be candidates for LHRH antagonist therapy.

ACKNOWLEDGMENT

I thank Johnson C. Fong for supplying the computer simulation shown in Fig. 1.

REFERENCES

1. Karten, M.J. and Rivier, J.E. Gonadotropin-releasing hormone analog design. Structure-function studies toward the development of agonists and antagonists: rationale and perspectives. Endocr. Rev., 7, 44 (1986)
2. Vickery, B.H. and Nestor, J.J., Jr. LHRH analogues: development and mechanism of action. Sem. Reprod. Endocrinol., in press (1986)
3. Nestor, J.J., Jr. Historical review of LHRH antagonists. In "LHRH Analogues: Contraceptive and Therapeutic Applications. Part 2", Vickery, B.H. and Nestor, J.J., Jr. (Eds.), MTP Press, Lancaster, 1987, in press.

4. Mais, V., Kaser, R.R., Cetel, N.S., Rivier, J., Vale, W. and Yen, S.S.C. The dependency of folliculogenesis and corpus luteum function on pulsatile gonadotropin secretion in cycling women using a gonadotropin-releasing hormone antagonist as a probe. J. Clin. Endocrinol. Metab., 62, 1250 (1986)

5. Pavlou, S.N., Wakefield, G.B. and Kovacs, W.J. LHRH antagonists in normal men. In "LHRH Analogs: Contraceptive and Therapeutic Applications. Part 2", Vickery, B.H. and Nestor, J.J., Jr. (Eds.), MTP Press, Lancaster, in press (1987)

6. Karten, M.J., Hook, W.A., Siraganian, R.P., Coy, D.H., Folkers, K., Rivier, J.E. and Roeske, R.W. In vitro histamine release with LHRH analogs. In "LHRH and Its Analogs: Contraceptive and Therapeutic Applications. Part 2", Vickery, B.H. and Nestor, J.J., Jr. (Eds.), MTP Press, Lancaster, in press (1987)

7. Morgan, J.E., O'Neil, C.E., Coy, D.H., Hocart, S.J. and Nekola, M.V. Antagonistic analogs of luteinizing hormone-releasing hormone are mast cell secretagogues. Int. Arch. Allergy Appl. Immunol., 80, 70 (1986)

8. Roeske, R., Chaturvedi, N.C., Hrinyo-Paulina, T. and Kowalczuk, M. LHRH antagonists with low histamine release activity. In "LHRH and Its Analogs: Contraceptive and Therapeutic Applications. Part 2", Vickery, B.H. and Nestor, J.J., Jr. (Eds.), MTP Press, Lancaster, in press (1987)

9. Roeske, R.W., Chaturvedi, N.C., Rivier, J., Vale, W., Porter, J. and Perrin, M. Substitution of Arg^5 for Tyr^5 in GnRH antagonists. In "Peptides: Structure and Function", Deber, C.M., Hruby, V.J. and Kopple, K.D. (Eds.), Pierce Chemical Co., Rockford, 1985, p. 561.

10. Rivier, J.E., Porter, J., Rivier, C.L., Perrin, M., Corrigan, A., Hook, W.A., Siraganian, R.P. and Vale, W.W. New effective gonadotropin-releasing hormone antagonists with minimal potency for histamine release in vitro. J. Med. Chem., 29, in press (1986)

11. Heber, D., Dodson, R., Swerdloff, R.S., Channabassavaiah, K. and Stewart, J.M. Pituitary receptor site blockade by a gonadotropin-releasing hormone antagonist in vivo: mechanism of action. Science, 216, 420 (1982)

12. Clayton, R.N. and Catt, K.J. Gonadotropin-releasing hormone receptors: characterization, physiological regulation and relationship to reproductive function. Endocr. Rev., 2, 186 (1981)

13. Sharpe, R.M. and Fraser, H.M. Leydig cell receptors for luteinizing hormone-releasing hormone and their modulation by administration or deprivation of the releasing hormone. Biochem. Biophys. Res. Commun., 95, 256 (1980)

14. Bramley, T.A., Menzies, G.S. and Baird, D.T. Specific binding of gonadotrophin-releasing hormone and an agonist to human corpus luteum homogenates: characterization, properties and luteal phase levels. J. Clin. Endocrinol. Metab., 61, 834 (1985)

15. Bramley, T.A. and Menzies, G.S. Subcellular fractionation of the human corpus luteum: distribution of GnRH binding sites. Molec. Cell. Endocr., 45, 27 (1986)
16. Eidne, K.A., Flanagan, C.A. and Millar, R.P. Gonadotropin-releasing hormone binding sites in human breast carcinoma. Science, 229, 989 (1985)
17. Iwashita, M., Evans, M.I. and Catt, K.J. Characterization of a gonadotropin-releasing hormone receptor site in term placenta and chorionic villi. J. Clin. Endocrinol. Metab., 62, 127 (1986)
18. Hsueh, A.J.W. and Jones, P.B.C. Extrapituitary actions of gonadotropin-releasing hormone. Endocr. Rev., 2, 437 (1981)
19. Hsueh, A.J.W. and Ling, W.C. Effect of an antagonistic analog of gonadotropin-releasing hormone upon ovarian granulosa cell function. Life Sci., 25, 1223.
20. Hsueh, A.J.W. Direct effects of gonadotropin-releasing hormone on testicular Leydig cell functions. Ann. N.Y. Acad. Sci., 383, 249 (1982)
21. Miller, W.R., Scott, W.N., Morris, R., Fraser, H.M. and Sharpe, R.N. Growth of human breast cancer cells inhibited by a luteinizing hormone-releasing hormone agonist. Nature, 313, 231 (1985)
22. Siler-Khodr, T.M., Khodr, G.S., Vickery, B.H. and Nestor, J.J., Jr. Inhibition of hCG, αhCG and progesterone release from human placental tissue in vitro by a GnRH antagonist. Life Sci., 32, 2741 (1983)
23. Nekola, M.V. and Coy, D.H. Direct and indirect inhibition of ovulation in rats by an antagonist of luteinizing hormone-releasing hormone. Endocrinology, 116, 756 (1985)
24. Corbin, A. and Beattie, C.W. Inhibition of the pre-ovulatory proestrous gonadotropin surge, ovulation and pregnancy with a peptide analogue of LH-RH. Endocr. Res. Commun., 2, 1 (1975)
25. Nekola, M.V. and Coy, D.H. LHRH antagonists in females. In "LHRH and Its Analogs: Contraceptive and Therapeutic Applications", Vickery, B.H., Nestor, J.J., Jr., and Hafez, E.S.E. (Eds.), MTP Press, Lancaster, 1984, p. 125.
26. Kenigsberg, D. and Hodgen, G.D. Ovulation inhibition by administration of weekly gonadotropin-releasing hormone antagonist. J. Clin. Endocrinol. Metab., 62, 734 (1986)
27. Balmaceda, J.P., Schally, A.V., Coy, D. and Asch, R.H. The effects of an LHRH antagonist ([N-Ac-D-Trp^{1,3},D-p-Cl-Phe^2,D-Phe^6,D-Ala^{10}]LH-RH) during the preovulatory period in the rhesus monkey. Contraception, 24, 275 (1981)
28. Vickery, B.H., McRae, G.I. and Goodpasture, J.C. Clinical uses of LHRH analogs in dogs. In "LHRH and Its Analogs: Contraceptive and Therapeutic Applications. Part 2", Vickery, B.H. and Nestor, J.J., Jr. (Eds.), MTP Press, Lancaster, in press (1987)
29. Vickery, B.H. Pharmacology of LHRH antagonists. In "Pharmacology and Clinical Uses of Inhibitors of Hormone Secretion and Action", Furr, B.J.A. and Wakeling, A. (Eds.), Bailliere Tindall, London, 1987, p. 385

30. Cetel, N.S., Rivier, J., Vale, W. and Yen, S.S.C. The dynamics of gonadotropin inhibition in women induced by an antagonistic analog of gonadotropin-releasing hormone. J. Clin. Endocrinol. Metab., 57, 62 (1983)

31. Hardt, W., Schmidt-Gollwitzer, K., Nevinny-Stickel, J. and Schmidt-Gollwitzer, M. Progress in the contraceptive use of the LHRH agonist buserelin by intermittent medication with withdrawal bleeding induced by a progestational agent. Geburtschilfe Frauenheilkd., 42, 874 (1982)

32. Lemay, A., Faure, N., Labrie, F. and Fazekas, A.T.A. Inhibition of ovulation during discontinuous intranasal luteinizing hormone-releasing hormone agonist dosing in combination with gestagen-induced bleeding. Fertil. Steril., 43, 868 (1985)

33. Rivier, C., Rivier, J. and Vale, W. Antireproductive effects of a potent GnRH antagonist in the female rat. Endocrinology, 108, 1425 (1981)

34. Rivier, C., Rivier, J. and Vale, W. Effects of gonadotropin-releasing hormone agonists and antagonists on reproductive function. J. Med. Chem., 26, 1545 (1983)

35. McRae, G.I., Vickery, B.H., Nestor, J.J., Jr., Bremner, W.J. and Badger, T.M. Biological evaluation of a highly potent LHRH antagonist. In "LHRH and Its Analogs: Contraceptive and Therapeutic Applications", Vickery, B.H., Nestor, J.J., Jr. and Hafez, E.S.E. (Eds.), MTP Press, Lancaster, 1984, p. 137.

36. Nishi, N., Arimura, A., de la Cruz, K.G. and Schally, A.V. Termination of pregnancy by sheep anti-LHRH gammaglobulin in rats. Endocrinology, 98, 1024 (1976)

37. Concannon, P.W. Effect of hypophysectomy and of LH administration on luteal phase plasma progesterone levels in the beagle bitch. J. Reprod. Fert., 58, 407 (1980)

38. Okkens, A.C., Dieleman, S.J., Bevers, M.M., Lubberink, A.A.M.E. and Willemse, A.H. Influence of hypophysectomy on the lifespan of the corpus luteum in the cyclic dog. J. Reprod. Fert., 77, 187 (1986)

39. Vickery, B.H. and McRae, G. Effect of a synthetic prostaglandin analog on pregnancy in the beagle bitch. Biol. Reprod., 22, 438 (1980)

40. Fraser, H.M., Abbott, M., Laird, N.C., McNeilly, S., Nestor, J.J., Jr. and Vickery, B.H. Effects of an LH-releasing hormone antagonist on the secretion of LH, FSH, prolactin and ovarian steroids at different stages of the luteal phase in the stumptailed macaque (Macaca arctoides) J. Endocrinol. 111, 83 (1986)

41. Fraser, H.M., Baird, D.T., McRae, G.I., Nestor, J.J., Jr. and Vickery, B.H. Suppression of luteal progesterone secretion in the stumptailed macaque by an antagonist analogue of luteinizing hormone releasing hormone. J. Endocrinol., 104, R1 (1985)

42. Fraser, H.M., Nestor, J.J., Jr. and Vickery, B.H. Suppression of luteal function by an LHRH antagonist during the early phase in the stumptailed macaque monkey and the effects of subsequent administration of hCG. Endocrinology, in press (1987)

43. Moudgal, N.R., MacDonald, G.J. and Greep, R.O. Role of endogenous primate LH in maintaining corpus luteum function in the monkey. J. Clin. Endocrinol. Metab., 35, 113 (1972)

44. Groff, T.R., Madhwa Raj, H.G., Talbert, L.M. and Willis, D.L. Effects of neutralization of luteinizing hormone on corpus luteum function and cyclicity in Macaca fascicularis. J. Clin. Endocrinol. Metab., 59, 1054 (1984)

45. Hutchison, J.S. and Zeleznik, A.J. The rhesus monkey corpus luteum is dependent on pituitary gonadotropin secretion throughout the luteal phase of the menstrual cycle. Endocrinology, 115, 1780 (1984)

46. Skarin, G., Nillius, S.J. and Wide, L. Failure to induce abortion of early human pregnancy by high doses of a superactive LRH agonist. Contraception, 26, 457 (1982)

47. Tolis, G., Comaru-Schally, A.M., Mehta, A.E. and Schally, A.V. Failure to interrupt established pregnancy in humans by D-Tryptophan-6-luteinizing-hormone-releasing-hormone. Fertil. Steril., 36, 241 (1981)

48. Siler-Khodr, T.M., Khodr, G.S., Vickery, B.H. and Nestor, J.J., Jr. Inhibition of hCG, αhCG and progesterone release from human placental tissue in vitro by a GnRH antagonist. Life Sci., 32, 2741 (1983)

49. Siler-Khodr, T.M., Khodr, G.S., Rhode, J., Vickery, B.H. and Nestor, J.J., Jr. Gestational age related inhibition of placental hCG, αhCG and steroid hormone release in vitro by a GnRH antagonist. Placenta, in press (1986)

50. Siler-Khodr, T.M., Kuehl, T.J. and Vickery, B.H. Effects of a GnRH antagonist on hormonal levels in the pregnant baboon and on fetal outcome. Fertil. Steril., 41, 448 (1984)

51. Siler-Khodr, T.M., Kuehl, T.J. and Vickery, B.H. Action of a GnRH antagonist in the pregnant baboon. 32nd Ann. Meet. Soc. Gynec. Invest., Phoenix, Arizona. Abstract (1985)

52. Siler-Khodr, T.M. and Khodr, G.S. Content of luteinizing hormone-releasing factor in the human placenta. Am. J. Obstet. Gynecol., 130, 216 (1978)

53. Currie, A.J., Fraser, H.M. and Sharpe, R.M. Human placental receptors for luteinizing hormone-releasing hormone. Biochem. Biophys. Res. Commun., 99, 332 (1981)

54. Petrie, E.C., Matsumoto, A.M., Nestor, J.J., Jr., Vickery, B.H., Gross, K., Southworth, M.B. and Bremner, W.J. Preclinical studies with LHRH antagonists. In "Male Contraception: Advances and Future Prospects", Zatuchni, G.I., Goldsmith, A., Spieler, J.M. and Sciarra, J.J. (Eds.), Harper and Row, Philadelphia, 1986, p. 361.

55. Rivier, C. and Vale, W. Hormonal secretion in male rats chronically treated with [D-Trp^6,Pro^9-NHEt]-LRF. Life Sci., 25, 1065 (1979)

56. Rivier, C., Rivier, J. and Vale, W. Antireproductive effects of a potent GnRH antagonist and testosterone propionate on mating behavior and fertility in the male rat. Endocrinology, 108, 1998 (1981)

57. Rea, M.A., Marshall, G.R., Weinbauer, G.F. and Nieschlag, E. Testosterone maintains pituitary and serum FSH and spermatogenesis in gonadotrophin-releasing hormone antagonist-suppressed rats. J. Endocrinol., 108, 101 (1986)

58. Bhasin, S., Fielder, T.J., Peacock, N. and Swerdloff, R.S. Testosterone selectively increases serum FSH but not LH in GnRH antagonist treated male rats: evidence for differential regulation of LH and FSH secretion. Endocrinology, 118, 499A (1986)

59. Vickery, B.H., McRae, G.I., Donahue, D.J., Roberts, B.B. and Worden, A.C. Suppression of testicular function in dogs with a highly potent LHRH antagonist. J. Androl., 6, 48P (1985)

60. Burgos-Briceno, L.A., Schally, A.V., Bartke, A. and Asch, R.H. Inhibition of serum luteinizing hormone and testosterone with an inhibitory analog of luteinizing hormone-releasing hormone in adult male rhesus monkeys. J. Clin. Endocrinol. Metab., 59, 601 (1984)

61. Akhtar, F.B., Weinbauer, G.F. and Nieschlag, E. Acute and chronic effects of a gonadotrophin-releasing hormone antagonist on pituitary and testicular function in monkeys. J. Endocrinol., 104, 345 (1985)

62. Weinbauer, G.F., Surmann, F.J., Akhtar, F.B., Vickery, B.H. and Nieschlag, E. Inhibition of male reproductive functions under long-term sustained release of a LHRH antagonist in a nonhuman primate. J. Steroid. Biochem., 20, 1410 (1984)

63. Weinbauer, G.F., Surmann, F.J., Akhtar, F.B., Shah, G.V., Vickery, B.H., and Nieschlag, E. Reversible inhibition of testicular function by a gonadotropin hormone-releasing hormone antagonist in monkeys (Macaca fascicularis). Fertil. Steril., 42, 906 (1985)

64. Adams, L.A., Bremner, W.J., Nestor, J.J., Jr., Vickery, B.H. and Steiner, R.A. Primate studies with a new potent gonadotropin releasing hormone (GnRH) antagonist. J. Androl., 6, P78 (1985)

65. Adams, L.A., Bremner, W.J., Nestor, J.J., Jr., Vickery, B.H. and Steiner, R.A. Suppression of plasma gonadotropins and testosterone in adult male monkeys (Macaca fascicularis) by a potent inhibitory analog of gonadotropin-releasing hormone. J. Clin. Endocrinol. Metab., 62, 58 (1986)

66. Heckel, N.J. and MacDonald, J.H. The rebound phenomenon of the spermatogenic activity of the human testis following the administration of testosterone propionate. Fertil. Steril., 3, 49 (1952)

67. Pavlou, S.N., DeBold, C.R., Island, D.P., Wakefield, G., Rivier, J., Vale, W. and Rabin, D. Single subcutaneous doses of a luteinizing hormone-releasing hormone antagonist suppress serum gonadotropin and testosterone levels in normal men. J. Clin. Endocrinol. Metab., 63, 303 (1986)

68. Pavlou, S.N., Wakefield, G.B., Island, D.P., Hoffman, P.G., LePage, M.E., Chan, R.L., Nerenberg, C.A. and Kovacs, W.J. Suppression of pituitary-gonadal function by a potent new luteinizing hormone-releasing hormone antagonist in normal men. J. Clin. Endocrinol. Metab., in press (1986)

69. Redding, T.W. and Schally, A.V. Inhibition of mammary tumor growth in rats and mice by administration of agonistic and antagonistic analogs of luteinizing hormone-releasing hormone. Proc. Natl. Acad. Sci. U.S.A., 80, 1459 (1983)

70. Miller, W.R., Scott, W.N., Morris, R., Fraser, H.M. and Sharpe, R.M. Suppression of the growth of a human breast cancer cell line by LHRH and an agonist analogue. Nature, 313, 231 (1985)

71. Redding, T.W., Coy, D.H. and Schally, A.V. Prostate carcinoma tumor size in rats decreases after administration of antagonists of luteinizing hormone-releasing hormone. Proc. Natl. Acad. Sci. U.S.A., 79, 1273 (1982)

72. Schally, A.V., Redding, T.W. and Comaru-Schally, A.M. Inhibition of prostate tumors by agonistic and antagonistic analogs of LHRH. The Prostate, 4, 545 (1983)

73. Waxman, J., Man, A., Hendry, W.F., Whitfield, H.N., Besser, G.M., Tiptaft, R.C., Paris, A.M. and Oliver, R.T. Importance of early tumor exacerbation in patients treated with long acting analogues of gonadotrophin-releasing hormone for advanced prostatic cancer. Brit. Med. J., 291, 1387 (1985)

74. Kahan, A., Delrieu, F., Amor, B., Chiche, R. and Steg, A. Disease flare induced by D-Trp⁶-LHRH analogue in patients with mestastatic prostate cancer. Lancet, 1, 971 (1984)

75. Kerbrat, P., Toussaint, C., Gedjuin, D. and Lobel, B. Aggravation of obstructive renal insufficiency by prostate cancer under treatment with a gonadorelin agonist. Presse Med., 15, 165 (1986)

76. Deghenghi, R. and Misset, J.L. Disease flare induced by luteinizing hormone-releasing hormone analogues in cancer patients. Lancet, 2, 1302 (1984)

77. Boumier, P., Koeger, A.C. and Camus, J.P. Dramatic aggravation of prostatic cancer at the onset of treatment with an LHRH agonist. Presse Med., 14, 1200 (1985)

78. De Quijada, M.G., Redding, T.W., Coy, D.H., Torres-Aleman, I. and Schally, A.V. Inhibition of growth of a prolactin-secreting pituitary tumor in rats by analogs of luteinizing hormone-releasing hormone. Proc. Natl. Acad. Sci. U.S.A., 80, 3485 (1983)

79. Redding, T.W. and Schally, A.V. Inhibition of growth of the transplantable rat chondrosarcoma by analogs of hypothralamic hormones. Proc. Natl. Acad. Sci. U.S.A., 80, 1078 (1983)

80. Schally, A.V. LH-RH analogs in contraception and cancer. In "LHRH and Its Analogs: Basic and Clinical Aspects", Labrie, F., Belanger, A. and Dupont, A. (Eds.), Elsevier Science Publishers, B.V., Amsterdam, 1984, p. 3.

81. Redding, T.W. and Schally, A.V. Inhibition of growth of pancreatic carcinomas in animal models by analogs of hypothalamic hormones. Proc. Natl. Acad. Sci. U.S.A., <u>81</u>, 248 (1984)

82. Smith, R.D. and Edgren, R.A. Elevated blood pressure following LHRH antagonists in rats. Contraception, <u>25</u>, 395 (1982)

83. Schmidt, F., Sundaram, K., Thau, R.B. and Bardin, C.W. [Ac-Nal(2)^1,4FD-Phe^2,D-Trp^3,D-Arg^6]-LHRH, a potent antagonist of LHRH produces transient edema and behavioral changes in rats. Contraception, <u>29</u>, 283 (1984)

84. Bouchard, P., Blondet, C., Spitz, I., Brailly, S., Jouannet, P. and Schaison, G. Sperm suppression by long acting GnRH agonist therapy in men: critical effect of testosterone substitution and duration of therapy. Endocrinology, <u>118</u>, 498A (1986)

85. Bremner, W.J. and Steiner, R.A. A potential male contraceptive: luteinizing hormone-releasing hormone (LHRH) antagonist plus testosterone. Clin. Res., <u>34</u>, 642A (1986)

14

Suppression of Plasma Gonadotropins, Testosterone and Sperm Production in Adult Male Monkeys by a Potent Inhibitory Analog of LHRH

W.J. BREMNER, L.A. ADAMS and R.A. STEINER

Veterans Administration Medical Center (III), 1660 South Columbian Way, Seattle, WA 98108, USA

INTRODUCTION

Suppression of circulating levels of reproductive hormones is desirable in some clinical situations, such as the treatment of precocious puberty and steroid-dependent neoplasms and the control of male and female fertility. Synthetic inhibitory analogs of LHRH are being developed as potential therapeutic agents for use in these circumstances, and as a prelude to human trials have been tested for their ability to inhibit reproductive function in a variety of animal models. Only limited information is available concerning the effects of these agents in male non-human primates [1-5].

In the present studies we examined acute and chronic effects of administration of the LHRH antagonist analog [N-Ac-D-Nal(2)^1, D-pCl-Phe^2, D-Trp^3, D-hArg(Et$_2$)^6, D-Ala^{10}] LHRH (RS-68439) to adult male macaques. The initial phase of this study was designed to assess the effect of a single injection of antagonist on circulating levels of reproductive hormones in both castrate and intact monkeys. Since administration of this compound to men is likely to involve a regimen of single daily injections, we were particularly interested in identifying a dose of antagonist that would suppress testosterone levels for 24 hours. The subsequent phase of the study was conducted to determine whether suppression of gonadotropins and testosterone in intact animals could be sustained for a period of weeks by daily injections of the antagonist. Finally, we have initiated studies of the long-term effects of the antagonist on spermatogenesis.

Animals

Sexually mature male crab-eating macaques, Macaca fascicularis, weighing 4.5-9.0 kg, were used in these experiments [4]. The animals were housed in individual cages under controlled conditions of light (on at 0600 h; off at 1800 h), heat (25.5 ± 1°C), and relative humidity (65%). Exp I was performed in castrate (n=8) and intact (n=7) animals. Exp II was performed in intact (n=12) animals. Exp III was performed in intact (n=5) animals.

Drugs

The LHRH antagonist (RS-68439) used in this study was [N-Ac-D-Nal(2)^1, D-pCl-Phe^2,D-Trp^3, D-hArg(Et$_2$)^6, D-Ala^{10}] LHRH (RS68439; Syntex Research, Palo Alto, CA). In Exp I, the compound was diluted in 0.15 M saline and kept frozen until used. In Exp II and III, the diluent was 0.0-2 M acetate buffer, pH 5.0, with 0.9% benzyl alcohol added as preservative; the solution was refrigerated until used.

Experimental Design

Exp I: castrate animals. Administration of the antagonist was begun one week after insertion of the venous catheter. Each animal received a single bolus iv injection of RS-68439 at doses of 0 (vehicle; n=8), 5 (n=8), 50 (n=8), 250 (n=3), and 500 (n=8) µg/kg; doses were given in pseudorandom order, separated by one-week intervals. Three blood samples (1 ml/sample) were obtained at 30-min intervals beginning at -1, +4, +8, +24, +48, and +72 hours relative to RS-68439 or vehicle administration; equal aliquots of plasma from each of the three samples were pooled for analysis of LH and FSH.

Exp I: intact animals. Each animal received single sc injections of antagonist at doses of 0 (vehicle; n=7), 5 (n=7), 50 (n=7), 250 (n=5), and 500 (n=7) µg/kg administered in pseudorandom order at one-week intervals. Blood samples were obtained at -0, +6, and +24 hours relative to RS-68439 or vehicle administration and consisted of a single 5-ml sample drawn by venipuncture of a femoral, cephalic, or saphenous vein while maintaining the animal under sedation with 20-30 mg ketamine hydrochloride (Park-Davis, Morris Plains, NJ).

Exp II: intact animals. Twelve intact animals received sc injections of a single daily dose of RS-68439 for 21 days. Injections were given between 1200-1300 hours to animals anesthetized with ketamine, and a single 5-ml blood sample was drawn by venipuncture immediately before RS-68439 administration on days 0, 1, 7, 14, and 21. RS-68439 was administered at doses of 0 (vehicle), 50, 100, or 250 µg/kg; each dose was given to three animals.

Exp III: intact animals. Following a 12-week control period, five animals received daily injections of 750 µg/kg of antagonist and testosterone-containing Silastic implants designed to maintain normal serum testosterone levels. The treatment period was 16 weeks. Sperm counts (electroejaculation) and serum testosterone levels were determined every two weeks during the control and treatment periods.

Blood Handling and Hormone Assays

Blood was centrifuged immediately after collection, and the plasma was stored at -20°C until analyzed for testosterone, LH, and FSH. Plasma testosterone levels in intact animals were determined by RIA, as described previously [4,6]. The sensitivity of the testosterone assay was less than 0.1 ng/ml, and the intra- and interassay coefficients of variations (CVs) were 5.1% and 9.8%, respectively. Plasma levels of LH in castrate animals were measured by RIA, as described by Peckham and Tontala [7] The reference preparation was rhesus pituitary LH (WP-XV-20); purified cynomolgus pituitary LH was used for radioiodination, and the antiserum was rabbit anti-hCG (R13). The sensitivity of the assay was 64 ng/ml, and the interassay CV was 13.0% at 75% binding. Plasma LH levels in intact animals were measured with a mouse Leydig cell bioassay [8], which had intra- and interassay CVs of 6% and 18%, respectively. The sensitivity of the assay was 0.3 µg/ml when samples were run at a 20-µl volume (Exp I) and 0.6 µg/ml when samples were run at a 10-µl volume (Exp II). The reference preparation was monkey pituitary gonadotropin LER 1902-2. FSH levels in castrate animals were determined by RIA with the method of Hodgen et al

218

[9]. The reference preparation was monkey pituitary gonadotropin cyn-FSH-RP1. Human FSH was used as the tracer and the primary antiserum was antiovine FSH (H-31), prepared in rabbits and used at a final dilution of 1:150,000. The interassay CV was 10% at a binding of 33%, and the sensitivity of the assay was 12.5 ng/ml. All samples from an individual animal were analyzed at the same time.

Data Analysis

The amount of hormone present in the plasma at each postinjection time point was compared to the preinjection control value for a particular animal, and the percentage of control value was calculated. One-way analysis of variance was performed on log-normalized data and used in conjunction with a Student's one-tailed t test to identify significant (P $\leq$ 0.05) decreases in hormone levels over time.

Effects in Castrate Animals

Plasma LH levels were markedly reduced by 4 hours after a single injection of 5, 50, 250, or 500 μg/kg RS-68439 (Fig.1). LH levels reached nadir values

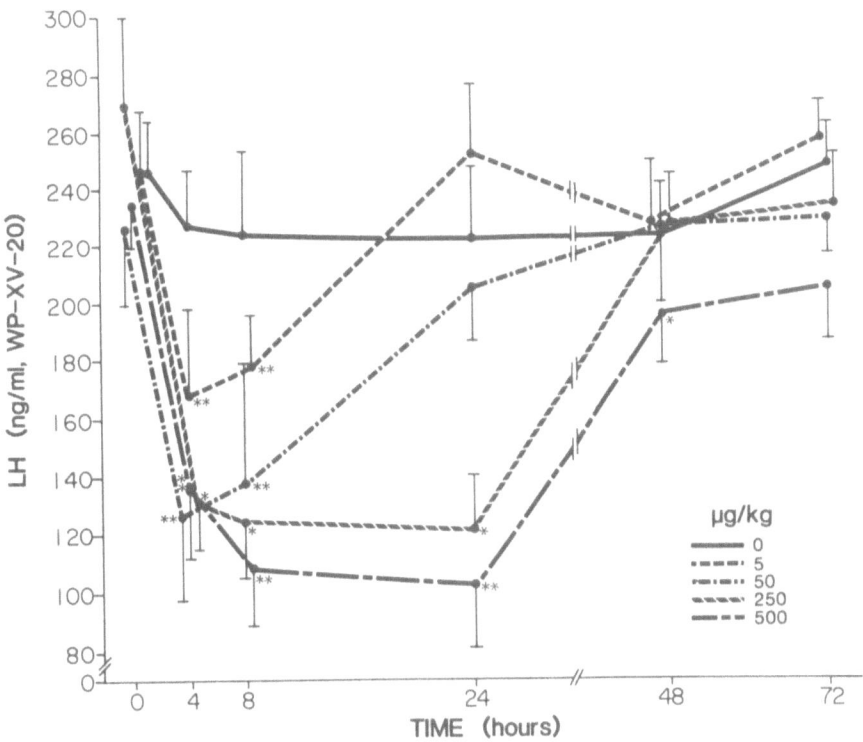

FIGURE I. Mean ($\pm$ SEM) plasma LH levels in castrate animals before and after iv injection of RS-68439. *, P $\leq$ 0.05; **, P $\leq$ 0.01 (RS-68439 treatment vs. preinjection). Reproduced from Adams et al/J. Clin. Endocrinol Metab., 62,58 (1986). Used by permission of the Endocrine Society.

219

by 8 hours after administration of 250 or 500 µg/kg doses, remained at these values for 24 hours, and had returned to 85% of the preinjection values by 48 hours. LH levels were reduced for 8 hours by 5 and 50 µg/kg RS-68439 and returned to 98% or more of control values by 24 hours after injection. Vehicle injections did not result in significant suppression of LH at any time point.

Plasma FSH levels were reduced by 4 hours after administration of each dose of antagonist (Fig. 2). Injections of 250 or 500 µg/kg RS-68439 maximally suppressed FSH levels for 24 hours ≤ 0.01), and 5 or 50 µg/kg RS-68439 suppressed FSH maximally for 8 hours.

The maximal degree of FSH suppression was comparable to that of LH at each dose, but FSH levels recovered more slowly than did LH levels after administration of 50, 250, and 500 µg/kg RS-68439. FSH levels were not significantly suppressed at any time after vehicle administration.

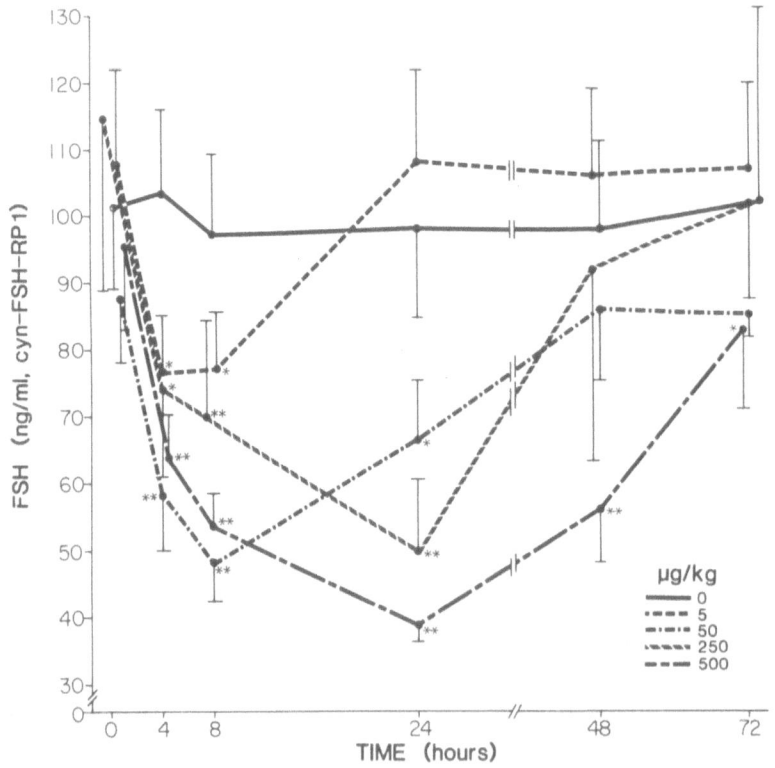

FIGURE 2.   Mean (±SEM) plasma FSH levels in castrate animals before (0 hours) and after iv injection of RS-68439. *, P ≤ 0.05; **, P ≤ 0.01 (for RS-68439 treatment vs. preinjection value). Reproduced from Adams et al/J. Clin. Endocrinol. Metab., 62,58 (1986). Used by permission of the Endocrine Society.

Effects of Single Injection in Intact Animals

Plasma testosterone levels declined markedly 6 hours after administration of 50, 250, or 500 µg/kg RS-68439 (Fig. 3). The two higher doses sustained this inhibition of testosterone at levels that were less than 30% of preinjection values at 24 hours. Neither vehicle nor 5 µg/kg RS-68439 significantly reduced plasma testosterone levels.

Plasma LH levels decreased 6 hours after administration of each dose of the antagonist. Maximal inhibition was evident 24 hours after administration of 250 or 500 µg/kg antagonist, and doses of 5 and 50 µg/kg maintained a slight inhibition of LH levels for this period of time. In animals receiving vehicle, LH levels were elevated at 6 and 24 hours, presumably because the samples were collected during spontaneous episodes of LH release.

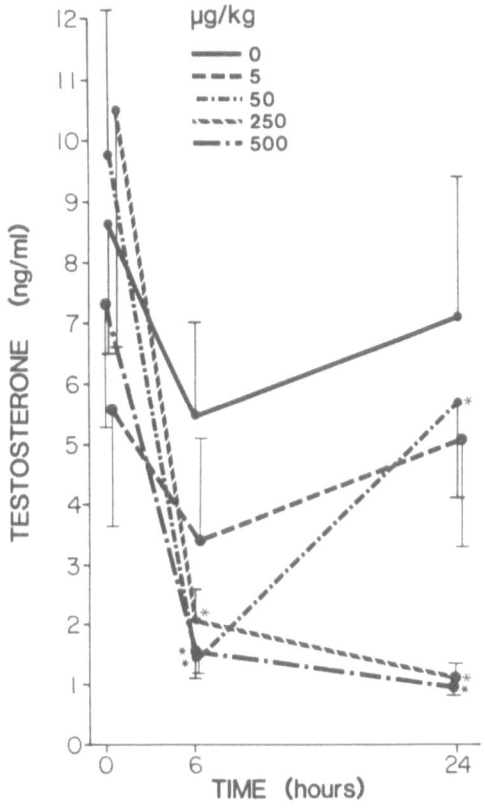

FIGURE 3. Mean (± SEM) plasma testosterone levels in intact animals before and after sc injection of RS-68439. *, P ≤ 0.05 (for RS-68439 treatment vs. preinjection value). Reproduced from Adams et al/J. Clin. Endocrinol. Metab. 62,58 (1986). Used by permission of the Endocrine Society.

Effects of Repetitive Daily Injection

Plasma testosterone decreased to near-castrate levels 24 hours after administration of 250 μg/kg RS-68439 and this suppression was sustained for the ensuing 20 days of treatment (Fig. 4). Daily injections of 0, 50, or 100 μg/kg RS-68439 did not suppress testosterone either acutely (24 hours) or chronically (three weeks).

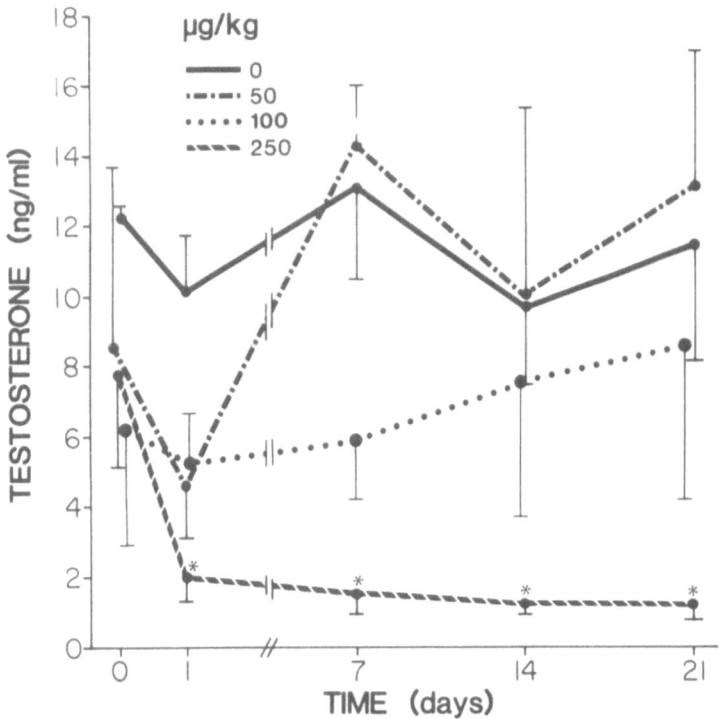

FIGURE 4. Mean (± SEM) plasma testosterone levels in intact animals receiving daily sc injections of RS-68439. *, P ≤ 0.05 (for RS-68439 treatment vs. preinjection value). Reproduced from Adams et al/J. Clin. Endocrinol. Metab. 62,58 (1986). Used by permission of the Endocrine Society.

Plasma LH levels were below the limit of detectability of the bioassay by 24 hours after administration of 250 μg/kg RS-68439 and were also undetectable in samples obtained after 21 days of treatment. Daily injections of vehicle did not lower plasma LH levels at either 24 hours or three weeks.

Supplementation with Testosterone

The Silastic implant containing testosterone exerted the desired effect of maintaining serum testosterone at normal levels despite daily injections of 750 μg/kg of antagonist. In this hormonal milieu of pituitary gonadotropin suppression exerted by the antagonist and normal serum testosterone levels maintained by the implant, all five animals were consistently azoospermic between 12 and 16 weeks on the experimental regimen.

DISCUSSION

In the present studies we evaluated the response of the reproductive axis to RS-68439 administration in both intact and castrate primates. The advantages of studying this compound in the castrate model include the fact that the pituitary and hypothalamus are released from inhibitory negative feedback effects normally exerted upon them by testicular hormones. This allows demonstration of the time course and degree of action of the antagonist specifically on pituitary function, without the confounding factors of changing gonadal feedback and possible direct gonadal effects of the peptide.

A single injection of this potent LHRH antagonist produced a marked dose-related reduction of plasma LH and FSH levels in castrate animals within 4 hours and sustained this effect for at least 24 hours. FSH levels returned to preinjection values more slowly than did LH levels; although the mechanism whereby LH and FSH may be differentially sensitive to suppression is not clear, our observations are consistent with those made in ovariectomized monkeys that LH levels recovered from suppression by an antagonist 24 hours earlier than did FSH levels [10].

A single injection of RS-68439 reduced testosterone and LH levels in a dose-related manner for 24 hours in intact animals, and daily injections of the compound for 21 days maintained suppression of LH and testosterone for that period of time. The fact that the degree of testosterone suppression effected by this compound was identical at 24 hours and 21 days suggests that this primate system does not become refractory to the effects of the antagonist over a period of weeks.

When the antagonist was administered for 16 weeks and testosterone levels in serum were maintained at a normal level by testosterone implants, all five animals became azoospermic. This interesting result implies that the degree of gonadotropin suppression produced by the antagonist is sufficient to eliminate spermatogenesis despite the possibility of direct stimulatory effects of testosterone on the testis.

Other workers tested this antagonist in castrate Macaca fascicularis and found that single injections of 200, 500, or 1000 µg/kg reduced plasma LH and FSH levels by 12 hours and maximally suppressed both gonadotropins by 24 hours after administration [3]. Continuous administration of the compound to intact male monkeys for a period of months resulted in androgen deficiency and severe oligospermia or azoospermia [3]. Although LH levels remained low for a longer period of time after single dose administration of 1000 µg/kg antagonist (96 hours) than after 200 or 500 µg/kg antagonist, the maximal degree of LH suppression was the same for all three doses. Our data also indicate that 250 and 500 µg/kg doses suppress LH to the same extent; these observations identify the lowest dose of antagonist that maintains LH suppression when administered once daily. Other inhibitory analogs of LHRH also suppress gonadotropin secretion in monkeys; however, they differ in potency, which may in part reflect species differences in sensitivity. For example administration of 200 µg/kg of the LHRH antagonist [N-Ac-Δ^3Pro^1, D-pF-D-Phe^2, D-Trp^{3,6}] LHRH to castrate male rhesus monkeys reduced plasma LH, but had no effect on FSH levels [1]. A similar dose (250 µg/kg) of the antagonist used in the present study reduced both gonadotropins for 48 hours and had a more profound suppressive effect on LH levels. A single injection of 5 µg/kg of the LHRH antagonist [N-Ac-D-pCl-Phe^{1,2}, D-Trp^3, D-Arg^6, D-Ala^{10}]LHRH to intact male rhesus monkeys promptly reduced serum LH and testosterone levels [2] and maintained inhibition of testosterone for 24 hours. In our animals, testosterone levels had returned to preinjection values 24 hours after administration of 5 µg/kg antagonist.

The results of these and other studies demonstrate the ability of antagonist analogs of LHRH to suppress gonadotropin and testosterone levels and sperm production [3] for a period of days to weeks. The immediate decline of reproductive hormone levels after antagonist administration circumvents the problems associated with agonist treatment and supports the use of these compounds as therapeutic agents in clinical situations requiring long term suppression of gonadal function. The ability of the antagonist combined with testosterone to completely suppress spermatogenesis in our studies [5] while maintaining normal serum testosterone levels suggests that this combination may be useful in male contraceptive development.

ACKNOWLEDGMENTS

The authors thank Connie Nosbisch, Pamela Kolb, Patricia Gosciewski, Florida Flor, and Lorraine Shen for their expert technical assistance and Elaine Rost, Donna Sawin, and Lynn Guthrie for preparation of the manuscript. We are grateful to Dr. Donald Clifton for his help with statistical analyses and to the staff of the Regional Primate Research Center at the University of Washington for their excellent animal care. Thanks to the NICHHD and NIADDK for gonadotropin assay preparations and to WHO for testosterone assay reagents.

This work was supported by Contract NOI-HD-4-2801 from the Contraceptive Development branch, NICHHD, by NIH Grants HD-12629, RR-00166, and ROI-HD-12625, and by a grant from the Veterans Administration. Portions of this chapter were published previously (J. Clin. Endocrinol. Metab. 62,58 1986) and are used with the permission of the Endocrine Society.

REFERENCES

1. Pineda, J.L., Lee, B.C., Spiliotis, B.E., Vale, W., Rivier, J., Brown, T.J. and Bercu, B.B. Effect of LHRH antagonist [Ac-Δ^{2}Pro^1,pF-D-Phe^2,D-Trp^{3,6}] LHRH on pulsatile gonadotropin secretion in the castrate male primate. J. Clin. Endocrinol. Metab., 56,420 (1983).
2. Burgos-Briceno, L.A., Schally, A.V., Bartke, A. and Asch, R.H. Inhibition of serum luteinizing hormone and testosterone with an inhibitory analog of luteinizing hormone-releasing hormone in adult male rhesus monkeys. J. Clin. Endocrinol. Metab., 59,601 (1984).
3. Weinbauer, G.F., Surmann, F.J., Akhtar, F.B., Shah, G.V., Vickery, B.H. and Nieschlag, E. Reversible inhibition of testicular function by a gonadotropin-releasing hormone antagonist in monkeys (Macaca fasicularis). Fertil. Steril., 42,906 (1984).
4. Adams, L.A., Bremner, W.J., Nestor, J.J., Vickery, B.H. and Steiner, R.A. Suppression of plasma gonadotropins and testosterone in adult

male monkeys (<u>Macaca fascicularis</u>) by a potent inhibitory analog of gonadotropin-releasing hormone. J. Clin. Endocrinol. Metab., <u>62</u>, 58 (1986).

5. Bremner, W.J. and Steiner, R.A. A potential male contraceptive: luteinizing hormone releasing hormone (LHRH) antagonist plus testosterone (T). Clin. Res. <u>34</u>, 642A (1986).

6. Matsumoto, A.M. and Bremner, W.J. Modulation of pulsatile gonadotropin secretion by testosterone in man. J. Clinic. Endocrinol. Metab., <u>58</u>, 609 (1984).

7. Peckham, W.D. and Tontala, F.G. A new radioimmunoassay for monkey luteinizing hormone (Abstract). Biol. Reprod., [Suppl 1], <u>24</u>, 193 (1981).

8. Steiner, R.A. and Bremner, W.J. Endocrine correlates of sexual development in the male monkey, <u>Macaca fascicularis</u>. Endocrinology, <u>109</u>, 14 (1981).

9. Hodgen G.D., Wilks, J.W., Vaitukaitis, J.L., Chen, HC., Papkoff, H. and Ross, G.T. A new radioimmunoassay for the follicle-stimulating hormone in macaques: ovulatory menstrual cycles. Endocrinology, <u>99</u>, 137 (1976).

10. Balmaceda, J.P., Coy, D.H., Schally, A.V. and Asch R.H. Temporal changes in FSH and LH concentrations following the administration of a potent LHRH inhibitory analogue [N-Ac-D-Trp^{1,3}, D-p-Cl-Phe^2,D-Ala^{10}]-LHRH to oophorectomized rhesus monkeys. Acta Eur. Fertil., <u>14</u>, 249 (1983).

15
LHRH Antagonists and Female Reproductive Function

H.M. FRASER

MRC Reproductive Biology Unit, Centre for Reproductive Biology,
37 Chalmers Street, Edinburgh, Scotland

INTRODUCTION

Early studies using LHRH antagonists were sometimes confounded by use of analogues of low potency which, because they were administered at insufficient dosage, gave incomplete blockade of the LHRH receptors. With the development of antagonists of greater potency, some early negative observations have required revision. With current studies, one must still take account of the degree of gonadotropin suppression achieved and the length of time for which each dose is effective as both parameters could influence the immediate outcome and return to normal ovarian function.

This review will focus on the major advances in uses of LHRH antagonists during the last three years to elucidate the role of LHRH and the pituitary gonadotropins during the various stages of the reproductive cycle in the female primate. This has been achieved by blocking the LHRH receptor for 1-6 days during the periods of follicle selection, and maturation of the dominant follicle and the pre-ovulatory LH surge. The same approach has been used to investigate the various stages of the luteal phase and early pregnancy.

CONTROL OF FOLLICULAR MATURATION

Early follicular development and selection

Detailed studies on measurement of serum LH and FSH profiles during the follicular phase in the monkey and in women [1-4] reveal a rise in FSH, during the last few days of the luteal phase as progesterone concentrations fall, which is maintained until estradiol and inhibin from the developing follicles exert their negative feedback action. These levels of FSH, together with pulses of LH occurring at a frequency of every 90 min - 2 hours are responsible for follicles undergoing recruitment to be selected for maturation, but the relative roles of these hormones throughout this process is incompletely understood. That LHRH is essential for follicular development has been established from studies in which the hypothalamic stimulation has been suppressed chronically in monkeys by pituitary stalk section [5], placing lesions in the arcuate nucleus to prevent LHRH release [6] and LHRH immunoneutralization [7]. Chronic daily administration to monkeys of 40 ug [N-Ac-D- Trp^{1,3},D-pCl-Phe^2,D-Phe^6,D-Ala^{10}] LHRH per Kg per day or 1000 ug [Ac-pCl-Phe^{1,2},D-Trp^3, D-Arg^6,D-Ala^{10}] LHRH antagonist/Kg/day beginning during the early follicular phase and continuing throughout the cycle also blocks follicular development as shown by low serum concentrations of estradiol [8,9], although in some monkeys an occasional 'breakthrough' rise in estradiol can be observed [9].

It should be possible to use this antagonist-induced 'medical hypophysectomy' to elucidate the relative roles of LH and FSH during the various stages of follicular development using exogenous LH or FSH [9,10]. For example, comparison of effects of administration of pure FSH or FSH plus LH to antagonist-treated monkeys revealed that follicular development and dominance could be induced just as effectively with FSH alone [9].

Administration of 200 ug [N-Ac-D-Trp^{1,3},D-pCl-Phe^2, D-Phe^6, D-Ala^{10}]/Kg/day LHRH antagonist from days 1-6 of the cycle in rhesus monkeys [11] or of 80 ug [Ac- ^{3}-Pro^1,D-pF-Phe^2, D-Trp^{3,6}] LHRH per Kg twice daily for 3 days (days 2-5) of the cycle in women [12] resulted in a fall in serum concentrations of LH, FSH and estradiol. The detailed changes in gonadotropins were not investigated in the rhesus monkey study. In women the administration of 80 ug/kg antagonist twice daily attenuated, but did not abolish, LH pulses and suppressed FSH output by only 22%, yet still suppressed estradiol secretion. The extended length of the follicular phase (2.4 days) was not significantly different from control cycles. Six day treatment of the monkeys extended the follicular phase by 9 days [11]. The delay in ovulation appears to be equivalent to the duration of antagonist-induced suppression of gonadotropin suggesting that the suppression of gonadotropin causes the demise of the follicles undergoing selection and new follicles must then be selected from those in the process of recruitment.

The prospects of using LHRH antagonist-induced FSH suppression during the period of follicle recruitment as a contraceptive by causing a defective luteal phase are not supported by these results. Instead of the follicles continuing to develop into an abnormal corpus luteum, recruitment and selection of new follicles leads to normal luteal function [11,12].

Considerable interest has focused on the process of follicular selection of the dominant follicle which occurs around day 7. This time point may be optimal for selective interference leading to contraceptive applications.

When 80 ug [Ac- ^{3}-Pro^1,D-pF-Phe^2,D-Trp^{3,6}] LHRH/Kg twice daily was administered for 3 consecutive days around this period, to women [12] or 300 ug [N-Ac-D-Nal(2)^1,D-pCl-Phe^2, D-Trp^3,D-hArg(Et2)^6 D-Ala^{10}] LHRH per Kg per day to stumptailed macaque monkeys, the resultant fall in serum LH and FSH concentrations lead to an abrupt fall in levels of estradiol which are normally rising at this point (Fig 1). This fall appears to be a reflection of the functional demise of the follicle selected for ovulation. The length of the following follicular phase in the stumptailed macaques was 17.8 + 0.6 days (mean + SEM, n=8) from the first antagonist injection. Since the 3-day treatment suppressed gonadotropins for 5 days, the following 12 day period proceeding the next ovulation indicates that follicular recruitment must be re-enactivated. Repeated administration of [Ac-pCl-Phe[1,2], D-Trp[3],D-Arg[6],D-Ala[10]] LHRH as a single large dose (5 mg/kg) every seventh day in rhesus monkeys for a 4 week period was associated with rises in serum estradiol to mid-follicular phase levels but prevented ovulation. It has been suggested that this regimen could be developed for contraception with intermittent administration of a progestagen to counteract effects of 'unopposed estrogen' on the endometrium [13].

The dominant follicle and the pre-ovulatory period

From the ease with which follicular selection can be inhibited, it might appear likely that administration of an LHRH antagonist in the few days prior to ovulation could also induce atresia of the dominant follicle. Our data in the stumptailed macaque, however, suggest the follicle is relatively autonomous at this time. In 4 of 5 monkeys, 300 µg [N-Ac-D-Nal(2)[1],D-pCl-Phe[2],D-Trp[3], D-hArg(Et$_2$)[6], D-Ala[10]] LHRH/kg/day administered for 3 days caused only a transitory decline in serum estradiol. The LH surge occurred 2 days later and was followed by a luteal phase of normal duration (Fig. 1). This differential effect agrees with similar observations after injection of LHRH antibodies in macaques [14]. Some of the earlier detailed studies on effects of LHRH antagonists given at this time which showed failure to affect ovulation may have been successful had treatment started earlier in the follicular phase [15]. It is likely that by the late follicular phase stage the dominant follicle has accumulated sufficient receptor bound gonadotropin to continue through the final stages of maturation [16] while other growing follicles become atretic. It may also be supported by low serum levels of FSH remaining after antagonist.

There is a report that administration of 200µg [N-Ac-D-Trp[1,3],D-pCl-Phe[2],D-Phe[6],D-Ala[10]] LHRH/Kg to rhesus monkeys on a daily basis from days 10-14 of the cycle caused delay of ovulation in five of seven monkeys for 6-10 days [17]. However in the 2 monkeys which ovulated on schedule, it is stated that 'treatment was started when estradiol values were already ascending'. This suggests that in the other monkeys treatment was started prior to the last few pre-ovulatory days. The 6-10 day delay in ovulation after 5 days antagonist treatment suggests ovulation of follicles already selected for maturation at the time of treatment but held in suspension by incompletely suppressed gonadotropins.

Estrogen-induced LH surge

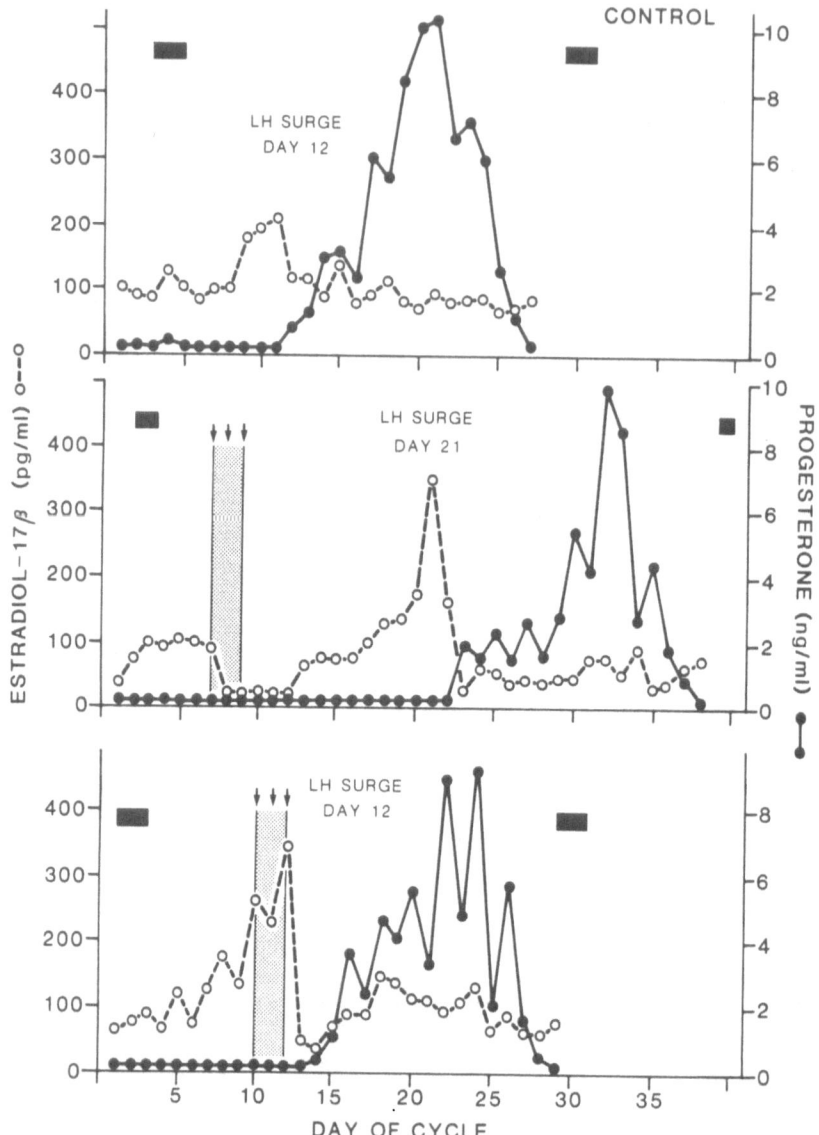

FIGURE 1   Effect of 3 daily s.c. injections of 300 ug, [N-Ac-D-Nal
            (2)[1],D-pCl-Phe[2],D-Trp[3],D-hArg(Et$_2$)[6],
            D-Ala[10]] LHRH antagonist/Kg body weight (arrows),
            administered starting day 7 (middle) or day 10 (bottom)
            of the follicular phase, on the serum concentrations of
            estradiol-17B and progesterone during the menstrual
            cycle of the stumptailed macaque. The top panel shows a
            typical control cycle, bars show menstrual bleeding.

During the period immediately prior to the LH surge the pituitary also seems much more resistant to receptor blockade by LHRH antagonist. The ability of the hypothalamo-pituitary axis to produce an LH surge may be tested by administering 40-50 ug/Kg estradiol benzoate to ovariectomized monkeys or intact monkeys during the early follicular phase. This will induce an LH surge within 48 hours. In monkeys chronically deprived of LHRH by lesions in the arcuate nucleus [6], active immunization against LHRH [7] or chronic LHRH antagonist administration [18] the LH surge is blocked. However, it is important to distinguish the effects of chronic deprivation of LHRH for several days or weeks with the function of the pituitary after acute LHRH receptor blockade.

To investigate the role of LHRH during the LH surge it is appropriate to have normal LHRH stimulation until the time of oestrogen administration. When this was investigated in monkeys with lesions in the arcuate nucleus in whom normal gonadotropin concentrations had been re-initiated by regular pulses of exogenous LHRH, it was observed that the LHRH could be stopped 24h prior to estrogen administration and still an LH surge could be induced [19]. This suggests that estrogen can induce an LH surge by acting on an LHRH primed pituitary [6,19]. This conclusion has been supported by experiments using passive LHRH immunoneutralization [14,20], but disputed by Norman et al [21] who claim some endogenous LHRH is being released. It should be remembered that the LHRH/oestrogen primed pituitary is particularly sensitive to LHRH stimulation. The number of pituitary LHRH receptors may also be increased [22], making it difficult to negate the actions of the endogenous hormone completely. Administration of 2000 ug [Ac-pCl-Phe[1,2],D-Trp[3],D-Arg, D-Ala[10]] LHRH per Kg per day to intact cynomologus monkeys for 4 days prior to injection of estradiol benzoate does abolish the LH surge [13], but there are no reports of effectiveness of delaying adminstration of antagonist to the time of estrogen injection in intact monkeys. This has been investigated in ovariectomized rhesus monkeys. In these animals the elevated serum concentrations of LH are initially suppressed by the negative feedback effects of estradiol, with a positive feedback occurring after 36-48 hours. Co-administration of [N-Ac-D-p-Cl-Phe[1,2],D-Trp[3],D-Arg[6],D-Ala[10]] LHRH or [N-Ac-D- Nal (2)[1],pF-D-Phe[2],D-Trp[3],D-Arg[10]] LHRH with the estradiol reinforced the negative feedback effect [23, 24]. Although the authors claim that continued administration of antagonist caused inhibition of the expected LH surge it is clear that LH still rises while antagonist is still being administered. While these results demonstrate a hypothalamic LHRH influence on the magnitude of the LH surge, a direct pituitary effect of estrogen still appears to be a significant component.

From the physiological point of view, measurement of LHRH in hypophysial portal blood of ovariectomized rhesus monkeys treated with estradiol benzoate has demonstrated an increased frequency and amplitude of LHRH pulses during the LH surge [25]. During the menstrual cycle, the increase in LH pulse frequency towards the late follicular phase and during the LH surge also implies an increase in LHRH pulse frequency [1-3].

Administration of LHRH antagonists during the late follicular phase does not appear to be a feasible contraceptive application. The dominant follicle appears to have a degree of autonomy, and the primed pituitary can be induced to release sufficient LH to produce ovulation. Even if the LH surge could be blocked, regular exposure of the endometrium to pre-ovulatory levels of estradiol in the absence of progesterone rises would be unacceptable. Prevention of follicular rupture and discharge of the ovum in the presence of normal steroid profiles might make a successful regimen. The occurrence of this situation after antagonist has been suggested [15] and requires further investigation.

LUTEAL PHASE

It has been known for many years that as the luteal phase progresses LH pulse frequency decreases and amplitude increases. More recently detailed evaluation of these changes and their relationship to progesterone secretion has been explored in studies in the rhesus monkey [26,27], stumptailed macaque monkey [28] and in women [29]. These studies have revealed that during the early luteal phase LH pulse frequency is highest, with low amplitude and high basal value (Fig. 2) but with no apparent relationship to progesterone secretion; the progesterone concentrations are low and without episodic pattern. During the mid luteal phase, the majority of LH pulses are associated with progesterone pulses, although some progesterone rises do not appear to be associated with an LH pulse.

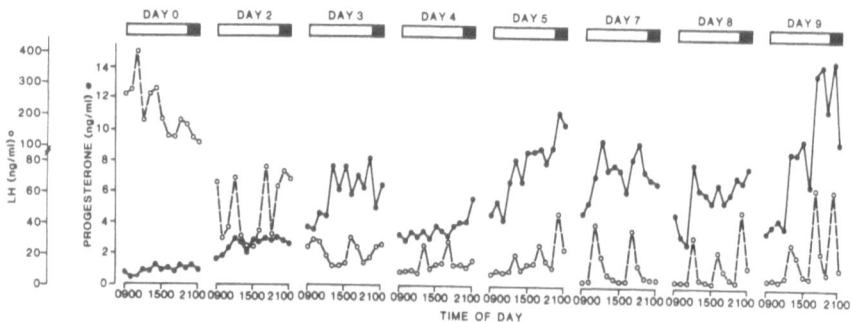

FIGURE 2   Serum concentrations of bioactive LH (0) and progesterone (0) in blood collected at hourly intervals on different days of the luteal phase in the stumptailed macaque. The day of the LH surge has been taken as day 0. Each set of daily data was obtained from a different monkey. Bars show lighting conditions (lights on, open bars; lights off, solid bars). Reproduced from Fraser et al J. Endocrinol III 83, (1986) [28] (by permission).

232

As the late luteal phase is entered the LH pulses are infrequent, but are of high amplitude and are followed by elevated levels of circulating progesterone.

The relationship between LH pulses and progesterone secretion during the mid-to-late luteal phase strongly indicate that the corpus luteum is being governed largely by acute changes in pituitary LH release at this time. The absence of a correlation between LH pulses and progesterone during the early luteal phase still leaves open the possibility that the corpus luteum is autonomous of LH at this time or is maximally stimulated by the high basal LH. Studies in which the LHRH signal is blocked during different stages of the luteal phase are beginning to unravel this relationship.

The role of LHRH and the pituitary gonadotropins in the control of the corpus luteum in primates and in women has been the subject of controversy. Most studies have indicated that LH is required for normal luteal function. Studies using antibodies to human chorionic gonadotrophin (hCG) or ovine LH to neutralize LH during the early luteal phase in monkeys demonstrated a shortening of cycle length [30,31]. Also, in rhesus monkeys with hypothalamic lesions in which ovulation had been induced with exogenous LHRH, and then this stimulation stopped during the luteal phase, serum concentrations of progesterone declined [32]. Investigations of hypophysectomized women treated with LH or hCG for different periods after ovulation suggested that, while the quota of LH required for ovulation could maintain progesterone secretion for a few days, the further daily administration of LH was necessary for normal luteal function [33]. In contrast, evidence that luteal function is independent of continued pituitary luteotrophic support has been provided by observations in rhesus monkeys hypophysectomized 1 day after ovulation [34]. The result was supported by further studies in which LH release was suppressed by blocking the LHRH receptor by daily administration of 200 µg [N-Ac-D-Trp^{1,3},D-pCl-Phe^1, D-Phe^6,D-Ala^{10}] LHRH/Kg/day throughout the luteal phase [35]. In both experiments progesterone secretion continued as normal.

The situation is complicated by the possibility that the dependence of the corpus luteum on the pituitary may change with age, there being an initial phase during which progesterone production is maintained by the LH produced by the mid-cycle surge, after which it becomes dependent on further LH secretion from the pituitary gland [36,37].

In a series of experiments in the stumptailed macaque involving single injections of 300 µg [N-Ac-D-Nal(2)^1,D-pCl-Phe^2, D-Trp^3, D-hArg(Et$_2$)^6,D-Ala^{10}] LHRH/Kg at different stages of the luteal phase we established firstly that when administered during the mid to late luteal phase, when the positive relationship between LH and progesterone is apparent, then suppression of LH was followed by a marked fall in serum progesterone secretion [38]. When the antagonist was given in the mid luteal phase, progesterone concentrations recovered once the effect of antagonist had worn off but were permanently suppressed when treatment was given on day 10.

Continued administration of LHRH antagonist twice daily from the
mid luteal phase until menses caused a sustained fall in serum
progesterone concentrations in cynomologus monkeys [39] and in
women [12].

When possible differential effects of selective gonadotropin
withdrawal were investigated by administering sufficient LHRH
antagonist to block LH release for a 24 hour period at different
stages of the luteal phase we found that even the early corpus
luteum is largely dependent upon LH [28] (Fig. 3). These findings
agree with a study in rhesus monkeys with hypothalamic lesions in
which ovulation had been induced with exogenous LHRH. When LHRH
stimulation was stopped during the luteal phase, serum progesterone
levels fell prematurely after stopping LHRH in either the early or
mid-luteal phases [32].

After a single injection of LHRH antagonist, although serum
progesterone concentrations fell to low values during the 24 hour
period, progesterone levels remained above baseline, particularly
in monkeys treated during the early luteal phase. This could be
the result of incomplete block of LH release, a degree of luteal
autonomy or a prolonged effect of previous exposure to LH being
capable of maintaining a basal release of progesterone in the
absence of further LH release. The latter explanation is the most
likely for the observations made during the early luteal phase.
Withdrawal of exogenous LHRH from monkeys with hypothalamic lesions
caused serum progesterone levels to fall more rapidly in the
mid-luteal phase (day 7) than in the early luteal phase (day 3).
In the latter case subnormal but detectable levels of progesterone
persisted for 2-3 days [32]. The failure of the study of Balmaceda
et al [35] to suppress luteal function with [N-Ac-D-Trp^{1,3},
D-pCl-Phe^1,D-Phe ^{6},D-Ala^{10}] LHRH was probably due to
incomplete suppression of LH and shows that the corpus luteum can
continue to function under subnormal levels of hormonal support.

The recovery in progesterone secretion and normal luteal length
after a single administration of [N-Ac-D-Nal(2)^1,D-pCl-Phe^2,
[D-Trp^3,D-hArg(Et$_2$)^6,D-Ala^{10}] LHRH antagonist during the
early or mid luteal phase shows that while progesterone secretion
is dependent on LH, the viability of the corpus luteum can be
preserved during this period of deprivation. The dependence of the
early corpus luteum on LH has been demonstrated more convincingly
by administering the same dose of this LHRH antagonist for 3
consecutive days beginning 1-5 days after the LH surge. All 8
stumptailed macaques demonstrated a progressive decline in serum
concentrations of LH FSH, estradiol and progesterone (e.g. Fig.4)
and premature menses. In 7 of the monkeys, progesterone
concentrations remained at follicular phase levels for the
remainder of the luteal phase, while in the remaining monkey a
normal luteal profile re-emerged after the last injection of LHRH
antagonist.

These studies showed that 3 daily injections of LHRH antagonist
during the early luteal phase can suppress luteal function. They
do not prove that premature luteal regression or luteolysis has

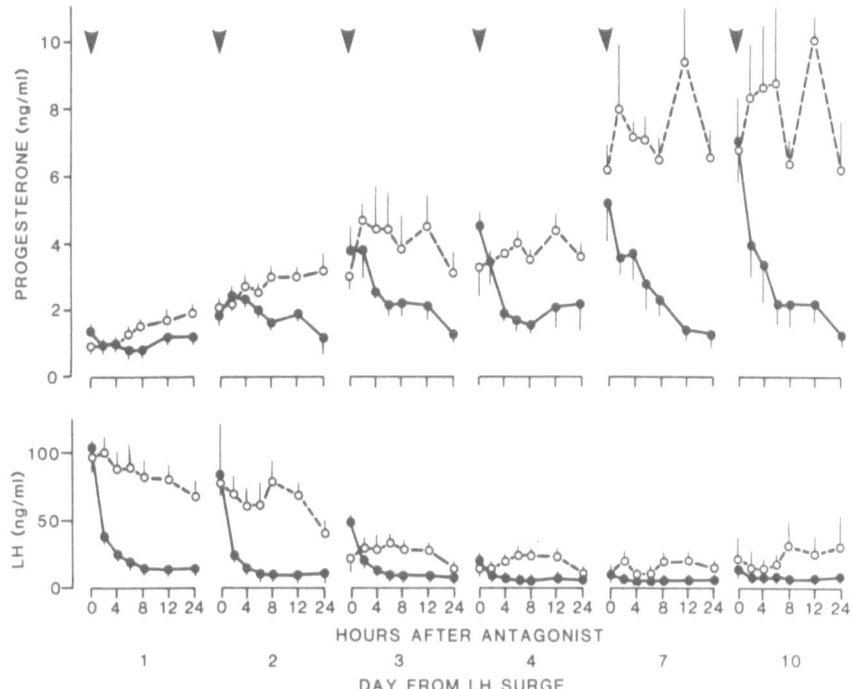

FIGURE 3   Effect of a single s.c. injection of vehicle alone (0)
or 300 ug [N-Ac-D-Nal(2)[1],D-pCl-Phe[2],
D-Trp[3],D-hArg (Et$_2$)[6], D-Ala[10]] LHRH /Kg body
weight (0) on different days of the luteal phase in the
stumptailed macaque on serum concentrations of bioactive
LH and progesterone. Values are means ± S.E.M. (n = 4-6
per group). Arrows show times of antagonist injection.
Reproduced from Fraser et al J. Endocrinol III 83,
(1986) [28] (by permission).

been induced. To test luteal function after antagonist and to
mimic the rescue of the corpus luteum during a fertile cycle and
assess the contraceptive effects of antagonist treatment, hCG in
ascending daily doses of 30,60,90,180 and 360 IU were administered
starting on day 7 of the luteal phase. Ten monkeys received 3
daily injections of 300 µg [N-Ac-D-Nal(2)[1],D-pCl-Phe[2],
D-Trp[3],D-hArg(Et$_2$)[6],   D-Ala[10]]   LHRH/Kg   beginning   on   days
1-6 from the LH surge.

In controls receiving hCG injections alone serum progesterone
concentrations were elevated to 15-20 ng/ml. In 3 monkeys in which
the antagonist administration did not commence until day 5 or 6,
the hCG overcame the suppressive effect of the antagonist.
However, in the remaining 7 monkeys in which antagonist
administration began on days 1-4, the hCG caused only a small
progesterone rise (maximal ranges 1.8 - 4.9 ng/ml), around 20% of
that observed in control monkeys receiving hCG (Fig. 4). These
results show that LH withdrawal has a deleterious effect upon the

235

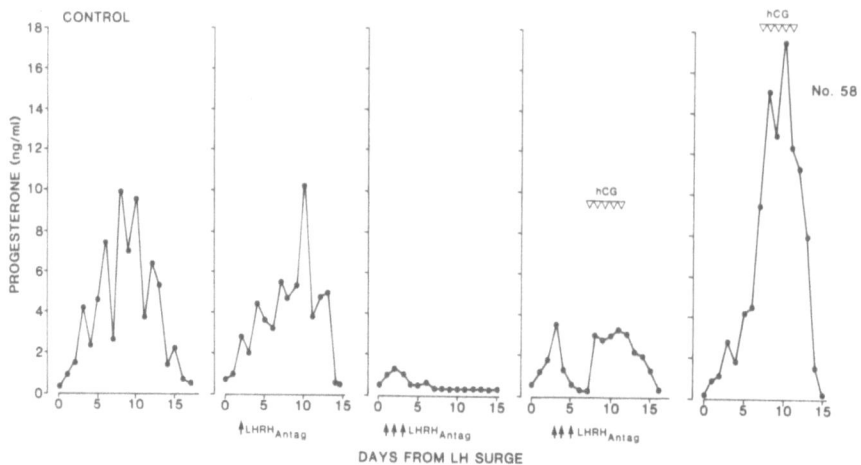

FIGURE 4   Serum progesterone concentrations during a control cycle
of an individual stumptailed macaque and during
treatment cycles in which the effects of early luteal
phase s.c. administration of 300ug [N-Ac-D-Nal(2)^1,D-
pCl-Phe^2,D-Trp^3,D-hArg(Et$_2$)^6,D-Al^{10}]   LHRH/Kg
body weight were studied either as (a) a single
injection (b) 3 consecutive daily injections (c) 3 daily
injections followed by sc injections of ascending
amounts of hCG from day 7 of the luteal phase. The
panel on the right shows effect of the hCG injections
alone. Arrows show times of hormone administration.

ability of the corpus luteum to respond to hCG, but treatment with
antagonist must start by day 4 of the luteal phase, otherwise the
hCG can overcome the effect.   The exact nature of the luteal
insufficiency induced has yet to be established.

In rhesus monkeys with lesions in the arcuate nucleus in whom
ovulation has been induced by exogenous LHRH pulses, withdrawing LH
support by stopping pulses during the early luteal phase resulted
in normal progesterone secretion when pulses were re-initiated
within 3 days [40].   The 3 days of LHRH antagonist administration
in the stumptailed macaque appears to suppress gonadotropins for
4-5 days, suggesting that a 3 day period is the maximum time the
corpus luteum can be deprived of LH and recover.

EARLY PREGNANCY

The relative roles of pituitary LH and placental chorionic
gonadotropin (CG) in the establishment and maintenance of very
early pregnancy have not been clearly defined.   One difficulty is
that removal of the pituitary support to the corpus luteum may be

counteracted by CG produced by the trophoblast. Eventually, pregnancy becomes independent of luteal support. It has been shown that pregnant rhesus monkeys can be ovariectomized as early as day 15 after ovulation and pregnancy can continue [41]. In women, the maintenance of pregnancy is dependent on the corpus luteum, as a source of progesterone, for 5 weeks [42].

If LHRH antagonists could be administered during very early pregnancy (e.g. a few days after a missed period) to cause luteal regression and a deleterious effect on placental CG production they might form a useful approach to fertility control. This would avoid disruption of the cycle or problems with steroid profiles which would be associated with chronic administration, and reduce exposure to antagonist.

Unfortunately, such experiments are difficult to perform since it is difficult to determine positively that pregnancy is established. Furthermore, it is likely that CG would rescue the corpus luteum. Intriguingly, it has been shown that the human placenta produces a peptide with LHRH-like propeties and addition of LHRH antagonist to placental cultures in vitro reduces production of hCG [43]. It has been suggested that administration of an LHRH antagonist might interfer with CG production in vivo, producing a deleterious effect on placental function. In a pilot study, [N-Ac-Pro^1,D-pCl-Phe^2, D-Nal(2)^{3,6}] LHRH antagonist at a dose of 5 mg/day was administered by infusion to baboons at 35-45 days of gestation for 7 days, i.e. when the ovary is no longer required for continuation of pregnancy. No abortions occurred but the animals showed evidence of reduction in placental steroid production and 2 of the 3 animals delivered still born infants [44]. It may be that since placental LHRH appears to be structurally different from hypothalamic LHRH, different structural analogs of LHRH may be required for effective placental blockade. Also, the degree of uptake of LHRH analogs by the placenta has not been established. LHRH antagonists should be useful tools in establishing the role of the pituitary during early pregnancy and the possible function of placental LHRH. However, it may be that their period of effectiveness in causing disruption of, pregnancy would be very limited and thus it is unlikely that they will be developed as contraceptives. Furthermore, the introduction of antiprogesterones combined with low dose prostaglandins for non-surgical termination of very early pregnancy is likely to satisfy the requirements for fertility regulation of this nature.

INVESTIGATION OF HYPOTHALAMO PITUITARY FUNCTION

The availability of an LHRH antagonist which effectively blocks LHRH receptors on the pituitary gonadotroph allows investigation of modulatory influences at the level of the pituitary. For example, the inter-relationships between LHRH release from the hypothalamus and prolactin release from the pituitary lactotrophs suggested by reports of co-incident pulses of LH on prolactin in women [45] and in the rhesus monkey [27] may be studied.

Studies in vitro suggest that LHRH stimulation of the gonadotroph may induce a stimulatory signal to the lactotroph [46].

Such a dual stimulation seems to be contradicted by the hypothesis that the LHRH precursor peptide from the hypothalamus is capable of reducing prolactin release [47]. If the LHRH and LHRH precursor were released concomitantly one would expect a decline in prolactin associated with LH release.

After administration of LHRH antagonist during the luteal phase no changes in serum prolactin levels were apparent [27]. This suggests that activation of the LHRH receptor and associated post-receptor events are not an important mediator of prolactin release. However, since prolactin release is under influence of several hypothalamic and extrahypothalamic factors it could be argued that changes induced by the antagonist may have influenced prolactin release or that any effects have been rapidly compensated.

CONCLUSIONS

Continued daily administration of LHRH antagonist beginning during the early-mid follicular phase of the menstrual cycle can suppress follicular development and ovulation. Short-term LHRH antagonist administration during the early follicular phase inhibits further development of follicles being recruited, while administration during the mid- follicular phase induces atresia of the follicle(s) undergoing selection. After stopping treatment the ovaries are inactive until recovery of pituitary function after which there appears to be a full period of follicular recruitment and maturation prior to ovulation. If antagonist administration is delayed until the last few days of maturation of the dominant follicle and continued towards the expected pre-ovulatory LH surge, the pituitary-ovarian axis becomes more resistant to inhibition by antagonist and the same treatment may fail to prevent the LH surge and ovulation.

As the luteal phase is entered, the ovary once again becomes vulnerable to LHRH antagonist-induced gonadotropin withdrawal. LHRH antagonist treatment during all stages of the luteal phase causes suppression of serum progesterone levels. The corpus luteum can survive suppression for up to 3 days if gonadotropin support is withdrawn during the early luteal phase, while the mid-late luteal phase is more susceptable. Even during the early luteal phase, antagonist administration for 3 consecutive days causes sustained suppression of luteal progesterone production and premature menstruation. This causes a much reduced response to subsequent hCG administration in macaques.

In terms of clinical application, long-term administration of LHRH antagonists to suppress ovarian function is unlikely to offer much advantage over use of agonists for contraceptive application. However, the ability of LHRH antagonist to cause blockade of selective events during the menstrual cycle is unique. The availability of antagonists for clinical trials should stimulate investigation in this area.

For treatment of estrogen-dependent disorders, the LHRH antagonists offer the advantage in that the initial stimulation of estradiol secretion observed with LHRH agonists is avoided. However, if agonist treatment is initiated during the luteal phase, this stimulation is not seen [48]. This, together with the efficacy of long-term low-dose agonist depot formulations makes hard competition for the more expensive LHRH antagonists. The LHRH antagonists may be more appropriate for short-term pituitary suppression as for induction of ovulation using gonadotropins, the treatment of polycystic ovarian desease and in the investigation of the premenstrual syndrome.

Finally, studies with LHRH antagonists in monkeys and man should provide information on the activity of the hypothalamic LHRH pulse generator. Studies incorporating inhibin and the LHRH precursor hormone should in addition help in the comprehensive understanding of the function of the hypothalamo-pituitary-ovarian axis.

ACKNOWLEDGEMENTS

I am grateful to Drs. B.H. Vickery and J.J. Nestor Jr. (Syntex) for gifts of $[N-Ac-D-Nal(2)^1, D-pCl-Phe^2, D-Trp^3, D-hArg(Et_2)^6, D-Ala^{10}]$ LHRH used in the studies on stumptailed macaques described in this chapter.

REFERENCES

1. Crowley, W.F., Filicori, M., Spratt, D.I. and Santoro, N. The physiology of gonadotropin-releasing hormone (GnRH) secretion in men and women. Rec. Prog. Horm. Res., 41, 473 (1985).
2. Djahanbakhch, O., Warner, P., McNeilly, A.S. and Baird, D.T. Pulsatile release of LH and oestradiol during the periovulatory period in women. Clin. Endocrinol. 20, 579 (1984).
3. Marshall, J.C., Kelch, R.P., Sauder, S.E., Barkan, A. and Reame, N.E. Pulsatile gonadotropin-releasing hormone (GnRH) studies of puberty and the menstrual cycle. In "Endocrinology" Proc. 7th Int. Cong. Endocrinol, Excerpta Media, Conf. series, Amsterdam.
4. Goodman, A.L. and Hodgen, G.D. The ovarian triad of the primate menstrual cycle. Rec. Prog. Horm. Res., 39, 1 (1983).
5. Vaughan, L., Carmel, P.W., Dyrenfurth, I., Frantz, G., Antunes, J.L. and Ferin, M. Section of the pituitary stalk in the rhesus monkey. 1. Endocrine Studies. Neuroendocrinology 30, 70 (1980).
6. Knobil, E. The neuroendocrine control of the menstrual cycle. Rec. Prog. Horm. Res. 36, 53 (1980).
7. Fraser, H.M. Active immunization of stumptailed macaque monkeys against luteinizing hormone releasing hormone, and its effect on menstrual cycles, ovarian steroids and positive feedback. J. Reprod. Immunol. 5, 173 (1983).
8. Balmaceda, J.P., Borghi, M.R., Burgos, L., Pauerstein, C., Schally, A.V. and Asch, R.H. The effects of chronic administration of LH-RH agonists and antagonists on the menstrual cycle and endometrium of the rhesus monkey. Contraception, 29, 83 (1984).

9. Kenigsberg, D., Littman, B.A., Williams, R.F. and Hodgen, G.D. Medical hypophysectomy: II Variability of ovarian response to gonadotropin therapy. Fertil. Steril., 42, 116 (1984).

10. Kenigsberg, D., Littman, B.A. and Hodgen, G.D. Induction of ovulation in primate models. Endocr. Rev., 7, 34 (1986).

11. Borghi, M.R., Neisvisky, R., Balmaceda, J.P., Coy, D.H. and Schally, A.V. Administration of LHRH analogs delays ovulation without affecting the luteal function in rhesus monkeys. Fertil. Steril., 40, 678 (1983).

12. Mais, V., Kazer, R.R., Cetel, N.S., Rivier, J., Vale. W. and Yen, S.S.C. The dependency of folliculogenesis and corpus luteum function on pulsatile gonadotrophin secretion in cycling women using a gonadotropin releasing hormone antagonist as a probe. J. Clin. Endocrinol. Metab. 62, 1250 (1986).

13. Kenigsberg, D. and Hodgen, G.D. Ovlation inhibition by administration of weekly gonadotropin-releasing hormone antagonist. J. Clin. Endocrinol. Metab., 62, 734 (1986).

14. Fraser, H.M., McNeilly, A.S., Abbott, M. and Steiner, R.A. The effect of LHRH immunoneutralization on follicular development, the LH surge and luteal function in the stumptailed macaque. J. Reprod. Fert., 76, 299 (1986).

15. Wilks, J.W., Folkers, K., Humphries, J. and Bowers, C.Y. Effect of (D-Phe2,Pro3,D-Phe6) LH-RH, an antagonist, on preovulatory gonadotropin secretion in the rhesus monkey. Biol. Reprod., 23, 1 (1980).

16. Zeleznik, A.J., Battelli, A.F. and Kubik, C.J. Ovarian responses in macaques to pulsatile infusion of FSH and LH. Society for the Study of Reproduction, Ithaca, Abst. 327 (1986).

17. Balmaceda, J.P., Schally, A.V., Coy, D. and Asch, R.H. The effects of an LHRH antagonist ([N-Ac-D-Trp1,3, D-p-Cl-Phe2, D-Phe6;Ala10]-LH-RH) during the preovulatory period in the rhesus monkey. Contraception, 24, 275 (1981).

18. Kenigsberg, D., Littman, B.A. and Hodgen, G.D. Medical hypophysectomy: I. Dose-response using a gonadotropin-releasing hormone antagonist. Fertil. Steril., 42, 112.

19. Wildt, L., Hausler, A., Hutchinson, J.S., Marshall, G. and Knobil, E. Estradiol as a gonadotrophin releasing hormone in the rhesus monkey. Endocrinology, 108, 2011 (1981).

20. McCormack, J.T., Plant, T.M., Hess, D.L. and Knobil, E. The effect of luteinizing hormone releasing hormone (LHRH) antiserum administration on gonadotrophin secretion in the rhesus monkey. Endocrinology, 100, 663 (1977).

21. Norman, R.L., Gliessman, P., Lindstrom, S.A., Hill, J. and Spies, H.G. Reinitiation of ovulatory cycles in pituitary stalk- sectioned rhesus monkeys: evidence for a specific hypothalamic message for the preovulatory release of luteinizing hormone. Endocrinology, 111, 1874 (1982).

22. Adams, T.E., Norman, R.L. and Spies, H.G. Gonadotrophin-releasing hormone receptor binding and pituitary responsiveness in estradiol primed monkeys. Science, 213, 1388 (1981).

23. Asch, R.H., Balmaceda, J.P., Borghi, M.R., Neisvisky, R. and Coy, D.H. Suppression of the positive feedback of estradiol benzoate on gonadotropin secretion by an inhibitory analog of luteinizing hormone-releasing hormone (LHRH) in oophorectomized rhesus monkey. J. Clin. Endocrinol. Metab., 57., 367 (1983).

24. Norman, R.L., Rivier, J., Vale, W. and Spies, H.G. Inhibition of estradiol-induced gonadotropin release in ovariectomized rhesus macaques by a gonadotropin-releasing hormone antagonist. Fertil. Steril., 45, 288 (1986).

25. Levine, J.E., Norman, R.L., Gliessman, P.M., Oyama, T.Y., Bangsberg, D.R. and Spies, H.G. In vivo gonadotropin-releasing hormone release and serum luteinizing hormone measurements in ovariectomized, estrogen-treated rhesus macaques. Endocrinology, 117, 711 (1985).

26. Ellinwood, W.E., Norman, R.L. and Spies, H.G. Changing frequency of pulsatile luteinizing hormone and progesterone secretion during the luteal phase of the menstrual cycle of rhesus monkeys. Biol. Reprod., 31, 714 (1984).

27. Healy, D.L., Schenken, R.S., Lynch, A., Williams, R.F. and Hodgen, G.D. Pulsatile progesterone secretion: its relevance to clinical evaluation of corpus luteum function. Fertil. Steril., 41, 114 (1984).

28. Fraser, H.M., Abbott, M., Laird, N.C., McNeilly, A.S., Nestor, J.J. and Vickery, B.H. Effects of an LHRH antagonist on the secretion of LH, FSH, prolactin and ovarian steroids at different stages of the luteal phase in the stumptailed macaque (macaca arctoides). J. Endocrinol., 111, 83-90.

29. Filicori, M., Butler, J.P. and Crowley, W.F. Neuroendocrine regulation of the corpus luteum in the human. Evidence for pulsatile progesterone secretion. J. Clin. Invest., 73, 1638 (1984).

30. Moudgal, N.R., MacDonald, G.J. and Greep, R.O. Role of endogenous primate LH in maintaining corpus luteum function in the monkey. J. Clin. Endocrinol Metab., 35, 113 (1972).

31. Groff, T.R., Madhwa, Raj, H.G., Talbert, L.M. and Willis, D.L. Effects of neutralization of luteinizing hormone on corpus luteum function and cyclicity in Macaca fascicularis. J. Clin. Endocrinol. Metab., 59, 1054 (1984).

32. Hutchison, J.S. and Zeleznik, A.J. The rhesus monkey corpus luteum is dependent on pituitary gonadotropin secretion throughout the luteal phase of the menstrual cycle. Endocrinology, 115, 1780 (1984).

33. Van de Weile, R.L., Bogumil, J., Dyrenfurth, I., Ferin, M., Jewelerwicz, R., Warren, M., Rizkallah, T. and Mikhail, G. Mechanisms regulating the menstrual cycle in women. Rec. Prog. Horm. Res., 26, 63 (1970).

34. Asch, R.H., Abou-Samra, M., Braunstein, G.D. and Pauerstein, C.J. Luteal function in hypophysectomized rhesus monkeys. J. Clin. Endocrinol. Metab. 55, 154 (1982).

35. Balmaceda, J.P., Borghi, M.R., Coy, D.H., Schally, A.V. & Asch, R.H. Suppression of postovulatory gonadotropin levels does not affect corpus luteum function in rhesus monkeys. J. Clin. Endocrinol. Metab., 57, 866 (1983).

36. Rothchild, I. The regulation of the mammalian corpus luteum. Rec. Prog. Horm. Res., 37, 183 (1981).

37. Wilks, J.W. and Noble, A.S. Steroidogenic responsiveness of the monkey corpus luteum to exogenous chorionic gonadotropin. Endocrinology, 112, 1256 (1983).

38. Fraser, H.M., Baird, D.T., McRae, G.I., Nestor, J.J. and Vickery, B.H. Suppression of luteal progesterone secretion in the stumptailed macaque by an antagonist analogue of luteinizing hormne releasing hormone. J. Endocrinol., 104, R1 (1985).

39. Collins, R.L., Sopelak, V.M., Williams, R.F. and Hodgen, G.D. Induction of luteolysis and menstruation by a GnRH antagonist in primates. Society for Gynecological Investigation, San Francisco, Abst. 117 (1984).

40. Hutchison, J.A. and Zeleznik, A.J. The corpus luteum of the primate menstrual cycle is capable of recovering from a transient withdrawal of pituitary gonadotropin support. Endocrinology 117, 1043 (1985).

41. Goodman, A.L. and Hodgen, G.D. Corpus luteum-conceptus-follicle relationships during the fertile cycle in rhesus monkeys: Pregnancy maintenance despite early luteal removal. J. Clin. Endocrinol Metab., 49, 469 (1979).

42. Csapo, A.I., Pulkkinen, M.O. and Wiest, W.G. Effects of luteectomy and progesterone replacement therapy in early pregnant patients. Am. J. Obstet. Gynecol., 115, 759 (1973).

43. Siler-Khodr, T.M., Khodr, G.S., Vickery, B.H. and Nestor, J.J. Inhibition of hCG, hCG and progesterone release from human placental tissue in vitro by a GnRH antagonist. Life Sci., 32, 2741 (1983).

44. Siler-Khodr, T.M., Kuehl, T.J. and Vickery, B.H. Effects of gonadotropin releasing hormone antagonist on hormonal levels in the pregnant baboon and on fetal outcome. Fertil. Steril., 41, 448 (1984).

45. Braund, W., Roeger, D.C. and Judd, S.J. Synchronous secretion of luteinizing hormone and prolactin in the human luteal phase: neuroendocrine mechanisms. J. Clin. Endocrinol. Metab., 58, 293 (1984).

46. Denef, C. and Andries, M. Evidence for paracrine interaction between gonadotrophs and lactotrophs in pituitary cell aggregates. Endocrinology, 112, 813 (1983).

47. Nikolics, K., Mason, A.J., Szonyi, E., Ramachandran, J. and Seeburg, P.H. A prolactin inhibiting factor within the precursor for human gonadotropin-releasing hormone. Nature, 316, 511 (1985).

48. Fraser, H.M. and Sandow, J. Suppression of follicular maturation by infusion of a luteinizing hormone releasing hormone agonist starting during the late luteal phase in the stumptailed macaque monkey. J. Clin. Endocrinol. Metab., 60, 579 (1985).

SECTION 5

BASIC CLINICAL STUDIES

16
LHRH Antagonists in Normal Men

S.N. PAVLOU, G.B. WAKEFIELD and W.J. KOVACS

Division of Endocrinology, Department of Medicine,
Vanderbilt University, AA-4206, Medical Center North Nashville,
TN 37232, USA

INTRODUCTION

During the last few years contraceptive research has focused on LHRH agonistic analogues because of their ability to inhibit gonadal function through a complex mechanism of pituitary desensitization [1-4]. However, in spite of our initial optimism, LHRH agonists do not completely and reliably suppress spermatogenesis [5-9]. Attention has therefore shifted to the investigation of potent antagonistic analogues of the hormone. Antagonistic analogues would be of considerable theoretic advantage in that not even transient stimulation of pituitary gonadotropin secretion would occur when such agents are used. Animal studies with LHRH antagonists have already shown that these analogues are more effective in inhibiting gonadal function and spermatogenesis than are agonists [10-16]. Until now such antagonists have been of relatively low potency. However, new LHRH antagonists have recently been synthesized that are potent enough to be evaluated in humans [12-14].

SINGLE DOSES OF THE 4F-ANTAGONIST

Early studies of LHRH antagonists in men were performed using analogues of relatively low potency, given at doses as high as 90 mg [17-19]. Results of these studies showed that basal gonadotropin levels were not affected, but that gonadotropin responses to 25 µg of LHRH were blocked.

The 4F-Antagonist ([Ac-Δ^3Pro^1, 4F-D-Phe^2, D-Trp^{3,6}]LHRH), synthesized by Drs. J. Rivier and W. Vale, [20] decreases gonadotropin levels in postmenopausal women when given at a dose of 80 µg/kg body weight (BW) [21]. We evaluated the ability of single doses of the 4F-Antagonist to suppress serum gonadotropin and testosterone levels in six normal men [22]. The 4F-Antagonist was given subcutaneously at four doses: 40, 80, 160 and 320 µg/kg BW, and serum levels of immunoreactive (IR) LH and FSH, bioactive (bio) LH and testosterone were measured over the subsequent 18 hours.

The number of LH pulses (mean ± SE) for all men decreased ($\underline{P}$ <0.001) from 3.5 ± 0.2 during the 6-h control period to 1.3 ± 0.2 during the first 6 h after sc injection of the antagonist. Mean LH pulse amplitude also decreased ($\underline{P}$ <0.001) from 3.0 ± 0.2 to 1.0 ± 0.1 mIU/ml. There was no dose related change in the number or amplitude of LH pulses after the four different doses.

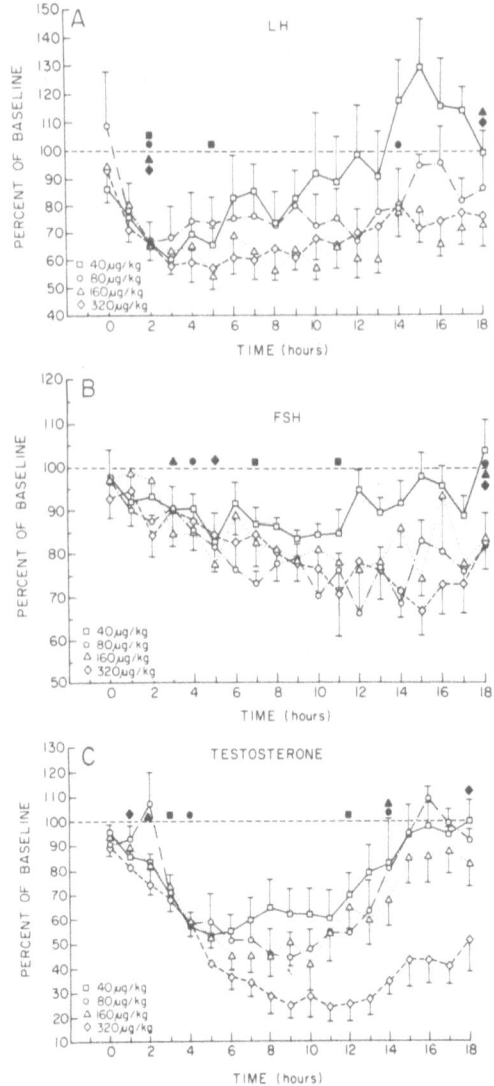

FIGURE 1 Mean (⁺ SEM) serum levels expressed as percent of mean baseline levels of LH (A), FSH (B) and testosterone (C). The 4F-antagonist was given subcutaneously at time 0. Points between closed symbols represent values different (P <0.05) from baseline for the respective doses.

After each of the four doses, serum LH, FSH and testosterone declined. Figure 1 shows the changes in mean levels of FSH, LH and testosterone expressed as percent of mean control baseline levels.

LH bioactivity for all subjects decreased ($\underline{P}$ <0.0001) after dosing with the 4F-antagonist. Bioactive LH levels decreased more than those of IR-LH, resulting in a decrease of the ratio of bioactive to immunoreactive LH (B/I).

Serum levels of LH fell rapidly within the first 2 hours after administration of the 4F-Antagonist, similar to results in postmenopausal women given 80 µg/kg of the same antagonist [21] and in rats and monkeys given other LHRH antagonists [10-16]. The different doses caused a similar rate of decline and maximum decrease of LH levels, perhaps due to the rather narrow range of doses used. However, the duration of suppression of LH levels was dose dependent. The responsivity of the pituitary to the endogenous hypothalamic LHRH appeared to be decreased for at least 6 h, as evidenced by the decrease in number of LH pulses, LH pulse amplitude, and LH bioactivity. The magnitude of suppression of serum FSH was less than that for LH, and its nadir occurred later.

Serum testosterone followed the same pattern of decrease as that of serum IR-LH with a two hour delay. However, fractional declines in testosterone levels were greater than those of IR-LH. The duration of testosterone suppression increased in a dose-related fashion to at least 18 hours at the two highest doses. However, serum testosterone levels started to return to normal 10 and 12 hours after the 160 and 320 µg/kg doses, respectively. In order to maintain long-term testosterone suppression, this analog would have to be given at fairly high doses more than once daily or by a continuous delivery system, such as a subcutaneous implant or microcapsule formulation. Whether delivery of such large amounts of material these routes is feasible is not known. This underscores the importance of developing more potent LHRH antagonists.

MULTIPLE DOSE ADMINISTRATION OF THE 4F-ANTAGONIST

The 4F-Antagonist, given at single doses, suppressed serum gonadotropin and testosterone levels but its duration of action was not longer than 8-12 hours, even with the higher doses used. Therefore, in the next series of experiments, we administered this analogue as a continuous subcutaneous infusion to three normal men for 72 hours. The infusion was initiated with a bolus dose of 80 µg/kg and then continued at a rate of 13.33 µg/kg/hour. A LHRH challenge test (50 µg iv) was performed during baseline control period, and at 6, 12, 24, 48, 72 and 96 hours. As shown in Figure 2 there was a moderate decrease in FSH and LH levels during the antagonist infusion, but there was a response to every LHRH test. This response was smaller during the first 12 hours, and thereafter there was no difference between the LHRH response during the treatment.

The 4F-antagonist was also given to three normal men as a sc injection of 100 µg/kg every 6 h for seven days (Figure 3). Serum FSH levels decreased during the first 4 days from 5.9 ± 0.2 mIU/ml during control to 3.7 ± 0.2 ($P < 0.001$) followed by a progressive increase reaching a maximum of 5.4 ± 0.7 mIU/ml on day 5. Serum LH decreased ($\underline{P} < 0.001$) during the first 2 days of treatment from 9.6 ± 0.4 mIU/ml to 5.3 ± 0.3 but then started rising to 8.5 ± 1.4 on day 5. Serum testosterone levels

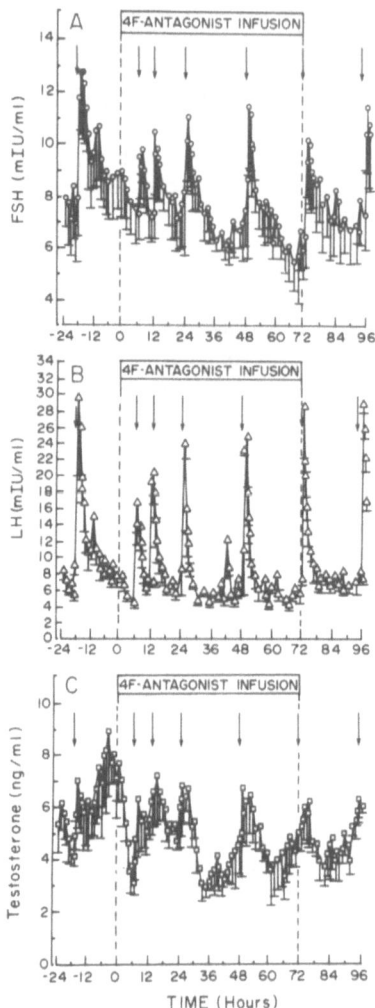

FIGURE 2 Mean (+ SEM) serum levels of FSH (A), LH (B), and testosterone (C) in three men who were given the 4F-antagonist infusion. The arrows show the times of a 50 μg iv bolus of LHRH.

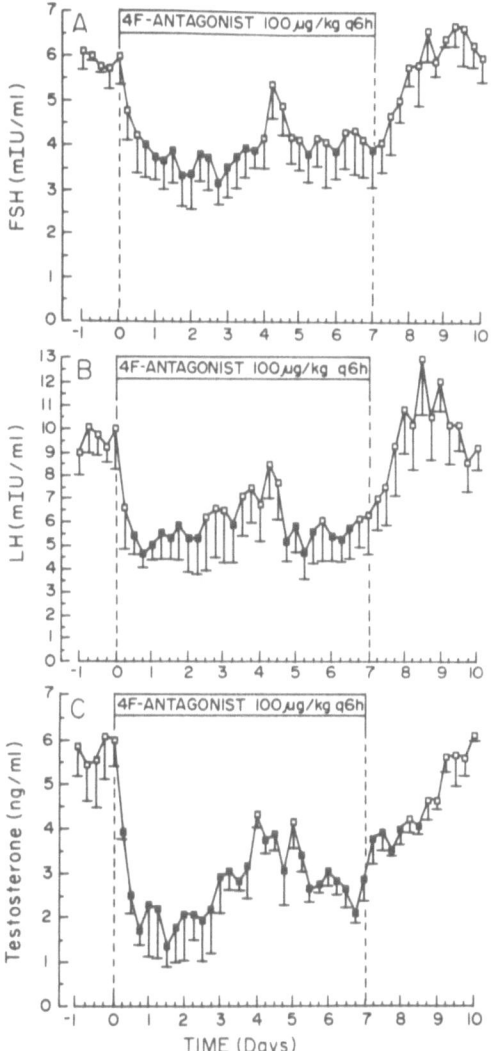

FIGURE 3 Mean (⁺ SEM) serum level of FSH (A), LH (B), and testosterone (C) in three men who received 100 μg/kg sc every 6 h of the 4F-antagonist for seven days. Blood samples were drawn during treatment just prior to antagonist injection. Closed symbols represent values different ($\underline{P} < 0.05$) from baseline.

reflected those of LH, falling ($\underline{P}$ < 0.001) from 5.8 ± 0.3 ng/ml during control to 1.9 ± 0.2 during the first 3 days and reaching a nadir of 1.3 ± 0.4 on day 2. Suppression was incomplete and levels rose to 4.3 ± 0.3 ng/ml on day 4. All FSH, LH and testosterone serum levels returned to control levels during the 72-h period after the end of treatment.

A possible explanation of gonadotropin and testosterone escape could be increased endogenous LHRH secretion from the hypothalamus which would eventually overcome the effects of the antagonist. Consequently, the LH-induced increase in testosterone would serve as negative feedback to the hypothalamus to decrease its activity and thereby render the LHRH antagonist more effective.

It is conceivable that higher doses, or more potent LHRH antagonist analogs, would be more effective in competing with endogenous LHRH and thus preventing this increase in FSH, LH and testosterone. Therefore, in the next studies we used a more potent LHRH antagonist, detirelix (RS-68439), [N-Ac-D-Nal(2)^1, D-pCl-Phe^2,D-Trp^3, D-hArg(Et$_2$)^6, D-Ala^{10}] LHRH, developed by Syntex Research.

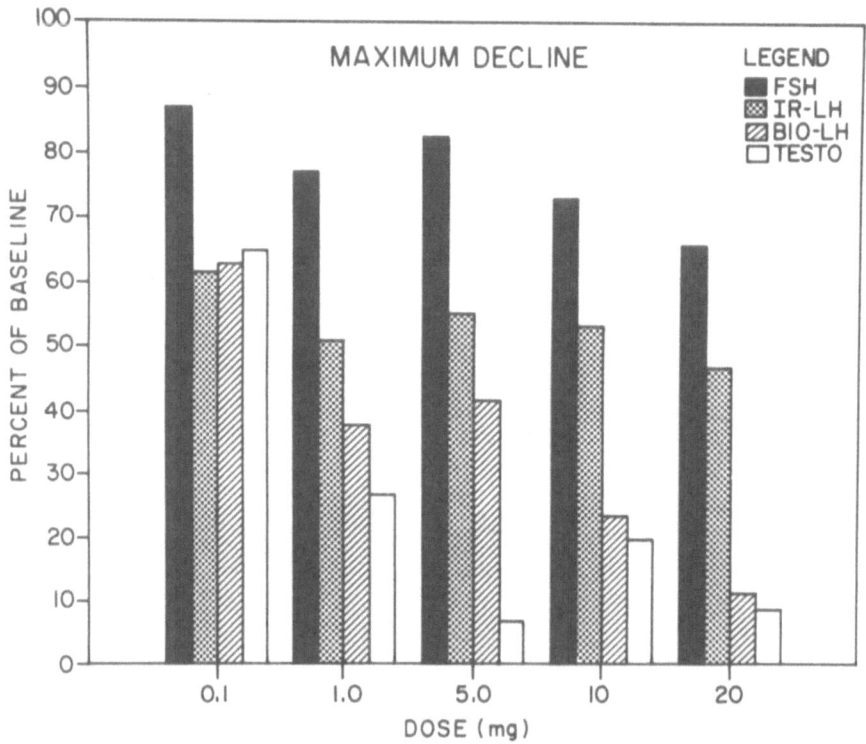

FIGURE 4 Maximum decline achieved in FSH, IR-LH, bio-LH and testosterone, as percent of mean control baseline, after the administration of the LHRH antagonist.

250

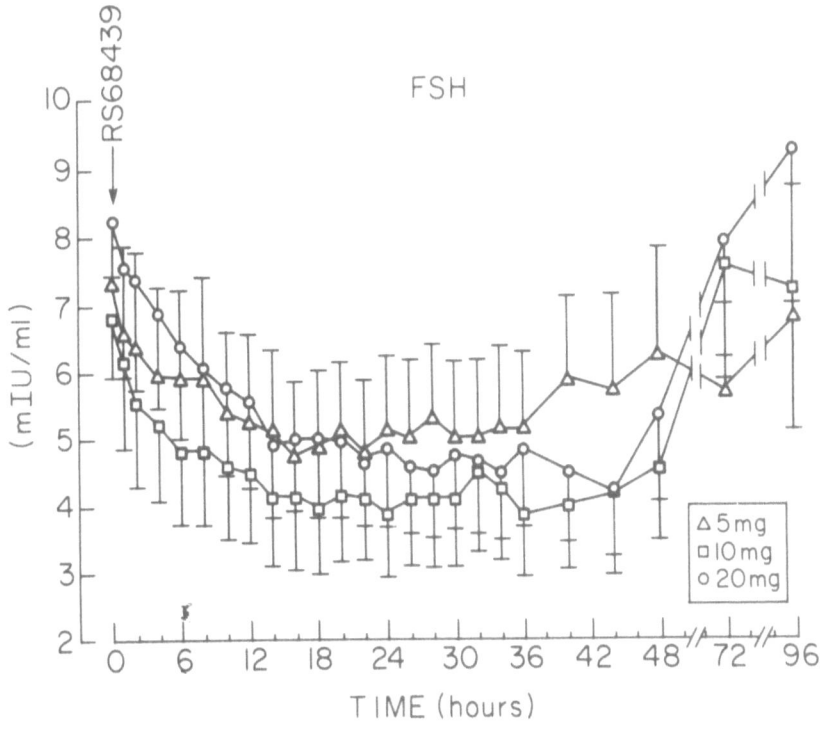

FIGURE 5 Serum FSH levels (mean ⁺ SEM) after a single dose of 5, 10 or 20 mg of detirelix (RS-68439) antagonist in nine normal men. Detirelix was given by a sc injection at time 0.

SINGLE DOSES OF DETIRELIX, A NEW LHRH ANTAGONIST

In the first study with this new LHRH antagonist seven dose levels of 0.001, 0.01, 0.1, 1, 5, 10 and 20 mg were given, one dose per subject. Six men received the first six doses and two men received the 20 mg dose.

Serum IR-LH levels decreased rapidly within the first 2 to 4 h following the administration of detirelix and reached a nadir of 3.15 mIU/ml with the highest dose. The decrease in bio-LH was more pronounced than that of IR-LH, falling from 1.2 mg/ml at baseline to 0.16 mg/ml of LH I-2 at 24 hours. This dissociation was most evident with higher doses; the B/I ratio decreased by 72% after administration of the 20 mg dose. Serum testosterone levels decreased between 12 and 24 hours reaching a mean nadir of 0.5 mg/ml after administration of the 20 mg dose and remained suppressed for at least 24 hours in both subjects. IR-FSH fell only by 30%, even with the 20 mg dose (Fig 4). IR-LH decreased by about 50% after all doses. In contrast, the decrease in bio-LH was dose

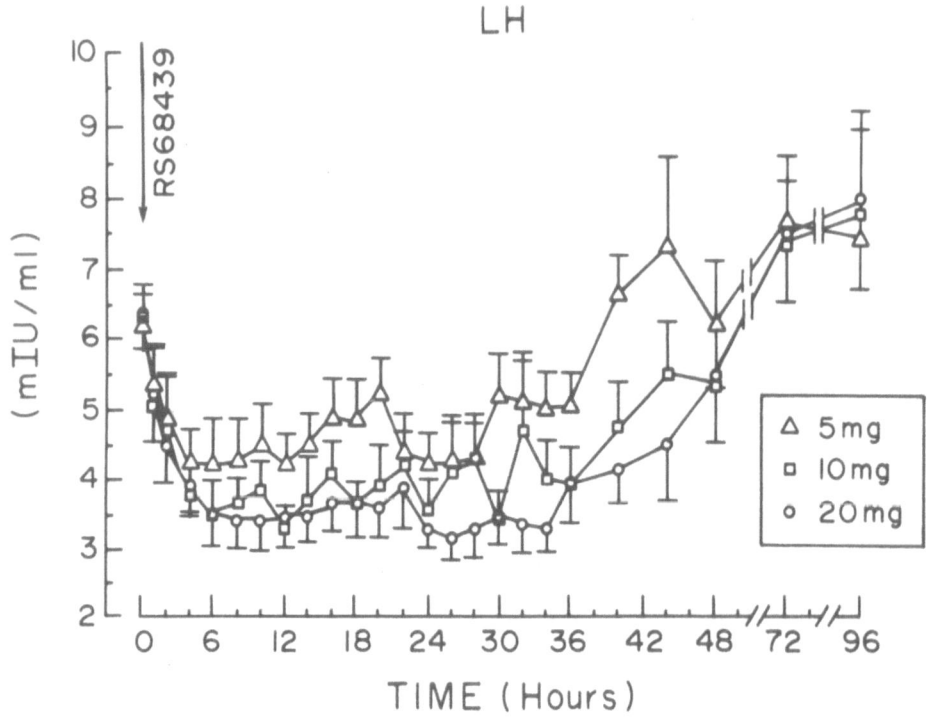

FIGURE 6 Serum LH levels (mean $^+$ SEM) after a single dose of 5, 10 or 20 mg of detirelix (RS-68439) antagonist in nine normal men. Detirelix was given by a sc injection at time 0.

dependent and reached a nadir of 12% of baseline after the 20 mg dose. Testosterone decline reflected closely the bio-LH response and fell to less than 10% after the higher doses. The duration of hormonal suppression was also clearly dose related. There was a good correlation between dose and area under the response curve for IR-LH (r=0.86 p <0.001), IR-FSH (r=0.8 p <0.03) and testosterone (r=0.95 p <0.001).

Three effective doses (5, 10 and 20 mg) were chosen and were given to nine normal men. Each subject received all three doses randomly, at least seven days apart. FSH decrease was not dose-dependent and reached a nadir approximately 12 hours after the administration of the antagonist (Fig 5). FSH levels had not returned to baseline at 48 hours with the two higher doses. Serum LH decreased rapidly within the first 2 to 4 hours and remained suppressed for up to 36 hours (Fig 6). Then a return to baseline levels was observed following a small rebound which persisted for up to 96 hours.

Serum testosterone levels, decreased by 4 to 6 hours after the LHRH antagonist administration (Fig 7). After the initial decrease a spontaneous escape was observed between 12 and 28 hours with a peak between 20 and 22 hours. This was more evident with the lower doses. Subsequently, testosterone levels decreased again and after the 20 mg dose, fell to the same levels as the initial decrease. Testosterone levels had not returned to baseline even 96 hours after the 10 and 20 mg doses.

The nadir of serum immunoreactive levels of FSH, LH and testosterone after the 3 doses of detirelix are shown in Table 1.

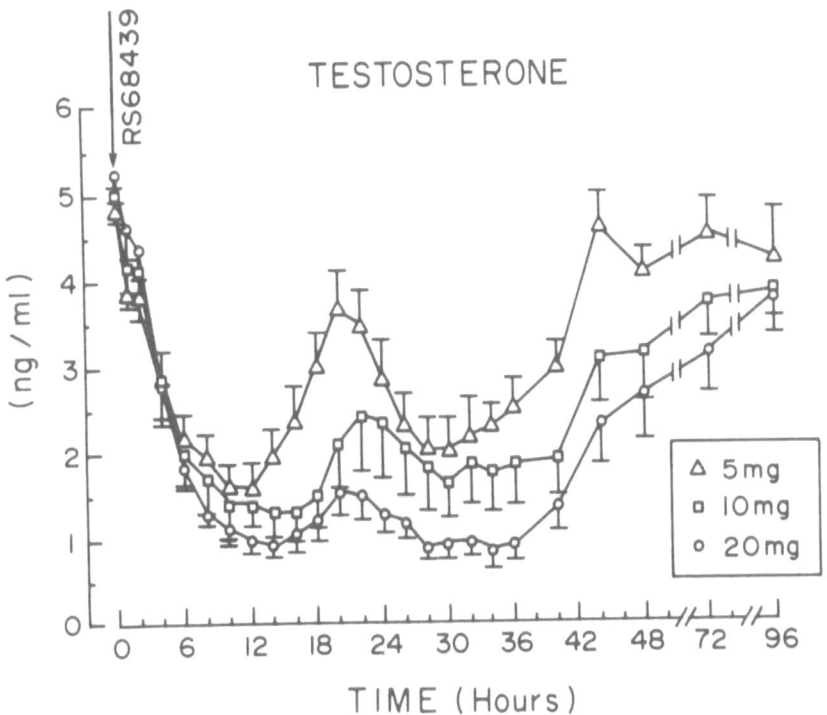

FIGURE 7 Serum testosterone levels (mean + SEM) after a single dose of 5, 10 or 20 mg of detirelix (RS-68439) antagonist in nine normal men. Detirelix was given by a sc injection at time 0.

Table 1. Nadir of serum FSH, LH, and testosterone after administration of detirelix

Dose (mg)	FSH (mIU/ml)	LH (mIU/ml)	Testosterone (ng/ml)
Baseline	6.9 ± 0.5	6.2 ± 0.3	5.1 ± 0.2
5	4.4 ± 1.1	3.3 ± 0.4	1.3 ± 0.3
10	3.6 ± 0.9	2.9 ± 0.3	0.9 ± 0.3
20	4.1 ± 0.9	2.7 ± 0.3	0.6 ± 0.1

FSH levels declined by approximately 40% and LH serum levels by 55%. In contrast, the decrease in testosterone was dose-dependent and reached a nadir of 0.6 ng/ml representing almost a 90% decrease after the 20 mg dose. LH reached its nadir earlier than FSH or testosterone. It took approximately 30 hours for FSH or testosterone to achieve their lowest levels with the higher doses.

Serum immunoreactive detirelix levels after subcutaneous injection of the 5, 10 and 20 mg doses rapidly reached a maximum; detectable concentrations were still present 7 days later. Representative pharmacokinetic of this antagonist are shown in Table 2.

Table 2. Pharmacokinetics of detirelix in man

DOSE (mg)	C_{max} (ng/ml)	T_{max} (h)	$T_{1/2}$ (h)
5	38 ± 4.6	1.3 ± 0.2	52 ± 6.5
10	67 ± 4.8	1.9 ± 0.3	43 ± 4.3
20	118 ± 11	2.2 ± 0.4	41 ± 2.5

Data are expressed as mean ± SEM

Because maximum concentration was reached at 2 to 4 hours, half-time calculations for all doses were based on extrapolated serum levels beginning after 4 hours. The half-life of this analogue was 41 to 52 hours and appeared to be somewhat longer with the smallest dose.

These results indicate that detirelix suppressed serum levels of immunoreactive FSH, LH and testosterone. Testosterone decrease was more pronounced than that of serum FSH or LH. Serum testosterone levels remained below 1 mg/ml for up to 36 hours after administration of 20 mg of detirelix. The half-life of this LHRH antagonist in humans was

254

approximately two days. The dissociation between serum gonadotropin levels and testosterone could be explained by the decrease of the ratio of bioactive to immunoreactive levels that we have observed for both FSH and LH.

CONCLUDING REMARKS

LHRH antagonists, and in particular detirelix, produce reversible suppression of the pituitary-gonadal axis in man. Serum testosterone levels, following this new, potent LHRH antagonist administration decreased to levels below 1 ng/ml and remain suppressed for up to 36 hours. Based on short term studies, they appear to be safe and free of side effects other than a minimal local erythema at the injection site.

REFERENCES

1. Pelletier, G., Cusan, L., Auclair, C., Kelly, P.A., Desy, L., and Labrie, F. Inhibition of spermatogenesis in the rat by treatment with [D-Ala[6], Des-Gly-NH$_2$[10]] LHRH ethylamide. Endocrinology, 103, 641 (1978)
2. Tcholakian, R.K., De La Cruz, A., Chowdhury, M., Steinberger, A., Coy, D.H., and Schally, A.V. Unusual antireproductive properties of the analog [D-Leu[6],Des-Gly-NH$_2$[10]]-lutenizing hormone-releasing hormone ethylamide in male rats. Fertil. Steril., 30, 600 (1978)
3. Smith, R., Donald, R.A., Espiner, E.A., Stronach, S.G., and Edwards, I.A. Normal adults and subjects with hypogonadotropic hypogonadism respond differently to D-Ser(TBU)[6]-LH-RH-EA[10]. J. Clin. Endocrinol. Metab. 48, 167 (1979)
4. Belanger, A., Labrie, F., Lemay, A., Caron, S., and Raynaud, J.P. Inhibitory effects of a single intranasal administration of [D-Ser(TBU)[6], des-Gly-NH$_2$[10]] LHRH ethylamide, a potent LHRH agonist on serum steroid levels in normal adult men. J. Steroid Biochem., 13, 123 (1980)
5. Linde, R., Doelle, G.C., Alexander, N., Kirchner, F., Vale, W., Rivier, J., and Rabin, D. Reversible inhibition of testicular steroidogenesis and spermatogenesis by a potent gonadotropic releasing hormone in normal men. N. Engl. J. Med., 305, 663 (1981)
6. Doelle, G.C., Alexander, A.N., Evans, R.M., Linde, R., Rivier, J., Vale, W., and Rabin, D. Combined treatment with an LHRH agonist and testosterone in man. J. Androl., 4, 298 (1983)
7. Pavlou, S., Interlandi, J.W., Wakefield, G., Rivier, J, Vale, W., and Rabin, D. Heterogeneity of sperm density profiles following 16-week therapy with continuous infusion of high dose LHRH analogue plus testosterone. J. Andrology, 7, 228, 1986.
8. Schurmeyer, T.H., Knuth, U.A., Freischem, C.W., Sandow, J., Akhtar, F., and Nieschlag, E. Suppression of pituitary and testicular function in normal men by constant gonadotropin-releasing hormone agonist infusion. J. Clin. Endocrinol. Metab., 59, 19 (1984)
9. Bhasin, S., Heber, D., Steiner, B., Handelsman, D.J., and Swerdloff, R. Hormonal effects of Gonadotropin-Releasing Hormone (GnRH) agonist in the human male: III Effects of long term combined

treatment with GnRH agonist and androgen. J. Clin. Endocrinol. Metab., 60, 998 (1985)

10. Rivier, C., Rivier, J., and Vale, W. Antireproductive effects of a potent gonadotropin-releasing hormone antagonist in the male rat. Science, 210, 93 (1980)

11. Heber, D., Dodson, R., Peterson, H., Channabasavaiah, K.C., Stewart, J.M., and Swerdloff, R.S. Counteractive effects of agonistic and antagonistic gonadotropin-releasing hormone analogs on spermatogenesis: site of action. Fertil. Steril., 41, 309 (1984)

12. McRae, G.I., Vickery, B.H., Nestor, J.J. Jr., Bremner, W.J., and Badger, T.M. Biological activity of a highly potent LHRH antagonist. In LHRH and its Analogs: Contraceptive and Therapeutic Applications. Vickery, H., Nestor, J.J. Jr., and Hafez, E.S.E. (Ed). MTP Press, Lancaster (1984) p. 137.

13. Rivier, C., Rivier, J., and Vale, W. Effect of a potent GnRH antagonist and testosterone propionate on mating behavior and fertility in the male rat. Endocrinology, 108, 1998 (1981)

14. Vickery, B.H., McRae, G., Nestor, J.J. Jr., and Bremner, W. Effects of a highly potent LHRH antagonist in rats, dogs and cynomolgus monkeys. J. Androl., 4, 37 (1983)

15. Weinbauer, G.F., Suzmann, F.J., Akhtar, F.B., Shah, G.V., Vickery, B.H., and Nieschlag, E. Reversible inhibition of testicular function by a gonadotropin hormone-releasing hormone antagonist in monkeys (Macaca fascicularis) Fertil. Steril., 42, 906 (1984)

16. Adams, L.A., Bremner, W.J., Nestor, J.J., Vickery, B.H., and Steiner, R.A. Suppression of plasma gonadotropins and testosterone in adult male monkeys (Macaca fascicularis) by a potent inhibitory analog of gonadotropin-releasing hormone. J. Clin. Endocrinol. Metab. 62, 58 (1986)

17. Gonzalez-Barcena, D., Kastin, A.J., Coy, D.H., Nikolics, K., and Schally, A.V. Suppression of gonadotropin release in man by an inhibitory analogue of luteinizing hormone-releasing hormone. Lancet, ii, 997 (1977)

18. Gonzalez-Barcena, D., Kastin, A.J., Schally, A.V., Coy, D.H., Vilchez-Martinez, J.A., Pedroza, E., Nikolics, K., and Seprodi, J. Inhibition of LHRH-induced LH and FSH release in man by synthetic competitive antagonistic LHRH analogs. Fertil. Steril., 29, 246 (1978)

19. Gonzalez-Barcena, D., Trevino-Ortiz, H., Gordon, F., Kastin, A.J., Coy, D.H., and Schally, A.V. Influence of LHRH agonists and antagonists on gonadotropin release in humans. Int. J. Fertil., 25, 185 (1980)

20. Rivier, C., and Vale, W. Temporal relationship between the abortifacient effects of GnRH antagonists and hormonal secretion. Biol. Reprod., 24, 1061 (1981)

21. Cetel, N.S., Rivier, J., Vale, W., and Yen, S.S.C. The dynamics of gonadotropin inhibition in women induced by an antagonistic analog of gonadotropin-releasing hormone. J. Clin. Endocrinol. Metab., 57, 62 (1983)

22. Pavlou, S.N., DeBold, C.R., Island, D.P., Wakefield, G., Rivier, J., Vale, W., and Rabin, D. Single subcutaneous doses of a LHRH antagonist suppress serum gonadotropin and testosterone levels in normal men. J. Clin. Endocrinol. Metab., 63(2):303, 1986.

17
Clinical Investigations of the Contraceptive and Therapeutic Potential of Nafarelin

S. E. MONROE, J. L. ANDREYKO and R. B. JAFFE

Reproductive Endocrinology Center, Department of Obstetrics,
Gynecology and Reproductive Sciences, University of California,
San Francisco, CA 94143, USA

INTRODUCTION

Chronic administration of superactive agonistic analogs
of LHRH decreases the secretion of gonadotropins and
secondarily disrupts gonadal function. These compounds
appear to be clinically useful in situations in which
reversible inhibition of gonadal function is desirable.
Consequently, LHRH analogs are being evaluated as
potential contraceptive agents and as treatment for
several clinical disorders including precocious puberty,
endometriosis, hirsutism, uterine leiomyomata, and
prostatic carcinoma [1–7]. One of the most clinically
useful analogs is nafarelin ([6-D-(2-naphthyl)alanyl]-
LHRH), a potent LHRH agonist that can be administered
intranasally, thus obviating the need for daily injections [8]. During the past several years we have
completed a series of studies to investigate possible
clinical uses of nafarelin in women. These studies can
be classified into 3 general categories: (1) characterization of the clinical pharmacology of nafarelin;
(2) assessment of its contraceptive potential; and (3)
assessment of its utility in the treatment of
endometriosis, hirsutism, and uterine leiomyomata.

CLINICAL PHARMACOLOGY OF NAFARELIN IN WOMEN

Initial clinical studies of nafarelin in women confirmed
in vitro and _in vivo_ animal studies which had shown that
this compound was an extremely potent LHRH agonist [9].
Single subcutaneous (SQ) doses of nafarelin acetate,
ranging from 1 to 100 μg in women, elicited a rapid
increase in serum concentrations of LH and FSH (Fig. 1).
The pattern of gonadotropin release after administration
of nafarelin was a function of both the dose and the
phase of the menstrual cycle. The pituitary gonadotropes were least sensitive to nafarelin stimulation
during the early follicular phase and most sensitive

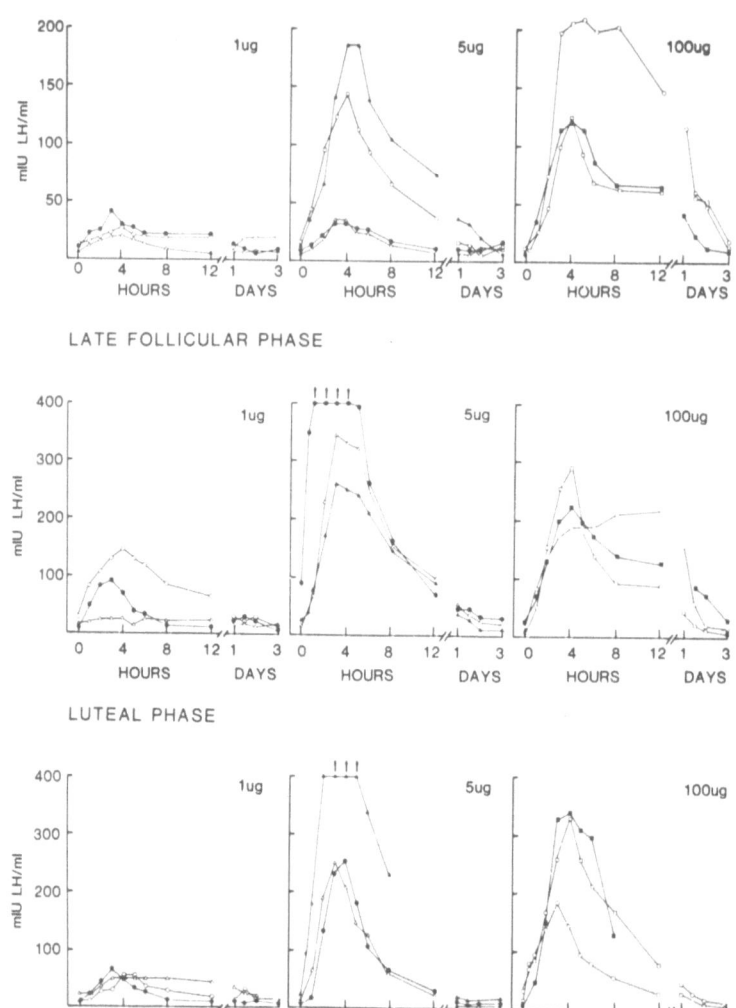

EARLY FOLLICULAR PHASE

LATE FOLLICULAR PHASE

LUTEAL PHASE

Figure 1   Serum concentrations of LH in individual
women   after a single SQ injection of 1,
5, or 100 μg of nafarelin acetate during
the early follicular, late follicular, or
luteal phase of the menstrual cycle. From
Monroe et al.   Fertil. Steril., 43:361
(1985), with permission.

during the late follicular and the luteal phases. Serum
LH and FSH concentrations reached peak levels 3 to 5
hours (h) after administration and gradually declined

thereafter. During the early follicular phase, there was a log dose-response relationship between the dose of nafarelin (1, 5, 20, and 100 μg) and the areas under the curves for LH and FSH (LH: r = 0.9; FSH: r= 0.87). A dose-response relationship for LH also was maintained for the 1 and 5 μg doses during the late follicular and the luteal phases. During these two periods, maximal responses were produced by the 5 μg dose. FSH release was similar to that described for LH, except that the quantity of FSH released was less in most instances.

The relationships between the SQ dose of nafarelin and its concentration in plasma at various times after injection are illustrated in Fig. 2. Nafarelin was

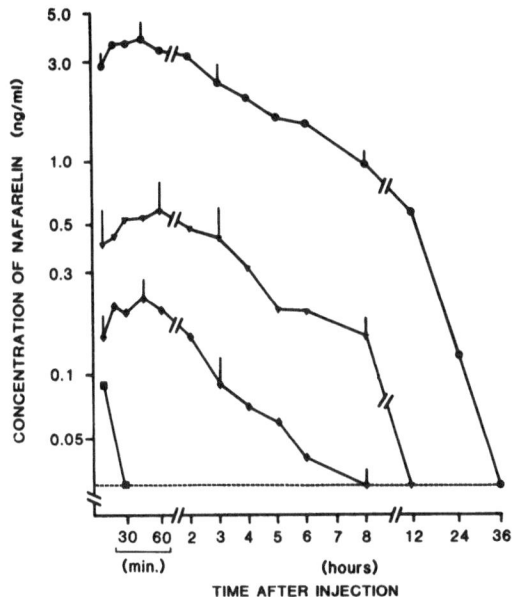

Figure 2   Mean (±SE) plasma levels of nafarelin after single SQ injections of 100 (● , n=9), 20 (▼ , n=2), and 5 (◆ , n=8) μg. Nafarelin could be detected in the plasma of only 1 of 9 women who received 1 μg (■). From Monroe et al. Fertil. Steril, 43:361 (1985), with permission.

detected in plasma within 10 minutes of SQ injection. The maximal plasma level was reached within 1 h and declined thereafter. Circulating levels of the agonist decreased below detectable limits (< 30 pg/ml) within 12 h after the 5 and 20 μg doses. After injection of the 100 μg dose, the LHRH agonist was still detectable in plasma 24 to 36 h after treatment. The plasma half-life was calculated to be 4 to 5 h. Nafarelin was detected in plasma in only 1 of 9 subjects who received the 1 μg dose.

Administration of nafarelin during the early follicular phase consistently delayed ovulation by a mean
(± SD) of 4.6 ± 1.7 days and prolonged the duration of
the menstrual cycle from a pretreatment length of 29.2
± 2.1 to 33.4 ± 4.0 days (P<0.001). When nafarelin was
administered shortly before or after ovulation, cycle
length was not altered consistently. Administration 5
to 10 days after ovulation resulted in a truncated
luteal phase. These observations suggest that the
hormonal events triggered by nafarelin during the early
follicular phase ablated or disrupted the events of the
ovarian cycle that had occurred prior to treatment.
Ovulation usually occurred about 2 weeks after this
"medical ablation" of the ovarian cycle suggesting that
a new follicular phase had been initiated.

STUDIES OF THE CONTRACEPTIVE POTENTIAL OF NAFARELIN

When it was recognized that chronic administration of
superactive agonistic analogs of LHRH had a paradoxical
or inhibitory effect on the secretion of LH and FSH,
several investigators initiated studies to assess the
contraceptive potential of these compounds [10, 11]. A
wide range of treatment schedules has been investigated
including administration of LHRH analogs for 1-3 days
during either the early follicular or luteal phases of
the menstrual cycle as well as daily administration for
up to 6 months [11-14]. We have investigated 3 treatment schedules by which nafarelin might be utilized as a
contraceptive. The approaches were: (1) assessment of
its luteolytic potential; and (2) assessment of its
capacity to inhibit ovulation when administered (a)
daily for 6 months, or (b) in an intermittent fashion
for 3 consecutive days during each of 4 consecutive
weeks.

Effects of Luteal Phase Administration of Nafarelin

Disruption of luteal function is an attractive and
potentially feasible method of contraception. This
approach might avoid some of the complications associated with the daily administration of LHRH analogs
(i.e. development of hypoestrogenemia and/or irregular
bleeding patterns). Therefore, we investigated the
luteolytic potential of prolonged administration of
nafarelin during the luteal phase [15]. Six women were
treated with 100 µg of analog by daily SQ injection for
10 days, beginning either 2 to 3 days or 5 to 7 days
after ovulation. Basal LH and FSH concentrations were
transiently elevated for 2 to 3 days after the onset of
treatment in all women. Serum LH and FSH subsequently
returned to levels similar to those observed during the

pretreatment control month although the normal premenstrual rise of FSH was not observed. There were no changes in mean estradiol (E_2) or progesterone (P) concentrations relative to control cycles. There also was no change in the length of the luteal phase during the treatment month.

In this study, a luteolytic effect of nafarelin could not be demonstrated in spite of pituitary desensitization to the analog and administration of extremely high doses for 10 days. We anticipated that daily treatment with 100 µg of nafarelin would decrease basal concentrations of LH and FSH since this dose was 20-fold that which produced a maximal gonadotropin response. Serum concentrations of LH and FSH during treatment, however, were not suppressed. Therefore, gonadotropin stimulation of the corpus luteum was not prevented. Other investigators have shown that administration of superactive agonistic analogs of LHRH for one to two days in the mid luteal phase of the cycle induces luteolysis [12]. Unfortunately, this luteolytic effect is reversed or prevented by human chorionic gonadotropin (hCG), thus permitting rescue of the corpus luteum if pregnancy were to occur [16].

Inhibition of Ovulation by Daily Intranasal Administration of Nafarelin

We investigated the effects of daily administration of nafarelin upon pituitary-ovarian function [17]. We designed our study to determine if a dose of nafarelin could be identified which would reliably block ovulation while only partially disrupting ovarian estrogen production. Thirty-two women with ovulatory menstrual cycles were treated with a low (125 µg, Gp I), intermediate (250 µg, Gp II), or high (1000 µg [500 µg b.i.d.], Gp III) dose of nafarelin acetate by intranasal spray for 6 months. Twenty-seven of the women completed treatment.

Serum hormone patterns during treatment. Mean serum concentrations of LH and FSH in the 27 women who completed the study are presented in Fig. 3. The data reflect gonadotropin levels immediately prior to the next dose of nafarelin (basal levels). In Gp I there was considerable variability in the degree of LH suppression. In the women receiving 250 and 1000 µg nafarelin acetate, mean basal LH concentrations declined (P<0.01) in a dose related fashion. Mean serum FSH concentrations decreased significantly (P<0.01) in all groups compared to early follicular phase FSH levels, although the magnitude of the change was small. In contrast to findings with LH, the magnitude and rapidity of the decline in FSH levels were relatively independent

261

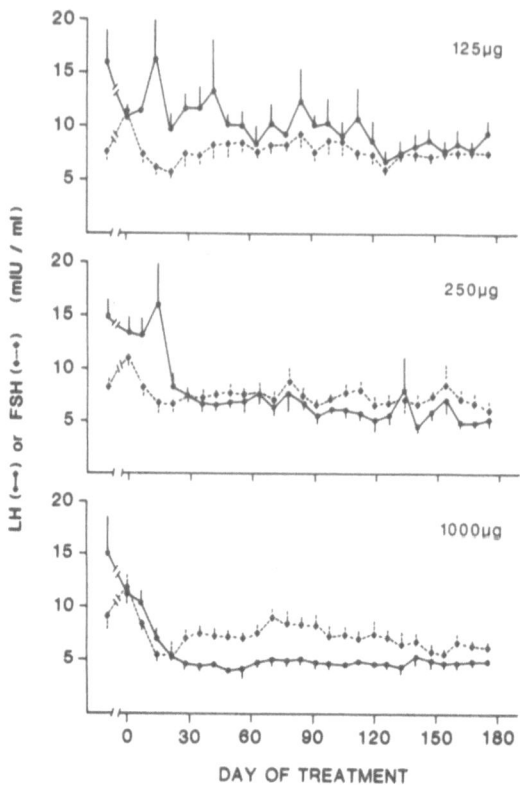

Figure 3   Mean (+SE) concentrations of LH and FSH in 27 women during administration of intranasal nafarelin acetate at doses of 125 (n=12), 250 (n=8), or 1000 (n=7) μg/day. Gonadotropin values are those immediately prior to the next dose of analog. From Monroe et al. J. Clin. Endocrinol. Metab. 63:1334 (1986), with permission.

of the dose of nafarelin. Consequently, the serum LH to FSH ratios declined as the dose increased.

The acute LH and FSH responses to nafarelin on days 1, 90, and 180 of treatment are shown in Fig. 4. The LH and FSH responses on the first day of treatment were proportional to the dose of nafarelin. Although mean gonadotropin levels declined during treatment, the pituitary gonadotropes were not completely desensitized to stimulation by the LHRH analog. Subsequent gonadotropin responses (days 90 and 180) varied inversely with the dose of nafarelin. In those women who received 500 μg twice daily, the gonadotropin responses were barely detectable on days 90 and 180 of treatment.

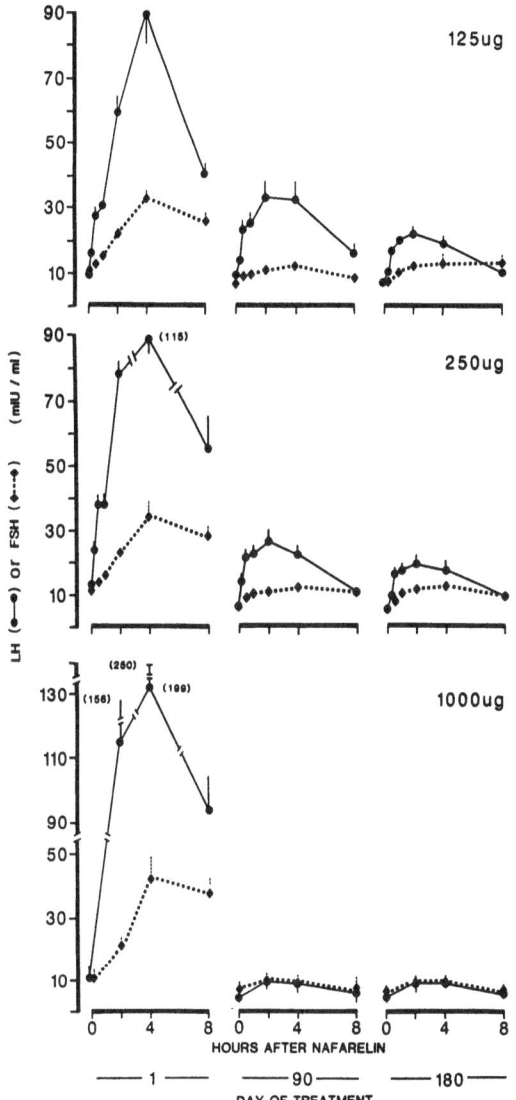

Figure 4   Mean (±SE) serum LH and FSH concentrations
before and 2, 4, and 8 h after intranasal
administration of 125, 250, or 500 µg nafarelin acetate on days 1, 90, and 180 of
treatment. From Monroe et al. J. Clin.
Endocrinol. Metab. <u>63</u>:1334 (1986), with
permission.

    Mean serum E_2 concentrations during treatment are
summarized in Fig. 5. The E_2 levels are those immediately before the next doses of nafarelin and are the
lowest concentrations during each 24 h period. During
the first 2 weeks of treatment, E_2 levels increased

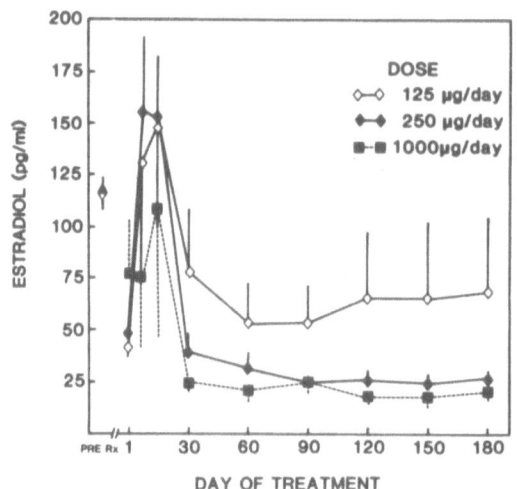

Figure 5   Mean (+SE) serum E_2 concentrations before
           and during the administration of nafarelin
           acetate at a dose of 125, 250, or 1000 µg
           per day.   From Monroe et al. J. Clin.
           Endocrinol. Metab. 63:1334 (1986), with
           permission.

markedly in all treatment groups.   By 1 month, mean
basal E_2 concentrations had declined to levels from
which they deviated relatively little.   In those women
receiving 250 µg nafarelin/day, serum E_2 levels were
low, with a mean E_2 value of approximately 25 pg/ml.
There was little variation in serum E_2 concentrations in
this group.   Mean E_2 levels in Gp III also were
uniformly low.   Acute E_2 responses to nafarelin on days
1, 90, and 180 are shown in Fig. 6. E_2 increased
markedly on day 1 in all groups.   After the initial
period of treatment, the acute E_2 responses were
inversely proportional to the dose of nafarelin.   Mean
serum concentrations 8 h after treatment with 125 or 250
µg nafarelin increased approximately 2-fold.   Those
women receiving 500 µg twice daily, however, exhibited
no acute E_2 responses.

Menstrual bleeding patterns and inhibition of ovulation.
There was considerable variation in menstrual bleeding
patterns in the 3 groups of women.   Although the pattern
of bleeding was not regular, it was well accepted by the
women.   In almost all instances, menstrual bleeding
during treatment was not associated with discomfort, and
blood loss was less than that which would normally have
occurred.   At the 125 µg dose, 5 of the 12 women who
completed 6 months of therapy developed amenorrhea by 60
days.   The remaining women in this group continued to

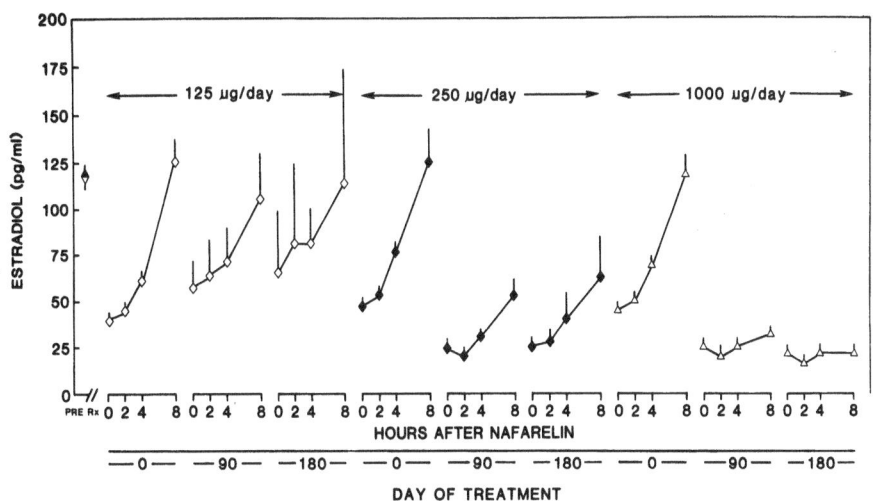

Figure 6   Acute serum E_2 responses (mean $\pm$SE) before and 2, 4, and 8 h after intranasal administration of 125, 250, or 500 µg nafarelin on treatment days 1, 90, and 180. From Monroe et al. J. Clin. Endocrinol. Metab. <u>63</u>:1334 (1986), with permission.

have episodes of uterine bleeding at approximately monthly or less frequent intervals. Seven of the 8 women who received 250 µg nafarelin for 6 months became amenorrheic. Six of the 7 women who received 1000 µg/day also developed amenorrhea within 60 days. The seventh woman had a single episode of bleeding after 5 months.

Serum P levels greater than 4 ng/ml suggested that ovulation had occurred. In Gp I, there were 4 instances in which serum P concentrations exceeded 4 ng/ml and 7 other instances in which serum P concentrations increased to levels of 2-4 ng/ml (Table 1). In Gp II, 2 women had one elevation of serum P to 2 ng/ml. Serum P concentrations in Gp III were uniformly below 2 ng/ml after the second week. All women had a rapid return of

Table 1: Effects of Nafarelin Administration on Ovarian Function

Dose (µg/day)	125	250	1000
Total No. of Rx months	73	58	44
No. of ovulations (progesterone, > 4 ng/ml)	4	0	0
No. of luteinizations (progesterone, 2-4 ng/ml)	7	2	0
Days (mean $\pm$ SE) to first ovulatory menses after stopping nafarelin	44 $\pm$ 5	48 $\pm$ 5	52$\pm$6

ovulatory menstrual function after discontinuance of nafarelin (Table 1). The interval of time to the first post treatment ovulatory menses (range, 24-77 days) did not correlate closely with the prior dose of nafarelin.

Endometrial histology. To assess the effects of treatment on the endometrium, biopsies were obtained at the end of treatment in 26 of the 27 women. In most instances, the histological pattern was that of a physiologically resting or early proliferative endometrium. In 6 women, the endometrium had become so scant that it was not possible to obtain adequate tissue for histological examination. There was no evidence of endometrial hyperplasia in any of the 26 women.

Complications and side-effects. All serum chemistries and blood indices (with one exception) were normal throughout the study. The exception was a tendency for total polymorphonuclear (PMN) leukocyte concentrations to fall in many of the women. The decline in PMN concentrations was not accompanied by any evidence of increased susceptibility to infection. Hot flashes were a frequent complaint. The prevalence and severity of hot flashes increased both with the duration of administration and with the dose of nafarelin. Thus, approximately 35% (Gp I), 65% (Gp II), and 100% (Gp III) of the women experienced hot flashes at some time. Most described them as being of moderate severity. None discontinued nafarelin because of this complaint. We did not assess the effects of decreased E_2 concentrations on bone density.

In conclusion, inhibition of pituitary-ovarian function by daily intranasal nafarelin administration is dose dependent. Gonadotrope sensitivity to 125 µg/day varies among women, and there is inconsistent disruption of follicular development and occasional ovulation. Daily doses of 250 or 1000 µg reliably inhibit ovulation, but also produce either a moderate (Gp II) or a marked (Gp III) reduction in serum E_2 concentrations. Further studies, in which the dose of nafarelin is adjusted according to individual patient sensitivity, may lead to the development of a clinically acceptable contraceptive which consistently prevents ovulation but only partially inhibits the secretion of ovarian E_2.

Alterations of Pituitary-Ovarian Function and Inhibition of Ovulation by Intermittent Nafarelin

To avoid or reduce the undesirable side-effects associated with daily administration of nafarelin, we investigated the effects of intermittent treatment upon pituitary-ovarian function. Nine women with normal ovulatory menstrual cycles each received 5 (n = 5) or 20

(n = 4) μg of nafarelin acetate by SQ injection for 3
consecutive days during each of 4 consecutive weeks
beginning on days 2 to 4 of their menstrual cycles. This
treatment schedule was based on earlier observations
that a single SQ injection of nafarelin during the
follicular phase delayed ovulation by 4-5 days. We
hypothesized that repeated intermittent administration
of an LHRH agonist would prevent ovulation. Intermittent nafarelin blocked ovulation in 7 of the 9 women
and ovulation was delayed by one week in an eighth
woman. Because of the intermittent treatment schedule,
there was only partial down-regulation or desensitization of pituitary gonadotropes during the 3 days of drug
administration (Fig. 7). Pituitary responsiveness to

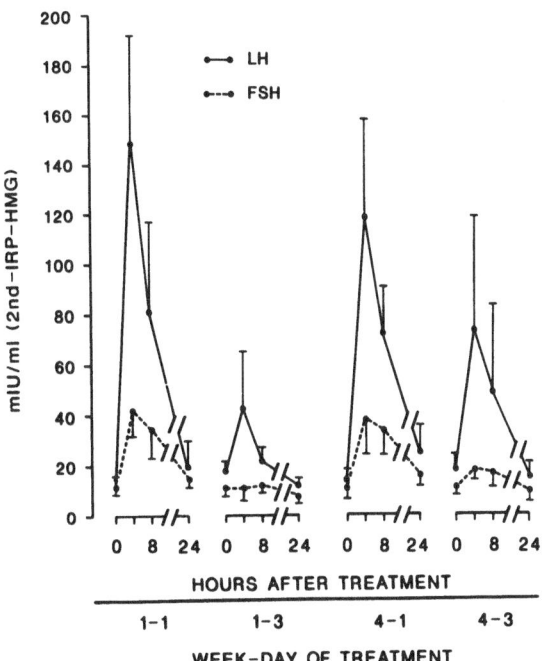

Figure 7   Mean (+SE) LH and FSH levels on days 1 and
            3 during weeks 1 and 4 of treatment
            following either 5 (n=4) or 20 (n=3) μg of
            SQ nafarelin acetate in the 7 women in whom
            ovulation was blocked.

the LHRH analog also returned to pretreatment levels
prior to the initiation of each weekly series of
treatments. Since serum levels of LH and FSH were not
suppressed, ovarian estradiol secretion was maintained
(Fig. 8). Mean serum levels of estradiol were slightly
greater on the third day of each treatment series than
those prior to the onset of treatment. This preliminary study demonstrates that intermittent administration
of a LHRH analog can block ovulation in a high percentage of women without significantly disrupting ovarian

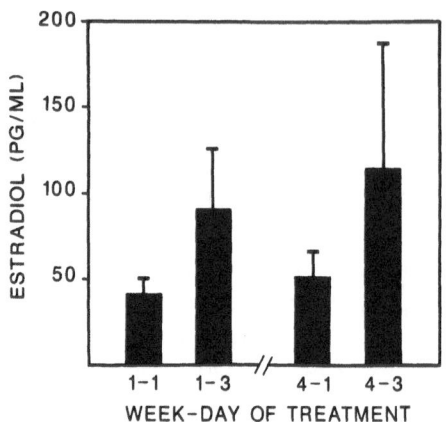

Figure 8   Mean (±SE) serum estradiol levels in the 7
women represented in fig. 7.

steroid secretion. Further studies utilizing intermittent or discontinuous LHRH may lead to the development of a treatment schedule in which ovulation can be
blocked reliably without significantly reducing ovarian
estradiol secretion.

THERAPEUTIC USES OF NAFARELIN IN WOMEN

Since chronic administration of superactive agonistic
analogs of LHRH disrupts gonadal function, these compounds appear to be useful for the treatment of disorders in which reversible inhibition of gonadal
function would be beneficial. LHRH analogs have been
used to treat precocious puberty, endometriosis,
hirsutism, uterine leiomyomata, and prostatic carcinoma
[1-7]. In this section, we describe our clinical
experience with nafarelin for the treatment of endometriosis [3], hirsutism [4], and uterine leiomyomata [6].

Endometriosis

Endometriosis is a common disease often associated with
dysmenorrhea, dyspareunia, pelvic pain, and infertility.
There is no uniformly successful treatment for endometriosis when the potential for future fertility must
be maintained. In this study, 8 women with endometriosis, 25-37 years of age, were treated with 500 μg
nafarelin acetate twice daily by intranasal spray for 6
months [3]. Endometriosis was documented and photo-
graphed at laparoscopy both prior to and at the completion of treatment. The severity of the endometriosis in
each patient was staged according to The American

Fertility Society classification [18]. No operative therapeutic procedures were performed during the staging laparoscopy. Women were examined and interviewed monthly for assessment of symptoms, and a severity profile of symptoms and physical findings was recorded.

Seven of the 8 women completed the 6 months of treatment and were surgically reexamined, 5 by laparoscopy and 2 by laparotomy. All had a decrease in their clinical staging and active disease scores after therapy ($P<0.02$; Table 2). Residual adhesions and a residual ovarian endometrioma accounted for most of the post treatment staging scores. No active endometrial implants were found after therapy in 5 of the 7 patients. All patients had complete loss or marked decrease in the painful symptoms of endometriosis during treatment. Most had significant symptomatic relief by 4 weeks of treatment, and improvement was maximal in all by 12 weeks of treatment (Table 2).

All women remained anovulatory during treatment. Vaginal bleeding during treatment was limited to spotting during the first month in 6 women and during the sixth month in one woman. Endometrial tissue obtained by biopsy at the conclusion of treatment was atrophic in one woman and proliferative in 3. In the remaining 3 women, sufficient tissue could not be obtained for histologic diagnosis. After the onset of treatment, concentrations of LH, determined in blood samples drawn immediately before nafarelin administration (basal concentrations), were elevated during the first 5 days of treatment but fell significantly within 2 weeks ($P<0.001$), and remained low throughout the treatment regimen. Mean basal FSH concentrations during the initial treatment period were not significantly elevated and fell significantly ($P<0.001$) within 2 weeks of the onset of treatment. After a transient increase in some patients during the initial month of treatment, mean E_2 concentrations decreased to <30 pg/ml by 4 weeks in all patients. Subsequently, E_2 elevations were observed in only one patient. After minimal elevations of serum P in some patients during the first few days, P levels remained below 0.5 ng/ml throughout the remainder of treatment.

All women developed symptoms of hypoestrogenemia. The major complaint was hot flashes, which became severe enough to necessitate decreasing the dose to 250 µg twice daily in 3 women. Other complaints included vaginal dryness in 4 women, mild transient headaches in five, and mild transient depression in 2. The effects of 6 months of hypoestrogenemia on bone density were not assessed. One patient was withdrawn from the study after 2 months of treatment because of the development of leukopenia. Subsequent WBC counts in this patient after treatment was discontinued remained at the lower limit of normal.

269

Table 2: Clinical Findings Prior to and Following Treatment with Nafarelin

Pt.	Extent of Disease				Severity Profile[c]	
	Total Disease[a]		Active Disease[b]			
	Before Rx	After Rx	Before Rx	After Rx	Before Rx	After Rx
1	34	31	7	4	8	2
2	16	6	5	0	8	3
3	3	1	3	1	2	1
4	2[d]	–	2[d]	–	11	4
5	7	2	4	0	8	3
6	28	22	5	0	4	3
7	10	5	9	0	7	1
8	1	0	1	0	2	0

[a]Stages within The American Fertility Society (AFS) Classifications are mild (1 to 5), moderate (6 to 15), severe (16 to 30), and extensive (31 to 54). Scores are based on size of endometriomas, implants of endometriosis, and severity of adhesions involving the peritoneum, the ovaries, and the fallopian tubes.

[b]Scores are derived by considering only active disease as reflected by endometrial implants.

[c]Scores are derived by grading and assigning a numerical value to the symptoms of dysmenorrhea, dyspareunia, and pelvic pain and the physical findings of pelvic tenderness and induration: absent = 0; mild = 1; moderate = 2; or severe = 3 (maximum score = 15).

[d]Treatment was discontinued after only 2 months, and follow-up laparoscopy was not performed.

Pretreatment and post treatment scores are significantly different: total disease, $P<0.02$; active disease, $P<0.02$; severity profile, $P<0.01$. Residual adhesions accounted for most of the post treatment total disease scores and residual induration for most of the post treatment severity profile scores.

The mean number of days from discontinuation of treatment until the first ovulatory menses was 47 ± 8 (SD) with a range of 36 to 57. All symptoms of hypoestrogenemia resolved during the first month after discontinuation of treatment. All women except one reported decreased or absent dysmenorrhea immediately after treatment. Recurrence of dysmenorrhea, however, either partial (n = 4) or complete (n = 2), occurred within 3 to 6 months after completion of treatment in 6 women. The recurrence of symptoms suggests that treatment induced a remission rather than a cure. The rate of recurrence in this study may be overestimated, however, because the study group consisted of patients who had severe endometriosis and had not benefitted from other therapies.

In summary, treatment of endometriosis with intranasal administration of nafarelin can: (1) decrease E_2 concentrations to approximately menopausal levels; (2) relieve symptoms of endometriosis; (3) cause disappearance of endometriotic lesions; and (4) is an alternative form of medical therapy for endometriosis. Clinical studies that involve a larger number of women with endometriosis are in progress to assess further the efficacy of nafarelin in the treatment of this disorder as well as the extent and reversibility of bone demineralization which may occur as a consequence of hypoestrogenemia.

Hirsutism

Hirsutism, the growth of excessive coarse terminal hairs, results from increased androgen production by either the ovaries or adrenal glands, or increased sensitivity of hair follicles to normal circulating androgen levels. Most frequently, increased androgen production is of ovarian origin and often associated with the polycystic ovarian (PCO) syndrome. In the PCO syndrome, elevated production of ovarian androgens is dependent upon gonadotropin stimulation. Suppression of LH secretion would be expected to reduce ovarian androgen production, and secondarily, reduce the formation of new terminal hairs. To investigate the therapeutic potential of nafarelin as a treatment for hirsutism, 6 women with this complaint, four of whom had the PCO syndrome, were treated with nafarelin acetate 1000 µg/day, by nasal spray, for 6 months [4]. Serum gonadotropin concentrations in all 6 patients were significantly suppressed by one month of treatment. Mean LH concentrations fell from 17.9 ± 4.6 (±SE) to 5.0 ± 0.5 mIU/ml (P<0.01) and FSH declined from 9.3 ± 0.7 to 7.2 ± 0.9 mIU/ml (P<0.05). Both remained at low levels throughout treatment. Serum androgen levels are shown in Fig. 9. Mean serum concentrations of testosterone (T) and androstenedione ($\Delta^4 A$) decreased significantly within one to 3 months of the onset of treatment and remained suppressed until nafarelin was discontinued. Serum E_2 and estrone (E_1) concentrations decreased significantly during treatment. E_2 decreased from 58.5 ± 7.4 to 28.2 ± 6.1 pg/ml (P<0.05) after 2 months. The mean serum E_2 level during the 6 months of therapy was 34.8 ± 3.1 pg/ml.

Clinically, the patients responded favorably in terms of hair growth. After 3 months all were shaving or using depilatories less often. They also noted that new hair growth was not as coarse as it had been previously.

271

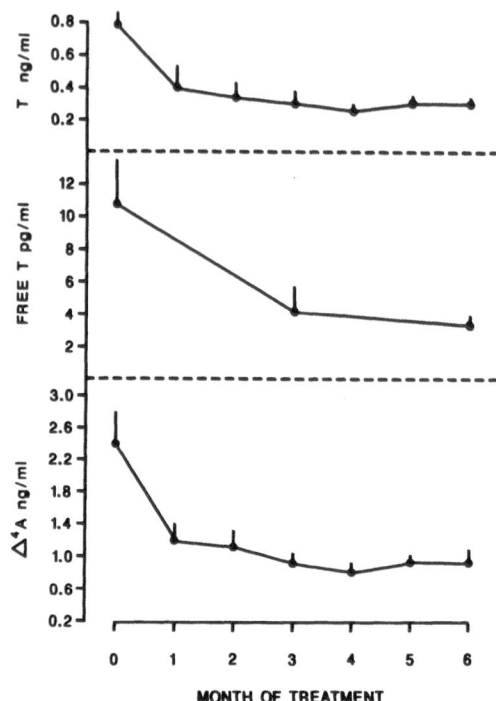

Figure 9   Mean ($\pm$SE) serum testosterone (T), free T, and androstenedione (Δ^4A) concentrations in 6 hirsute women before and during nafarelin treatment. From Andreyko et al. J. Clin. Endocrinol. Metab. 63:854 (1986), with permission.

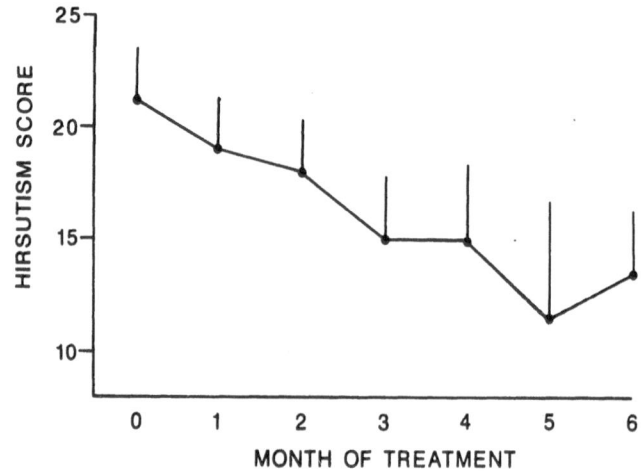

Figure 10   Mean ($\pm$SE) hirsutism scores in 6 women before and during treatment with nafarelin. From Andreyko et al. J. Clin. Endocrinol. Metab. 63:854 (1986), with permission.

Changes in hair growth also were assessed by the scale of Ferriman and Gallwey [19]. There was a significant improvement in the mean hirsutism score after 6 months of treatment (P<0.05), and remaining hairs were less pigmented and finer in quality (Fig. 10). In areas that were shaved by the investigator, new hair was very fine and, in most patients, regrew very slowly. Patients tolerated the medication well. Most had hot flashes but in no case did treatment have to be stopped.

This study demonstrates the capacity of nafarelin to maintain long term ovarian androgen suppression with resultant improvement in hair growth. One would anticipate that this effect would be apparent only as long as medication was continued, since androgen levels began to rise shortly after treatment was stopped. All patients in this study had normal pretreatment serum concentrations of dehydroepiandrosterone sulfate (DHAS), an indicator of adrenal androgen secretory activity. As expected, treatment had no significant effect on serum DHAS concentrations. Thus, one would anticipate that nafarelin would not be beneficial in treating hyper-androgenemia of adrenal origin. The beneficial effect of nafarelin treatment probably would be enhanced if women also received estrogen replacement during the period of pituitary-ovarian suppression. Estrogen replacement therapy would stimulate the production of sex hormone binding globulin (SHBG) by the liver. Increased serum concentration of SHBG would reduce further the concentrations of free or biologically active T. In addition, such treatment would decrease the incidence of hot flashes and reduce the potential risk of bone demineralization.

Uterine Leiomyomata

Uterine leiomyomata, interlacing whorls of smooth muscle and fibrous tissue within the myometrium, are common, benign uterine tumors which may present symptomatically as discomfort from an enlarging pelvic mass, heavy and irregular menstrual bleeding, or occasionally, infertility. Standard treatment for symptomatic leiomyomata has been surgical - either myomectomy or hysterectomy-depending on age and desire for childbearing. There is evidence that the growth of leiomyomata is stimulated by estrogen and/or progesterone. Myomata tend to enlarge in pregnancy, a high estrogen and progesterone state, and decrease in size after the menopause, when levels of these steroids are low. Receptors for both steroids also have been identified in tissue culture preparations of human myomata [20]. Therefore, there is increasing interest in the possibility of treating women with leiomyomata by medical as opposed to surgical means, particularly women in whom preservation of future fertility is desired. One approach which is being

273

investigated is to reduce ovarian estrogen and
progesterone production by chronic treatment with LHRH
analogs.

We have treated 11 women, aged 30 to 43 years, with
intranasal nafarelin acetate, (500 µg b.i.d.) for 6
months [6]. All were desirous of preserving future
fertility and all were symptomatic to the extent that
they would have undergone myomectomy had they not
received nafarelin treatment. Eight of the 11 had heavy
or irregular uterine bleeding. Ten of the 11 completed
6 months of treatment. During treatment there was a
significant reduction in serum gonadotropins and E_2.
The mean E_2 concentration decreased from a follicular
phase mean of 43 ± 8.3 to 19.8 ± 3.1 pg/ml (P<0.050) at
3 months and to 14.8 ± 2.2 pg/ml (P<0.01) at 6 months of
treatment. Mean seum T, Δ^4A and DHAS concentrations did
not change significantly during treatment.

Uterine size was monitored clinically by pelvic
examination and by magnetic resonance imaging (MRI)
[21]. Clinically, uterine size was estimated in terms
of equivalent uterine sizes at various weeks of pregnancy (i.e. gestational weeks). Eight of the 11 patients
had a decrease in overall uterine size by pelvic
examination. Prior to treatment, the mean ($\pm$ SE)
uterine size was $13.5 \pm .9$ gestational weeks (range 8-
20). At the completion of treatment, the mean size had
decreased to 8.2 ± 1.9 (range 0 (not pregnant) to 20).
The volume of individual leiomyomata, as well as overall
uterine size, were assessed by MRI (Fig. 11). The size

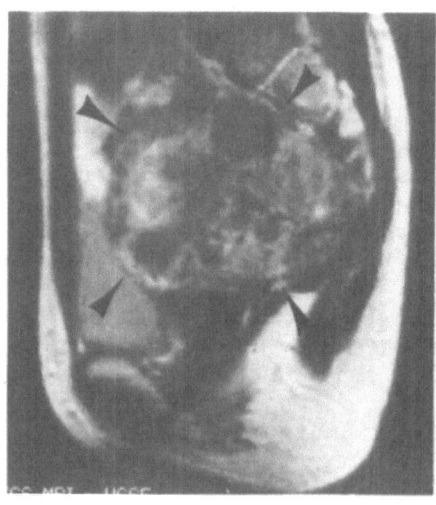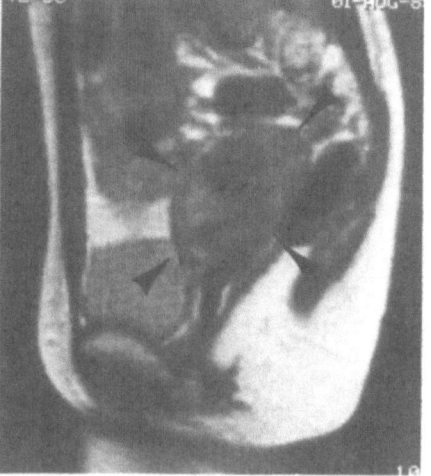

Figure 11   Magnetic resonance images of a myomatous
             uterus prior to (left panel) and following
             (right panel) 3 months of treatment with
             nafarelin. Both the total volume of the
             uterus (outlined by arrows) and individual
             myomata decreased in size.

of the largest leiomyoma in each woman decreased in 9 of the 11 patients. The mean ($\pm$SE) decrease was 48$\pm$9 percent.

Ten of the 11 patients developed amenorrhea by 90 days and none had further uterine bleeding after 120 days of treatment. Amenorrhea was an additional benefit of therapy since metrorrhagia had been a problem in 8 women prior to treatment. All women experienced hot flashes, but in no case were these so severe that treatment was discontinued. Four of the patients underwent myomectomy at the conclusion of the 6 month treatment period. In all cases, surgery was performed easily, with little intraoperative blood loss.

This study, like others [5,22], suggests that LHRH analogs, such as nafarelin, may be useful for the treatment of uterine leiomyomata. Such treatment rapidly reduced the heavy and irregular uterine bleeding often present in this disorder and reduced the size of the largest leiomyoma in 9 of the 11 women. In addition, treatment with nafarelin may facilitate the surgical removal of these growths at the time of myomectomy. Further clinical studies will be required to define the eventual role of this form of medical treatment in the management of this common disorder.

Concluding Remarks

These studies, as well as those of others, suggest that agonistic analogs of LHRH, such as nafarelin, are well-tolerated, clinically beneficial, potent endocrinologic agents which should prove to be useful additions to the therapeutic armamentarium. They have potential value as contraceptive agents, proven efficacy in the treatment of endometriosis, hirsutism, leiomyomata, and sexual precocity, and great promise for a variety of menstrual cycle-related disorders such as excessive vaginal bleeding and menstrual cycle-related migraine headaches, and in vitro fertilization programs for more controlled induction of follicular development. In addition, these compounds are useful probes for investigating the regulation of the hypothalamic-pituitary-gonadal axis.

Acknowledgments

These studies were supported, in part, by contracts No. 1-HD-0-2811 and No. 1-HD-3-2831 from the National Institute of Child Health and Human Development, Bethesda, Maryland. We thank Ms Carol Vandello for her assistance in the preparation of this chapter.

REFERENCES

1. Comite, F., Cutler, G.B. Jr., Rivier, J., Vale, W.W., Loriaux, D.L. and Crowley, W.F. Jr. Short-term treatment of idiopathic precocious puberty with a long-acting analogue of luteinizing hormone-releasing hormone. A preliminary report. N. Engl. J. Med., 305:1546 (1981).

2. Lemay, A., Maheux, R., Faure, N., Jean, C. and Fazekas, A.T.A. Reversible hypogonadism induced by a luteinizing hormone-releasing hormone (LH-RH) agonist (Buserelin) as a new therapeutic approach for endometriosis. Fertil. Steril., 41:863 (1984).

3. Schriock, E., Monroe, S., Henzl, M., and Jaffe, R. Treatment of endometriosis with a potent agonist of gonadotropin-releasing hormone. Fertil. Steril., 44:583 (1985).

4. Andreyko, J., Monroe, S. and Jaffe, R. Treatment of hirsutism with a GnRH agonist (nafarelin). J. Clin. Endocrinol. Metab., 63:854 (1986).

5. Maheux, R., Lemay, A., Merat, P. Use of intranasal luteinizing hormone-releasing hormone agonist in uterine leiomyomas. Fertil. Steril., 47:229 (1987).

6. Andreyko, J., Blumenfeld, Z., Marshall, L., Hricak, H., Cann, C. and Monroe, S. Treatment of uterine leiomyomata with a GnRH agonist. In Proceedings of the Society for Gynecologic Investigation, Toronto, March 19, 1986, Abstract 127.

7. Tolis, G., Ackman, D., Stellos, A., Mehta, A., Labrie, F., Fazekas, A.T.A., Comaru-Schally, A.M. and Schally, A.V. Tumor growth inhibition in patients with prostatic carcinoma treated with luteinizing hormone-releasing hormone agonists. Proc. Natl. Acad. Sci., USA 79:1658 (1982).

8. Nestor, J.J. Jr., Ho, T.L., Simpson, R.A., Horner, B.L., Jones, G.H., McRae, G.I. and Vickery, B.H. Synthesis and biologic activity of some very hydrophobic superagonist analogues of luteinizing hormone-releasing hormone. J. Med. Chem., 25:795 (1982).

9. Monroe, S.E., Henzl, M.R., Martin, M.C., Schriock, E., Lewis, V., Nerenberg, C. and Jaffe, R.B. Ablation of folliculogenesis in women by a single dose of gonadotropin-releasing hormone agonist: significance of time in cycle. Fertil. Steril., 43:361 (1985).

10. Linde, R., Doelle, G.C., Alexander, N., Kirchner, F., Vale, W., Rivier, J. and Rabin, D. Reversible inhibition of testicular steroidogenesis and spermatogenesis by a potent gonadotropin-releasing hormone agonist in normal men. N. Engl. J. Med. 305:663 (1981).

11. Nillius, S.J., Bergquist, C. and Wide, L. Inhibition of ovulation in women by chronic treatment with

a stimulatory LRH analogue. A new approach to birth control? Contraception, 17:537 (1978).

12. Casper, R.F. and Yen, S.S.C. Induction of luteolysis in the human with a long-acting analog of luteinizing hormone-releasing factor. Science, 205:408 (1979).

13. Bergquist, C., Nillius, S.J. and Wide, L. Long-term intranasal luteinizing hormone-releasing hormone agonist treatment for contraception in women. Fertil. Steril., 38:190 (1982).

14. Lemay, A., Faure, N., Labrie, F. and Fazekas, A.T.A. Inhibition of ovulation during discontinuous intranasal luteinizing hormone-releasing hormone agonist dosing in combination with gestagen-induced bleeding. Fertil. Steril., 43:868 (1985).

15. Schriock, E.D., Monroe, S.E., Martin, M.C., Henzl, M.R. and Jaffe, R.B. Effect on corpus luteum function of luteal phase administration of a potent gonadotropin-releasing hormone analog (nafarelin). Fertil. Steril., 43:844 (1985).

16. Bergquist, C., Nillius, S.J. and Wide, L. Luteolysis induced by a luteinizing hormone-releasing hormone agonist is prevented by human chorionic gonadotropin. Contraception, 22:341 (1980).

17. Monroe, S.E., Blumenfeld, Z., Andreyko, J.L., Schriock, E., Henzl, M.R. and Jaffe, R.B. Dose-dependent inhibition of pituitary-ovarian function during administration of a gonadotropin-releasing hormone agonistic analog (nafarelin). J. Clin. Endocrinol. Metab., 63:1334 (1986).

18. American Fertility Society: Classification of endometriosis. Fertil. Steril., 32:633 (1979).

19. Ferriman, D. and Gallwey, J.D. Clinical assessment of body hair growth in women. J. Clin. Endocrinol. Metab., 21:1440 (1961).

20. Tamaya, T., Fujimoto, J. and Okada, H. Comparison of cellular levels of steroid receptors in uterine leiomyoma and myometrium. Acta. Obstet. Gyneacol. Scand., 64:307 (1985).

21. Hricak, H., Lacey, C., Schriock, E., Fisher, M.R., Amparo, E., Dooms, G. and Jaffe, R. Gynecologic masses: value of magnetic resonance imaging. Am. J. Obstet. Gynecol., 153:31 (1985).

22. Healy, D.L., Lawson, S.R., Abbott, M., Baird, D.T. and Fraser, H.M. Toward removing uterine fibroids without surgery: subcutaneous infusion of a luteinizing hormone-releasing hormone agonist commencing in the luteal phase. J. Clin Endocrinol. Metab., 63:619 (1986).

18
LHRH Agonists and Antagonists: Therapeutic Possibilities for Premenstrual Syndrome

R.L. REID* and S.S.C. YEN**
*Division of Reproductive Endocrinology,
Department of Obstetrics and Gynaecology, Queen's University,
Kingston, Ontario, Canada, K7L 3N6;
**Division of Reproductive Endocrinology, Department of
Reproductive Medicine, University of California, La Jolla,
California, CA 92093, USA

INTRODUCTION

Premenstrual syndrome is the cyclic recurrence in the luteal phase of the menstrual cycle of a combination of distressing physical, psychological, and or behavioural changes of sufficient severity to result in deterioration of interpersonal relationships and/or interference with normal activities [1]. While the term 'premenstrual' provides a useful clinical descriptor to focus attention on the issue of illness related to the menstrual cycle, it should be noted that classical manifestations of premenstrual syndrome may occur in the absence of menstrual bleeding when ovarian cyclicity has been preserved at the time of hysterectomy [2] and in some anovulatory patients experiencing intermittent development and atresia of ovarian follicles [3].

Available estimates indicate that as many as 30 to 40 percent of women are sufficiently distressed by their premenstrual symptomatology to have sought help from their physician or have tried over-the-counter remedies. Approximately 5 to 10 percent of women of reproductive age range report premenstrual changes, though temporary, to be of a severe or disabling nature [4,5]. The symptoms most often linked to this degree of lifestyle disruption include fatigue, depression, anxiety, irritability, insomnia, and headaches. Premenstrual syndrome is known to span the complete age range from puberty until the menopause with many women reporting a worsening of symptoms in the later reproductive years [1].

CLINICAL MANIFESTATIONS

Symptoms experienced by most women with premenstrual syndrome will fall into one of four temporal patterns defined according to the onset and duration of manifestations with the vast majority experiencing patterns A and B (Fig. 1).

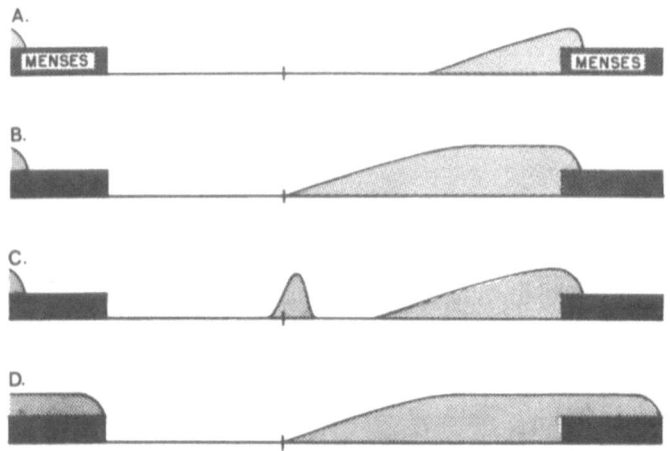

FIGURE 1   Schematic diagram showing variability in the onset and duration of premenstrual symptoms. (Reproduced from Reid, RL, Yen SSC,: Premenstrual syndrome. Clin. Obstet. Gynecol. 26:710, 1983 [6] (Harper and Row Publishers Inc., with permission).

A small group of patients will experience a transient recurrence of all their usual premenstrual symptomatology coincident with the abrupt drop in estradiol that occurs during the periovulatory period [7]. Since many of the symptoms ascribed to premenstrual syndrome are common to other conditions, such as chronic depression, attention to the timing of symptoms in relation to menstruation is of utmost importance in establishing a diagnosis.

The earliest symptoms of premenstrual syndrome include breast swelling and tenderness together with lower abdominal bloating and constipation. Though usually attributed to generalized fluid retention these symptoms often exist in the absence of weight gain or edema suggesting that local fluid shifts within the body may be involved. Marked fatigue, emotional lability, and depression may result in women sleeping longer or taking extra naps, devoting less energy to household chores, or having more frequent emotional outbursts over matters of minor importance. More severely affected individuals may become completely withdrawn from family and friends, choosing to physically isolate themselves, to relinquish parental responsibilities to the spouse, and to cancel social commitments. Uncommonly, recurrent suicidal thoughts and behaviour may be present. At times anxiety, tension, and anger predominate leading to physical unrest, irritability, and combativeness. Deterioration of interpersonal relationships, and perceived inefficiency at work, often precipitate feelings of personal inadequacy, hopelessness, and guilt.

Although some women report the dramatic lifting of inward tension and irritability several hours before the onset of menstrual flow, most experience relief from their distressing symptoms only after the second or third day of menstruation. Pelvic pain and menorrhagia are usually not features of premenstrual syndrome and suggest the need for full gynaecologic evaluation to rule out coexisting disorders.

Accounts from PMS sufferers indicate that persistence of such troublesome symptoms for extended periods of time may have a pronounced impact on, not only the affected individual, but also upon her family and career. These concerns, and the potential medical/legal impact of premenstrual syndrome, were recently reviewed [1,8].

PATHOPHYSIOLOGY OF PREMENSTRUAL SYNDROME

The pathophysiology of premenstrual syndrome is presently unknown. Though there is increasing evidence to indicate that the intensity of coexisting life stresses may play an important role in modifying the expression of premenstrual symptomatology it is clear that cyclic ovarian function is the sine qua non of this disorder.

Just how the diverse manifestations of premenstrual syndrome are linked to cyclic changes in ovarian steroid production is a matter of some controversy. It is likely that some manifestations of PMS are a direct effect of circulating steroids whereas other manifestations are mediated through changes in neurotransmitters within the brain. For example, breast tenderness and enlargement are likely the result of direct steroid effects on breast tissue and intralobular edema. The effect that gonadal steroids have on the regulation of behaviour, appetite, sleep, and temperature is surely more complex and probably involves a variety of neuro-transmitter systems within the brain [1].

Data supporting an obligatory role for ovarian secretion in the pathophysiology of premenstrual syndrome arise from several sources. It is known that premenstrual syndrome does not appear prior to activation of the hypothalamic-pituitary-ovarian axis at puberty. Premenstrual syndrome disappears during periods of hypogonadotropic amenorrhea that occur in women subjected to excessive stress of a physical, psychological, or nutritional nature. Thus amenorrheic marathon runners, and women with amenorrhea secondary to weight loss, experience relief from cyclic symptoms that they may have noted prior to the development of amenorrhea. Premenstrual syndrome will persist following hysterectomy if ovarian function remains intact and yet can be eliminated by surgical or natural menopause.

Sporadic reports of cyclic PMS-like symptoms in oophorectomized or postmenopausal woman must be viewed circumspectly in the absence of simultaneous hormonal measurements to rule out the possibility of incomplete ovarian resection or sporadic follicular recruitment. An alternative explanation for these reports might be that menopausal symptoms (due to inadequate hormone replacement) are being ascribed to PMS since there is considerable overlap of symptomatology in these two conditions (sleep disturbance, palpitations, hot flushes, depression, irritability, etc.) [9].

THERAPY WITH LHRH AGONISTS AND ANTAGONISTS

"At present, in the severest cases of this nature, temporary or permanent amenorrhea brought about by roentgen treatment (to the ovaries) appears to be the proper procedure".
(R. Frank, 1931) [10].

Frank, in one of the first publications on premenstrual syndrome, recognized the value of eliminating ovarian cyclicity in the control of severe premenstrual syndrome. Over the years ovariectomy has been employed sporadically for treatment of severe and intractable premenstrual syndrome, however, it is not surprising that this procedure has never been widely endorsed by the gynaecological community. Fears that acknowledging a surgical solution for premenstrual syndrome without a strict, widely accepted operational definition for this disorder might lead to overutilization of surgery when lesser interventions would suffice and concerns about the longterm impact of premature ovariectomy have been largely responsible for the limited utilization of a therapy which most gynaecologists have found effective for premenstrual syndrome at one time or another. We have had experience with oophorectomy (and concomitant hysterectomy) for treatment of severe PMS in 24 women who failed to get relief from available medical interventions and have documentation of dramatic and persisting relief from symptoms in these women when they are maintained on low dose estrogen replacement therapy [11].

The large number of PMS sufferers and the fact that many are young women who have yet to complete their reproductive careers means that counselling and medication must remain the primary mode of treatment for this disorder. To date, despite many claims to the contrary, there exists no single medical intervention that will assure relief to all women with PMS. Often treatment amounts to counselling and reassurance followed by a 'hit and miss' trial of a number of medications with supposed benefits for specific PMS manifestations.

Recently attention has turned to the possibility of developing an agent which could reversibly suppress ovarian activity without the adverse effects of synthetic steroids.

In examining the merits of any method of suppressing ovarian activity for premenstrual syndrome, several principles must be kept in mind:
1) Although elimination of cyclic ovarian function will remove the hormonal trigger for cyclic premenstrual symptomatology, attention to intervention through modification of the contribution of psychological stress to PMS should not be overlooked [12].

2) Maintenance of early follicular phase levels of estradiol is necessary to avoid supplanting premenstrual symptomatology with menopausal symptomatology occasioned by oversuppression of ovarian steroidogenesis. Chronic hypoestrogenism may be associated with increased risks of ischemic heart disease and osteoporosis [13,14].
3) Long term unopposed estrogenic stimulation of the endometrium resulting from anovulation incurs a risk of endometrial hyperplasia and/or malignancy that necessitates regular endometrial sampling or intermittent progestagen therapy [15].
4) A method of drug administration must be found to maximize patient acceptability.

One such agent, Danazol, employed in the treatment of endometriosis, affords dramatic relief from cyclic premenstrual symptomatology once amenorrhea is achieved. In our experience Danazol has proved to be highly effective as a diagnostic and therapeutic tool in premenstrual syndrome and is often an ideal short term treatment for crisis intervention. Danazol in dosages from 400-800 mg per day will effectively eliminate ovarian cyclicity in most women while maintaining early follicular phase levels of estradiol [16]. The cost, mild androgenic side effects (oilyness of skin, hirsutism, increased appetite, and weight gain), and adverse impact of Danazol on serum lipoproteins, however, are likely to preclude the longterm use of this agent in the treatment of PMS.

LHRH agonists and antagonists are other options that could reversibly suppress ovarian steroidogenesis in women with severe PMS and thereby afford temporary respite from the cyclic symptoms until fertility is desired.

PRELIMINARY RESULTS WITH LHRH AGONISTS

Muse et al. 1984 [17], working with one of us (SSCY), have published preliminary data on the use of LHRH agonists [D-SER (tBu)[6], Pro[9]-NHEt] LHRH in the treatment of premenstrual syndrome employing a double-blind cross-over design. Daily ratings of ten behavioural symptoms and five physical symptoms were obtained for a minimum of one cycle pre-treatment and for the duration of the six month trial. Each subject was taught to self administer 50 ug of the LHRH agonist, or an equal volume of saline as a placebo daily, in the double-blind cross-over trial. Employing this regimen most patients had menstrual bleeding at the end of the first month of agonist treatment and following completion of the three months

of agonist treatment. Because patients were informed
that either treatment could effect menstrual
cyclicity, it appeared unlikely that agonist induced
amenorrhea influenced the blindedness of patients
during the study interval. Only one patient had hot
flushes during the last two cycles of agonist
treatment. As expected, the LHRH agonist treatment
abolished cyclic fluctuations of steroid hormones
approximately two weeks after initiation of agonist
therapy (Fig. 2).

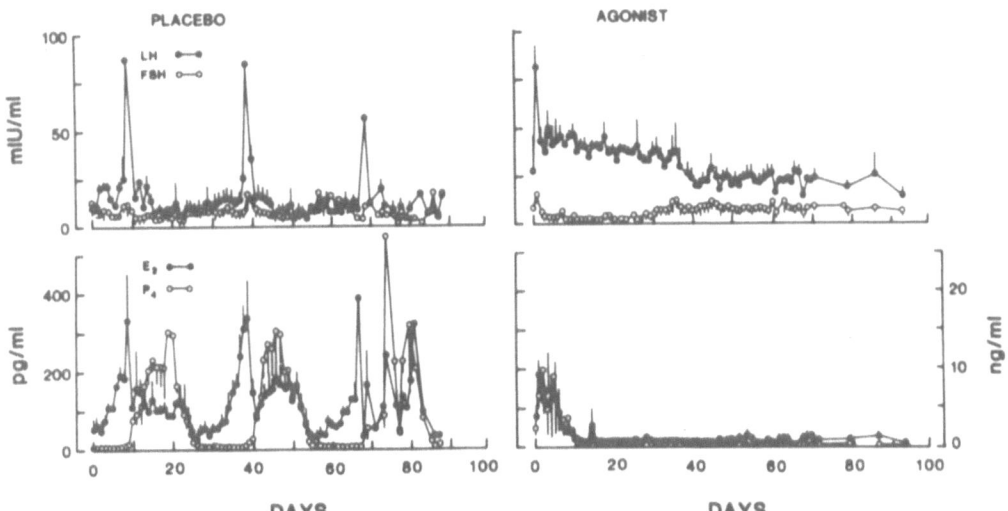

FIGURE 2   Mean concentrations (± S.E.) of Luteinizing
             Hormone (LH), Follicle Stimulating Hormone
             (FSH), Estradiol (E2), and Progesterone (P4)
             during 90 days of treatment with the GnRH
             Agonist. Data on placebo administration are
             standardized to peak LH values and the onset
             of menses. Data on GnRH-agonist treatment
             are normalized to the first day of
             administration. Reproduced with permission
             from Muse et al. N. Engl. J. Med. 311:1345
             (1984).

Those four women who received LHRH agonist treatment initially all ovulated within two weeks of crossing over to placebo therapy confirming the rapid reversibility of ovarian function with this treatment protocol.

The cyclic occurrence of premenstrual symptoms was abolished during treatment with the LHRH agonist (Fig. 3).

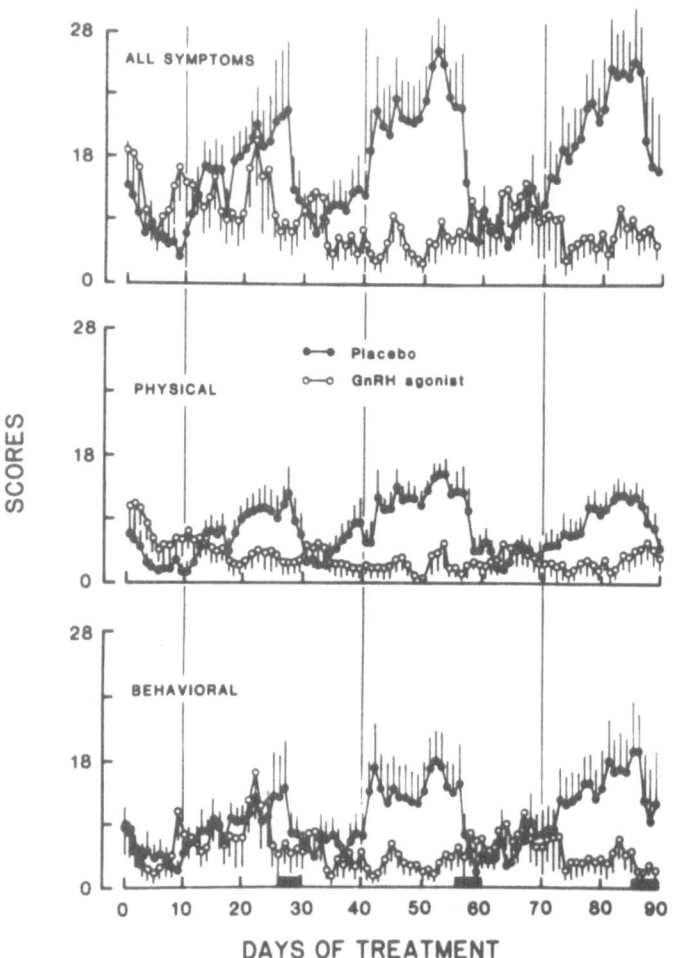

FIGURE 3   Mean Scores (± S.E.) for all 15 symptoms, 5 physical symptoms, and 10 behavioural symptoms, during GnRH-agonist treatment and placebo administration.   Reproduced with permission from Muse et al. N. Engl. J. Med. 311:1345 (1984).

Behavioural manifestations of premenstrual
syndrome were not attenuated during the first agonist
treatment cycle, most likely the result of continuing
ovarian steroid secretion (Fig. 2). Quantitative
assessment of the symptoms across the last two
treatment cycles employing transverse means for
symptoms scores during follicular and luteal phases
confirmed the significant benefit afforded by LHRH
agonist treatment (Fig. 4).

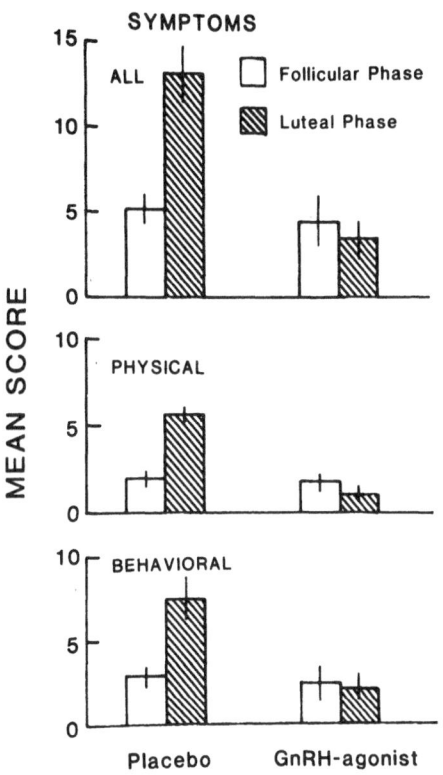

FIGURE 4   Transverse mean of scores (± S.E.) for 5
physical symptoms, 10 behavioural symptoms,
and all 15 symptoms during the last two
cycles of treatment. Luteal phase scores
were significantly lower (P<0.05) during
GnRH-agonist treatment than during placebo
administration. Reproduced with permission
from Muse et al. N. Engl. J. Med. 311:1345
(1984).

287

Bancroft et al [18] have used buserelin by nasal spray in 20 women suffering from PMS for periods up to two years. With dosages of 600 ug intranasally daily in three divided doses these authors achieved inconsistent ovarian suppression and, accordingly, the symptomatic response of PMS sufferers in their study was variable. In one case (Fig. 5) they did have very adequate suppression of ovarian follicular activity together with elimination of symptoms of irritability and swelling. When placebo was substituted for agonist in a blinded fashion there was a return of ovarian activity and prompt recrudescence of PMS symptomatology. Reinstitution of buserelin therapy was once again accompanied by relief from symptoms.

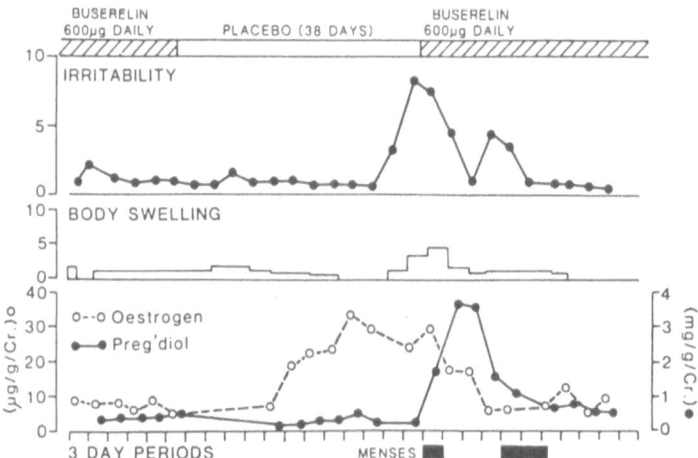

FIGURE 5   Single blind introduction of placebo for a 34 year old woman after 9 months of buserelin 600 ug daily. Reproduced with permission from Bancroft et al [18]. Proc. 13th Annual Meeting of the International Foundation for Biochemical Endocrinology Edinburgh, 1985, K.W. McKerns, G. Fink, A.J. Harmar (eds.), Plenum Press, New York.

Another patient studied by these authors showed clear cyclic exacerbation of breast tenderness and irritability which was effectively suppressed during buserelin treatment (Fig. 6). Because buserelin therapy was started in the late luteal phase there was slight aggravation of symptoms at the onset. Thereafter symptoms were almost eliminated in spite of a further period of follicular stimulation and incomplete corpus luteum activity.

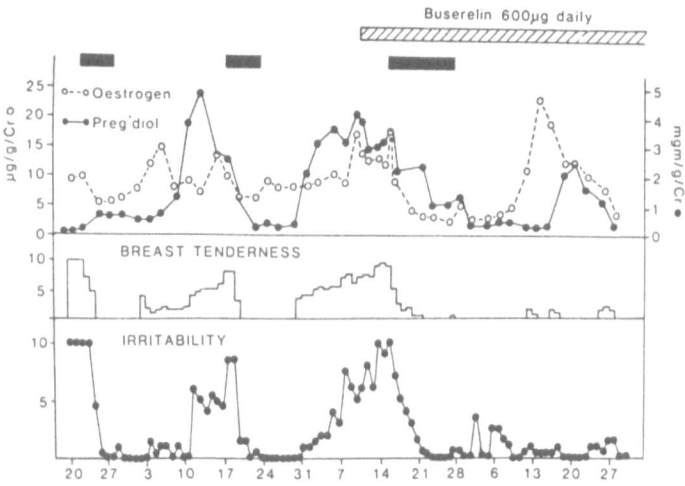

FIGURE 6   Buserelin therapy for severe premenstrual irritability and breast pain. Reproduced with permission from Bancroft et al. Proc. 13th Annual Meeting of the International Foundation for Biochemical Endocrinology, Edinburgh, 1985. K.W. McKerns, G. Fink, A.J. Harmar (eds.), Plenum Press, N.Y.

It is noteworthy, however, that some ovarian activity remained. The explanation for remission from symptoms, despite continuing ovulatory activity, is uncertain although reduced steroid secretion may have been responsible.

This latter study represents an effort to utilize a more acceptable means for drug administration than the daily subcutaneous injections required in the study by Muse et al [17]. A somewhat unpredictable response to intranasal buserelin in these studies, however, indicates that additional dosage forms must be examined to simply achieve effective ovarian suppression.

More potent super active agonists of GnRH, such as nafarelin intranasally on a once daily basis [19], or the intramuscular injection of long acting microcapsules containing LHRH agonist [20] in combination with cyclic gestagen-induced bleeding [21], may afford a reasonable combination of simplicity of administration, while maintaining early follicular phase levels of estradiol, and avoiding prolonged unopposed endometrial stimulation.

Potent GnRH antagonists [22], which may be administered on a weekly or monthly basis, may afford more prompt elimination of premenstrual symptomatology by avoiding the stimulatory phase associated with LHRH agonist usage. It will be essential that with both agonists and antagonists that dosage be titrated to avoid suppression of ovarian function to menopausal levels.

CONCLUSION

LHRH agonists and antagonists may afford relief for PMS sufferers by producing reversible suppression of cyclic ovarian function. Additional work is needed to develop an ideal method of administration which combines efficacy, patient acceptability, and a low risk of complications associated with insufficient or unopposed estrogen production.

REFERENCES

1. Reid, R.L. Premenstrual Syndrome. Current Problems in Obstetrics, Gynecology and Fertility, Vol. VIII, No. 2, February 1985.
2. Backstrom, C.T., Boyle, H., Baird, D.T. Persistence of symptoms of premenstrual tension in hysterectomized women. Brit. J. Obstet. Gynaecol., 88, 530 (1981).
3. Reid, R.L. and S.S.C. Yen. The premenstrual syndrome. Am J Obstet. Gynecol., 139, 85 (1981).
4. Coppen, A., Kessel, N. Menstruation and personality. Br J Psychiatry., 109, 711 (1963).
5. Wood, N.F., Most, A., Dery, G.K. Prevalence of perimenstrual symptoms. Am J Public Health, 72, 1257 (1982).
6. Reid, R.L., Yen, S.S.C. Premenstrual syndrome. Clin Obstet. Gynaecol., 26, 710 (1983).

7. Reid, R.L. Endogenous opioid activity and the premenstrual syndrome, Lancet 2, 786 (1983).
8. Ethical and Legal Implications of the Biobehavioural Sciences: Premenstrual Syndrome. B.E. Ginsburg, B.F. Carter (eds.), Plenum Press, New York, In Press.
9. Reid, R.L., Greenaway-Coates, A., Hahn, P.M., MacLellan, D., Graves, G., Casper, R.F. Menopausal-like hot flushes in women of reproductive age: A clue to the pathophysiology of premenstrual syndrome. Abstract, Combined Meeting American Fertility Society/Canadian Fertility and Andrology Society, Toronto, Ontario, Canada, 27 September - 2 October, 1986.
10. Frank, R.T. The hormonal causes of premenstrual tension. Arch. Neurol. Psychiatry, 26, 1053 (1931).
11. Reid, R.L. and Hahn, P.M. Ovariectomy: An unsung solution for severe and intractable premenstrual syndrome. In preparation.
12. Halas, C. Relief from premenstrual syndrome. Frederick Fell Publishers, New York, 1984.
13. Parrish, H.M., Carr, C.A., Hall, D.G., King, T. Time interval from castration in premenopausal women to development of excessive coronary atherosclerosis. Am. J. Obstet. Gynecol. 99, 155 (1967).
14. Ayers, J.W.T., Gidwani, G.P., Schmidt, R.N., Gross, M. Osteopenia in hypoestrongenic young women with anorexia nervosa. Fertil. Steril. 41, 224 (1984).
15. Schmidt-Gollwitzer, M., Hardt, W., Schmidt-Gollwitzer, K., von der Ohet, M., Nevinny-Stickel, J. Abstract, Influence of the LH-RH analogue buserelin on cyclic ovarian function and on endometrium. A new approach to fertility control? Contraception 23(2), 187 (1981).
16. Rannevik , G., and Thorell J.I. The influence of danazol on pituitary function and on the ovarian follicular hormone secretion in premenopausal women. Acta. Obstet. Gyneco. Scand. Suppl. 123, 89 (1984).
17. Muse, K.N., Cetel, N.S., Futterman, L.A., Yen, S.S.C. The premenstrual syndrome: Effects of "Medical Ovariectomy". N. Engl. J. Med. 311, 1345 (1984).
18. Bancroft, J., Boyle, H., Fraser, H. The use of an LHRH agonist in the treatment and investigation of the premenstrual syndrome. Proc. 13th Annual Meeting of the International Foundation for Biochemical Endocrinology, Edinburgh, 1985. K.W. McKerns, G. Fink, A.J. Harmar (eds.), Plenum Press, New York.

19. Gudmundsson, J.A., Nillius, S.J., Bergquist, C. Inhibition of ovulation by intranasal nafarelin, a new superactive agonist of GnRH. Contraception 30, 107 (1984).
20. Lahlou, N., Roger, M., Canlorbe, P., Chaussain, J.L., Faynaud, F., Toublanc, J.E., Schally, A.V. Plasma levels of D-TRP-6-LH (Decapeptyl) after intramuscular injection of long-acting microcapsules in children treated for precocious puberty. Paediatric Research, 19, 635 (1985).
21. Lemay, A., Faure, N., Labrie, F., Frazekas, A.T.A. Inhibition of ovulation during discontinuous intranasal luteinizing hormone-releasing agonist dosing in combination with gestagen-induced bleeding. Fertil. Steril. 43, 868 (1985).
22. Vickery, B.H. Comparison of the potential for therapeutic utilities with gonadotropin-releasing hormone agonists and antagonists. Endocrine Reviews 7, 115 (1986).

19
Early Clinical Studies with LHRH Antagonists in Women

Z. M. van der SPUY, L. PILLAY, F. HARDIE, M. van der WATT, T. de CHALAIN, H. KAPLAN, R. ROESKE* and R. P. MILLAR

Department of Obstetrics and Gynecology and MRC Regulatory
Peptides Research Unit, Department of Chemical Pathology, University
of Cape Town Medical School/Groote Schuur Hospital 7925 Observatory,
Cape; *Department of Biochemistry, Indiana University School of
Medicine, Indianapolis, USA

INTRODUCTION

Over the past few years LHRH agonist analogs have been increasingly used to down-regulate the pituitary and induce a state of hypogonadotropic hypogonadism. This form of endocrine manipulation has now become a feasible therapy option in a wide range of hormone-dependent diseases [1,2,3].

A number of gynecological disorders such as endometriosis and uterine leiomyomata have proven amenable to this method of treatment [4,5]. The ability to achieve medical castration by means of easily administered medical therapy also has offered us effective adjuvant therapy in hormone-dependent malignant disease such as prostatic and breast carcinoma [6,7]. In addition, LHRH agonist therapy is now an option for the treatment of abnormalities of gonadotropin secretion such as is seen in polycystic ovarian disease and precocious puberty [8,9].

The LHRH antagonist analogs offer potential therapeutic and investigative advantages over the agonists. The initial stimulation which follows agonist administration and precedes pituitary desensitization causes increased steroid hormone production which may be potentially harmful in some conditions. In addition, inhibition of gonadotropin by LHRH agonists may take weeks to achieve with resultant delay in the institution of effective therapy. In contrast, antagonist analogs cause immediate inhibition of gonadotropins by competition with endogenous LHRH for LHRH receptors. We describe here preliminary clinical experience with LHRH antagonist analogs.

LHRH ANTAGONIST ANALOGS

While considerable animal data are available, little work with antagonists has been done in humans. We have selected two LHRH antagonists, [N-Ac-D-Nal(2)^1, D-α-Me, pCl-Phe^2,D-Trp^3, D-Arg^6,D-Ala^{10}]LHRH (antagonist A) and [N-Ac-D-Nal(2)^1, D-α-Me, pCl-Phe^2,D-Trp^3, Lys(iPr)^5,D-Tyr^6,D-Ala^{10}]LHRH (antagonist B) for possible clinical use and have assessed their ability to suppress gonadotropins when administered either by the intravenous (iv) or subcutaneous (sc) route.

Both antagonist A and antagonist B had a similarly high anti-ovulatory ED_{100} of 1 ug/rat. However, antagonist A elicited a far greater histaminic response (ED_{50} 0.1 ug/ml) in mast cell cultures than antagonist B (ED_{50} 2.0 ug/ml). The sequence $Arg^6-X-Arg^8$ in antagonist A is known to induce high histaminic activity [10,11].

SIDE-EFFECTS

Varying doses of both peptides were administered to healthy volunteers and a wide spectrum of hematological and biochemical parameters which were monitored before and after administration remained unchanged.

Skin rashes developed in 3 women immediately after an iv dose of antagonist A, while a mild urticarial reaction was seen in one woman following antagonist B administration (iv). All rashes disappeared within 4 hours. Except for local tenderness and swelling at the injection site, no problems were encountered following sc administration of either antagonist. In all volunteers, blood pressure, pulse and temperature readings remained stable and there was no evidence of any systemic reaction to the peptides.

CLINICAL STUDIES

Thirty-two subjects have been studied. They were recruited from staff and patients at Groote Schuur Hospital and gave informed consent for the studies. Ethics Committee consent was obtained for all the studies described and consent for use of the LHRH antagonists was given both by the Medicines Control Council and the local Ethics Committee. Antagonist A was administered iv to nine subjects and sc to nine subjects. Antagonist B was administered iv to four subjects and sc to ten subjects.

Effect of antagonist and recovery of LHRH responsivity

Repeated doses of antagonist A, when administered by the intravenous route, resulted in suppression of luteinizing hormone (LH) to below the limit of detection of our assay with a less profound effect on follicle stimulating hormone (FSH). Prolactin concentrations were not affected (Figure 1).

When low doses of LHRH (10 ug) were administered at hourly intervals after the antagonist, there was a gradual increase in response, with increasing amounts of LH being secreted following each pulse (Figure 1). FSH secretion is also stimulated but to a lesser degree. Of interest is the prolactin response following antagonist and LHRH. While the antagonist fails to inhibit prolactin secretion, subsequent LHRH administration is able to stimulate prolactin secretion. This suggests that although exogenous LHRH can stimulate prolactin, endogenous LHRH does not play an important role in the control of prolactin secretion, since receptor occupancy by the antagonist does not affect prolactin secretion.

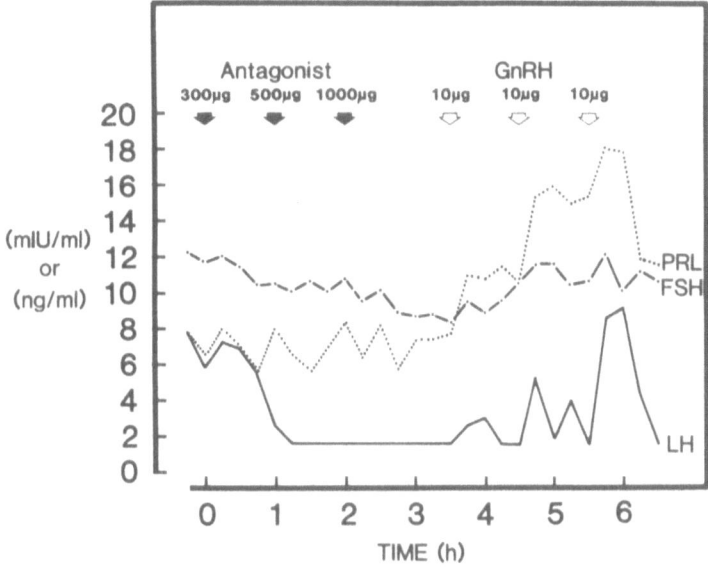

Figure 1. Effect of repeated iv administration of LHRH antagonist 6 (black arrows) on LH, FSH and prolactin during the luteal phase. Restoration of responsivity to 10 ug iv administration of LHRH (open arrows) was tested at hourly intervals, commencing two hours after the last injection of antagonist.

Response to a single subcutaneous dose of LHRH antagonist

Single subcutaneous doses of either antagonist were administered to subjects in an attempt to establish an effective dose for clinical studies.

LH levels were decreased after antagonist administration in the dose range 1-4 mg in the majority of subjects (9 out of 11) but FSH levels were less affected (Table 1). Some subjects did not demonstrate gonadotropin suppression following antagonist administration (e.g. J D after 2 mg antagonist B). This poor effect may be due to inadequate dosage or may indicate that repeated dosing may be required (see below). Infrequent sampling may also obscure effects as prior to antagonist administration may also result in sampling during the nadir.

Studies in postmenopausal subjects

Antagonists A and B were administered by the iv route to a number of postmenopausal subjects. All of these women had undergone

Table 1. Response to a single subcutaneous dose of LHRH antagonist

Dose/Subject	Age	Sex	Pre-Administration		Post-Administration (12 – 24 Hours)	
			LH	FSH	LH	FHS
Antagonist A						
1 mg (M.H.)	40	M	17.6	14.7	12.4	11.7
1 mg (M.K.)	22	M	9.4	7.1	4.2	5.5
1 mg (A.G.)	21	F	3.8	3.2	4.3	2.6
1.5 mg (K.R.)	24	F	41.8	9.3	28.8	7.9
2 mg (D.R.)	26	M	10.5	6.7	6.1	5.8
Antagonist B						
2 mg (J.K.)	22	M	19.0	5.4	14.6	4.7
2 mg (J.D.)	34	M	5.9	8.8	7.4	9.9
3 mg (A.K.)	22	F	25.0	9.2	15.5	8.2
3 mg (M.K.)	23	M	16.5	7.3	12.5	7.1
4 mg (R.M.)	32	M	23.9	3.7	19.7	3.3
4 mg (R.M.)	42	M	9.0	4.8	7.4	8.4

LH and FSH expressed as mIU/ml.

hysterectomy and bilateral oophorectomy at least 8 weeks earlier and had elevated gonadotropin levels with low peripheral estradiol concentrations.

A single iv dose caused maximum LH suppression by 2 – 3 hours and abolition of the pulsatile pattern of secretion, with subsequent restoration of pulsatile LH secretion and a return to pretreatment concentrations. Repeated iv doses of antagonist causes a decrease in LH concentration and abolition of pulsatility and a less marked fall in FSH during an eight hour study period (Figure 2). Prolactin concentrations were unaffected.

The doses employed did not reduce LH concentrations to undetectable levels in postmenopausal women. In three postmenopausal subjects given repeated iv doses of antagonist at a dose of 0.5 mg/hr for eight hours, there was a consistent inhibition of LH to a mean value more than 50% lower than basal, while FSH was not significantly affected (Figure 3).

Repeated daily sc antagonist administration for three weeks to a perimenopausal women with uncontrolled menorrhagia and fibroids resulted in an eventual fall of LH and FSH to less than 20% and 35% of the initial concentration, respectively, with a resultant decrease in estradiol. Despite the detection of substantial circulatory levels of LH and FSH by radioimmunoassay, ovarian steroidogenesis was suppressed, suggesting that although the circulating gonadotropins were immunologically active they had low biological activity. Rapid increases in LH and FSH occurred when antagonist treatment was withdrawn and this was accompanied by an increase in estradiol concentrations. During the 3 weeks of treatment, this patient who had had excessive, irregular vaginal

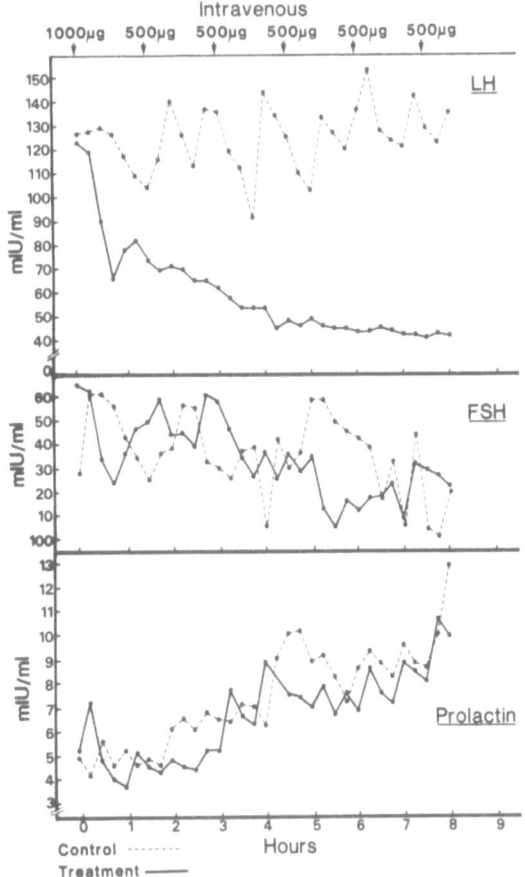

Figure 2. Effect of repeated iv administration of antagonist A to a subject post-oophorectomy (solid line). Dose and time of administration are indicated by arrows.

bleeding, requiring repeated blood transfusion, stopped menstruating, allowing time to optimize her pre-operative condition.

Studies during the luteal phase

Administration of antagonist A (iv) and antagonist B (sc) during the luteal phase of the menstrual cycle resulted in a suppression of LH baseline concentrations and an abolition of pulsatility. FSH concentrations suppressed later than did LH and often only exhibited a decline after a second dose. Twenty-four hours after repeated administration of antagonist, both estradiol and progesterone concentrations showed suppression; often to undetectable levels.

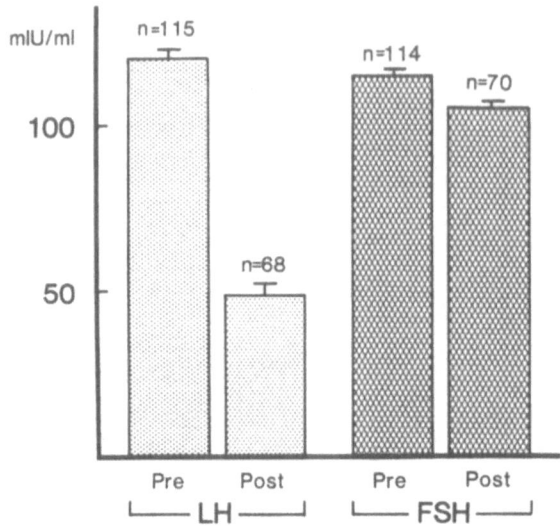

Figure 3. Plasma LH and FSH concentrations before and after
administration of 0.5 mg/hr antagonist A to three
postmenopausal women over eight hours. Data shows
the mean +SEM and a number of plasma samples.

Smaller doses of antagonist were required for gonadotropin
suppression in these women when compared with the postmenopausal
subjects and adequate suppression of ovarian function was possible
with repeated doses given 12 hours apart. Mean LH levels 3-8
hours after the first dose of antagonist were significantly lower
than initial levels while FSH was unchanged (Figure 4).

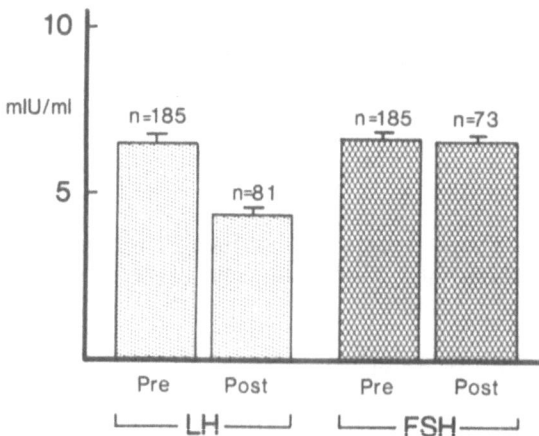

Figure 4. Plasma LH and FSH concentrations before and after
administration   of   2-3   mg   antagonist A   or
antagonist B to six women in the luteal phase.
Data shows the mean +SEM and number of plasma
samples.

298

CONCLUDING REMARKS

In women the decline in gonadotropin was accompanied by a decrease in peripheral estradiol and progesterone concentrations. Unlike the agonist analogs where microgram amounts are effective in achieving pituitary desensitization and concomitant decreased gonadal steroidogenesis, milligram quantities of antagonist are required to cause adequate inhibition. This is explained by their different mode of action, namely competition with endogenous LHRH for its receptors [12]. The removal of negative feedback by steroid hormones exacerbates the problem by increasing endogenous LHRH output.

Repeated dosage was required to maintain inhibition, and rapid onset of effect was demonstrated following both iv and sc administration. For clinical use, sc injection appears preferable since only local reaction has occurred using this route of administration.

In all our studies, LH was inhibited more rapidly and more profoundly than FSH. A similar effect was demonstrated when sheep were treated with LHRH antiserum with subsequent preferential inhibition of LH [13,14]. This phenomenon may be the result of LH being released directly from stores while FSH release is less regulated and is merely released in relation to biosynthetic rates. This notion is supported by the sluggish rise in FSH compared with LH which is seen following LHRH administration in hypogonadotropic subjects [15].

Alternatively, the differential LH and FSH response may be explained by the presence of FSH regulating factors other than LHRH. The β-dimers of inhibin recently described may play a role in the control of FSH secretion [16] or there may be novel forms of LHRH exerting an influence on FSH release [17].

In postmenopausal women, LH is initially suppressed to less than 40% of baseline and only after prolonged administration to less than 20% of baseline. Gonadotropin suppression in these women therefore requires fairly high doses of prolonged administration. There is the possibility that in these subjects non-LHRH regulators may be important in maintaining gonadotropin secretion and of these the most likely candidates are the LHRH-associated peptide (GAP) or further processed fragments of this molecule [18,19].

The studies reported here demonstrate a potential role for the antagonists in clinical practice, both in therapeutic regimens and as contraceptive agents. The rapid onset of action offers particular advantages both as investigative and therapeutic agents.

ACKNOWLEDGEMENTS

The studies described here were funded by the University of Cape Town, The Herman Caporn Fund, The National Cancer Association and The Medical Research Council.

REFERENCES

1. Schally, A.V., Kastin, A.J. and Coy, D.H. LH-releasing hormone and its analogues: Recent basic and clinical investigations. Int. J. Fertil., 20, 1 (1976).
2. Sandow, J. Clinical applications of LH-RH and its analogues. Clin. Endocrinol., 18, 571 (1983).
3. McLachlin, R.I., Healy, D.L. and Burger, H.G. Clinical aspects of LHRH analogues in gynaecology: a review. Brit. J. Obstet. Gynaecol., 93, 431 (1986).
4. Lemay, A., Maheux, R., Faure, N., Jean, C. and Fazekas, A.T.A. Reversible hypogonadism induced by a luteinizing hormone-releasing hormone (LH-RH) agonist (Buserelin) as a new therapeutic approach for endometriosis. Fertil. Steril., 41, 863 (1984).
5. Healy, D.L., Fraser, H.M. and Lawson, S.L. Shrinkage of a uterine fibroid after subcutaneous infusion of an LHRH agonist. Brit. Med. J., 289, 1267 (1984).
6. Allen, J.M., O'Shea, J.P., Mashiter, K., Williams, G. and Bloom, S.R. Advanced carcinoma of the prostate: treatment with a gonadotrophin releasing hormone agonist. Brit. Med. J., 286, 1607 (1983).
7. Klijn, J.G.M. and de Jong, F.H. Treatment with a luteinizing-hormone-releasing-hormone analogue (buserelin) in premenopausal patients with metastatic breast cancer. Lancet, 1, 1213 (1982).
8. Fleming, R., Haxton, M.J., Hamilton, M.P.R., McCune, G.S., Black, W.P., MacNaughton, M.C. and Coutts, J.R.T. Successful treatment of infertile women with oliogomenorrhoea using a combination of an LHRH agonist and exogenous gonadotrophins. Brit. J. Obstet. Gynaecol., 92, 369 (1985).
9. Stanhope, R., Adams, J. and Brook, C.G.D. The treatment of central precocious puberty using an intranasal LHRH analogue (buserelin). Clin. Endocrinol., 22, 795 (1985).
10. Foreman, J., and Jordan, C. Histamine release and vascular changes induced by neuropeptides. Agents and Actions, 13, 105 (1983).
11. Schmidt, F., Sundaram, K., Thau, R.B. and Bardin, C.W. [Ac-D-NAL(2)^1,4FD-Phe^2,D-Trp^3,D-Arg^6]LHRH, a potent antagonist of LHRH, produces transient edema and behavioral changes in rats. Contraception, 29, 282 (1984).
12. Conn, P.M., Hsueh, A.J.W., Crowley, W.F. jnr. Gonadotropin-releasing hormone: molecular and cell biology, physiology and clinical applications. Fed. Pro., 43, 2351 (1984).
13. Lincoln, G.A. and Short, R.V. Seasonal breeding: Nature's contraceptive. Rec. Prog. Horm. Res., 36, 1 (1980).
14. McNeilly, A.S., Fraser, H.M. and Baird, D.T. Effect of immunoneutralization of LH releasing hormone on LH, FSH and ovarian steroid secretion in the pre-ovulatory phase of the oestrous cycle in the ewe. J. Endocrinol., 101, 213 (1984).
15. Hurley, D.M., Brian, R., Outch, K., Stockdale, J., Fry, A., Hackman, C., Clarke, I. and Burger, H.G. Induction of ovulation and fertility in amenorrheic women by pulsatile

low-dose gonadotropin-releasing hormone. New Engl. J. Med., <u>310</u>, 1069 (1984).

16. Ling, N., Ying, S-Y., Ueno, N., Shimasaki, S., Esch, F., Hotta, M. and Guillemin, R. Pituitary FSH is released by a heterodimer of the β-subunits from the two forms of inhibin. Nature, <u>321</u>, 779 (1986).

17. Millar, R.P., Milton, R.C. de L., Follett, B.K. and King, J.A. Receptor binding and gonadotropin-releasing activity of a novel chicken gonadotropin-releasing hormone (His^5, Trp^7,Tyr^8) GnRH and a D-Arg^6 analog. Endocrinology, <u>119</u>, 224 (1986).

18. Nikolics, K., Mason, A.J., Szonyi, E., Ramachandran, J. and Seeburg, P.H. A prolactin-inhibiting factor within the precursor for human gonadotropin-releasing hormone. Nature, <u>316</u>, 511 (1985).

19. Millar, R.P., Wormald, P.J. and Milton, R.C. de L. Stimulation of gonadotropin release by a non-GnRH peptide sequence of the GnRH precursor. Science, <u>232</u>, 68 (1986).

20

Profertility Uses of LHRH Agonist Analogues

H. S JACOBS, R. PORTER, A. ESHEL and I. CRAFT*

The Middlesex Hospital Medical School and University College London,
Mortimer Street, London W1N 8AA, England.
*Humana Hospital Wellington, Wellington Place, London NW8, England

INTRODUCTION

We describe here our experience of using one of the superactive analogues of LHRH for induction of ovulation in humans for in vitro and for in vivo fertilization. Our studies have all been performed with the Hoechst compound, buserelin [D-Ser(tBu^6),Pro^9-NHEt] LHRH, given either as a nasal insufflation or by subcutaneous infusion. In the latter case miniaturised infusion pumps, originally designed for pulsatile delivery of native LHRH were used. The use of an LHRH analogue for suppression of endogenous gonadotrophin secretion, followed by stimulation of the ovaries with exogenous gonadotrophins, was first described by Fleming and his colleague in 1985 [1]. Before describing our studies and recording their results, it is necessary to give some background clinical physiology to provide their context.

INDUCTION OF OVULATION FOR IN VIVO FERTILISATION

So far as the use of a superactive analogue of LHRH for induction of ovulation for fertilization in vivo is concerned, our perception of the need for this treatment arose out of our experience of treating patients with the polycystic ovary syndrome with pulsatile native LHRH [2]. These patients, like indeed all the others we have treated with pulsatile LHRH, had been resistant to induction of ovulation with clomiphene. We found that the overall response to pulsatile LHRH of the patients with polycystic ovaries was disappointing: in contrast to the usual 85% cumulative rate of conception at 6 months obtained in patients with LHRH deficiency, in patients with polycystic ovary syndrome the cumulative conception rate at 6 months was only 55% [3]. When anovulatory cycles were eliminated from calculation of the cumulative conception rate, the figure then rose to 90%, indicating that these patients' infertility resulted entirely from a failure of ovulation and not from any other adverse factor. When the clinical and endocrine features of the patients who had failed to ovulate were compared with those of the patients who did ovulate, the only difference we could detect was in their body weight - those who ovulated regularly had a mean body mass index

(BMI, weight/height , normal range 20-25) of 20, those who ovulated variably had a mean BMI of 25 and those that were completely refractory to this treatment had a BMI exceeding 25 [4]. The type of response to LHRH was not however associated with any particular pattern of serum gonadotrophin, prolactin or androgen concentrations. These studies therefore defined a group of overweight, anovulatory patients with the polycystic ovary syndrome who were resistant to treatment with antioestrogens and to pulsatile LHRH and who therefore clearly needed induction of ovulation with gonadotrophins. They thus presented an opportunity to explore the value of suppression of endogenous gonadotrophin secretion during induction of ovulation with different gonadotrophin preparations.

When we analysed the outcome of the pregnancies in the patients with polycystic ovaries who had conceived on treatment with LHRH, we found a disappointingly high rate of early pregnancy loss [5], which we have defined as miscarriage occuring within 4 weeks of ovulation, as diagnosed by ultrasound. It has been known for many years that patients with the polycystic ovary syndrome often have raised basal levels of LH [6] and our own studies have shown that even when ovulation is induced with pulsatile LHRH, LH concentrations remain very high throughout the follicular phase [7]. Further analysis revealed that the patients who conceived on LHRH treatment and then suffered early pregnancy losses had had very high follicular phase serum LH concentrations in the conception cycles (over 12 U/L during the phase of maximum follicular growth), while those who conceived and carried their pregnancies to term had had follicular phase LH concentrations below 12 U/L. We have hypothesized that premature exposure of the ovaries to high LH concentrations during the phase of maximum follicular growth is deleterious to the developing oocyte(s) [8].

Our concept is based on the observation that throughout their life, oocytes are normally held in the dictyotene stage of their first meiotic division until just before ovulation. Up to this time progression through meiosis is inhibited by Oocyte Maturation Inhibitor [9], a peptide found in follicular fluid. The production or action of Oocyte Maturation Inhibitor is itself inhibited by the timely action of LH at mid-cycle [10], so ensuring ovulation of an egg matured at the appropriate time. There is a species specific interval between completion of the first meiotic division of oocytes ("oocyte maturation") and their fertilisation (24-36 hours in man), during which conditions for producing a normal embryo are optimal. If the interval is extended, either by premature oocyte maturation, as has been induced in pigs with HCG [11] or by delaying fertilisation, as has been done in rats [12], poor rates of fertilisation result and embryos that are produced survive poorly and usually abort. In humans, Guerrero and Rojas [13] have shown in a study of the outcome of artificial insemination with donor semen, in which of course the timing of insemination is accurately known, that extension of the interval between ovulation and artificial insemination is associated with a large increase in the rate of abortion of the ensuing pregnancies.

We hypothesise that, in women with polycystic ovaries, if the LH concentrations are very high early in the follicular phase, they penetrate the follicle, allow premature completion of oocyte maturation and so result in ovulation of an oocyte that is physiologically "aged". Such oocytes would be expected to fertilise poorly and to produce embryos that implant poorly and therefore abort early. This suggestion that inappropriate secretion of LH may impair

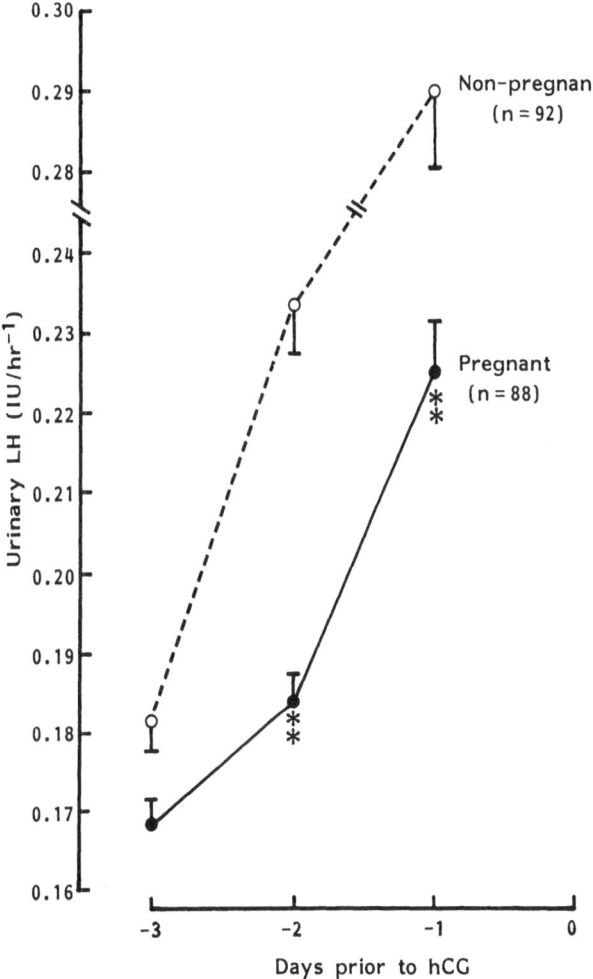

Figure I   Urinary LH excretion in women undergoing in vitro fertilisation and embryo transfer who became pregnant (●) compared with those who did not conceive (o).   Significant differences (p<0.01) are indicated by the asterisks.   Data of Howells et al 1985 reference 15, reproduced with permission of the authors and the editor of The Lancet.

fertilisation is compatible with the findings of in vitro fertilisation of human oocytes reported by Stanger and Yovich [14] and recently confirmed by Howles et al [15] (Figure 1). Whether the early pregnancy losses seen in in vivo and in vitro fertilisation associated with untimely secretion of high amounts of LH can be prevented is at present uncertain, but provides the context in which the following studies were undertaken.

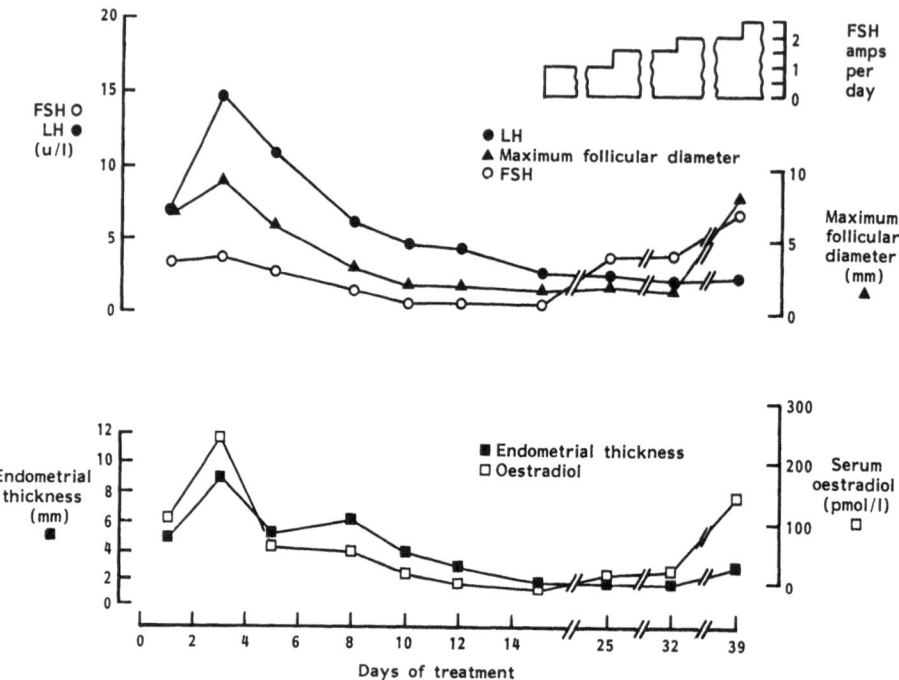

Figure 2   Relation of serum oestradiol and gonadotrophin concentrations to ovarian follicle diameter and uterine endometrial thickness in a patient treated with nasal buserelin who received FSH for induction of ovulation for in vivo fertilisation.

THE USE OF A SUPERACTIVE LHRH ANALOGUE FOR IN VIVO FERTILISATION

All of the patients in this study had in the past failed to ovulate on treatment with clomiphene. They had also all received treatment with pulsatile LHRH but only half of them had ovulated. All 13 received a subcutaneous infusion of buserelin (100 µg/day) and 4 also received 6 cycles of treatment with nasal buserelin (1200 µg/day). The day-to-day response to treatment was monitored by ultrasound assessment of the ovaries and uterus. In most cases we found excellent coincidence between regression of the follicles and endometrium and suppression of circulating gonadotrophin and oestradiol concentrations (Figure 2).

When this close relationship was not maintained, we found that suppression of gonadotrophins preceded the ultrasound evidence of regression of follicles and endometrium by up to 3 days. These results indicated that the ultrasound appearance provided a safe, if not always completely accurate, index of suppression of pituitary hormone secretion. When adequate suppression of endogenous gonadotrophin secretion was obtained (as judged in this way, usually after 2 – 4 weeks of treatment with the analogue, the longer periods in the more obese patients), the patients were then randomly allocated to induction of ovulation with HMG (pergonal, Serono, 75 IU LH, 75 IU FSH per ampoule) or with pure FSH (metrodin, Serono 75 IU FSH <1 IU LH per ampoule). When a dominant follicle, of diameter equal to or greater than 17 mm, was seen on ultrasound, an intramuscular injection of 10,000 IU of HCG was given. Treatment with buserelin was discontinued the following day. The results, to the time of writing, of induction of ovulation using this protocol are shown in Table 1.

Table I Results of induction of ovulation for in vivo fertilisation using pituitary desensitisation and gonadotrophic stimulation

Number of	Induction with HMG	Induction with FSH
Patients	8	5
Cycles	16	19
Overstimulations	4	5
Hyperstimulations	2	3
Anovulatory cycles	3	3
Ovulations	9	11
Pregnancies*	2	2

*Two additional pregnancies occurred in the first post-treatment cycle (for details see text)

Of the 13 patients so far treated, 5 had had very high follicular phase LH concentrations and several had had an early pregnancy loss on previous treatment with clomiphene or HMG. A total of 35 courses of ovulation induction have been given of which only 20 were ovulatory. Four pregnancies have resulted so far and

the results in relation to one are shown in Figure 3. This patient
had had two early pregnancy losses in the past. In the cycle in
which the second one occurred she was receiving HMG but not
buserelin. As may be seen in Figure 3, serum LH concentrations
were extremely high throughout the follicular phase of the cycle in
which conception occurred. HCG was given when the follicular
diameter of the single dominant follicle was 17 mm and a corpus
luteum was formed, accompanied by rising serum progesterone
concentrations. A miscarriage occurred 23 days after the injection
of HCG. Subsequently she received treatment with a subcutaneous
infusion of buserelin and induction of ovulation with HMG was
repeated. She conceived in the second cycle of this treatment and
has a continuing pregnancy. The follicular phase serum LH
concentrations in this conception cycle were 5 U/L or lower.

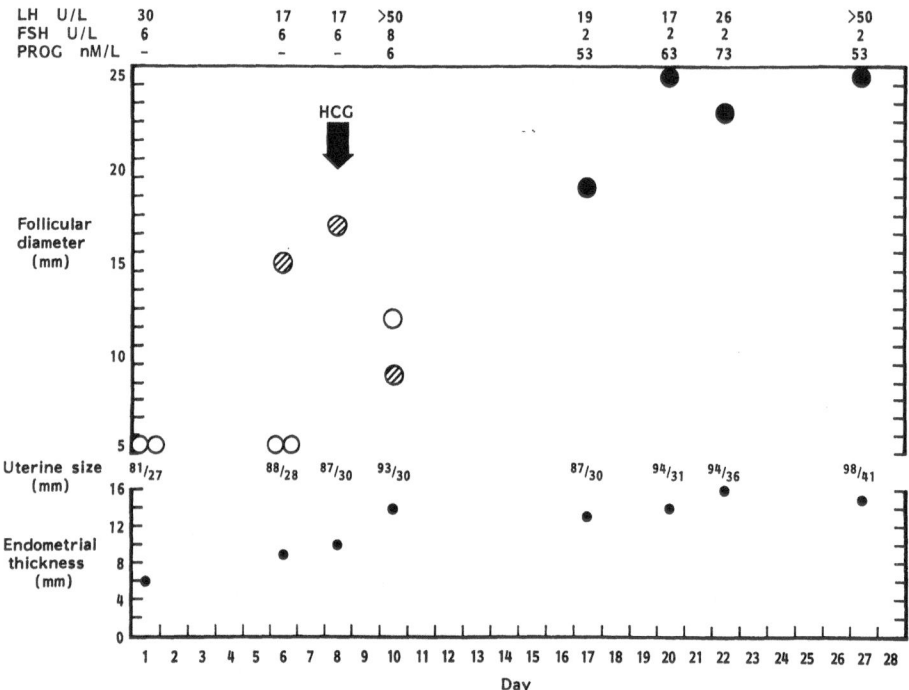

Figure 3   Endocrine and ultrasound data in a conception cycle
during treatment with HMG without buserelin. Serum LH
concentrations remained high during the phase of rapid follicle
growth. The patient ovulated after the injection of HCG and
conceived, but miscarried 23 days later.

Hyperstimulation (grade 1 to 2, using the usual WHO criteria)
[16] occurred in 5 courses of treatment and a further 9 courses were

308

abandoned (that is, the HCG was withheld) because of overstimulation of the ovaries (more than 3 follicles observed on ultrasound with a diameter of 15 mm or more).

Most of the patients given buserelin experienced a mild degree of flushing which passed off as soon as the treatment with gonadotrophins was started. We prefer the subcutaneous route of administration because it is more economical and also more efficacious (ie, suppression of ovarian follicles is more readily obtained than with the nasal route). The patients however preferred the nasal route of administration, a dilemma which may, of course, be resolved when long acting injectable preparations become available. We have routinely discontinued treatment with the LHRH analogue one day after the administration of HCG. Continuation beyond this time necessitates supplementary treatment with HCG to maintain the corpus luteum. Although the number of cases of hyperstimulation did fall when the analogue was continued into the luteal phase, none of the patients we treated in this way has in fact conceived.

So far we have found no difference in the responses obtained with stimulation with FSH and HMG, suggesting that the LH content of the ampoules of HMG has little if any deleterious effect on the ovary. Intriguingly, the high rate of ovarian over-stimulation (Table I) could not be attributed to overexposure of the ovaries to gonadotrophins per se, since endogenous pituitary gonadotrophins were suppressed by the LHRH analogue and the numbers of ampoules of exogenous gonadotrophin administered were no greater in the cycles in which exaggerated responses occurred compared with those in which uniovulation and/or pregnancy occurred. These results are therefore consistent with the idea that in patients with polycystic ovaries the sensitivity, and the fluctuations in the sensitivity, of the ovarian response to gonadotrophins are intrinsic properties of the polycystic ovary and are not caused by prevailing endogenous gonadotrophin concentrations. This conclusion is further supported by our finding no difference in the number of ampoules required to stimulate the ovaries in the cycles in which ovulation occurred compared with those in which the response was anovulatory.

In addition to the four pregnancies mentioned above, two others deserve special mention. They occurred in two of these 13 women with polycystic ovaries who had particularly long histories of infertility and resistance to all forms of induction of ovulation. Both had extremely high basal serum LH concentrations (50-60 U/L). Each had two cycles of treatment with subcutaenous buserelin, one receiving ovarian stimulation with HMG and the other with pure FSH. The serum LH concentrations were well suppressed during the administration of buserelin (below 8 U/L) and this suppression persisted after buserelin treatment was discontinued. In the next month both ovulated spontaneously, during which cycles the serum LH concentrations in the follicular phase were measured and remained in the normal range (though LH presumably rose at midcycle to cause ovulation). Both patients conceived and have carried these pregnancies to term. It seems that in these cases the high LH level was impairing fertilisation rather than causing miscarriage; moreover temporary administration of buserelin caused prolonged suppression of basal LH secretion but did not apparently prevent normal oestrogen-mediated positive feedback, an observation clearly of potentially great importance.

At the present time it is clear that we have too few data to test our basic hypothesis that treatment with a superactive analogue of LHRH will, by protecting the oocytes from premature stimulation by an inappropriately timed high concentration of endogenous LH, prevent the early pregnancy losses that typically complicate induction of ovulation for in vivo fertilisation in patients with polycystic ovaries. Sadly, there is no doubt, however, that this treatment contributes nothing at all to avoiding the extreme sensitivity to gonadotrophic stimulation of the polycystic ovary and it also contributes nothing to elimination of the fluctuations in ovarian sensitivity that characterised these patients.

We conclude, therefore, that the only role we can determine at present for LHRH analogues in induction of ovulation for in vivo fertilisation is suppression of inappropriately high serum LH concentrations, but clearly we have to await the acquisition of further information before reaching firm decisions about whether use of these analogues will reduce the rate of early pregnancy loss in patients with polycystic ovaries.

INDUCTION OF OVULATION FOR IN VITRO FERTILISATION

Whereas a major requirement of programmes of induction of ovulation for in vivo fertilisation is the production of a single appropriately matured oocyte, the major requirement of programmes of induction of ovulation for in vitro fertilisation is the development of multiple follicles and oocytes. This requirement results from the clear demonstration that the outcome of the in vitro fertilisation-embryo transfer procedure is directly related to the number of embryos replaced [17], typical figures being that 10% of transfers of one embryo result in pregnancy, 15% of transfers of two embryos and 19% of transfers of three embryos proving successful. Since the usual rate of in vitro fertilisation of human oocytes is about 80%, it is clear that at present at least about 4-5 mature eggs per cycle are required for the in vitro fertilisation and embryo transfer procedure to have a maximum chance of success. The need for large numbers of mature human oocytes is likely to increase with the advent of cryopreservation and of donation of oocytes and embryos.

The normal human cycle is uniovulatory. We have been impressed however by the high rates of multiple ovulation and conception reported in hypopituitary patients treated with exogenous gonadotrophins [18]. We therefore considered the use of a superactive analogue of LHRH to create a background of temporary hypogonadotrophic hypogonadism which might then permit the use of high doses of gonadotrophins for hyperstimulation of the ovaries. It was hoped that by physiologically isolating the ovaries from the pituitary one could avoid the oestrogen-mediated discharge of LH and so avoid unscheduled and premature ovulation and also perhaps influence the high rate of pregnancy failure that complicates all programmes of in vitro fertilisation and embryo transfer. The creation of temporary hypogonadotrophic hypogonadism also provides a number of additional scientific opportunities for the investigator – firstly, by creating a uniform endogenous endocrine environment, it permits direct comparison of the different preparations of exogenous gonadotrophins used to induce ovulation. Secondly, by providing the investigator with an opportunity for tight control of the extra ovarian endocrine environment, it creates a unique opportunity to examine endocrine control of the intra-follicular micro-environment of a single cell – that is, of the developing human oocyte. Finally, elimination of endogenous pituitary hormones permits assessment of the extent to which the ovarian response to gonadotrophic stimulation is determined by the nature of the exogenous gonadotrophins administered and to what extent it is determined by the intrinsic state of the ovaries.

THE USE OF A SUPERACTIVE LHRH ANALOGUE FOR IN VITRO FERTILISATION

We studied 42 patients [19]. In the past 39 had had at least 1 previous attempt at in vitro fertilisation and embryo transfer and the mean rate of oocyte recovery had been one per cycle. These women had therefore been classified as "poor responders". All of these patients had had their pre-treatment ovarian ultrasound images recorded photographically and the images were subsequently reviewed by a single observer who had had no direct contact with the programme. The ovaries were classified as polycystic (21 cases, including the 7 who had been originally referred for this clinical indication) or normal (non polycystic, 21 cases) according to the criteria of Adams et al [2].

Two treatment protocols were used (Figure 4). In the first "long" protocol, 17 patients received 26 cycles of treatment with buserelin from the first day of menstruation until there was ultrasonic confirmation of regression of all ovarian follicles to less that 5 mm in diameter and the endometrial echo had disappeared. The patients were then randomly allocated to induction of ovulation with either HMG or pure FSH. In the second shorter protocol (26 cycles), we took advantage of the initial agonistic phase of treatment with buserelin: the exogenous gonadotrophin preparations were started on day 4 of agonist treatment to supplement the increase in the endogenous hormone concentrations. In both protocols, the buserelin and gonadotrophic treatments were continued until follicle maturation was judged to have occurred [20] and approximately 36 hours later an injection of HCG was given to initiate oocyte maturation. Oocyte recovery was undertaken 36 hours later either laparoscopically, or transvesically using ultrasound guidance. The techniques of sperm preparation, in vitro fertilisation, embryo culture and transfer have been described elsewhere [21]. Embryo transfer was undertaken in 48 of these cycles.

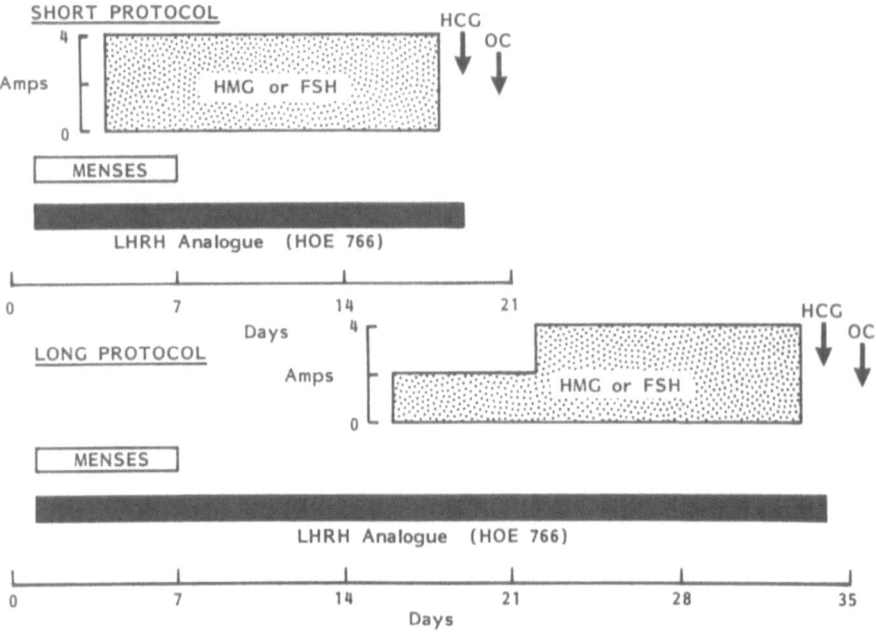

Figure 4   Diagramatic representation of the "short" and "long"
protocols of pituitary desensitisation and gonadotrophic stimulation
for in vivo fertilisation (HOE 766 = buserelin).

A variety of doses of buserelin were investigated (Figure 5)
and no differences were detected between doses of 30–1000 µg per
day given subcutaneously using the miniature infusion pumps
mentioned above, compared with 600 µg per day given in divided
doses intranasally.   During treatment with buserelin, the time taken
to complete ultrasound determined regression of ovarian follicles and
of endometrial growth was 15.5 ± 3.8 days and was independent of
the route of administration.   The duration of the phase of
gonadotrophic stimulation was shorter in the "short" protocol (13.7 ±
3. days) compared with that in the "long" protocol (17.1 ± 4.6 days,
p < 0.005), a difference that was also independent of the route of
administration of the analogue.   Patients in the "short" protocol
received the same number of ampoules of gonadotrophin as those in
the "long" protocol but they received them over a shorter period of
time.   We found no difference in the duration of treatment or in the
number of ampoules of gonadotrophins required in the group
receiving HMG compared with that receiving FSH and there was no
effect on the gonadotrophin requirement of the route of
administration of the analogue.   Finally, there was no difference in
the number of ampoules received by patients with ultrasonically
diagnosed polycystic ovaries compared with those who had ovaries

that were normal.

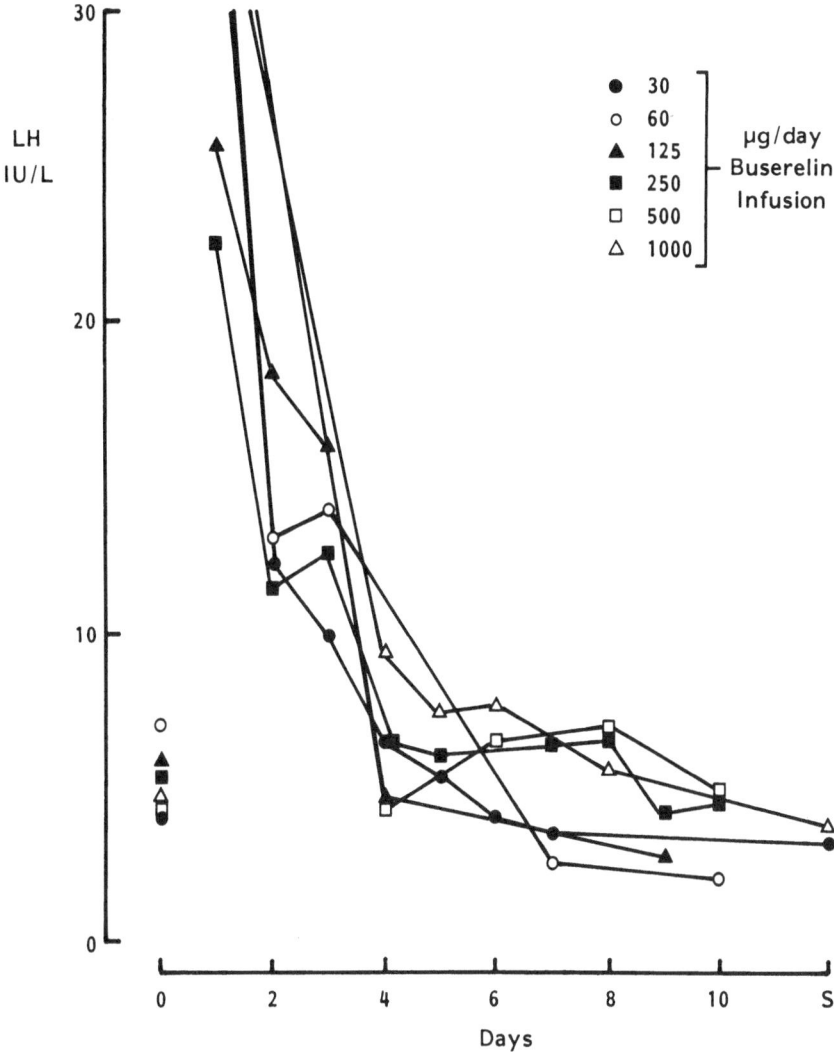

Figure 5 Serum LH concentrations before and during treatment with subcutaneous buserelin, up to the time of gonadotrophic stimulation (S). There were no differences in the responses during the agonist or the desensitisation phases, despite variations in dosage of buserelin from 30 to l00 μg per day.

The results are shown in Figures 6 and 7, from which it may be seen that while the number of oocytes recovered in the various treatment groups varied, the overall mean number of oocytes recovered (ll.l ± 6.6) was 10 times greater than that in all of the previous attempts at in vitro fertilisation in these patients. There

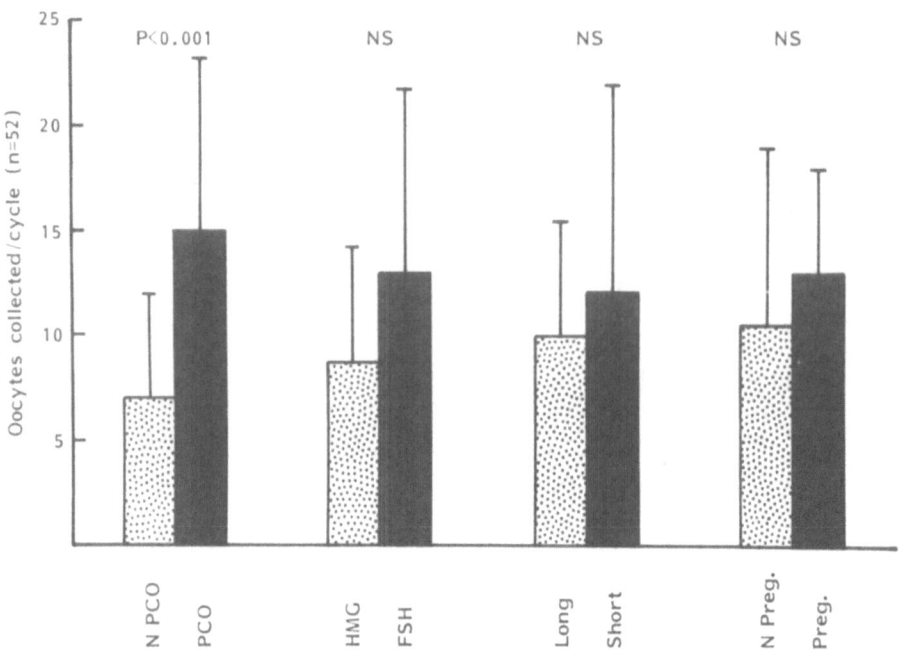

Figure 6 The response to treatment, expressed in terms of the mean (± standard deviation) number of oocytes obtained in relation to the protocol of pituitary desensitisation, the type of gonadotrophin used for stimulation, the clinical outcome (number of pregnancies) and the presence of ultrasound diagnosed polycystic ovaries (ns = differences that were not statistically significant).

was no significant difference between any of the treatment groups in the numbers of follicles aspirated or in the number of oocytes retrieved. The ovarian status however proved critical (Figure 7). More oocytes were collected from the group with polycystic ovaries (14.8 ± 8.5, (SD)) than from the group with normal ovaries (6.9 ± 5.1, p<0.001), despite the two groups receiving the same amount of gonadotrophic stimulation.

Ten clinical pregnancies were established (7 in the group with polycystic ovary disease and 3 in the non-polycystic group, 6 in the group treated with HMG, 4 in the group treated with FSH). Since these pregnancies occurred in subjects defined by their previous experience of in vitro fertilisation and embryo transfer as 'poor responders' they were all the more remarkable.

The majority of the patients described here experienced some hot flushes which, as in the patients treated for in vivo fertilisation, passed off rapidly as gonadotrophic stimulation was started. All but 6 experienced mild (grade 2) hyperstimulation but 4 developed grade

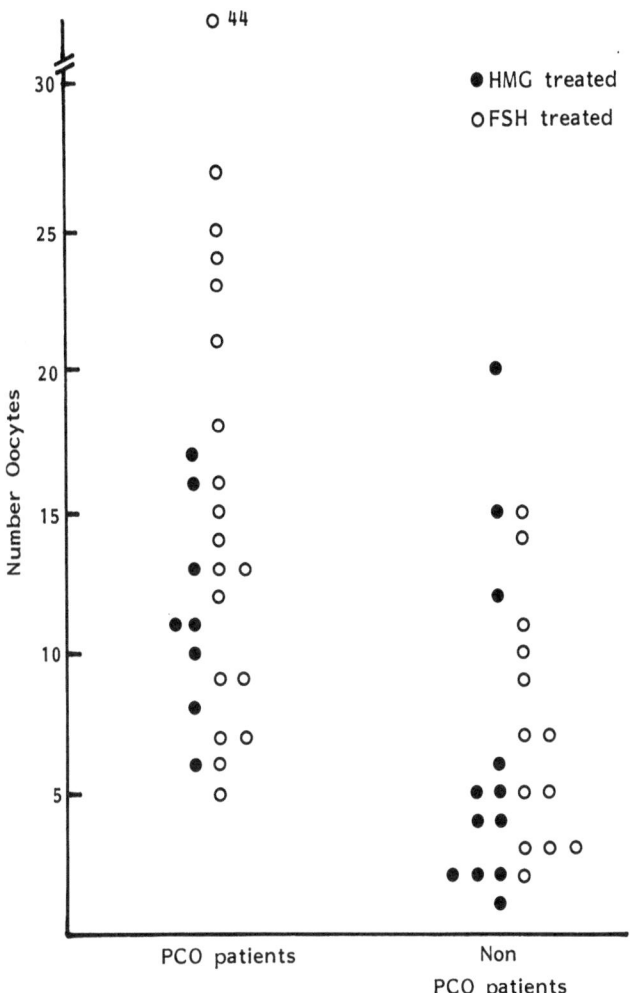

Figure 7 The number of oocytes collected from patients with ultrasonically diagnosed polycystic ovaries compared with the number in the patients without polycystic ovaries. The difference between these two groups was statistically significant (p < 0.001).

3 hyperstimulation. Although they required hospitalisation they all recovered on conservative treatment.

The results of this study of the use of buserelin for in vitro fertilisation seem very encouraging - in purely clinical terms this treatment converted a group of 42 patients resistant to induction of ovulation into one where one quarter conceived and the prognosis for the remainder with further courses of the same treatment looks excellent. Full evaluation of the impact of this treatment clearly needs a contemporary rather than an historical control group, but in our experience it is difficult to give such large doses of gonadotrophins to patients with intact cycles without provoking unscheduled ovulations – presumably in response to the large amounts of oestrogen produced by the large numbers of follicles that are stimulated. In many in vitro fertilisation and embryo transfer programmes, some 10 per cent of subjects ovulate before oocyte recovery can be scheduled [17], so causing a whole cycle of treatment to be lost. None of our subjects had a spontaneous LH surge resulting in ovulation, indicating that in this group of subjects the LHRH analogue had certainly blocked oestrogen-mediated positive feedback. The cost of such intensive gonadotrophic stimulation was of course the 4 patients (one of whom actually conceived) who developed grade 3 ovarian hyperstimulation.

As described in detail elsewhere [19] we found it necessary in these patients to give supplemental HCG in the luteal phase, a finding consistent with the results in the patients who, using buserelin for in vivo fertilisation, maintained LH suppression after the analogue was discontinued.

Elimination of the endogenous secretion of gonadotrophins permitted us to compare directly the effects of pure FSH and of HMG and here the study design has permitted us to draw firm conclusions – no difference in outcome could be seen between those treated with pure FSH compared with those treated with HMG. Since pure FSH is so much more expensive than HMG, we have discontinued its use for induction of ovulation for in vitro fertilisation for purely clinical indications. It remains, of course, a fascinating agent for scientific studies – for example, in these patients we were unable to find any reduction in the pre-HCG ("follicular phase") plasma progesterone concentrations in the patients given pure FSH compared with those given HMG [22]. Thus elimination of follicular phase LH stimulation of the ovary did not prevent premature, pre-ovulatory, luteinisation of the gonadotrophin stimulated follicles.

Finally, the use of buserelin in these studies allowed a controlled study of the ovarian response to identical regimens of gonadotrophin stimulation. The results depicted in Figure 7 clearly showed that the response of the polycystic ovaries was significantly greater than that of the normal ovaries, even when endogenous gonadotrophin stimulation had been suppressed and exogenous gonadotrophin stimulation equalised between the two groups. In a detailed analysis of the hormonal content of the follicular fluids obtained from these patients, we found that, while the follicular fluid testosterone concentration was in part determined by the nature of the gonadotrophic stimulation (higher in follicles in the women given HMG than in those given FSH), it was also determined by whether the fluid was obtained from polycystic or normal ovaries. In contrast to the concentrations of testosterone, however, follicular fluid concentrations of progesterone and of somatomedin-C were determined only by the ovarian status (higher in follicles obtained from normal than from polycystic ovaries) and not by the particular gonadotrophin used [23].

CONCLUDING REMARKS

At present, while the role of superactive analogues of LHRH for fertilisation in vivo is uncertain, we speculate that in the long term it will prove to be of considerable value for the patient suffering from the consequences of untimely secretion of large amounts of LH. For patients requiring induction of ovulation for in vitro fertilisation, at present we consider the main value of these analogues is in blocking oestrogen-mediated positive feedback, so permitting large quantities of exogenous gonadotrophic stimulation to be applied without the risk of ovulation prior to oocyte recovery. In clinical terms, the powerful ovarian stimulation permitted by such an agent has allowed treatment to succeed in a group of women previously refractory to induction of ovulation. It may be, however, that suppression of tonic secretion of LH in programmes of in vitro fertilisation will also prove advantageous, for the reasons that we have postulated for in vivo fertilisation, because both Stanger and Yovitch [14] and Howles et al [15] have reported that the outcome of in vitro fertilisation was significantly poorer in women with high rates of secretion of LH prior to oocyte recovery than in those with normal LH production (Figure 1). Such a speculation is certainly supported by results we have recently obtained in a patient with ultrasound diagnosed polycystic ovaries and high serum LH concentrations in whom two attempts at fertilising a total of 14 oocytes were unsuccessful but who, after ovulation was induced during treatment with buserelin, produced two eggs which fertilised and formed good embryos (Steptoe, Howles and Jacobs, unpublished observations).

ACKNOWLEDGEMENTS

Invaluable help in treating these patients and in analysing the results was provided by Miss Judy Adams and Mr W Smith and by Dr K Ahuja. It is a pleasure to thank Dr Patrick Magill of Hoechst UK for the gift of an Aloka ultrasound machine and for generous supplies of buserelin and Dr Ellis Snitcher of Serono UK for generous supplies of Metrodin.

REFERENCES

1. Fleming R., Haxton M. J., Hamilton M. P. R., McCune G.S., Black W. P., MacNaughton M. C. and Coutts J. R. T. Successful treatment of infertile women with oligomenorrhoea using a combination of an LHRH agonist and exogenous gonadotrophins. British Journal of Obstetrics and Gynaecology, 92, 369 (1985).

2. Adams J., Franks S. Polson D. W., Mason H. D., Abdulwahid N. A., Tucker M., Morris D. V., Price J. and Jacobs H. S. Multifollicular ovaries: clinical and endocrine features and response to pulsatile gonadotrophin releasing hormone. Lancet ii, 1375 (1985).

3. Armar N. A., Adams J. and Jacobs H. S. Induction of ovulation with gonadotrophin releasing hormone. In "Recent Advances in Obstetrics and Gynaecology", 15, J. Bonnar (Ed), Churchill Livingstone, Edinburgh and London, 1986 p. 259.

4. Abdulwahid N. A., Armar N. A., Adams J. and Jacobs H. S. Clinical and endocrine predictors of the response of patients with polycystic ovary syndrome to induction of ovulation with pulsatile LHRH therapy. Fertility and Sterility, in press (1986).

5. Armar N. A., Tan S. L., Adams J. and Jacobs H. S. Obstetric outcome of patients treated with LHRH. British Journal of Obstetrics and Gynaecology, in press.

6. McArthur J. W., Ingersoll F. M. and Worcester J. The urinary excretion of interstitial cell and follicle stimulating hormone activity by women with diseases of the reproductive system. Journal of Clinical Endocrinology and Metabolism, 18, 1202 (1958).

7. Abdulwahid N. A., Adams J., van der Spuy Z. M. and Jacobs H. S. Gonadotrophin control of follicular development. Clinical Endocrinology, 23, 613 (1985).

8. Armar N. A., Eshel A., Abdulwahid N. A., Tan S. L., Adams J., Franks S. and Jacobs H. S. Early pregnancy loss (EPL) in patients with ultrasonically diagnosed polycystic ovaries. Proceedings of 24th British Congress of Obstetrics and Gynaecology, 15-18 March 1980, Abstract 55, RCOG (1986).

9. Channing C. P., Anderson L. D., Hoover D. J., Kolena J., Osteen K. G., Pomerantz S. H. and Tanabe K.. The role of non-steroidal regulators in control of oocyte and follicular maturation. Recent Progress in Hormone Research, 38, 331 (1982).

10. Tsafriri A. and Pomerantz S.H. Oocyte maturation inhibitor. Clinics in Endocrinology and Metabolism, 15, 157 (1986).

11. Hunter R. H. F., Cook B. and Baker T.G. Dissociation of response to injected gonadotropin between the Graafian follicle and oocyte in pigs. Nature, 260, 156 (1976).

12. Austin C. R. The Egg. In "Reproduction in Mammals", 2nd Edition: No 1, Germ Cells and Fertilisation, C. R. Austin and R. E. Short (Eds.), Cambridge University Press, Cambridge, 1982, p.58.

13. Guerrero R. J. and Rojas O. I. Spontaneous abortion and ageing of human ova and spermatazoa. New England Journal of Medicine, 293, 573 (1975).

14. Stanger J. D. and Yovich J. L. Reduced in vitro fertilisation of human oocytes from patients with raised basal luteinising hormone levels during the follicular phase. British Journal of Obstetrics and Gynaecology, 92, 385 (1985).

15. Howles C. M., MacNamee M. C., Edwards R. G., Goswamy R. and Steptoe P. C. Effect of high tonic levels of luteinising hormone on outcome of in vitro fertilisation. Lancet, ii, 521 (1986).

16. Schenker J. G. and Weinstein D. Ovarian hyperstimulation syndrome: a current survey. Fertility and Sterility, 30, 255 (1978).

17. Steptoe P.C., Edwards R. G. and Walters D. E. Observations on 767 pregnancies and 500 births after human in vitro fertilisation. Human Reproduction, 1, 89 (1986).

18. Brown J. B. Gonadotropins. In "Infertility:Male and Female", Insler V. and Lunenfeld B. (Eds), Churchill Livingstone, Edinburgh, 1986, p. 359.

19. Porter R.N., Jacobs H. S., Smith W., Adams J., Ahuja K. and Craft I. Ovulation induction for in vitro fertilisation during suppression of gonadotrophins with buserelin. Submitted for publication 1986.

20. Smith W., Porter R., Ahuja K. and Craft I. Ultrasonic assessment of endometrial changes in stimulated cycles in an in vitro fertilisation and embryo transfer programme. Journal of IVF and ET, 1, 233 (1984).

21. Craft I. In vitro fertilisation: clinical methodology. British Journal of Hospital Medicine, 31, 90 (1984).

22. Porter R. N., Honour J. W., Holownia P., Craft I. and Jacobs H. S. The intrafollicular environment of the developing oocyte - gonadotrophic and ovarian determinants. Programme of 5th Joint Meeting of British Endocrine Societies, April 1986. Journal of Endocrinology, 108: Sup 79.

23. Honour J. W., Holownia P., Hill D. J., Porter R. N., Adams J. and Jacobs H. S. Steroid and IGF1 concentrations in the environment of the developing human oocyte - gonadotrophic and ovarian determinants. Programme of 7th Joint Meeting of British Endocrine Societies, November 1986. Journal of Endocrinology, 110, Sup, in press.

SECTION 6

CLINICAL TRIALS

21
Ovulation Induction with Pulsatile LHRH

S.J. ORY
Mayo Medical School, Mayo Foundation, Rochester, MN 55905, USA

INTRODUCTION

Shortly after LHRH was isolated, characterized and synthesized, clinical application to disorders of reproduction and sexual development was initiated. The early experiences with LHRH administered once or twice daily for induction of ovulation were largely unsuccessful.[1,2] The elucidation of the pulsatile release of LHRH by Knobil and colleagues[3] potentiated use of the agent in a physiologic manner and led to the development of successful ovulation induction regimens and pubertal maturation strategies.[4,5] The clinical efficacy of pulsatile LHRH therapy is currently well-documented and it has become an alternative therapy of choice for ovulation induction in patients with suspected hypothalamic suppression.[6-9] Pulsatile LHRH has been reported to be effective in widely variable circumstances including variations in means of administration,[6-9] routes of administration[6,9,10], dosages[6,7], and underlying disease states.[4,11] This paper will review the current experience of LHRH used for ovulation.

LHRH PHARMACODYNAMICS

Few direct data exist addressing normal LHRH pharmacodynamics in the human due to its episodic release in minute quantities into a sequestered and clinically inaccessible portal system. The relative absence of a highly sensitive radioimmunoassay for LHRH and its short half-life and very low levels in the peripheral circulation have further complicated clinical studies. LHRH is presumed to consistently produce release of LH and clinical studies investigating the pharmacodynamics of LH-RH have assessed this indirectly via peripheral serum LH determinations.

Crowley and colleagues have provided the most substantial normative data addressing LHRH therapy. They studied gonadotropin release dynamics in normal women and women with hypogonadotropic hypogonadism (HH), a putative endogenous LHRH deficiency[7,12] They performed frequent LH sampling inferring LHRH release and then developed models for physiologic frequency and dosage replacement in individuals with HH.

Several different patterns of abnormal LHRH release were identified suggesting considerable heterogeneity in the expression of HH. They studied individuals that appeared to have a total absence of LHRH secretion, abnormalities in the amplitude or frequency of LHRH release, and a nocturnal pattern of LH release similar to that seen in early puberty. The latter pattern was interpreted as being consistent with a developmental arrest. Following these studies, they attempted to re-establish normal ovulatory cycles in women with hypothalamic amenorrhea (HA) using doses of 25 ng/kg and 100 ng/kg. They determined that 25 ng/kg was a threshold dose; 80% of subjects responded. The higher dose was consistently effective in eliciting a response but more than one follicle was frequently detected at sonography suggesting a supraphysiologic effect. They concluded that optimum dose range for LHRH replacement appeared to be between 25 and 100 ng/kg as there is considerable variation in individual response.

Their data suggested that LHRH frequency of release varies markedly throughout the menstrual cycle. In the early follicular phase the frequency was approximately every 90 minutes and most subjects exhibited almost complete suspension of pulsatile release during sleep. During the midfollicular phase, the frequency increased to essentially a circhoral pattern, a concomitant decrease in amplitude occurred and the sleep entrained suspension of LH release disappeared. They noted marked slowing of the LH frequency after ovulation with a bimodal pattern of LH release with large LH pulses interspersed with smaller ones. This pattern became more pronounced in the midluteal phase and progesterone release became closely coupled to LH release at this time. At the end of the luteal phase, only one or two LH pulses were detectable in a 24 hour period.

CLINICAL EXPERIENCE

The principal advantage of LHRH therapy most often cited is that it represents the most physiologic therapy currently available for ovulation induction. If physiologic amounts of LHRH are replaced in a pulsatile fashion, the gonadotrophs are reactivated and the remainder of the reproductive system functions in a near normal manner. The most common adverse effects of other ovulation induction agents, ovarian hyperstimulation and multiple pregnancy, may be avoided. Similarly, since ovulation occurs at the appropriate time with an endogenous LH surge, the intensive surveillance required for timing of hCG administration in other ovulation induction regimens might be avoided. It was anticipated that significant cost savings might be achieved by avoiding some of the monitoring measures. Although LHRH therapy continues to hold great promise, some of these advantages have yet to be realized.

The fixed hypothalamic LHRH input defined by Knobil with unvarying frequency and amplitude of LHRH administration represents the minimal requirement of the pituitary and is adequate to permit ovulation and conception in the majority of patients with HH. Any potential benefit of ovulation induction regimens using varied doses and frequencies has yet to be clinically documented but their use may permit wider application of LHRH therapy to include other anovulatory patients who do not respond to fixed schedules. Currently it is clear that a variety of dosages, frequencies, and routes of administration are effective in inducing ovulation in patients with HH. In fact, ovulation may still occur if nocturnal pulses of LHRH are omitted or if therapy is only given at night.[13] The minimum requirement for ovulation has not been defined. A summary of the current clinical experience is presented in Table 1.

Table 1. Clinical experience with pulsatile LHRH for ovulation induction

Investigator	Dx	Pts.	Cycles	Ovulation (pts/cycles)	Preg/Multi/Abs	Route of Therapy	Dose (ug)	Frequency Minutes	Luteal Phase	Ref.
Leyendecker and and Wildt	HA	33	143	33/143	38/5/9	IV	2.5-20	90	hCG/GnRH	6
Miller et al.	HA	8	23	8/20	7/0/5	IV	1-5	96-120	hCG/GnRH	43
Berg et al.	HA	12	14	9/10	4/0/2	IV	20	90	hCG	44
	Pgst- Pgst+ 15		26	13/22	7/1/1	IV	20	90	hCG	
Crowley	HA	8	11	/9	3	IV	25ng/kg	60	GnRH	7
Jansen et al	HA	12	22	12/22	9/2	IV	2.5-5	90	hCG	45
Goerzen et al.	HA	6	10	6/10	4	IV	10	120¶	hCG	46
Bennink et al.	PCO	15	42	10/29	8	IV	10-20	90	GnRH	15
Rolland et al.	HA	18		/39	9/1/4	IV	5	90	GnRH	47
	PCO	4		/16	0	IV	5	90	GnRH	
	LPD	5		/18	0	IV	5	90	GnRH	
Schriock, Martin, & Jaffe	HA	14	24	13/23	7/0/2	IV	1.2-10	90	hCG	41
	PCO	10	17	6/10	1	IV	1-40	90-153	hCG	
	LPD	2	3	/3	0	IV	1.3	90	hCG	
Reid and Sauerbrei	HA	3	8	3/7	1	IV	2.5-5	90-120	hCG	13
		2	3	0/0		SC	5-10	120-180	hCG	
		3	8	2/2		SC	2-20	60-240‖	GnRH	
Jacobs et al.	HA	25	83	25/80	25/1/8	SC	10-25	90	hCG/GnRH	9
		3	6	3/6	3	IV	10-25	90	hCG/GnRH	
Tucker et al.	PCO	16	23	/7	3/0/0	SC	10-25	90	hCG/GnRH	48
		6	17	/11	2/0/2	IV	10-25	90	hCG/GnRH	
Hurley et al.	HA	14	36	14/30	13/0/2	SC	5-15	90	hCG	20
Skarin et al.	HA	19		17/55	12/1/3	SC	20	90	GnRH	8
Keogh et al.	HA	14		10/	6	SC	50-200	60-120	GnRH ug/day	49
Woodhouse et al.	HA	4	9	4/9	4	SC	2.5-15	90	GnRH	21
Seibel et al(19)	HA	7	10	/10	2	SC	20	120	GnRH	19
Ory	PCO	6	9	6/6		IV	1.2-2.5	90	Nothing	
	HA	5	8	5/6	1/0/2	IV	1.2-5	90	hCG	

Preg, pregnancies; Multi, multiple births; Abs, spontaneous abortions; HA, hypothalamic amenorrhea; PCO, polycystic, ovarian disease; LPD, luteal phase deficiency; Megalo, megalocystic disease; Pgst, progestin, Dx, diagnosis; Pt, patient.
¶ Self-administered 6 AM to midnight
‖ Daytime only
Modified and reproduced from Schriock, E.D. and Jaffe, R.B. Induction of ovulation with gonadotropin-releasing hormone. Obstet. Gynecol. Surv 41, 414 (1986).

Patient Selection

Although the United States Food and Drug Administration does not currently approve the use of LHRH for ovulation induction, it is used for this pupose in a number of research centers around the world. Its relative expense and limited clinical experience have

restricted its use thus far.   Patients being considered for
pulsatile LHRH therapy should undergo comprehensive endocrine
evaluations to elucidate the cause of anovulation and an
infertility assessment to exclude other possible causes of
infertility prior to beginning treatment.   It is critical to
exclude pituitary and ovarian failure before initiating therapy.
Many investigators elect to perform a dynamic LHRH stimulation
test prior to commencing pulsatile therapy to confirm the
integrity of the pituitary.   However, many patients who are
responsive to therapy require multiple boluses of LHRH to elicit
an initial response and a single injection test is usually not
helpful.

Most patients receiving LHRH have the diagnosis of HA. This
diagnosis is often difficult to establish but is suggested in
hypoestrogenic women with low serum gonadotropins and estrogen
levels.   There is often an antecedent history of vigorous
exercise, significant weight change or unusual emotional stress.
They usually do not have withdrawal bleeding following progestin
exposure but this response is inconsistent.

A more common cause of anovulation is polycystic ovary
syndrome (PCOS).   Women with PCOS usually have evidence of
greater endogenous estrogen production than do those with HA.
The clinical expression is highly variable and rarely are all the
typical   clinical   features   of   obesity,   hirsutism,
oligo-anovulation, glucose intolerance, enlarged cystic ovaries,
mild to moderate hyperandrogenemia and an elevated LH:FSH ratio
present in one patient. HA and PCOS may be thought to represent
different points on the spectrum of anovulation and it is often
difficult to distinguish the two.   Most investigators have
reported a poor response to pulsatile LHRH therapy in PCOS
patients   but   ovulation[14]   (Figure   1)   and   subsequent
pregnancy[15] has been reported. Although there is no consensus
regarding the underlying abnormality in PCOS, it is assumed that
endogenous LHRH release exists with a possible disturbance of
frequency and amplitude. If therapy could be made more effective
with additional adjustments in frequency and dosage, a much
larger group of patients would be available for therapy.
Currently, there is no available therapy which is consistently
effective for many of these women. Pulsatile LHRH therapy has
also been effective in inducing ovulation in women with
hyperprolactinemia[4]. These women usually have an associated
endogenous deficiency of LHRH that may be overridden with
therapy.   The LHRH deficiency is thought to be secondary to
abnormalities in common neuroregulatory pathways involving
dopamine.   It has been suggested that excessive prolactin may
also directly inhibit ovarian steriodogenesis and this effect
would probably not be affected by LHRH therapy.[16,17] This
phenomenon has not been observed in the treatment of
hyperprolactinemic women with LHRH.

LHRH ADMINISTRATION

326

Some investigators feel that a standard dose of LHRH is
sufficient for all patients[18]. Leyendecker notes that a
critical threshold for response may be variable due to
differences in various subjects endogenous LHRH production[6]. He
advocates determining the minimum effective dose and cites an
increased risk of exaggerated follicle development and multiple
gestation with inappropriately high doses. Most investigators
have used intravenous doses ranging from 1 to 20 mcg per bolus.

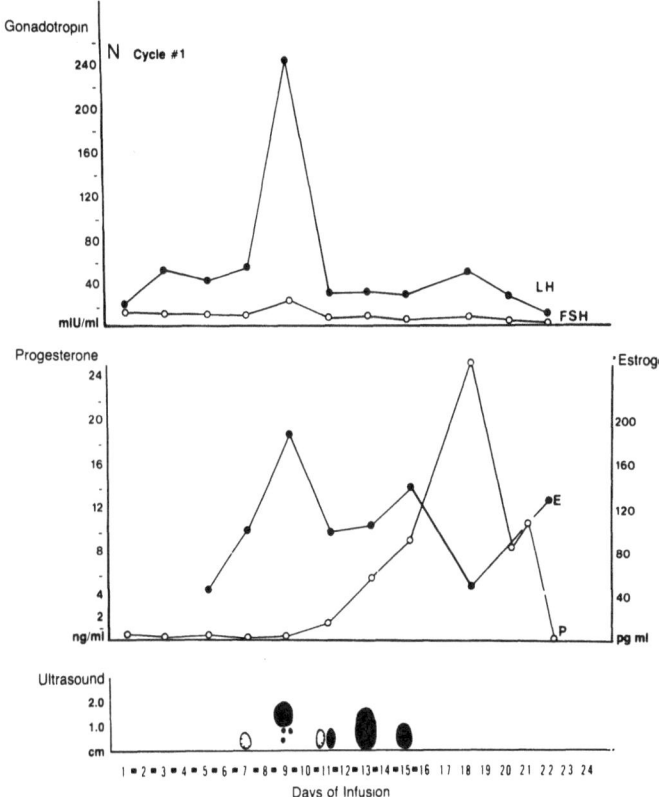

Figure 1.   Ovulation induction with pulsatile LHRH. The day of
            infusion is represented by the dotted line. Ovarian
            follicles in the right ovary are represented by the
            dark spaces, and in the left ovary by shaded spaces.
            Reproduced from Ory, S.J., et al., Fertil. Steril.,
            43:20, (1985) with permission.

Successful therapy with subcutaneous administration has been
achieved with doses ranging from 2.5 to 20 mcg[8,19-22].
   Most successful clinical protocols have relied on a 60 to 90
minute frequency of intravenous adminstration.   To date, no
studies have examined the clinical effect of varying the
frequency within the same cycle.

The initial limited experience with subcutaneous LHRH therapy was unsuccessful and it was postulated that the slower subcutaneous absorption produced an elevated LH:FSH ratio similar to that seen in patients with PCOS[23]. Subsequent studies using subcutaneous administration at 90 to 120 minute intervals in patients with HH have noted success rates comparable to intravenous regimens.[8,19-22] Subcutaneous administration has obvious advantages for use by ambulatory patients but may be less effective in patients with less complete hypothalamic suppression. Intravenous administration produces more clearly defined gonadotropin pulses which may represent more physiologic replacement, and may entail a shorter duration of therapy. A 1 mcg pulse of LHRH administered intravenously will produce a peak peripheral concentration of 200 to 260 pg/ml within 4 minutes and will be undetectable within 12 minutes of administration.[24] In addition to subcutaneous and intravenous routes, LHRH is absorbed via intramuscular, nasal and sublingual administration although the latter three have not been widely adopted in successful ovulation induction protocols.[1,25]

LHRH is currently marketed in the United States as a lyophilized powder as gonadorelin hydrochloride (Factrel, Ayerst Laboratories, New York, NY). It is dissolved in a sterile diluent prior to use and the dose administered is determined by its concentration in the diluent and the volume of each pulse administered. Stability and potency of LHRH are decreased when LHRH is in solution but biologic potency in solution is adequate for at least 3 days of therapy. Heparin is added to intravenous infusion solutions to prevent catheter occlusion with blood clots.

LHRH administration requires the use of a pulsatile infusion pump and there are currently three suitable models in the United States. The Auto Syringe (Travenol Laboratories, Inc., Hooksett, NH) delivers a pre-set bolus at programmed intervals by a motor-driven pump that advances a syringe plunger. The Zyklomat (Ferring GmbH, Kiel, FRG) and Pulsamat (Ferring Laboratories, Inc., Ridgewood, NJ) are peristaltic pumps with unique reservoirs and catheter systems. All of these pumps have documented reliability, are compact (particularly the Ferring models) but are expensive ($1000 to $1500). Other mechanical devices have also been successfully used.[14]

CLINICAL PROTOCOL

Most investigators begin pulsatile LHRH therapy within five days of the onset of menses if bleeding can be induced. Some patients are hospitalized briefly at the outset to allow them to become acquainted with the protocol and infusion system but this can be easily accomplished on an ambulatory basis as well. Many investigators prefer the subcutaneous route because of the added margin of safety, but there is now ample documentation of the safety of intravenous infusions conducted on an out-patient basis.[7,12]

We currently initiate out-patient intravenous LHRH therapy with a 5 mcg dose delivered every 90 minutes. All new patients are oriented as out-patients in the Clinical Research Center after undergoing a baseline pelvic sonogram (to exclude the presence of previous ovarian follicles), and serum determinations of LH, FSH, and estradiol. All patients are monitored with these tests three times a week; however, this frequency may be altered to accommodate individual circumstances. Patients are encouraged to keep basal body temperature charts, and pelvic exams are periodically performed to assess cervical mucus in conjunction with laboratory studies. We have recently begun to use a rapid qualitative urinary LH detection kit (OvuSTICKS, Monoclonal Antibodies, Inc., Mountain View, CA), to aid in the identification of the LH surge. It is sometimes difficult to ascertain when ovulation occurs and this last measure has been helpful in determining an optimal time to stop or alter the infusion. It is initiated after follicle formation is detected with ultrasound. The dose is increased to 10 mcg per pulse if no response is noted within 14 days of onset of therapy; therapy is discontinued if there is no evidence of follicle development within 21 days. LHRH therapy is reinitiated within 3 to 5 days of menses following an unsuccessful cycle.

Unlike patients receiving human menopausal gonadotropins who require close monitoring to avoid ovarian hyperstimulation and multiple pregnancy, individuals receiving LHRH characteristically initiate appropriately timed endogenous LH surges and usually avoid multiple follicle development. The purpose of monitoring patients receiving LHRH is to insure a normal clinical response.

Luteal Phase Support

Normal luteal function is thought to be dependent on continued LH secretion and its absence is associated with a short luteal phase or luteal phase deficiency.[26] Some recent studies have challenged this notion. Normal corpus luteum function has been maintained in hypophysectomized monkey, presumably without a source of gonadotropins.[27] Luteinized granulosa cells have been reported to continue to produce progesterone in vitro without either LH or FSH.[28] However, more direct evidence supports the role of LH in luteal function. Abrupt cessation of pulsatile LHRH infusions in rhesus monkeys with massive median eminence lesions results in premature onset of menses[29] as does administration of LH antisera in the midluteal phase.[30]

Currently, most investigators believe that a source of LH or a surrogate LH is essential for successful LHRH therapy in HH patients. Luteal phase deficiency has been noted to occur in anovulatory patients treated with pulsatile LHRH when therapy has been stopped following ovulation[31] and continuing pulsatile infusion without varying dose or frequency after ovulation.[32,33] Pulsatile LHRH therapy has also been successfully employed to treat luteal phase deficiency.[24]

The hypothetical adverse effect of a single, fixed dose and frequency regimen for LHRH administration may be due to the failure to use a slower frequency in the luteal phase. Alternatively, it has been suggested that LHRH directly suppresses ovarian steroidogenesis[34].

Luteal phase support has usually been accomplished by continuing the pulsatile infusion at the same rate used in the follicular phase[6,22] or administering hCG 1000 to 2500 units intramuscularly at 3 or 4 day intervals through the luteal phase.[6,9,12] Despite theorectical objections, these approaches have generally been clinically successful. Other investigators have elected to treat with progesterone suppositories 25 mg daily and have documented its effectiveness.[35] However, vaginal progesterone absorption may not be consistent and may be inadequate in some patients. Optimal recommendations have not yet been formulated and potential undesireable affects may be associated with all of these regimens. We are currently using hCG injections 2500 units intramuscularly every 3 days for luteal support.

SIDE EFFECTS

A major advantage of pulsatile LHRH therapy has been a much lower incidence of adverse effects than is associated with other forms of ovulation induction. As experience increases, however, more untoward effects are being reported. Few data are available addressing the incidence of these events.

Phlebitis, hematoma formation, and pain at the needle insertion site are the most commonly reported side effects. Febrile episodes have been noted during therapy but there are no reports of sepsis or other major complications to date. Both IgG and IgE anti-LHRH antibodies have been found in men and women receiving LHRH therapy and this may occur in as many as 3 percent of subjects.[36,37] Two women with HA were noted to have antibodies prior to initiation of therapy.[37] No clinical sequelae other than failure to respond to LHRH therapy were noted.

Although ovarian hyperstimulation and multiple pregnancies can usually be avoided with LHRH therapy if small doses are employed, they have been reported.[38-40] Both of these occurrences appear to be related to the dose of LHRH administered and are more likely in patients with PCOS rather than HA. Two patients with PCOS developed ovarian hyperstimulation with 5 mcg and 10 mcg pulses subsequently avoided hyperstimulation and ovulated when a lower dose (25 ng/kg/pulse) was used.[41] Multiple follicle development has been deliberately induced with 10 mcg pulses in women with normal ovulatory cycles.[42] This regimen may prove to be useful in in vitro fertilization program protocols to increase the number of available oocytes.

CONCLUSIONS

The long-term risks of LHRH therapy have not been assessed. LHRH receptors are widely distributed throughout the body and extra-pituitary effects may result from therapy. Spontaneous abortions have been reported after successful LHRH therapy; the incidence of congenital abnormalities following therapy is unknown.[8,22]

Pulsatile LHRH infusion therapy is a safe effective modality for inducing ovulation in patients with HH who do not respond to clomiphene citrate. Its future use will be limited by its relative cost and the amount of effort required of the patient. However, these factors may be lessened if less intensive monitoring produces clinically acceptable results.

The recent data addressing LHRH pharmacodynamics in normal women and those with hypothalamic dysfunction may enable women with HH to be treated more efficiently and may potentiate the development of more effective regimens to treat patients with PCOS and hyperprolactinemia. Additional studies addressing the merit of variable frequency and dose regimens, various routes of administration, and requirements for luteal phase support should lead to improved results.

LHRH treatment continues to be investigational therapy. Although the initial experience has been generally favorable, an accurate appraisal of risks, specifically those of antibody formation, spontaneous abortion, congenital abnormalities and affects on extra-target organs, remains to be performed. For these reasons and to permit more efficient compilation of data, use of LHRH for ovulation induction should be confined to an institutional research setting.

REFERENCES

1. Akande, E.O., Carr, P.J., Dutton, A., Bonner, J., Corker, C.S., MacKinnon, P.C.B. and Robinson, D. Effect of synthetic gonadotropin-releasing hormone in secondary amenorrhea. Lancet, 2, 112 (1972).
2. Zarate, A., Canales, E.S., Soria, J., Gonzalez, A., Schally, A.V. and Kastin, A.J. Further observations on the therapy of anovulatory infertility with synthetic luteinizing hormone-releasing hormone. Fertil. Steril., 25, 3 (1974).
3. Knobil, E., Plant, T.M., Wildt, L., Belchetz, P.E. and Marshall, G. Control of the rhesus monkey menstrual cycle: Permissive role of hypothalamic gonadotropin-releasing hormone. Science 207, 1371 (1980).
4. Leyendecker, G., Struve, T. and Plotz, E.J. Induction of ovulation with chronic intermittent (pulsatile) administration of LHRH in women with hypothalamic and hyperprolactinemic amenorrhea. Arch. Gynecol., 229, 177 (1980).
5. Valk, T.W., Corley, K.P., Kelch, R.P. and Marshall, J.C.: Hypogonadotropic hypogonadism. Hormonal response to low dose pulsatile administration of gonadotropin-releasing hormone. J. Clin. Endocrinol. Metab., 51, 730 (1980).
6. Leyendecker, G. and Wildt, L. Induction of ovulation with pulsatile administration of GnRH in hypothalamic amenorrhea.

J. Steroid Biochem., 20, 1382 (1984).

7. Crowley, W.F., Jr., Filicori, J. and Spratt, D. The physiology of gonadotropin-releasing hormone (GnRH) secretion in men and women. Rec. Prog. Horm. Res., 41, 473 (1985).

8. Skarin, G., Nillius, S.J. and Wide, L. Pulsatile subcutaneous low-dose gonadotropin-releasing hormone treatment of anovulatory infertility. Fertil. Steril., 40, 454 (1983).

9. Jacobs, H.S., Adams, J., Franks, S., Cell, C., Leonard, R., Masson, W.P., Morris, D.V., Sutherland, I. and Van-Der-Spuy, Z.M. Induction of ovulation with LHRH--problems, indications and contraindications. J. Steroid Biochem., 20, A36 (1984).

10. Hanker, J.P., Bohnet, H.G. and Schreider, H.P.L. Nasal spray assisted pulsatile LHRH in the treatment of hypothalamic amenorrhea. Neuroendocrinol. Lett., 2, 269 (1980).

11. Bringer, J., Hedon, B., Jaffiol, C., Cristol, C., Nicolau, S., Orsetti, A., Orsetti, A., Bressot, N. Viala, J.L., Mirouze, J. Influence of the frequency of gonadotropin-releasing hormone (GnRH) administration of ovulatory responses in women with hypothalamic anovulation (H.A.) and polycystic ovarian syndrome (P.C.O). Proceedings of 7th Int. Congr. Endocrinol., Excctpra Medica, Amsterdam, 1984, p. 470 Congr. Ser. 652 (Abstract).

12. Santoro, N., Filicori, M. and Crowley, W.F., Jr. Hypogonadotropic disorders in men and women: Diagnosis and therapy with pulsatile gonadotropin-releasing hormone. Endocr. Rev. 7, 11 (1986).

13. Reid, R.L., and Sauerbrei, E. Evaluation of techniques for induction of ovulation in out-patients employing pulsatile gonadotropin releasing hormone. Am. J. Obstet. Gynecol., 148, 648 (1984).

14. Ory, S.J., London, S.N., Tyrey, L., and Hammond, C.B. Ovulation induction with pulsatile gonadotropin-releasing hormone administration in patients with polycystic ovarian syndrome. Fertil. Steril., 43, 20 (1985).

15. Bennink, H.J.T., Weber, H.W., Alsbach, G.P.J., and Thijssen, J.H.H. Induction of ovulation by pulsatile intravenous administration of GnRH in polycystic ovarian disease. Proceedings of 7th Int. Cong. Endocrinol., Excerpta Medica, Amsterdam, 1984, p. 470 Congr. Ser. 652 (Abstract).

16. McNatty, K.P., Neal, P. and Baker, T.G. Effect of prolactin on the prodution of progesterone by mouse ovaries in vitro. J. Reprod. Fert., 47, 155 (1976).

17. Wang, C., Hsueh, A.J.W., and Erickson, G.F. Prolactin inhibitor of estrogen production by cultured rat granulosa cells. Mol. Cell. Endocrinol., 20, 135 (1980).

18. Berg, D., Mickan, H., Michael, S., Doring, K., Gloning, K., Janicke, F. and Rjosk, H.K. Ovulation and pregnancy after pulsatile administration of gonadotropin releasing hormone. Arch. Gynaekol., 233, 205 (1983).

19. Seibel, J.M., Kamrava, M., MacArdle, C., and Taymor, M., Ovulation induction and conception using subcutaneous luteinizing hormone-releasing hormone. Obstet. Gynecol., 61,

292 (1983).

20. Hurley, D.M., Brian, R., Outeh, K., Stockdale, J., Fry, A., Hackman, C., Clarke, I. and Burger, H.G. Induction of ovulation and fertility in amenorrheic women by pulsatile low-dose gonadotropin-releasing hormone. N. Engl. J. Med., 310, 1069 (1984).

21. Woodhouse, N.I.J., Niles, N., and Othman, H.L. Hypothalamic hypogonadism: induction of ovulation and pregnancy by subcutaneous pulsatile injections of gonadotropin releasing hormone. Horm. Res., 20, 172 (1984).

22. Mason, P., Adams, J., Morris, D.V., Tucker, M., Price, J., Voulgaris, Z., Van der Spuy, Z.M., Sutherland, I., Chambers, G.R., and White, S. Induction of ovulation with pulsatile luteinizing hormone-releasing hormone. Br. Med. J., 288, 181, (1984).

23. Reid, R.L., Leopold, G.R. and Yen, S.S.C. Induction of ovulation and pregnancy with pulsatile luteinizing hormone releasing factor: dosage and mode of delivery. Fertil. Steril. 36, 553 (1981).

24. Liu, J.H. and Yen, S.S.C. The use of gonadotropin-releasing hormone for the induction of ovulation. Clin. Obstet. Gynecol. 27, 975 (1984).

25. London, D.R., Batt, W.R., Lynch, S.S., Marshall, J.C., Owusu, S., Robinson, W.R. and Stephenson, J.M. Hormonal responses to intranasal luteinizing-hormone releasing hormone. J. Clin. Endocrinol. Metab., 37, 829 (1973).

26. Vande Wiele, R.L., Bogumil, J., Dyrenfurth, I., Ferin, M., Jewelewica, R., Warren, M., Rizkallah, T. and Mikhail, G. Mechanisms regulating the menstrual cycle in women. Rec. Prog. Horm. Res., 26, 63 (1970).

27. Asch, R.H., Moustopha, A.S., Braunstein, G. and Pauerstein, C.J. Luteal function in hypophysectomized rhesus monkeys. J. Clin. Endocrinol. Metab., 55, 154 (1982).

28. Channing, C.P. Influences of the in vivo and in vitro hormonal environment upon luteinization of granulosa cells in tissue culture. Rec. Prog. Horm. Res., 26, 589 (1970).

29. Hutchison, J.S., and Zeleznik, A.J. The rhesus monkey corpus luteum is dependent on pituitary gonadotropin secretion throughout the luteal phase of the menstrual cycle. Endocrinology, 115, 1780 (1984).

30. Groff, T.R., Raj, H.G.M., Talbert, L.M., and Willis, D.L. Effects of neutralization of luteinizing hormone on corpus luteum function and cyclicity in Macaca fascicularis. J. Clin. Endocrinol. Metab., 59, 1504 (1984).

31. Weinstein, F.G., Seibel, M.M., and Taymor, M.L. Ouvlation induction with subcutaneous pulsatile gonadotropin-releasing hormone: the role of human chorionic gonadotropin in the luteal phase. Fertil. Steril., 41, 546 (1984).

32. Nillius, S.J. and Wide, L., Gonadotropin-releasing hormone treatment for induciton of follicular maturation and ovulation in amenorrheic women with anorexia nervosa. Br. Med. J., 3, 405 (1975).

33. Casas, P.R.F., Badano, A.R., Aparicio, N., Lencioni, L.J.,

Berli, R.R., Badano, H., Biccoca, C. and Schally, A.V. Luteinizing hormone-releasing hormone in the treatment of anovulatory infertility. Fertil. Steril. 26, 549 (1979).

34. Sheehan, K.L., Casper, R.F. and Yen, S.S.C., Luteal phase defect induced by an agonist of luteinizing hormone-releasing factor. Science, 215, 170 (1982).

35. Berger, N.G., and Zacur, H.A. Exogenous progesterone for luteal support following gonadotropin releasing hormone ovulation induction: case report. Fertil. Steril, 44, 133 (1985).

36. Lindner, J., McNeil, L.W., Marney, S. Conway, M., Rivier, J., Vale, W. and Rabin, D. Characterization of human anti-luteinizing hormone-releasing hormone (LRH) antibodies in the serum of a patient with isolated gonadotropin deficiency treated wtih synthetic LRH. J. Clin Endocrinol. Metab. 52, 267 (1981).

37. Meakin, J.L., Keogh, E.J., and Martin, C.E. Human anti-luteinizing hormone releasing hormone in patients treated with synthetic luteinizing hormone releasing hormone. Fertil. Steril., 43, 811 (1985).

38. Schoemaker, J., Simons, A.H.M, van Osnabrugge, J.C., Lugtenburg, C., and Van Kessel, H. Pregnancy after prolonged pulsatile administration of luteinizing hormone-releasing hormone in a patient with Clomiphene resistant secondary amenorrhea. J. Clin. Endocrinol. Metab., 52, 882 (1981).

39. Bogchelman, D., Lappohn, R.E., and Janssens, J. Triplet pregnancy after pulsatile administration of gonadotropin releasing hormone. Lancet, 2, 45 (1982).

40. Leyendecker, G., and Wildt, L. Induction of ovulation wtih chronic intermittent (pulsatile) administration of GnRH in women with hypothalamic amenorrhea. J. Reprod. Fert., 69, 397 (1983).

41. Schriock, E.D., and Jaffe, R.B. Induction of ovulation with gonadotropin-releasing hormone. Obstet Gynecol Surv., 41, 414 (1986).

42. Liu, J.H., Durfee, R., Muse, K., and Yen, S.S.C. Induction of multiple ovulation by pulsatile administration of gonadotropin-releasing hormone. Fertil Steril, 40, 18, 1983.

43. Miller, D.S., Reid, R.L., Cetel, N.S., Rebar, R.W., and Yen, S.S. Pulsatile administration of low-dose gonadotropin-releasing hormone. J. Am. Med. Assoc., 250, 2937 (1983).

44. Berg, D., Mickan, H., Michael, S., Doring, K., Gloning, K., Janicke, F. and Rjosk, H.K. Ovulation and pregnancy after pulsatile administration of gonadotropin releasing hormone. Arch. Gynaekol, 233, 205 (1983).

45. Jansen, R.P.S., Handelsman, D.J. and Boylan, L.M. Induction of ovulation with pulsatile intravenous injections of gonadotropin-releasing hormone (GnRH). Proceedings of 7th Int. Congr. Endocrinol., Excerpta Medica, Amsterdam, 1984, p. 470, Congr. Ser. 652, (Abstract).

46. Goerzen, J., Corenblum, B., Wiseman, D., and Taylor, P.J.

Ovulation induction and pregnancy in hypothalamic amenorrhea using self-administered intravenous gonadotropin-releasing hormone. Fertil. Steril. 41, 319 (1984).

47. Rolland, R., Lorijn, R.H.W., and Willemsen, W.N.P. Chronic intermittent administration of gonadotropin-releasing hormone (LHRH) in infertile women with different cycle abnormalities. J. Steroid Biochem. 20, 1402 (1984).

48. Tucker, M., Adams, J., Mason, W.P., Morris, D.V., Franks, S., and Jacobs, H.S.   Multiple   cystic   ovarian   disease. Proceedings of 7th Int. Cong. Endocrinol., Excerpta Medica, Amsterdam, 1984, p. 470, Congr. Ser. 652, (Abstract).

49. Keogh, E. J., Carati, C., Meakin, J., et al.   Clinical application of pulsatile gonadotropin-releasing hormone (GnRH). 7th International Congress of Endocrinology, Quebec City, Canada, 1984.

22
Treatment of Endometriosis by Nasal Administration of Nafarelin

M.R. HENZL[1,2] **and S.E. MONROE**[2]

[1]Syntex Research, 3401 Hillview Avenue, Palo Alto, CA 94304, USA;
[2]University of California, San Francisco, CA 94143, USA.

INTRODUCTION

Endometriosis, the ectopic location of endometrial tissue, may have an incidence up to 6% of all women of reproductive age. Patients present with symptoms ranging from chronic pelvic pain, to dyspareunia to infertility. Up to 50% of infertile women may have associated endometriosis. The condition ameliorates during pregnancy and spontaneously resolves at the menopause and after oophorectomy. There is however no uniformly successful therapy for endometriosis when future fertility is desired. Treatment has included conservative surgery, combination high dose oral contraceptives taken continuously for 6 months (induced pseudo-pregnancy) and more recently, danazol, an androgenic isoxazole derivative of 17α-ethinyl testosterone. While daily doses of 400-800 mg for 6 months of this steroid lead to clinical and objective improvement in up to 70% of cases, approximately 85% of patients experience troublesome side effects including weight gain, reduced breast size, acne and hirsutism [1-4].

The availability of highly potent agonist analogs of LHRH has led to a new form of therapy based on induction of a temporary "pseudomenopause" or "medical oophorectomy" [5-13]. Long-term administration of these agents inhibits ovulation and at higher doses serum estrogen levels are reduced to menopausal concentrations [14-17]. The mechanism of this paradoxical effect of LHRH agonists may be mediated via a down-regulation and desensitization of the pituitary LHRH receptors leading to a reduction or alteration of the pattern of gonadotropin secretion. It has also been reported that the bioactive:immunoreactive ratio of secreted LH may be substantially reduced [18,19].

The present chapter reviews our preliminary experiences with nafarelin ([D-Nal^2)^6]LHRH) administered intranasally in a double-blind, double-placebo, multicenter phase III clinical trial. This trial was initiated following encouraging results in a pilot study with 8 patients [20].

337

PREREQUISITES TO SUCCESSFUL TREATMENT OF ENDOMETRIOSIS

In designing a treatment regimen for endometriosis we reasoned that the dose of the LHRH agonist must be adequate to rapidly (1) induce amenorrhea, (2) substantially decrease circulating levels of estrogens and, in particular (3) cause a sufficiently profound degree of down-regulation of the pituitary-ovarian axis to prevent the acute stimulation of ovarian steroidogenesis that follows the initial doses of the agonist.

Clinical pharmacology studies [17] showed that nafarelin given by a nasal spray, after an initial period of stimulation, suppressed ovarian steroidogenesis in a dose-dependent fashion (Fig. 1).

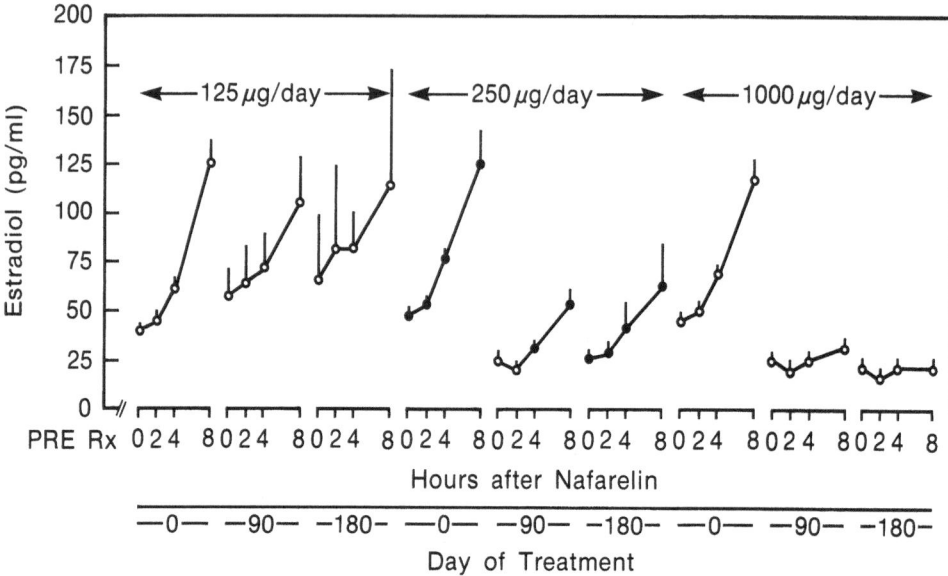

FIGURE 1. Nafarelin suppresses estradiol in women in a dose-related manner.

Dose levels of 250 µg per day or more gave basal (pre-dosing) levels of estradiol in the menopausal range. However, more detailed evaluation of these responses, immediately following the nasal insufflation, revealed a further difference between single administration of 250 µg per day of nafarelin and 500 µg administered morning and evening. A transient, acute estradiol response continued throughout the entire 6 month treatment period in subjects receiving 250 µg per day; in those administered the higher dose, the acute response was abolished (Fig. 2).

MULTICENTER STUDY WITH NAFARELIN

In this study patients with endometriosis were randomized to receive daily, either 400 or 800 µg of nafarelin by nasal spray

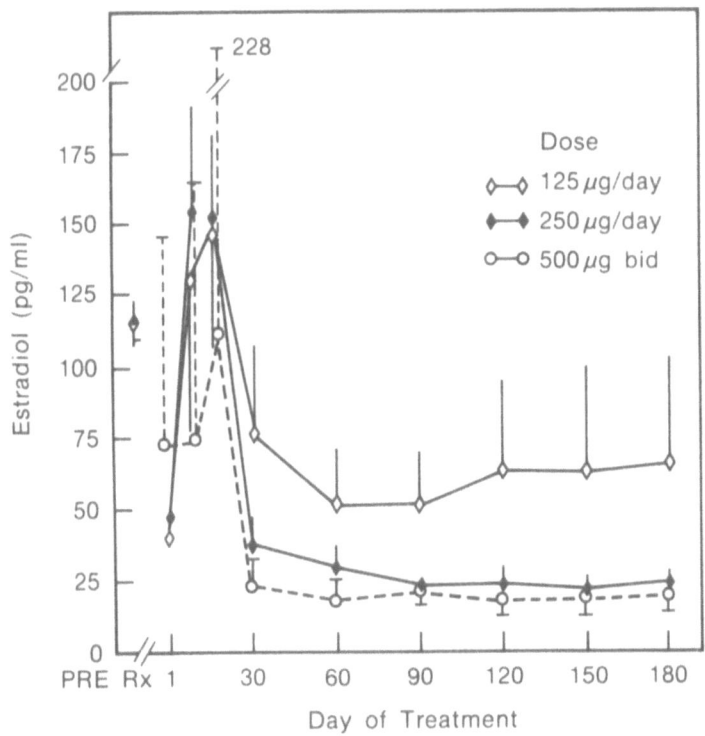

FIGURE 2. Acute estradiol responses to 125, 250 and 1000 μg of
nafarelin on days 1, 90, and 180 of treatment. Mean
(± S.E.)

along with placebo oral tablets or 800 mg danazol orally along
with placebo nasal spray [21]. The treatment lasted 6 months,
with 3 and 12 months post-treatment follow-up.

Of 238 patients currently enrolled in the study, pre- and
post-treatment laparoscopies have been compared in 201 patients.
Symptoms of endometriosis have been analyzed in 203 patients.
Timing of menstruation following treatment cessation has been
established in 122 patients.

Hormonal effects

Estradiol concentrations in blood were monitored at regular
intervals. As can be seen from Figure 3 there was a relationship
between the estradiol levels and amenorrhea for both danazol and
nafarelin. Danazol treatment, through a direct suppression of
estradiol secretion, leads to a gradual accumulation of numbers of
patients with amenorrhea. Although both doses of nafarelin caused
an initial elevation of estradiol levels this effect was

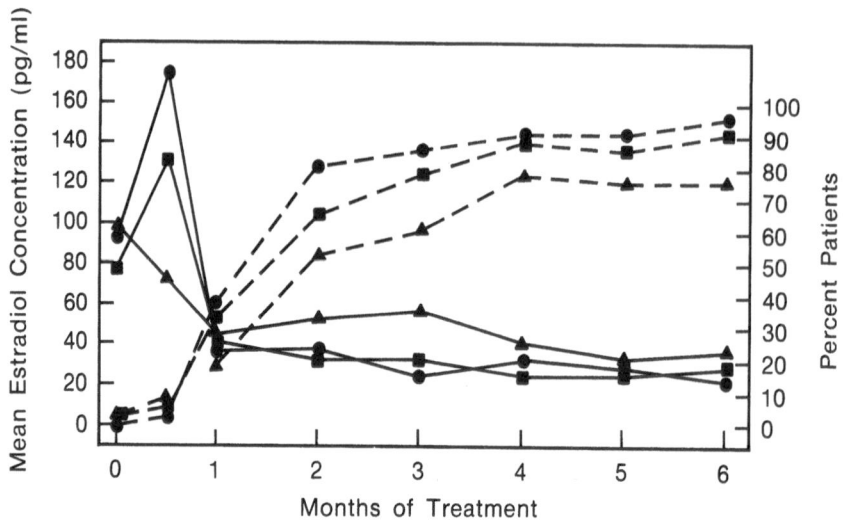

FIGURE 3.   Mean   estradiol   concentrations   and   percent   of
amenorrheic   patients   during   nafarelin   and   danazol
treatment.

transient, followed by estradiol suppression and development of amenorrhea.

Subjective symptoms

The patients were questioned monthly regarding the subjective symptoms of endometriosis (dysmennorrhea, dyspareunia and menstrual cycle-independent pelvic pain). They also had a pelvic examination to assess induration and/or pelvic tenderness. Each of these symptoms was scored as mild, moderate or severe. The scores were then summed to give a composite index of severity score. There was a continuous decrease of the mean severity score through the treatment (Fig. 4), reflecting the decrease in circulating levels of estradiol and the development of amenorrhea.

The improvement in subjective symptoms was still apparent at the first menstrual bleeding after completing treatment, although the recurrence of dysmenorrhea in a few patients caused a slight rise in the mean severity score.

Further analysis of the data established that about 90% of nafarelin treated patients improved clinically versus 80% of patients receiving danazol (Fig. 5). Ten to 15% of patients treated with nafarelin had no change or worsened; this figure was 20% for danazol treatment. The difference between treatments was not statistically significant.

Another important parameter is the magnitude of improvement in these subjective symptoms. There was an impressive shift from high pretreatment severity score to low on-treatment scores with nafarelin (Fig. 6). Of the 70 patients analyzed so far 30 became symptomless.

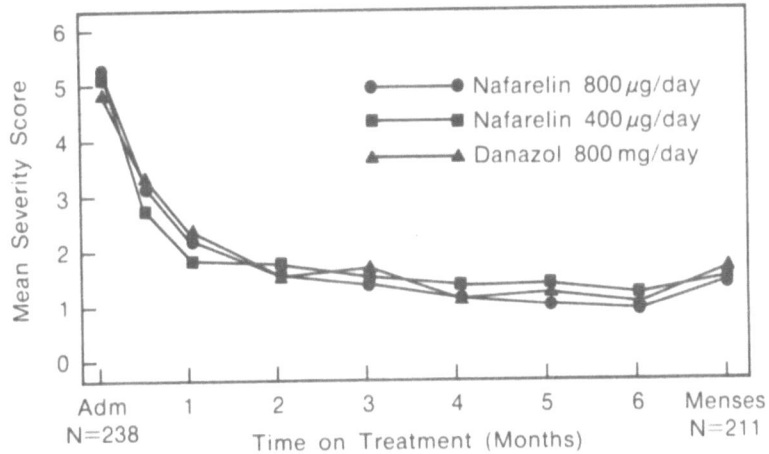

FIGURE 4.   Mean severity score for symptoms of endometriosis under
treatment with nafarelin or danazol.

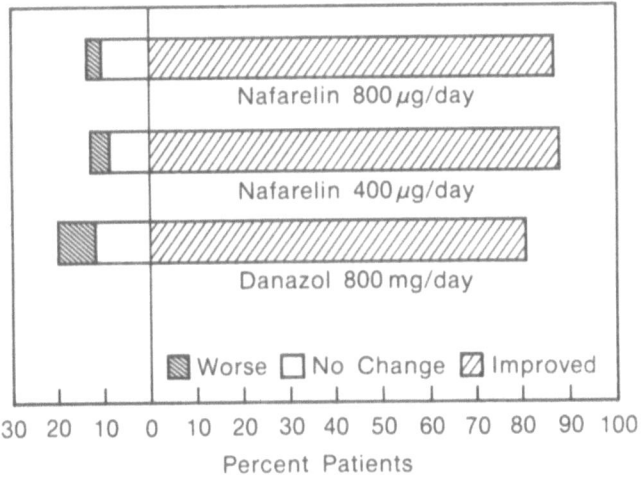

FIGURE 5.   Change of symptoms of endometriosis from pretreatment.

Effects on extent of endometriotic implants

The improvement of the symptoms of endometriosis is most likely
the consequence of arrest of growth and/or regression of the
endometriotic implants.   The extent of ectopic endometrial growth
pre- and post-treatment in this series has been staged by the
American Fertility Society recommended classification [22].   Both
nafarelin and danazol treatments were highly effective and gave a

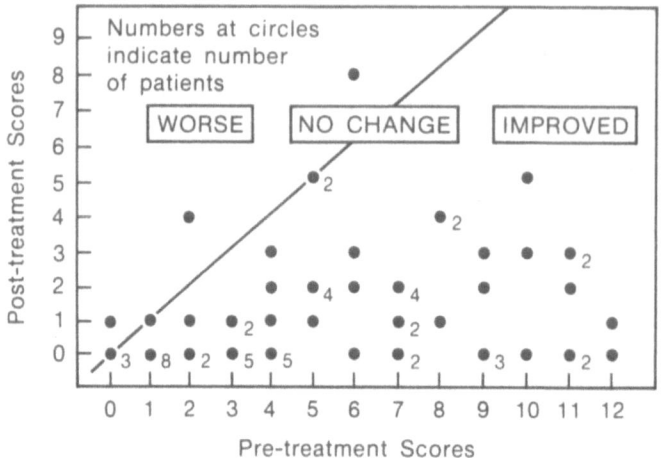

FIGURE 6. Scores of symptoms of endometriosis. Change from pretreatment values in individual patients treated with 400 µg/day of nafarelin (n = 70).

statistically significant (p<0.01) decrease in staging scores (Fig. 7). Some endometriotic foci completely disappeared. The percentage of patients who showed regression or arrest of spread

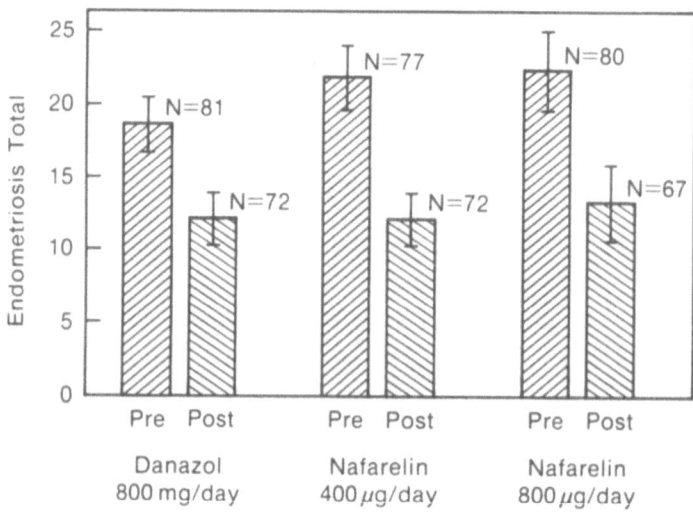

FIGURE 7. Pre- vs. post-treatment laparoscopic staging of endometriosis (American Fertility Society Classification) Mean ± S.E.

Table 1. Occurrence of pregnancy in endometriosis patients attempting to conceive following treatment with nafarelin or danazol.

	Treatment	No. of Pregnancies	Time to Pregnancy After Treatment Completion (Months)		
			Range	Mean	Median
1.	Danazol 800 mg/day	11	1-6	2.8	2
2.	Nafarelin 400 µg/day	12	1-8	4.6	4
3.	Nafarelin 800 µg/day	17	0-13	5.0	7

of endometriosis by laparoscopic examination was high for all three treatments.

Pregnancy following treatment

The ultimate proof of efficacy of therapy for endometriosis, at least in those patients presenting for infertility, is the occurrence of pregnancy after completion of treatment. So far, 40 patients have conceived: 11 who had received danazol; 12 after nafarelin at 400 µg per day and 17 after 800 µg per day of nafarelin.

Side effects

In general the side effects of nafarelin were indirect and due to induction of a pseudomenopause; side effects with danazol reflected its androgenic properties (Table 2). Hot flashes were the most prominent side effect. The incidence with nafarelin treatment was dose-related, being 76% and 92% for the lower and higher dose respectively. However, regardless of treatment regimen, hot flashes were well-tolerated by the patients.

Twice as many patients on danazol reported weight gain, edema or myalgia than on nafarelin. Seborrhea and hirsutism were somewhat more common for danazol. Vaginitis (due to hypoestrogenism) and rhinitis (associated with the nasal route of administration) were more frequent on nafarelin treatment.

A subpopulation of these patients has been evaluated for change in bone mineral content resulting from the hypoestrogenic state [23]. Twentytwo of the women treated with nafarelin (n = 14, 400 µg/day; n = 8, 800 µg/day) were compared to 13 women receiving danazol. Spinal trabecular bone mineral content was measured using the technique of quantitated computed tomography. Blinded evaluations were made at entry into the

Table 2. Incidence of side effects associated with nafarelin or danazol treatment of endometriosis.

Side Effects*	Treatment	
	Nafarelin**	Danazol†
Hot flashes	84%	39%
Weight gain	20%	52%
Edema	18%	36%
Myalgia	26%	47%
Seborrhea	16%	25%
Hirsutism	8%	13%
Vaginitis	18%	5%
Rhinitis	12%	4%

*Patients reporting side effects at any time of study.
**n = 155
†n = 80

study, at 3 and 6 months of treatment and 3 or 6 months after stopping therapy.

Bone mineral content was equivalent for all groups at entry. Six months of treatment with nafarelin caused loss of bone mineral content, but not in a dose-related fashion (7.7% and 6.9% for low and high dose, respectively). Patients on danazol gained an average of 4.2% over the course of treatment. Three months after stopping nafarelin, the decrease in bone mineral content was halved and in a small number of patients who have completed 6 months follow-up, bone recovery is essentially complete. It thus appears that the hypoestrogenism induced by nafarelin treatment, essential for the successful treatment of endometriosis, produces rapid bone loss (equivalent to that following ovariectomy) but that this loss is equally rapidly reversed after completion of the recommended course of treatment.

CONCLUDING REMARKS

The dependency of endometriosis on cyclical changes in ovarian steroids, particularly estradiol, makes suppression of ovarian steroidogenesis the appropriate therapeutic approach. Results of this and other studies have shown that the induction of a temporary hypogonadotropic-hypogonadism with LHRH agonists, such as nafarelin, is an effective treatment for remission of endometriosis with temporary side effects that occur as a consequence of their mechanism of action. The major side effect, hot flashes, rapidly disappears after completion of the therapy, and is well-tolerated by the patients, presumably weighed against the therapeutic benefit.

It appears that nafarelin administered by the nasal route provides a viable alternative to the current treatment modalities for endometriosis.

ACKNOWLEDGMENTS

This study was made possible by the dedicated work of the following investigators who rightfully are regarded as co-authors of this contribution.

Adamson, G. David	Palo Alto, CA
Ayers, Jonathan	Ann Arbor, MI
Bergquist, Christer	Falun, Sweden
Burry, Kenneth	Portland, OR
Buttram, Veasy C.	Houston, TX
Corson, Stephen L.	Philadelphia, PA
Coulam, Carolyn	
Field, Charles	Rochester, MN
Hale, Ralph	Honolulu, HI
Hanson, Fred	Davis, CA
Jacobson, Jan	Sodertalje, Sweden
Jones, Kirtly P.	Salt Lake City, UT
Moghissi, Kamran	Detroit, MI
Moore, Donald	Seattle, WA
Scommegna, Antonio	Chicago, IL
Soderstrom, Richard	Seattle, IL
Stewart, Gary	Sacramento, CA
Trobough, Gerald	Los Gatos, CA
Yuzpe, A. Albert	London, Ontario

The authors appreciate the contributions to this study of the:

Clinical Study Coordinator, Myrleen F. Fisher, RN and of

Biostaticians, Philip Carusi, MS and
                Long Kwei PhD,
                All of Syntex Research, Palo Alto, CA

REFERENCES

1. Barbieri, R.L. and Ryan, K.G. Danazol: endocrine pharmacology and therapeutic application. Am. J. Obstet. Gynecol., 141, 453 (1981)

2. Barbieri, R.L., Evans, S. and Kistner, R.W. Danazol in the treatment of endometriosis: analysis of 100 cases with a four year follow-up. Fertil. Steril., 37, 737 (1982)

3. Biberoglu, K.O. and Behrman, S.J. Dosage aspects of danazol therapy in endometriosis: short-term and long-term effectiveness. Am. J. Obstet. Gynecol., 139, 645 (1981)

4. Buttram, V.C., Jr., Belue, J.B. and Reiter, R. Interim report of a study of danazol for the treatment of endometriosis. Fertil. Steril., 37, 478 (1982)

5. Meldrum, D.R., Chang, R.J., Lu, J., Vale, W., Rivier, J. and Judd, H.L. "Medical oophorectomy" using a long-acting GnRH agonist: a possible new approach to the treatment of endometriosis. J. Clin. Endocrinol. Metab., 54, 1081 (1982)

6. Meldrum, D.R., Pardridge, W.M., Karow, W.G., Rivier, J., Vale, W. and Judd, H.L. Hormonal effects of danazol and medical oophorectomy in endometriosis. Obstet. Gynecol., 62, 480 (1983)

7. Shaw, R.W., Fraser, H.M. and Boyle, H. Intranasal treatment with luteinizing hormone-releasing hormone agonist in women with endometriosis. Brit. Med. J., 287, 1667 (1983)

8. Lemay, A., Maheux, R., Faure, N., Jean, C. and Fazekas, A.T.A. Reversible hypogonadism induced by a luteinizing hormone-releasing hormone (LH-RH) agonist (buserelin) as a new therapeutic approach for endometriosis. Fertil. Steril., 41, 863 (1984)

9. Pring, D.W., Maresh, M. and Fraser, A.C. Luteinizing hormone-releasing hormone agonist in women with endometriosis. Brit. Med. J., 287, 1718 (1983)

10. Steingold, K.A., Lu, J.K., Randle, D., Moore, J.G., Judd, H.L. and Meldrum, D.R. Treatment of endometriosis with a long-acting GnRH analog - a blinded evaluation. Proc. 32nd Ann. Meet. Soc. Gynec. Invest., Phoenix, Arizona (1985)

11. Zorn, J.R., Tanger, Ch., Roger, M., Grenier, J., Comaru-Schally, A.M. and Schally, A.V. Therapeutic hypogonadism induced by a delayed-release preparation of microcapsules of D-Trp-6-luteinizing hormone-releasing hormone: a preliminary study in eight women with endometriosis. Int. J. Fert., 31, 11 (1986)

12. Anonymous. LHRH analogues in endometriosis. Lancet, Nov. 1, 1016 (1986)

13. McLachlan, R.I., Healy, D.L. and Burger, H.G. Clinical aspects of LHRH analogues in gynaecology: a review. Brit. J. Obstet. Gynaecol., 93, 431 (1986)

14. Nillius, S.J., Bergquist, C. and Wide, L. Inhibition of ovulation in women by chronic treatment with a stimulatory LRH analogue. A new approach to birth control? Contraception, 17, 537 (1978)

15. Gudmundsson, J.A., Nillius, S.J. and Bergquist, C. Inhibition of ovulation by intranasal nafarelin: a new super-active agonist of GnRH. Contraception, 30, 107 (1984)

16. Brenner, P.F., Shoupe, D. and Mishell, D.R. Ovulation inhibition with nafarelin acetate administration for six months. Contraception, 32, 531 (1985)

17. Monroe, S.E., Blumenfeld, Z., Andreyko, J.L., Shriock, E., Henzl, M.R. and Jaffe, R.B. Dose-dependent inhibition of pituitary-ovarian function during administration of a GnRH agonistic analog (nafarelin). J. Clin. Endocrinol. Metab., 63, 1334 (1986)

18. Chiang, R-S., Barnes, R.B., Shoupe, D. and Lobo, R.A. Dose-related changes in LH bioactivity with intranasal GnRH agonist administration. Contraception, 32, 347 (1985)

19. Meldrum, D.R., Tsao, Z., Monroe, S.E., Braunstein, G.D., Sladek, J., Lu, J.K.H., Vale, W., Rivier, J., Judd, H.L. and Chang, R.J. Stimulation of LH fragments with reduced bioactivity following GnRH agonist administration in women. J. Clin. Endocrinol. Metab., 58, 755 (1984)

20. Shriock, E., Monroe, S.E., Henzl, M. and Jaffe, R.B. Treatment of endometriosis with a potent agonist of gonadotropin-releasing hormone (nafarelin). Fertil. Steril., 44, 583 (1985)

21. Henzl, M.R., Monroe, S.E. Carson, S.L. and Moghissi, K. Management of endometriosis with nasal dosing of a GnRH agonist-nafarelin. Endocrinology, 118, 26A (1986)

22. American Fertility Society: Classification of endometriosis. Fertil. Steril., 32, 633 (1979)

23. Cann, C.E., Henzl, M., Burry, K., Andreyko, J., Hanson, F., Adamson, D. and Trobough, G. Reversible bone loss is induced by GnRH agonists. Endocrinology, 118, 24A (1986)

23
Effects of Naferelin in
Precocious Puberty

J.L KIRKLAND and T.H. LIN
Department of Pediatrics, Baylor College of Medicine,
Houston, TX 77030, USA

INTRODUCTION

Pubertal development in children results from an activation of the
hypothalamic-pituitary-gonadal axis so that gonadal secretions produce secondary sexual development. The current concept of normal
pubertal development is that tonic inhibition from an unknown
neural pathway prevents activation of the hypothalamic-pituitary
axis during the prepubertal years [1]. Pubertal development then
results from a gradual diminishment of this inhibitory control.
Several investigators have suggested that the pineal gland may
be involved in the inhibition of the hypothalamic-pituitary axis
throughout childhood [2,3]. A recent report suggested that the
inhibitory substance might be melatonin [4,5]. The onset of physical signs of secondary sexual development may be the sequel of
numerous other subtle biochemical alterations such as changes in
biological potency of gonadotropins, nocturnal release of gonadotropins, and increase in amplitude and frequency of gonadotropin
release [1,6,7]. The subsequent activation of the gonad by peripheral LH and FSH is thought to proceed through membrane receptors
at the target organ. Adrenarche and pubarche in children are
activated in a manner similar to that of the pituitary release of
gonadotropins [1]. That is, the anterior pituitary gland releases
a hormone which causes the adrenal gland to secrete sex steroid
hormones. This hormone was isolated from dogs and humans recently
and is being investigated further [8].
  Precocious puberty is defined as the onset of secondary sexual
development in boys before nine or ten years of age and in girls
before eight years of age [9-11]. The etiology of precocious
puberty in many children is related to central nervous system damage, for example, that which might occur from acute trauma, infec-
tions, or tumors [9-11]. However, the etiology in most females
and some males is unknown. The puberty which results from activation and maturation of the hypothalamic-pituitary-gonadal axis is
defined as gonadotropin-dependent precocious puberty. Other forms
of precocious puberty may result from gonadotropin-independent processes such as familial precocious puberty or McCune-Albright
Syndrome.

The most significant effects of precocious puberty are the physiological sequelae of secondary sexual development (i.e., menses, breast development, pubic hair, axillary hair, and tall stature) in a child and the subsequent osseous maturation which occurs so that the bone age exceeds the chronologic age. Although the child is tall compared to peers during childhood, adult height frequently is diminished secondary to early osseous maturation. The adult heights reported in previous summaries were less than five feet in more than 50% of children with precocious puberty [12]. The most significant reduction in adult stature occurs when the onset of puberty starts at a very early age [12].

The major drugs which have been used to treat precocious puberty have included Depo-Provera, a long acting form of medroxyprogesterone, which is a progestational agent [13,14]; Cyproterone Acetate, an antiandrogen and antigonadotropic agent [15,16], and Danazol, an antigonadotropic agent [17]. The clinical results of these medications have produced a diminishment and regression of some signs of precocious puberty and menses. However, these drugs do not prevent premature closure of the epiphyses and subsequent short stature, and adverse side effects have been observed using these agents to treat precocious puberty in children [18-27].

Several years ago continuous infusion of LHRH was discovered to depress the secretion of pituitary gonadotropins [28]. The pharmacological properties of the LHRH agonistic analogues suggested that similar gonadotropin responses might occur when daily treatment with analogues was substituted for continuous infusion of LHRH [29].

These characteristics of LHRH analogues have led to their clinical use in females with breast cancer and males with prostatic carcinoma [30,31]. Another use of these agents has been for the treatment of precocious puberty [32-47].

The LHRH analogues administered in clinical studies have had numerous structural modifications in the native decapeptide. The first studies in children in the United States involved [D-Trp[6], Pro[9]-NHEt]LHRH [32]. The initial studies in children in Europe were performed with [D-Trp[6]]LHRH [34]. Two other compounds have been used subsequently by investigators in North America. These include [D-Ser(tBu)[6],Pro[9]-NHEt]LHRH, buserelin, and [D-Nal(2)[6]] LHRH, nafarelin. The increased biological potency and prolonged half life of some of these analogues have permitted administration by the intranasal route. This facilitates the use of the drug in children.

The information that follows summarizes our experience with nafarelin administered intranasally as treatment for gonadotropin dependent puberty and compares the results with other LHRH analogues. The average dose of nafarelin in these studies was 25 µg/kg administered in three divided dosages per day. Differences in our results from those of other investigators may be related to analogue structure, mode of administration, and dose. The results are preliminary in that long term evaluation must demonstrate a beneficial effect in final adult height and an absence of side effects.

EFFECTS OF NAFARELIN ON GONADOTROPINS

The effects of LHRH analogues on gonadotropins have been measured by several methods. Pescovitz et al. [45] have demonstrated that basal serum levels of gonadotropins are decreased following treatment with an analogue administered subcutaneously while Stanhope et al. [43] have demonstrated elevated basal levels using an analogue intranasally. Our results with nafarelin administered intranasally for six months do not reveal differences in pretreatment and treatment levels of gonadotropins obtained in the basal state for either sex. Another method used to assess the pharmacological actions of these analogues is stimulation of the pituitary gland to release LH and FSH using the native decapeptide, LHRH, while under treatment. Untreated children in advanced stages of puberty usually have a peak response within 60 minutes. However, the peak responses of LH and FSH to the native decapeptide are diminished following several months of treatment with the analogues [32,38,44-47]. We have utilized nafarelin itself as a stimulant to determine suppressability of the pituitary response following treatment. The peak responses of serum levels of LH and FSH are decreased significantly following treatment as indicated in Table 1.

Table 1. The effects of nafarelin on serum gonadotropin levels following analogue stimulation (200µg intranasally). Asterisk denotes statistical significance at p <.01.

	Pretreatment	Month 6
Females (n=15)		
Peak FSH (miu/ml)	19.4 ± 2.2	3.7 ± 0.5*
Peak LH (miu/ml)	53.0 ± 12.4	6.1 ± 0.8*
Males (n=3)		
Peak FSH (miu/ml)	5.8 ± .8	1 ± 0
Peak LH (miu/ml)	21.8 ± 8.2	5.7 ± 2.7

We have assessed also the effects of nafarelin on urinary gonadotropins. This method allowed us to avoid sampling errors which might exist with isolated determinations of serum LH and FSH. The results are depicted in Figure 1. The pretreatment levels of urinary gonadotropins were elevated for prepubertal children but decreased during treatment. The LH levels remained slightly above the prepubertal levels in both sexes at six months but the FSH levels returned to prepubertal values in both. The discrepancy between LH and FSH responses during treatment has been observed by others [44,46] measuring serum levels of gonadotropins. The cause is unknown.

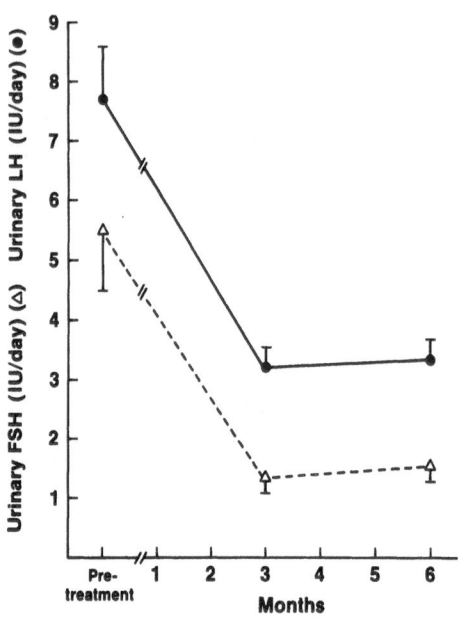

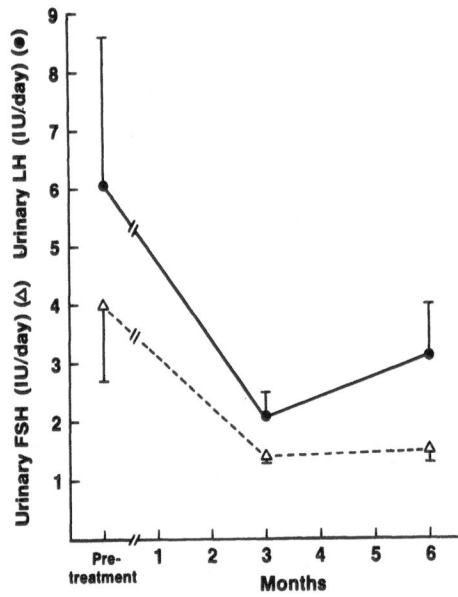

FIGURE 1   The effects of nafarelin on urinary gonadotropins in females (upper panel) and males (lower panel). Prepubertal levels of urinary LH are less than 3.0 IU/d while FSH are less than 2.4 IU/d. Levels of gonadotropins at 3 and 6 months differed statistically (p less than .01) from pretreatment levels. The data are expressed as the mean ±SEM.

The biological effects of intranasal nafarelin on gonadotropins may be assessed by measurements of testicular size. Figure 2 depicts the changes in testicular volume that occurred in males during one year of treatment. These results are similar to those which have utilized LHRH analogues by the subcutaneous route [45, 46].

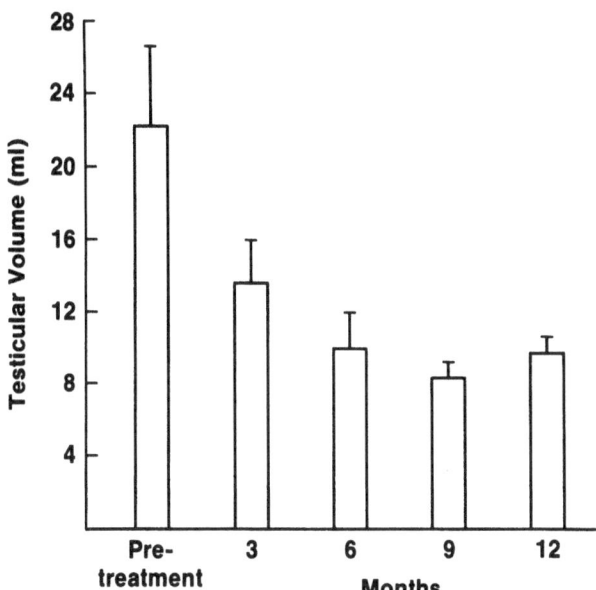

FIGURE 2   The effects of nafarelin on testicular volume after 12 months of treatment. Treatment values were statistically different (p less than .01) from pretreatment values. The data are expressed as the mean ± SEM.

EFFECTS OF NAFARELIN ON GONADAL SEX STEROIDS

The effects of LHRH analogues on the sex steroid hormones, estradiol and testosterone, have been impressive. Numerous investigators have demonstrated a rapid reduction in these hormones following treatment [35,44-47]. Figure 3 illustrates the changes in sex steroid hormones in children with precocious puberty when treated intranasally with nafarelin. Luder et al [38] used an analogue administered intranasally in female children with precocious puberty. The reduction in serum levels of estradiol were similar to those reported here but the levels were not reduced to prepubertal ones. Stanhope et al. [43] used an LHRH analogue intranasally but did not measure serum levels of estradiol. However, reductions were observed in the sizes of the uterus and ovary following treatment, implying a reduction in estradiol levels.

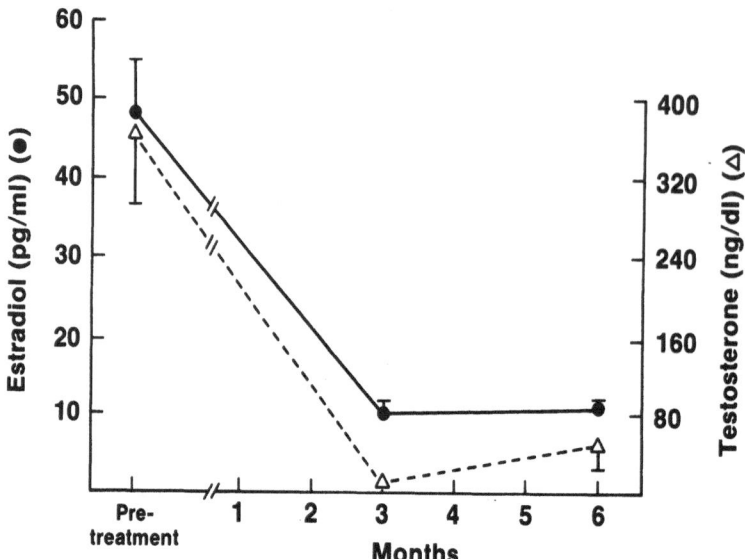

FIGURE 3   The effects of nafarelin on estradiol and testosterone
            levels. Prepubertal levels of estradiol are less than
            15 pg/ml while testosterone levels are less than 60 ng/
            dl. Levels during treatment differed statistically (p
            less than 0.1) from pretreatment levels. The data are
            expressed as the mean ±SEM.

        Other investigators have assessed the changes in the vaginal
mucosa following treatment [33-35]. This has been performed by
rating the degree of estrogenicity of the vaginal cells by the
vaginal maturation index (VMI). High scores signify more estrogen
effect whereas low scores indicate less estrogen effect. Figure
4 illustrates the effects of nafarelin on the VMI of children with
precocious puberty. Another method of assessing estrogen effect
is to measure the change in basal and parabasal cells. A higher
percentage would indicate a diminished effect of estrogen on the
target tissue. Figure 4 also indicates those changes. Breast
tissue decreased in girls treated subcutaneously with the analogues
[45]. However, our studies with nafarelin have revealed an arrest
of breast development but no significant regression as measured
by Tanner Staging.

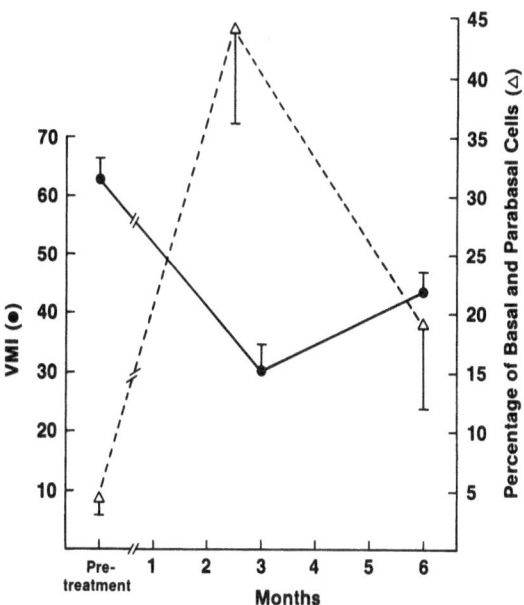

FIGURE 4   The effects of nafarelin on the vaginal cytology.   Values of the VMI and the percentage of basal and parabasal
cells differed statistically (p less than .01) from pretreatment values.   The data are expressed as the mean ±
SEM.

EFFECTS OF LHRH ANALOGUES ON GROWTH

Growth in children with precocious puberty is characterized by a
rapid growth velocity for chronologic age, advanced bone age for
chronologic age, and a shorter than normal adult height [9,11].
Previous treatment regimens frequently were able to diminish the
physical signs of puberty such as breast development and menses, but
growth and bone maturation continued at a rapid rate. LHRH analogues have altered the natural course of growth in children with precocious puberty in three ways, which are: a decrease in the rapid
growth velocity; a decrease in the rapid rate of osseous maturation,
and an increase in the predicted height after treatment. The biological mechanisms whereby these three changes occur are uncertain,
but may be secondary to the stimulatory effects that sex steroid
hormones have on growth hormone secretion and somatomedin formation.
The decrease in the rapid growth velocity may be explained by the
findings of Harris et al. [48] who demonstrated that children with
precocious puberty have values of somatomedin which are increased
for the degree of sexual development as well as the bone and chronologic age. The somatomedin levels decreased to levels consistent
with bone age and not chronologic age following treatment with LHRH

355

analogues. The growth velocity following treatment in most children
appears to correlate better with bone age as opposed to the chronologic age of the child. The effects of nafarelin treatment on
growth velocity are illustrated in Figure 5.

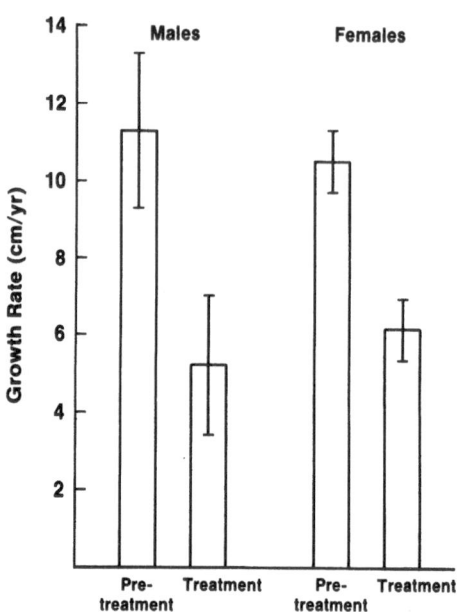

FIGURE 5   The effects of nafarelin on growth rates. Values were
determined for at least 6 months and expressed as yearly
rates. Values during treatment differed statistically
(p less than .01) from pre-treatment values. The data
are expressed as the mean ±SEM.

    The decrease in the rapid advancement of bone age has been ob-
served in several long term studies [33,45,48]. Most treated
children in these studies have bone age changes which are comparable
to the changes in their chronological age, or even less advancement
in bone age during long term therapy [33,45,48]. The effects of
intranasal nafarelin on the ratio of the change in bone age to the
change in chronological age during a one year treatment period was
.63 for females and .48 for males. The resulting decreased growth
rates and decreased degrees of osseous maturation have led to
changes in the predicted heights for treated children. Boepple et
al. [46] found an approximate 8 cm increase in predicted height,
while Mansfield et al. [35] have demonstrated an approximate 3 cm
increase in predicted height using an analogue administered subcutaneously. The changes in predicted height with nafarelin administration are demonstrated in Figure 6.

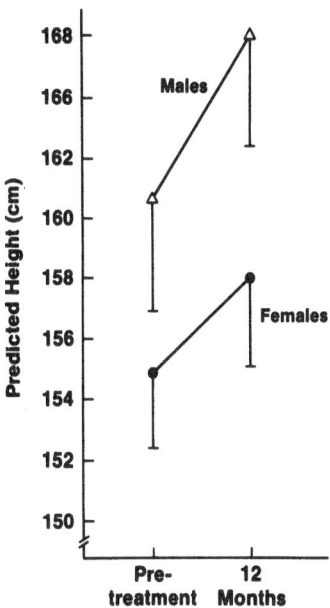

FIGURE 6   The effects of nafarelin on predicted heights following
            12 months of treatment.   The data are expressed as the
            mean ±SEM.

EFFECTS OF LHRH ANALOGUES ON NON-GONADAL SEX STEROID HORMONES, PUBARCHE, AND ADRENARCHE

The effects of LHRH analogues on adrenal secretory products have
been determined in children with precocious puberty. The possibility existed that peripheral effects of the analogues might alter the
production or secretion of sex steroid hormones by the adrenal
gland. However, the levels of dehydroepiandrosterone and delta 4
androstenedione in most females with precocious puberty have not
been altered, although some investigators have reported slight
changes [35,37,49]. The clinical effects of the LHRH analogues on
pubarche and adrenarche have been determined also. Most investigators report that the staging of pubic hair by the Tanner method
does not change, although some have reported mixed responses [35,37,
43]. The consensus appears to be that children with advanced pubarche and adrenarche continue to proceed with this aspect of their
sexual development, while those that do not have significant pubarche and adrenarche do not continue to develop. This aspect of
sexual development and effect of analogues has not been investigated
fully in males because of the difficulty in determining the source
of androgens.

EFFECTS ON CHILDREN WITH GONADOTROPIN INDEPENDENT PUBERTY

Gonadotropin-independent puberty includes forms of puberty which do not originate from stimulation of the gonads by gonadotropins in the classical manner. These include clinical entities such as McCune-Albright Syndrome and familial forms of precocious puberty in males. Several investigators have reported their findings in children with gonadotropin-independent precocious puberty in which attempts have been made to treat with the LHRH analogues. As expected, the results have indicated that this form of precocious puberty does not respond to treatment with LHRH analogues [50,51].

SIDE EFFECTS

Side effects have been minimal to non-existent in most children treated with the analogues. Some children have experienced vaginal bleeding for several days probably secondary to estrogen withdrawal [33,44,46]. Our studies using nafarelin have included an assessment of urinary, hematological, and liver function studies. No abnormalities have been recorded.

SUMMARY AND CONCLUSIONS

Treatment of gonadotropin-dependent precocious puberty in children has been complicated previously because of a lack of medications which would permit a child to obtain genetically determined adult height. The initial studies of LHRH analogues suggest that they may be effective in preventing adult short stature in children with precocious puberty as well as decreasing or stabilizing the signs of puberty. The analogues produce a reduction in the biological effects of gonadotropins, probably through a reduction of their secretion or a lack of periodicity, as well as a reduction in the secretion of gonadal sex steroid hormones. They also produce a reduction in the growth velocity and rate of osseous maturation. The preliminary data suggest that final adult height will be greater. Further studies are required to document the long term safety and effects of these new drugs and to determine if these analogues will be useful in other situations such as delaying puberty in children with genetic short stature.

ACKNOWLEDGEMENTS

This research was supported by NIH MO1 RR00188 and FD-R-000097. The authors would like to thank Mrs. Jana Grana for secretarial support.

358

REFERENCES

1. Grumbach, M.M. The neuroendocrinology of puberty. Hosp. Pract., 15, 51 (1980).
2. Ariens-Kappers, F. A survey of advances in pineal research. In "The Pineal: Anatomy and Biochemistry", R.J. Reiter (Ed.), CRC Press, Boca Raton, 1981, p. 1.
3. Kitay, J.I. Pineal lesions and precocious puberty: a review. J. Clin. Endocrinol Metab., 14, 622 (1954).
4. Silman, R.E., Leone, R.M., Hooper, R.L., and Preece, M.A. Melatonin, the pineal gland and human puberty. Nature, 282, 301 (1979).
5. Waldhauser, F., Weiszenbacher, G., Frisch, H., Zeitlhuber, U., Waldhauser, M., and Wurtman, R.J. Fall in nocturnal serum melanbuin during prepuberty and pubescence. Lancet, 1, 362 (1984).
6. Eisenberg, E. Toward an understanding of reproductive function in anorexia nervosa. Fertil. Steril., 36, 543 (1981).
7. Styne, D.M., Kaplan, S.L., and Greenbach, M.M. Plasma glycoprotein hormone-subunit in the neonate and in prepubertal and pubertal children: Effects of luteinizing hormone-releasing hormone. J. Clin. Endocrinol. Metab., 50, 450 (1980).
8. Parker, L.N., Lifrak, E.T., and Odel, W.D. A 60,000 molecular weight human pituitary glycopeptide stimulates adrenal androgen secretion. Endocrinology, 113: 2092 (1983).
9. Wilkins, L. "The Diagnosis and Treatment of Endocrine Disorders in Childhood and Adolescence," 3rd ed., Charles C. Thomas, Springfield, IL, 1965.
10. Seckel, H.P.G. Precocious sexual development in children. M. Clin. North Am., 30, 183 (1946).
11. Sigurjonsdotter, T.T., and Hayles, A.B. Precocious puberty (A Report of 96 Cases). Am. J. Dis. Child., 115, 309 (1968).
12. Cloutier, M.D., and Hayles, A.B. Precocious puberty. Adv. Pediatr., 17, 125 (1970).
13. Kuppermann, H.S., and Epstein, J.A. Medroxyprogesterone acetate in the treatment of constitutional sexual precocity. J. Clin. Endocrinol. Metab., 22, 456 (1962).
14. Kaplan, S.A., Ling, S.M., and Irani, N.G. Idiopathic isosexual precocity (Therapy with Medroxyprogesterone). Am. J. Dis. Child., 116, 591 (1968).
15. Rager, K., Huenger, R., Gusta, D., and Bierich, J.R. The treatment of precocious puberty with cyproterone acetate. Acta. Endocrinol., 74, 399 (1973).
16. Werder, E.A., Murset, G., Zachmann, M., Brook, C.G.D., and Prader, A. Treatment of precocious puberty with cyproterone acetate. Pediatr. Res., 8, 248 (1974).
17. Lee, P.A., Thompson, R.G., Migeon, C.J., and Blizzard, R.M. The effect of danozol in sexual precocity. Johns Hopkins Med. J., 137, 265 (1975).
18. Smith, C.S., Harris, F. Preliminary experience with danazol in children with precocious puberty. J. Int. Med. Res., 5: Suppl. 3, 109 (1977).
19. Richman, R.A., Underwood, L.E., French, F.S., and Van Wyk, J.J. Adverse effects of large doses of medroxyprogesterone (MPA) in Idiopathic Isosexual Precocity. J. Pediatr., 79, 963 (1971).

20. Lemli L., Aron, M., and Smith, D.W. The action of depo-provera in 3 girls with idiopathic isosexual precocity: decrease in estrogen effect without urinary gonadotropin reduction. J. Pediatr., 65, 888 (1964).

21. Sadeghi-Nejad, A., Kaplan S.L., and Grumbach, M.M. The effect of medroxyprogesterone acetate on adrenocortical function in children with precocious puberty. J. Pediatr., 78, 616, 1971.

22. Smith, C.S., and Harris, F. The role of danazol in the management of precocious puberty. Postgrad. Med. J., 55, Suppl. 5, 81 (1979).

23. Mathews, J.H., Abrams, C.A.L., and Morishima, A. Pituitary-adrenal function in ten patients receiving medroxyprogesterone acetate for true precocious puberty. J. Clin. Endocrinol. Metab., 30, 653 (1970).

24. Camacho, A.M., Williams, D.L., and Montalvo, J.M. Alterations of testicular histology and chromosomes in patients with constitutional sexual precocity treated with medroxyprogesterone acetate. J. Clin. Endocrinol. Metab., 34, 279 (1972).

25. Jeffcote, W.J., Edwards, C.R.W., Rees, L.H., and Besser, G.M. Cyproterone acetate. Lancet, 2, 1140 (1976).

26. Von Muhlendahl, K.E., Korth-Schutz, S., Muller-Hess, R., Helge, H., and Weber, B. Cyproterone acetate and adrenocortical function. Lancet, 1, 1160 (1977).

27. Heinz, F., Teller, W.M., Fehm, H.L., and Joos, A. The effect of cyproterone acetate on adrenal corticol function in children with precocious puberty. Eur. J. Pediatr., 128, 81 (1978).

28. Rabin, D., and McNeil, L.W. Pituitary and gonadal desensitization after continuous luteinizing hormone-releasing hormone infusion in normal females. J. Clin. Endocrinol. Metab., 51, 873 (1980).

29. Linde, R., Soelle, G.C., Alexander, N., Kirchner, F., Vale, W., Rivier, J., and Rabin, D. Reversible inhibition of testicular steroidogenesis by a potent gonadotropin-releasing hormone agonist in normal man. An approach toward the development of a male contraceptive. N. Engl. J. Med., 305, 663 (1981).

30. Labrie, F., Belanger, A., Cusan, L., Seguin, C., Pelletier, G., Kelly, P.A., Lefebvre, F.A., Lemay, A., and Raynaud, J.P. Antifertility effects of LHRH agonists in the male. J. Androl., 1, 209 (1980).

31. Harvey, H.A., Lipton, A., and Max, D.T. LHRH analogs for human mammary carcinoma. In "LHRH and Its Analogs: Contraceptive and Therapeutic Applications," B.H. Vickery, J.J. Nestor, Jr., and E.S.E. Hafez (Eds.), MTP Press, Boston, 1984, p. 329.

32. Crowley, W.F., Comite, F., Vale, W., Rivier, J., Loriaux, D.L., and Cutler, G.B. Therapeutic use of pituitary desensitization with a long-acting LHRH agonist: A potential new treatment for idopathic precocious puberty. J. Clin. Endocrinol. Metab., 52, 370 (1981).

33. Comite, F., Cutler, G.B., Rivier, J., Vale, W., Loriaux, D.L., and Crowley, W.F. Short-term treatment of idiopathic precocious puberty with a long-acting analogue of luteinizing-releasing hormone. N. Engl. J. Med., 305, 1546 (1981).

34. Laron, Z., Kauli, R., Zeev, Z.B., Comaru-Schally, A.M., and Schally, A.V. D-TRP[6]-analogue of luteinising hormone-releas-

ing hormone in combination with cyproterone acetate to treat precocious puberty. Lancet, <u>2</u>, 955 (1981).

35. Mansfield, M.J., Beardsworth, D.E., Loughlin, J.S., Crawford, J.D., Bode, H.H. Rivier, J., Vale, W., Kushner, D.C., Crigler, J.F., and Crowley, W.F. Long-term treatment of central precocious puberty with a long-acting analogue of luteinizing hormone-releasing hormone. N. Engl. J. Med., <u>309</u>, 1286 (1983).

36. Beardsworth, D., Wierman, M., Mansfield, J., Crawford, J., Crigler, J., Bode, H., Kushner, D., and Crowley, W. Use of an LHRH agonist in the treatment of males with central precocious puberty. Pediatr. Res., <u>18</u>, 164A (Abstract) (1984).

37. Kauli, R., Pertzelan, A., Ben-Zeev, Z., Prager Lewin, R., Kaufman, H., Comaru Schally, A.M., Schally, A.V., and Laron, Z. Treatment of precocious puberty with LHRH analogue in combination with cyproterone acetate - further experience. Clin. Endocrinol. (Oxf), <u>20</u>, 377 (1984).

38. Luder, A.S., Holland, F.J., Costigan, D.C., Jenner, M.R., Weilgosz, G., and Fazeekas, ATA. Internasal and subcutaneous treatment of central precocious puberty in both sexes with a longacting analog of luteinizing hormone-releasing hormone. J. Clin. Endocrinol. Metab., <u>58</u>, 966 (1984).

39. Comite, F., Pescovitz, O.H., Reith, K.G. Dwyer, A.J., Hench, K., McNemar, A., Loriaux, D.L, and Cutler, G.B. Leutinizing hormonereleasing hormone analog treatment of boys with hypothalamic hamartoma and true precocious puberty. J. Clin. Endocrinol. Metab., <u>59</u>, 888 (1984).

40. Lin, T., LePage, M.E., Henzl, M., Kirkland, J.L. Intranasal LHRH analogue treatment of idiopathic central precocious puberty in Girls. Pediatr Res., <u>19</u>, 633 (Abstract) (1985).

41. Beyer, P., Eibs, H., Schmidt-Gollwitzer, M., Weber, B., and Helge, H. Intranasal treatment of precocious puberty (PP) with a long-acting LH-RH analogue. Pediatr. Res., <u>19</u>, 634 (Abstract) (1985).

42. Stephure, D.K., Silverman, B.L., Conte, F.A., Rosenthal, S.M., Kaplan, S.L., and Grumbach, M.M. Treatment of precocious puberty (TPP) with an intranasal (IN) luteinizing hormone releasing factor (LRF) agonist (A). Pediatr. Res., <u>19</u>, 193A (Abstract), 1985.

43. Stanhope, R., Adams, J., and Brook, C.G.D. The treatment of central precocious puberty using an intranasal LHRH analogue (Buserelin). Clin. Endocrinol., <u>22</u>, 795 (1985).

44. Styne, D.M., Harris, D.A., Egli, C.K., Conte, F.A., Kaplan, S.L., Rivier, J., Vale, W., and Grumbach, M.M. Treatment of true precocious puberty with a potent luteinizing hormone-releasing factor agonist: effect on growth, sexual maturation, pelvic sonography, and hypothalamic-pituitary-gonadal axis. J. Clin. Endocrinol. Metab., <u>61</u>, 142 (1985).

45. Pescovitz, O.H., Comite, F., Hench, K., Barnes, K., McNemar, A., Foster, C., Kenigsberg, D., Loriaux, D.L., and Cutler, G.B. The NIH experience with precocious puberty: diagnostic subgroups and response to short-term luteinizing hormone releasing hormone analogue therapy. J. Pediatr., <u>108</u>, 47 (1985).

46. Boepple, P.A., Mansfield, M.J., Wierman, M.E., Rudlin, C.R., Bode, H.H., Crigler, J.F., Jr., Crawford, J.D., and Crowley, W.F. Use of a potent, long acting agonist of gonadotropin-releasing hormone in the treatment of precocious puberty. Endocr. Rev., 7, 24 (1986).

47. Comite, F., Cassorla, F., Barnes, K.M., Hench, K.D., Dwyer, A., Skerda, M.C., Loriaux, D.L., Cutler, G.B., and Pescovitz, O.H. Luteinizing hormone releasing hormone analogue therapy for central precocious puberty. JAMA, 255, 2613 (1986).

48. Harris, D.A., Vliet, G.V., Egli, C.A., Grumbach, M.M., Kaplan, S.L., Styre, D.M., and Vainsel, M. Somatomedin-C in normal puberty and in true precocious puberty before and after treatment with a potent luteinizing hormone-releasing hormone agonist. J. Clin. Endocrinol. Metabol., 61, 152 (1985).

49. Wierman, M., Beardsworth, D., Crawford, J., Crigler, J., Bode, H., Kushner, D., and Crowley, W. Adrenarche and growth during LHRH administration. Pediatr. Res., 18, 179A (Abstract), 1984.

50. Wierman, M.E., Beardsworth, D.E., Mansfield, M.J., Badger, T.M., Crawford, J.D., Crigler, J.F., Bode, H.H., Loughlin, J.S., Kushner, D.C., Scully, R.E., Hoffman, W.H., and Crowley, W.F. Puberty without gonadotropins. A unique mechanism of sexual development. N. Engl. J. Med., 312, 65 (1985).

51. Comite, F., Shawker, T.H., Pescovitz, O.H., Loriaux, D.L., and Cutler, G.B. Cyclical ovarian function resistant to treatment with an analogue of luteinizing hormone-releasing hormone in McCune-Albright syndrom. N. Engl. J. Med., 311, 1032 (1984).

24

Pharmacokinetics, Metabolism and Clinical Studies with Buserlin

J. SANDOW, and W. Von RECHENBERG

Hoechst Ag, Pharmacology H 821, D-6230 Frankfurt/Main 80,
Federal Republic of Germany.

INTRODUCTION

LHRH agonists are a new group of antigonadotrophic agents with
highly specific action on the gonadal system, a remarkable biological tolerance, absence of serious side effects, and a wide spectrum
of clinical indications [1, 2]. The LHRH agonist studied by our
group, [D-Ser(tBu)[6],Pro[9]-NHEt]LHRH (buserelin) was synthetized in
1974, and has been investigated as a peptide contraceptive [3-5], in
oestrogen-dependent disorders such as endometriosis and leiomyoma
uteri [6, 7], in the endocrine management of hormone-dependent
tumours [8-11], and in precocious puberty [12, 13].

PRECLINICAL STUDIES

Pituitary suppression

The preclinical studies on mechanisms of action in experimental animals were performed to develop optimal treatment regimens. Single
daily doses (14-28 days s.c.) in rats, dogs, guinea pigs and monkeys
induced a reduction in the secretory capacity for testosterone, or
inappropriate ovulation and luteolysis. The reasons were partial desensitization of LH release, and effects on gonadal receptors in the
testes or ovary [14, 15]. Buserelin binds to pituitary receptors
with high affinity leading to high and sustained concentrations in
anterior pituitary tissue. An increased plasma level is maintained
by resistance to enzyme degradation [16, 17]. Buserelin binding [20]
initiates the internalization of hormone-receptor complexes and
causes a loss of receptors by intracellular proteolysis, which cannot be compensated by de novo synthesis of receptor protein. Pituitary desensitization and receptor loss explain the suppression of
oestrogen- and testosterone secretion in hormone-dependent tumours
[18, 20]. There are marked differences in the species response to
buserelin, depending on factors such as the length of the ovarian
cycle, sensitivity of the corpus luteum, the rate of metabolism, and
the persistence of intact buserelin in the circulation. The predomi-

nant site of action during sustained release of buserelin [18, 20, 21] is pituitary desensitization followed by inhibition of gonadotrophin secretion and synthesis. Due to its slow rate of inactivation, buserelin acts like a desensitizing LHRH infusion.

Effects on steroidogenesis

Submaximal gonadotrophin release after buserelin injection reduces the testicular LH/hCG receptors. This inhibition of the secretory capacity of the Leydig cells is supported by secondary mechanisms enhancing the decrease in testosterone secretion. In rats, a local regulatory system in the Leydig cells is physiologically responsive to LHRH-like peptide factors secreted by the Sertoli cells [20, 27]. This paracrine system participates in the antifertility effects of buserelin, but the evidence for similar mechanisms in the human is controversial [19, 28]. A direct action of buserelin on steroidogenic enzymes in the testes has been established in rats. During long-term treatment by injection, the capacity to secrete testosterone is severely restricted, whereas the secretory capacity for progesterone is markedly enhanced. Such changes in the ratio of C_{21}/C_{19}-steroids after single dose treatment with LHRH, buserelin or hCG and have been referred to as steroidogenic lesions [17, 20]. Androgen biosynthesis is disrupted at the level of the 17-hydroxylase and 17,20-desmolase. Progesterone becomes the major product of steroidogenesis, and there is also an increased formation of 5-alpha-pregnane-3,20-dione, a progesterone metabolite inhibiting the activity of the 17,20-desmolase [15] in a similar way as progesterone. To obtain consistent changes in the ratio of C_{21}/C_{19}-steroids, buserelin injections must be administered daily. Treatment twice per week activates rather than reduces testosterone secretion. The initial testosterone stimulation in male animals can be neutralized by an androgen receptor blocker during the first week of buserelin treatment. This procedure significantly accelerates the weight decrease of the androgen-dependent organs.

Inhibition of spermatogenesis

The treatment with LHRH agonists inhibits spermatogenesis and testosterone secretion [21, 26]. With regard to precocious puberty, it is not known whether long-term treatment will impair fertility at adulthood. As an animal model for temporary inhibition of sexual development, we treated rats at an early stage of sexual maturation with daily injections or infusions of buserelin (5 µg/day s.c.). Weight development of androgen-dependent organs was markedly retarded, and these rats were unable to mate with females. The secretory capacity for testosterone in vitro was very low. After treatment, the rats underwent normal sexual maturation and had all become fertile within 8-16 weeks. Despite focal areas of tubular atrophy, in about 5 % of tubules examined, transient inhibition of sexual maturation in male rats does not impair development of spermatogenesis and subsequent fertility [22].

In adult rats, after submaximal gonadotrophin stimulation by hCG, LHRH or buserelin, acute histological changes are found, characterized by increased capillary permeability, local exudation, oedema, and the appearance of multinucleated giant cells [15]. Such changes may be related to acutely increased testicular temperature, they are also found in rats with experimental cryptorchidism. Buserelin has a local effect on testicular blood flow and capillary permeability both in intact rats, and in hypophysectomized rats [23]. The adult rat displays a reaction to prolonged buserelin treatment different from that of other species. After daily buserelin injections (2.5-12.5/ug/kg s.c.) for 6-12 months, there is a gradual reduction in fertility. and partial inhibition of spermatogenesis, with focal areas of tubules devoid of germinal epithelium. At high buserelin doses (300-500/ug/kg s.c. once daily) the germinal epithelium may entirely disappear, only Sertoli cells remaining. At lower doses (2.5-12.5/ug/kg s.c.), marked Leydig cell hyperplasia is induced [15], similar to the effect of daily hCG injections [24]. This histological reaction may be due to incomplete pituitary suppression. The buserelin-induced changes are associated with a fibrous induration in the atrophic testes. In contrast to spermatogenesis, Leydig cell function recovers completely even after 12 months of treatment, and the steroidogenic lesion disappears. Inhibition of spermatogenesis by buserelin is fully reversible in the dog [25], the monkey [21], and in humans after 12 weeks of treatment by infusion with a daily dose of 118-230/ug [26]. In adult rats, spermatogenesis does not recover completely after long-term treatment. These species differences may be due to different intratesticular paracrine regulatory mechanisms. The rat has testicular LHRH receptors with high binding affinity, which regulate steroidogenesis even after hypophysectomy [27] whereas such receptors and actions have not been found in the human testes [19, 28].

Suppression of ovarian function

When buserelin is given by daily injections to juvenile or adult rats, reduced uterine weight is explained by inappropriate ovulation, with a predominance of corpora lutea. The oestrogen secretion is reduced by a decrease in the number of follicles, because ovulation and luteinization are accelerated. When buserelin infusions (5/ug/day) are administered starting at 35 days of age, pituitary function is inhibited as demonstrated by the extremely low gonadotrophin tissue content. The weight development of the uterus and the ovaries is retarded, and a true delay of sexual maturation is achieved. After treatment, the pubertal development is resumed, and all previously treated rats become fertile. The therapeutic results in precocious puberty [78] indicate that sexual development is inhibited by injections, and by multiple daily doses of the buserelin nasal spray [13, 29, 77]. The rat model does not reflect the therapeutic situation, because a high dose injection of buserelin can induce ovulation of immature follicles at any time of the oestrus cycle and even during pregnancy.

A reliable approach to ovarian suppression is the sustained release of buserelin [30, 34]. In adult rats, infusion (5/ug/day

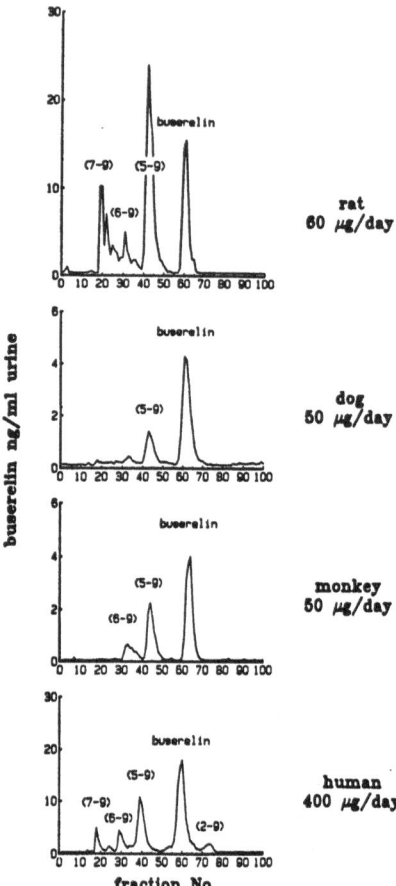

FIGURE 1 Urinary metabolites of buserelin in the rat, dog, monkey
and human. Separation by HPLC and determination by specific radioimmunoassay for buserelin.

s.c. for 14 days) greatly reduced the pituitary content of LH and
FSH, and indirectly (by suppression of oestrogen secretion), lowered
the content of growth hormone and prolactin. Buserelin implants suppressed proliferation of the vaginal epithelium and endometrium, and
reduced weight of the uterus and ovaries to low levels [31]. A luteolytic potential has been discussed for many LHRH agonists [32].
In immature rats primed with gonadotrophins (PMSG and hCG), buserelin induced luteolysis, and a post-coital contraceptive effect was
observed in adult rats and rabbits. No teratogenicity was found, but
the animals had an increased incidence of fetal resorption, due to
the luteolytic effect.

Studies on inhibition of ovulation were performed in adult
female guinea pigs exposed to fertile males for 90 days. The animals
were protected from pregnancy by 4-16/ug/kg buserelin per day
(s.c.). Suppression of ovarian function was investigated in monkeys.
The results are similar to the contraceptive effects confirmed in
the human, but significant differences in the dose-requirement are
found. The sensitivity to buserelin suppression is lower in monkeys

366

than in humans. In female stumptail macaques (macaca arctoides), buserelin 4/ug daily (s.c.) suppressed ovulation in the majority of animals, but did not prevent intermittent oestradiol increases. In some monkeys, the antiovulatory dose had to be increased to 20/ug per day (s.c.) for a consistent effect. The contraceptive effect was rapidly reversible, oestradiol rises and ovulatory cycles with appropriate progesterone elevations occurred within 30-50 days after treatment. There were no secondary hormonal effects on thyroid or adrenal function [33]. The suppression during sustained release of buserelin is related to the consistent reduction in pituitary LHRH receptor binding capacity. During buserelin infusion (50/ug/day s.c.), follicular maturation was blocked for periods of 90 days [34]. Implantations of minipumps during the luteal phase of the cycle, when follicular maturation for the next cycle is about to begin, caused only a small rise in oestradiol. When implantations were delayed until the early follicular phase, the initial oestradiol stimulation was much more pronounced. This indicates that in endometriosis, the treatment should start during the luteal phase when the undesirable endometrial activation is minimal.

Pharmacokinetics and metabolism

The enhanced suppressive potential of buserelin in comparison with LHRH (gonadorelin) is explained by the low rate of inactivation of buserelin in vivo. In rats, studies with ^{125}I-buserelin indicate a long-lasting accumulation in pituitary tissue (biological target organ), and an increased accumulation of ^{125}I-labelled metabolites in liver and kidney. Inactivation by pyroglutamyl-peptidase, chymotrypsin-like enzymes and neutral endopeptidases results in the formation of biologically inactive metabolites, which were identified in organ tissues, and in serum or urine. Serum and urine concentrations of buserelin are measured by highly specific radioimmunoassay procedures. The serum concentrations reached during LHRH infusion under steady state conditions are low, and only a small fraction of immunoreactive LHRH is found in the urine. The serum concentrations of buserelin during infusion are much higher, elimination after the end of infusion is prolonged ($T_{1/2}$ 60-80 min). After buserelin infusion, 25-30 % of the dose are found in the urine of rats, in comparison with 0.002 % of the dose after infusion of LHRH. Intact buserelin and buserelin metabolites in serum and urine can be separated by high performance liquid chromatography (HPLC), and radioimmunoassay (RIA) with a specific buserelin antiserum as the detection method. This antiserum (AS-639) detects intact buserelin and all C-terminal metabolites including the (7-9)tripeptide. Serum protein binding of buserelin is about 15 %, whereas a much higher protein binding has been reported for nafarelin. The rates of absorption from different drug formulations and sites of administration, and the drug concentrations during treatment with sustained release formulations were determined [16, 35, 36]. Serum concentrations of buserelin were detectable after injection of 15/ug i.v. After buserelin 500-1000/ug s.c., the serum concentration reached a maximum after 30-60 min and remained detectable for 6-8 hours, the half-life estimate was 75-85 min. During maintenance therapy with buserelin nasal spray, the urinary excretion of immunoreactive buserelin was dose-related, 3 x 300/ug to 8 x 300/ug/day [16, 31]. In long-term treatment by infusions or implants, the daily release rate was conveniently monitored by the urinary buserelin excretion. The urinary buserelin/creatinine ratio was dose-dependent during infusion of 50-400/ug/day in women, and provided reference values for the evaluation of sustained release formulations.

The metabolism of buserelin in different species was evaluated by the pattern of urinary metabolites (Fig. 1). In the rat, buserelin is metabolized to a higher extent than in the dog, monkey and human. The metabolites found in serum and in the urine are similar, consisting of intact buserelin together with smaller peaks of the (5-9)pentapeptide, (6-9)tetrapeptide, and (7-9)tripeptide. In the serum of dogs, and in human serum there is almost entirely intact buserelin (90-95 %), and a small fraction of the (5-9)pentapeptide. In rat serum, much higher amounts of the (5-9)pentapeptide are circulating. This correlates with the rapid loss of biological activity in rat serum after buserelin injection, whereas the decrease of the immunoreactive buserelin is more delayed. In the urine, the fraction of intact buserelin in the rat was 22.5 %, whereas in the dog, 70.2 % were identified as intact buserelin. Conversely, the main metabolite of buserelin, the (5-9)pentapeptide was present to 44.2 % in the rat urine, and to 22.4 % in the urine of dogs. Excretion of buserelin metabolites in bile is much higher than excretion of immunoreactive LHRH after a similar dose, the material consists almost exclusively of the biologically inactive (5-9)pentapeptide. High bile/serum ratios of 60-80 are reached indicating an active secretion process. The fraction excreted with bile does not contribute to the serum concentration by enterohepatic circulation.

CLINICAL STUDIES

When the potential of LHRH agonists for treatment of steroid-dependent disorders was recognized in 1975, studies on pituitary desensitization in women, and in men indicated, that the suppressive effect on gonadotrophin secretion was independent of the presence of the gonads [1]. The therapeutic requirements were adjusted by selecting different dose ranges and regimens depending on the clinical objectives. The early availability of nasal spray formulations for LHRH and buserelin was a significant improvement for long-term therapy [36]. In the contraceptive trials, the principle of suppressing ovulation in a reversible manner was established by injection studies at doses of 5-10/ug/day s.c. [37]. It was recognized that such regimens would only be practical with self-administered contraceptive medication using the nasal spray formulation.

Contraception

The antigonadotrophic and contraceptive potential of LHRH agonists has attracted much attention because male and male reproduction are susceptible to the reversible suppression of pituitary function [25, 38, 39]. The advantage of this approach is the excellent biological tolerance and absence of side effects, which makes LHRH agonists preferable for indications of medical contraception, where oestrogen-containing steroid preparations have an increased risk or where drug interactions limit efficacy of oral contraceptives. The suppression of pituitary responsiveness in normal women [3] suggested several contraceptive regimens. A practical approach is to control ovulation by administering a buserelin nasal spray once daily beginning with menstruation as the natural index of ovarian cyclicity. This "continuous" regimen is effective [4], but the absence of luteal progesterone rises requires secretory transformation of the endometrium by a progestagen to establish a regular bleeding pattern. Reduction of pituitary sensitivity by the buserelin nasal spray requires several days. Follicles which begin to develop during the preceding luteal phase are stimulated and an initial oestrogen rise is found, which corresponds to the normal physiology of the menstrual cycle and constitutes a protective mechanism against the development of osteoporosis. This contraceptive regimen is "discontinuous", with intervals of 7 days between treatment cycles of 21 days, and a progestagen medication between days 16-21.

Two bioequivalent nasal spray formulations have been used (300 or 400/ug/day). In early studies, the 400/ug nasal spray was administered daily for more than 200 days. Treatment was well accepted and consistent inhibition of ovulation was achieved [3, 4, 41]. There is a wide range of ovarian responses to pituitary suppression. In one group of women, the contraceptive medication with buserelin may induce prolonged periods of low oestrogen secretion and early amenorrhoea. A second group of women responds with intermittent oestrogen rises and a third group with relatively high oestradiol responses. The individual susceptibility to pituitary-ovarian suppression became apparent in many studies with uninterrupted daily administration. Bleeding patterns were unpredictable, although dysfunctional uterine bleeding was not observed [4, 38, 41]. The oestradiol levels decreased gradually, and the endometrial changes ranged from atrophy to mild hyperplasia, which remained within the range of endometrial changes observed during the normal menstrual cycle [4]. The occurrence of hot flushes during buserelin contraception was highly variable. Some authors reported transient hot flushes in 20 % of users, whereas in other studies, the contraceptive regimen was well tolerated without subjective symptoms of oestrogen deficiency. This problem may depend on the subjective evaluation in the clinical interview. Experience with high dose buserelin regimens in endometriosis indicates, that hot flushes decrease with time of use, and may respond to transient low dose clonidine medication. Buserelin nasal spray contraception was well accepted, the women using this method were willing to continue with their regimen. Regimens with progestagen medication to achieve regular secretory transformation of the endometrium ("discontinuous" peptide contraception) have used the buserelin nasal spray (300/ug/day) from day 1-21 of the menstrual cycle. The progestagen dose and treatment period are adjusted to ensure secretory transformation [5, 42, 43]. The dose requirements may be lower than in menopausal women, where a pharmacological oestrogen dose to prevent osteoporosis has to be balanced against the progestagen dose. Studies have been performed with norethisterone acetate [42] and with medroxyprogesterone ace tate [5]. The period of 7 days without buserelin medication between two cycles allows for maturation of follicles, which are then exposed to gonadotrophin stimulation during the next cycle. These oestrogen rises decrease with progressive time of medication, but remain sufficient to ensure prostagen-induced bleeding [43].

A critical aspect of the contraceptive efficacy is to administer the nasal spray for a sufficient period to ensure pituitary suppression. In a regimen of 1-2 weeks, follicular maturation is only transiently inhibited and delayed ovulation may occur [44]. Attempts to disrupt follicular development by short-term treatment are unreliable, because a sufficient reduction in pituitary sensitivity to endogenous LHRH is only achieved after 7-10 days of daily use. Contraception by a buserelin nasal spray without a progestagen may have its importance in post-partum contraception, where a steroid compound is undesirable because of its excretion into mother's milk and absorption by the infant. Preliminary studies indicate that LHRH and buserelin are excreted into milk in small concentrations, which do not induce LH release in infants. The amounts of immunoreactive buserelin found in mother's milk after the buserelin nasal spray 600/ug (equivalent to 10/ug s.c.) are minute, and do not stimulate LH release from the neonate's pituitary, although infants are responsive to LHRH test injections until 3 months after birth [45]. Oral activity in the adult is negligible, buserelin 5 mg (p.o.) does not stimulate LH release. Other contraceptive approaches based on inducing luteolysis at different stages of the luteal phase have failed, because the corpus luteum is protected by the early hCG rise of pregnancy [40, 46]. It has also been impractical to disrupt the cycle by single high dose administration [46], early follicular treatment [44], or high dose treatment in early pregnancy [47].

Endometriosis

Suppression of follicular maturation and prolonged periods of induced amenorrhoea provide relief from symptoms of the disease. The daily administration of a buserelin nasal spray or the injection of a sustained release preparation has practical advantages. In endometriosis, reversible inhibition of follicular maturation is limited to 6-12 months of therapy, to prevent the late development of osteoporosis. The symptoms of endometriosis are caused by hormone-dependent cyclic changes in dystopic endometrium, with local complications due to the bleeding associated with proliferation and shedding after secretory transformation. The local sequelae are formations of adhesions, scars and cystic tumours. The disease is progressive, but responds to inhibition of oestrogen secretion. A sustained block of follicular maturation is achieved by starting suppression during the luteal phase of the menstrual cycle, thus intercepting follicular development at its earliest stages [34, 50]. Throughout treatment, a state of pseudomenopause is maintained, and hot flushes are frequently experienced. Buserelin treatment is devoid of androgenic side effects encountered with danazol, or side effects associated with pituitary suppression by progestagens. Treatment with buserelin is highly effective in endometriosis [6, 7], but there is marked

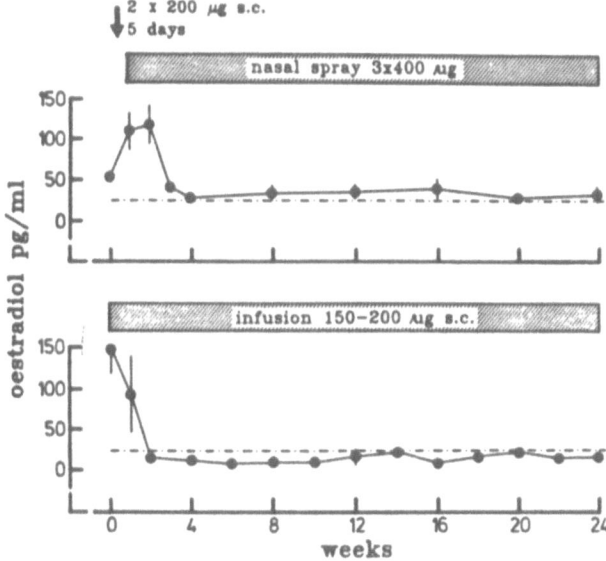

FIGURE 2   Treatment of endometriosis with buserelin injections
(2 x 200/ug s.c.) followed by nasal spray (3 x 400/ug/
day), or by infusion (150-200/ug/day). Broken line indicates castrate-like range of serum oestradiol concentrations.

variability in the dose requirement for oestrogen suppression [49].
The majority of patients is suppressed by the buserelin nasal spray
(3 x 300/ug/day, equivalent to 30/ug s.c.), a small group requires a
higher daily dose [10, 68]. This group may benefit from sustained-
release formulations to improve control of oestrogen secretion. Pituitary suppression is accelerated (Fig. 2) by initial high dose injections (2 x 200/ug s.c. for several days) or infusion (150-200/ug
s.c./day) from external osmotic minipumps [50]. Long-term infusion
studies with 50-400/ug/day (s.c.) have established the dose requirements for sustained release from buserelin implants [50, 51].
    The major advantage of buserelin in endometriosis is the speci-
fic action and absence of metabolic and androgenic side effects.
Since LHRH agonists do not interact with endometrial receptors for
steroids, a combined therapy with progestagens could be envisaged
because of the dual sites of action on the endometrium and on the
enhancement of pituitary suppression by progestagens. In the long-
term management of endometriosis, there is a gradual tendency to
recurrence after temporary suppression of ovarian function. To avoid
new manifestations, repeated treatment courses are advisable, together with surgical intervention to remove accessible endometriotic
tissue, and long-standing lesions progressed to a hormone-refractory
stage. In a study by Minaguchi [52], dose adjustment in patients
with symptoms of endometriosis by buserelin nasal spray 900-

1200/ug/day consistently blocked oestradiol secretion. Thus, treatment with LHRH agonists together with surgical intervention in severe or long-lasting endometriosis may be suitable to restore fertility, and control new manifestations of the disease. The extent of bone mineral loss during treatment courses of up to one year remains to be studied, its early rapid phase can be controlled by calcium supplementation or calcitonin injections.

Leiomyoma uteri

The temporary suppression of oestrogen secretion by buserelin at high doses can induce regression of leiomyoma uteri (uterine fibroids), by depriving the myoma of its growth stimulus [53-55]. This regression has also been observed with other LHRH agonists [55]. A reduction in size of the leiomyoma facilitates surgery, and hysterectomy in young women may be avoided or postponed if pregnancy is desired. Persistent and effective oestrogen suppression is achieved by buserelin infusion (200-400/ug/day s.c.), or by biodegradable sustained release formulations, administered at 4-6 weeks intervals. The response of myomas of different size to suppression is variable [84], the regression depends on the oestrogen receptor binding capacity in the tissue, and on the different anatomical locations. The initial stimulation phase is reduced by high dose injections or infusions, and enhancement of pituitary suppression by cyproterone acetate during this phase is advisable. The clinical index of efficacy is the absence of breakthrough bleeding, and the reduction in the size of the myoma assessed by ultrasonography. As in endometriosis, oestrogen suppression is temporary and reversible, resulting in a tendency to recurrent growth at the end of therapy. In long-term management, multiple treatment courses or post-treatment surgery may be required. The high dose buserelin treatment can provide rapid relief of symptoms such as meno/metrorrhagia and may preserve fertility by facilitating surgical correction.

Other gynaecological indications

Transient suppression of pituitary function is suitable to improve the efficacy of gonadotrophin therapy in infertile women [56, 57]. Inhibition of inappropriate androgen secretion in the polycystic ovarian syndrome has been investigated [58, 59], and studies on the effects of buserelin in the premenstrual syndrome have been performed [60], to elucidate the role of medical contraception in this disorder. In these indications, the highly specific action, extremely good biological tolerance, reversibility and absence of teratogenicity suggested the exploration of LHRH agonists as a diagnostic or therapeutic approach.

Hormone-dependent tumours

Treatment with LHRH agonists is highly effective in the suppression of testosterone secretion in hormone-dependent prostate carcinoma, and oestrogen secretion in premenopausal mammary carcinoma. This treatment can replace orchiectomy or ovariectomy during the initial management of the disease, and establish whether the patient would benefit from surgical castration. In prostate carcinoma, the regression of tumour and metastatic tissue after orchiectomy in hormone-sensitive tumours is established since many years. Testosterone secretion can be blocked by high dose injections of LHRH agonists (buserelin, leuprolide, nafarelin, Decapeptyl$^{(TM)}$, Zoladex$^{(TM)}$), and by sustained release formulations currently under clinical investigation [31, 62]. Long-term treatment is facilitated by the buserelin nasal spray 3 x 400 /ug/day [8, 64]. Numerous studies have established similar rates of remission as after orchiectomy [63-65]. The initial rise in serum testosterone during the stimulation phase should be neutralized by an androgen receptor blocker, e.g. cyproterone acetate 3 x 50 mg p.o. starting 7 days before agonist treatment, and continuing during the first 4 weeks of treatment. This protective measure is particularly important because an initial disease flare can occur during the stimulation phase [66]. Remarkable acute symptoms have been reported in orchiectomized treated with one androgen dose to synchronize cell proliferation for cytostatic therapy. An urgent matter for investigation are the potential long-term benefits of removing not only the testicular source of androgens, but also to neutralize the remaining stimulatory effect of adrenal androgens, by combining LHRH agonists or orchiectomy with androgen receptor blockers, e.g. cyproterone actetate, flutamide or Anandron$^{(TM)}$. Such regimens have been investigated with different LHRH agonists and androgen receptor blockers [67, 68]. In the studies with buserelin, a clear advantage of the initial protection by cyproterone acetate has been established [68]. Previous experience with long-term cyproterone acetate treatment immediately after orchiectomy has been inconclusive. Further studies on long-term survival rates after neutralization of adrenal androgens are required before the benefit of this therapy can be evaluated in comparison with suppression of testicular androgens alone. Treatment is significantly facilitated by new long-acting formulations, to be administered at intervals of 4 weeks by s.c. implantation [62, 82]. A sustained release formulation of buserelin (disk-shaped tablet 6 x 2 mm for surgical implantation) has been used at a single dose of buserelin 5 mg and a dose interval of 4 weeks. The implant material (polyhydroxybutyric acid) has an excellent tissue tolerance, but rates of biodegradation are lower than with conventional polylactide/glycolide copolymers. This disk implant can be removed to control its duration of action. A injectable buserelin implant containing a dose of 3 mg administered at a dose interval of 4-6 weeks has been effective to maintain suppression in patients with prostate carcinoma.

In premenopausal mammary carcinoma, the suppression of oestrogen secretion is of significant benefit to defer ovariectomy until hormone responsiveness has been established [69-71]. The buserelin nasal spray is unsatisfactory for long-term suppression because of the high dose requirement. The therapeutic objective, to block oestradiol secretion can be achieved by buserelin nasal spray 2400 /ug/ day (equivalent to 80 /ug s.c.), but injections of 2 x 1000 /ug/day (s.c.) provide better control [71]. The optimal regimen is sustained release at a higher rate than in prostate carcinoma. The role of LHRH agonists in postmenopausal women is controversial. Clinical experience indicates a low rate of response in postmenopausal women treated with leuprolide [72], and buserelin [73], in contrast to the beneficial response in premenopausal women [70, 71]. On the other hand, buserelin has direct effects of oestrogen-dependent mammary tumour cell lines in vitro [69, 74], and some mammary tumours contain specific receptors for LHRH agonists [75]. Important problems for the future are to neutralize the initial stimulation phase of oestrogen secretion, using an oestrogen-receptor blocker in a similar regimen as in prostate carcinoma, and to investigate whether additional benefits of hormone treatment result from direct effects on mammary tumour cells. The dose requirements for clinical management of mammary carcinoma are high, suppression of oestrogen secretion is achieved by 100-400/ug/day (s.c. infusion), whereas maintenance doses for testosterone suppression are 30-50/ug/day (s.c. from implants).

Precocious puberty

Sexual maturation can be delayed by treatment with LHRH agonists. Pubertal development is resumed after treatment and the prognosis for fertility is favourable. Fertility of animals temporarily suppressed with buserelin is not impaired when they reach sexual maturity [15, 22]. Idiopathic precocious puberty is caused by early activation of endogenous LHRH secretion. Suppression of gonadotrophin secretion by down-regulation of LHRH receptor capacity has to be maintained until the appropriate age for puberty. The treatment therefore should be easy to administer, without metabolic side effects and without problems of compliance. Studies with the buserelin nasal spray at doses of 3-8 x 400/ug/day have been successful [12, 13, 29, 92], the dose requirement is higher in girls than in boys [91]. Frequently, the effective dose has to be raised by administering s.c. injections (4-20/ug/kg daily). Thus, the treatment by nasal spray is envisaged for the temporary delay of sexual maturation in older children, where psychosocial adjustment to the age group is desirable [8]. In precocious puberty of young children, to normalize growth velocity and enhance the final height, long-acting sustained release formulations are preferable to avoid the compliance problems of a treatment extending over a period of 6-10 years. Preliminary experience with the LHRH agonist, [D-Trp[6],Pro[9]-NHEt]LHRH with regard to the effect on growth velocity and final height is encouraging [78], a final assessment will only be possible when long-term studies with sustained release formulations have been evaluated. The risk of developing neutralizing antibodies during long-term buserelin treatment is negligible, in numerous clinical studies no antibodies have been detected either against buserelin, or against endogenous LHRH [79].

Benign prostate hypertrophy

In buserelin-treated patients with prostate carcinoma, the beneficial effect on urinary obstruction is often spectacular, but studies in benign prostate hypertrophy have been disappointing, because the size of the prostate was not reduced in the patients. In management of the predominantly adenomatous type of benign prostate hypertrophy, agonist treatment may be considered as a temporary measure providing relief before surgical intervention by the urologist. In experimental animals, involution of normal or hyperplastic prostate tissue is readily achieved [25, 81]. Despite the differences in histopathology in dogs and in the human, a size reduction of hormone-responsive adenomatous tissue could be expected. This treatment is always associated with predictable side effects (loss of libido and potency). The clinical decision whether to consider buserelin treatment depends on the age and sexual activity of the patient, and on a risk-benefit analysis of removing urinary obstruction by transurethral resection of the adenoma.

Male contraception

Reversible methods based on inducing functional changes in the testicular system are highly desirable. Significant progress towards a male contraceptive has been made by inducing azoospermia in monkeys by buserelin minipump infusions, with subsequent androgen substitution to restore male reproductive behaviour. In human males, it is difficult to achieve azoospermia because spermatogenesis can be restored by substitution with testosterone esters in hypogonadotrophic hypogonadism. During injection studies with LHRH agonists [2], a decrease in sperm density and motility was found. In the rhesus monkey, daily injections of buserelin (up to 200/ug/day s.c.) were ineffective, although the testicular volume decreased during treatment, whereas infusion (50/ug/day s.c.) induced azoospermia [21] within 4-6 weeks. A transitory period of androgen deficiency was mandatory for a consistent effect on spermatogenesis. In a human contraceptive method, transient androgen deficiency (hot flushes, loss of libido and potency) may have to be accepted before starting testosterone substitution. A contraceptive regimen was investigated in normal men [26], by infusing buserelin from external minipumps (118-230/ug/day s.c.). Serum testosterone and of gonadotropin sensitivity to LHRH test injections were suppressed, but the effect on spermatogenesis was inconsistent. This may be due to the early substitution of testosterone when symptoms of androgen deficiency occurred. Buserelin infusion (400/ug/day s.c.) and testosterone substitution also did not induce azoospermia [80], a result which can be attributed to the maintenance of spermatogenesis by testosterone. During investigations of sustained release preparations it will be mandatory to delay testosterone supplementation until azoospermia has been achieved.

Sustained release studies

The use of LHRH agonists depends on different delivery systems specifically designed for short-term use, long-term reversible use, and permanent suppression of pituitary-gonadal function. Short treatment periods by injection formulations have the advantage that a high dose can be administered. For long-term reversible use, the nasal spray formulations are optimal, because they can be self-administered at daily doses sufficient to inhibit ovulation, or block follicular maturation [31, 36]. The buserelin nasal spray formulations are fully effective in long-term androgen suppression, if administered 3-times per day. When long-term compliance is of critical importance, e.g. in precocious puberty, or when high dose requirements are established, e.g. in mammary carcinoma, sustained release formulations are required. They can be administered by s.c. injection of implants as previously demonstrated with steroids [83], or as a suspension of microcapsules. Such buserelin formulations have been effective for 8-23 weeks in rats, dogs and monkeys after single doses of 2.6-3 mg [82], and are presently under clinical investigation. The therapeutic options have been enlarged by the different dosage forms that can be adjusted to the requirements of each therapeutic indication in the wide spectrum from contraception to hormone-dependent tumours.

REFERENCES

1. Sandow, J. Clinical applications of LHRH and its analogues. Clin. Endocrinol., 18, 571 (1983).
2. Sandow, J. Therapeutic use of LHRH analogs in reproductive disorders. In "Andrology: Infertility and Sterility", J.D. Paulson, A. Negro-Vilar, E. Lucena and L. Martini (Eds.), Academic Press, New Jersey, 1986, p. 15.
3. Nillius, S.J., Bergquist, C. and Wide, L. Inhibition of ovulation in women by chronic treatment with a stimulatory LRH analogue: a new approach to birth control? Contraception, 17, 537 (1978).
4. Schmidt-Gollwitzer, M., Hardt, W. and Schmidt-Gollwitzer, K. Risks and benefits of LHRH agonists as antifertility agents. In "LHRH and its Analogues", B.H. Vickery, J.J. Nestor, Jr., and E.S.E. Hafez (Eds.), MTP Press, Boston, 1984, p. 243.
5. Lemay, A., Faure, N., Labrie, F. and Fazekas, A.T.A. Inhibition of ovulation during discontinuous intranasal luteinizing hormone-releasing hormone agonist dosing in combination with gestagen induced bleeding. Fertil. Steril., 43, 868 (1985).
6. Lemay, A. and Quesnel, G. Potential new treatment of endometriosis - reversible inhibition of pituitary-ovarian function by chronic intranasal administration of a LHRH agonist. Fertil. Steril., 38, 376 (1982).
7. Shaw, R.W., Fraser, H.M. and Boyle, H. Intranasal treatment with luteinizing hormone releasing hormone agonist in women with endometriosis. Brit. Med. J., 287, 1667 (1983).
8. Borgmann, V., Hardt, W., Schmidt-Gollwitzer, M., Adenauer, H. and Nagel, R. Sustained suppression of testosterone production by the luteinising-hormone releasing-hormone agonist buserelin in patients with advanced prostate carcinoma. Lancet, 1097 (1982).

9. Labrie, F., Dupont, A., Belanger, A., Lacoursiere, Y., Raynaud, J.P., Gareau, J., Fazekas, A.T.A., Sandow, J., Monfette, G., Girard, J.G., Emond, J. and Houle, J.G. New approach in the treatment of prostate cancer: complete instead of only partial removal of androgens. Prostate, 4, 579 (1983).
10. Waxman, J.H., Wass, J.A.H., Hendry, W.F., Whitfield, H.N., Besser, G.M., Malpas, J.S. and Oliver, R.T.D. Treatment with gonadotrophin releasing hormone analogue in advanced prostatic cancer. Brit. Med. J., 286, 1309 (1983).
11. Wenderoth, U.K. and Jacobi, G.H. Gonadotropin-releasing hormone analogues for palliation of carcinoma of the prostate. A new approach to the classical concept. World J. Urol., 1, 40 (1983).
12. Luder, A.S., Holland, F.J., Costigan, D.C., Jenner, M.R., Wielgosz, G. and Fazekas, A.T.A. Intranasal and subcutaneous treatment of central precocious puberty in both sexes with a long-acting analog of luteinizing hormone-releasing hormone. J. Clin. Endocrinol. Metab., 58, 966 (1984).
13. Stanhope, R., Adams, J. and Brook, C.G.D. The treatment of central precocious puberty using an intranasal LHRH analogue (buserelin). Clin. Endocrinol., 22, 795 (1985).
14. Sandow, J. The regulation of LHRH action at the pituitary and gonadal receptor level: a review. Psychoneuroendocrinology, 8, 277 (1983).
15. Sandow, J., Engelbart, K. and von Rechenberg, W. The different mechanisms for suppression of pituitary and testicular function. Med. Biol., 63, 192 (1985).
16. Sandow, J., Seidel, H.R., Krauss, B. and Jerabek-Sandow, G. Pharmacokinetics of LHRH agonists in different delivery systems. International Symposium on "Hormonal manipulation of cancer: peptides, growth factors and new (anti)steroidal agents", Rotterdam, June 4.-6., 1986 (in press).
17. Clayton, R.N. and Catt, K.J. Gonadotropin-releasing hormone receptors: characterization, physiological regulation, and relationship to reproductive function. Endocr. Rev., 2, 186 (1981).
18. Sandow, J. Inhibition of pituitary and testicular function by LHRH analogues. In "Progress towards a male contraceptive", S.L. Jeffcoate, and M. Sandler (Eds.), John Wiley & Sons Ltd., London, 1982b, p. 19.
19. Huhtaniemi, I., Nikula, H. and Rannikko, S. Treatment of prostatic cancer with a gonadotropin-releasing hormone agonist analog: acute and long-term effects on endocrine functions of testis tissue. J. Clin. Endocrinol. Metab., 61, 698 (1985).
20. Sandow, J. and Beier, B. LHRH agonists - mechanism of action and effect on target tissues. In "Therapeutic prinicples in the management of metastatic prostatic cancer", EORTC Genitourinary Group Monograph 2, Part A, F.H. Schröder, and B. Richards (Eds.), Alan Liss, New York, 1985, p. 121.

377

21. Akhtar, F., Marshall, G.R., Wickings, E.J. and Nieschlag, E. Reversible induction of azoospermia in rhesus monkeys by constant infusion of a gonadotropin-releasing hormone agonist using osmotic minipumps. J. Clin. Endocrinol. Metab., 56, 534 (1983).

22. Sandow, J., Engelbart, K., von Rechenberg, W. and Krauss, B. Reversible inhibition of sexual maturation in male rats. Acta Endocrinol. (Suppl.), 102, 138 (1983).

23. Damber, J.E., Berg, A. and Daehlin, L. Stimulatory effect of an LHRH-agonist on testicular blood flow in hypophysectomized rats. Int. J. Androl., 7, 236 (1984).

24. Christensen, K.A. and Peacock, K.C. Increase in Leydig cell number in testes of adult rats treated chronically with an excess of human chorionic gonadotropin. Biol. Reprod., 22, 383 (1980).

25. Sandow, J. Gonadotropic and antigonadotropic actions of LHRH analogues. In "Neuroendocrine perspectives", R.M. McLeod, and E.E. Müller (Eds.), Elsevier Biomedical Press, Amsterdam, 1982a, p. 335.

26. Schürmeyer, Th., Knuth, U.A., Freischem, C.W., Sandow, J., Akhtar, F.B. and Nieschlag, E. Suppression of pituitary and testicular function in normal men by constant gonadotropin-releasing hormone agonist infusion. J. Clin. Endocrinol. Metab., 59, 19 (1984).

27. Kerr, J.B. and Sharpe, R.M. Effects and interactions of LH and LHRH agonists on testicular morphology and function in hypophysectomized rats. J. Reprod. Fertil., 76, 175 (1986).

28. Schaison, G., Brailly, S., Vuagnat, P. et al. Absence of a direct inhibitory effect of the gonadotropin-releasing hormone (GnRH) agonist D-Ser(TBU)^6,des-Gly-NH$_2$ GnRH ethylamide (buserelin) on testicular steroidogenesis in men. J. Clin. Endocrinol. Metab., 58, 885 (1984).

29. Stanhope, R., Adams, J. and Brook, C.G.D. Disturbances of puberty. Clin. Obstet. Gynaecol., 12, 557 (1985).

30. Rechenberg v., W., Sandow, J., Hahn, M., Kille, S. and Klante, G. Suppression of oestradiol secretion by continuous infusion of an LHRH agonist (buserelin). Acta Endocrinol. (Suppl.), 102, 136 (1983).

31. Sandow, J., Fraser, H.M. and Geisthövel, F. Pharmacology and experimental basis of therapy with LHRH agonists in women. In "Gonadotropin down-regulation in gynaecological practice", R. Rolland, D.R. Chadha, and W.N.P. Willemsen (Eds.), Alan Liss Inc., New York, 1986, p. 1.

32. Bex, F.J. and Corbin, A. LHRH and analogs - reproductive pharmacology and contraceptive and therapeutic utility. In "Frontiers in Neuroendocrinology", Vol. 8, L. Martini, and W. Ganong (Eds.), Raven Press, New York, 1984, p. 85.

33. Fraser, H.M. Effect of treatment for one year with a luteinizing hormone-releasing hormone agonist on ovarian thyroidal, and adrenal function and menstruation in the stumptailed monkey (macaca arctoides). Endocrinology, 112, 245 (1983).

34. Fraser, H.M. and Sandow, J. Suppression of follicular maturation by infusion of a luteinizing hormone-releasing hormone agonist starting during the late luteal phase in the stumptailed macaque monkey. J. Clin. Endocrinol. Metab., 60, 579 (1985).

35. Sandow, J., Jerabek-Sandow, G., Krauss, B. and von Rechenberg, W. Pharmacokinetic and antigenicity studies with LHRH analogues. In "Future Aspects in Contraception", Part 2, "Female Contraception", B. Runnebaum, T. Rabe, and L. Kiesel (Eds.), MTP Press Ltd., Boston, 1985c, p. 129.

36. Petri, W., Seidel, R. and Sandow, J. A pharmaceutical approach to long-term therapy with peptides. In "LHRH and its analogues", F. Labrie, A. Belanger, and A. Dupont (Eds.), Elsevier Science Publishers B.V., 1984, p. 63.

37. Baumann, R., Kuhl, H., Taubert, H.D. and Sandow, J. Ovulation inhibition by daily i.m. administration of a highly active LHRH analog (D-Ser(TBU)^6-LHRH(1-9)nonapeptide-ethylamide). Contraception, 21, 191 (1980).

38. Sandow, J., Engelbart, K. and von Rechenberg, W. Contraceptive action of LHRH and analogues in animals and in humans. In "Secretion and Action of Gonadotropins", B. Runnebaum, T. Rabe, L. Kiesel, and W.E. Merz (Eds.), Springer Verlag, Heidelberg, 1984, p. 19.

39. Thau, R.B. Luteinizing hormone-releasing hormone (LHRH) and its analogs for contraception in women: a review. Contraception, 29, 143 (1984).

40. Bergquist, C., Nillius, S.J. and Wide, L. Effects of a luteinizing hormone-releasing hormone agonist on luteal function in women. Contraception, 287 (1980a).

41. Bergquist, C., Nillius, S.J. and Wide, L. Peptide contraception in women. Inhibition of ovulation by chronic intranasal LRH agonist therapy. Contraception, 31, 111 (1985).

42. Kuhl, H., Jung, C. and Taubert, H.-D. Contraception with an LHRH agonist: effect on gonadotrophin and steroid secretion patterns. Clin. Endocrinol. 21, 179 (1984).

43. Schumacher, T., Zwirner, M., Unterberg, H., Pohl, C., Keller, E. and Schindler, A.E. Effects of the LHRH-analogue buserelin given discontinuously as a contraceptive on ovarian cycle and lipometabolism. Neuroendocrinol. Lett., 6, 267 (1984).

44. Skarin, G., Nillius, S.J. and Wide, L. Early follicular phase luteinizing hormone-releasing hormone agonist administration - effects on follicular maturation and corpus luteum function in women. Contraception, 25, 31 (1982).

45. Tapanainen, J., Koivisto, M., Huhtaniemi, I., Vihko, R. Effect of gonadotropin-releasing hormone on pituitary-gonadal function of male infants during the first year of life. J. Clin. Endocrinol. Metab. 55, 689 (1982).

46. Bergquist, C., Nillius, S.J. and Wide, L. Luteolysis induced by a luteinizing hormone-releasing hormone agonist is prevented by human chorionic gonadotropin. Contraception, 22, 341 (1980b).

47. Skarin, G., Nillius, S.J. and Wide, L. Failure to induce abortion of early human pregnancy by high doses of a superactive LRH agonist. Contraception, 26, 457 (1982).

379

48. Lemay, A., Maheux, R., Faure, N., Jean, C. and Fazekas, A.T.A. Reversible hypogonadism induced by luteinizing hormone releasing hormone (LHRH) agonist (buserelin) as a new therapeutic approach for endometriosis. Fertil. Steril., 41, 863 (1984).

49. Hardt, W. and Schmidt-Gollwitzer, M. Sustained gonadal suppression in fertile women with the LHRH agonist buserelin. Clin. Endocrinol., 19, 613 (1983).

50. Lemay, A., Maheux, R., Jean, C. and Faure, N. Efficacy of different modalities of LHRH agonist (buserelin) administration on the inhibition of the pituitary-ovarian axis for the treatment of endometriosis. In "Gonadotropin down-regulation in gynaecological practice", R. Rolland, D.R. Chadha, and W.N.P. Willemsen (Eds.), Alan Liss Inc., New York, 1986, p. 157.

51. Geisthövel, F., Rieger, B., Geyer, H., Peters, F. and Sandow, J. Effect of long-term subcutaneous infusion of a GnRH agonist (buserelin) on pituitary and ovarian function. Acta Endocrinol. (Suppl.), 111, 90 (1986)

52. Minaguchi, H., Uemura, T. and Shirasu, K. Clinical study on finding optimal dose of a potent LHRH agonist (buserelin) for the treatment of endometriosis - multicenter trial in Japan. In "Gonadotropin Down-Regulation in Gynecological Practice", R. Rolland, D.R. Chadha, and W.N.P. Willemsen (Eds.), Alan Liss, Inc., New York, 1986, p. 211.

53. Healy, D.L., Fraser, H.M. and Lawson, S.L. Shrinkage of a uterine fibroid after subcutaneous infusion of a LHRH agonist. Br. Med. J., 289, 1267 (1984).

54. Maheux, R., Guilloteau, C., Lemay, A., Bastide, A. and Fazekas, A.T.A. Luteinizing hormone-releasing hormone agonist and uterine leiomyoma: a pilot study. Am. J. Obstet. Gynecol., 152, 1034 (1985).

55. Filicori, M., Hall, D.A., Loughlin, J.S., Rivier, J., Vale, W. and Crowley, W.F. A conservative approach to the management of uterine leiomyoma: pituitary desensitization by a luteinizing-releasing hormone analogue. Am. J. Obstet. Gynecol., 147, 726 (1983).

56. Bettendorf, G., Braendle, W. and Sprotte, C. Gonadotropin stimulation during LHRH-analogue-induced inhibition of pituitary function. Geburtshilfe Frauenheilk., 45, 431 (1985).

57. Fleming, R., Haxton, M.J., Hamilton, M.P.R., McCune, G.S., Black, W.P., MacNaughton, M.C. and Coutts, J.R.T. Successful treatment of infertile women with oligomenorrhoea using a combination of an LHRH agonist and exogenous gonadotrophins. Br. J. Obstet. Gynaecol., 92, 369 (1985).

58. Fleming, R., Black, W.P. and Coutts, J.R.T. Effects of LH suppression in polycystic ovary syndrome. Clin. Endocrinol., 23, 683 (1985).

59. Mongioi, A., Maugeri, G., Macchi, M., Calogero, A., Vicari, E. and Coniglione, F. Effect of gonadotrophin-releasing hormone analog (GnRH-A) administration on serum gonadotrophin and steroid levels in patients with polycystic ovarian disease. Acta Endocrinol., 111, 228 (1986).

60. Bancroft, J. and Backstrom, T. Premenstrual syndrome. Clin. Endocrinol., 22, 313 (1985).

61. Schally, A.V., Comaru-Schally, A.M. and Redding, T.W. Anti-tumor effects of analogs of hypothalamic hormones in endocrine-dependent cancers. Proc. Soc. Exp. Biol. Med., 175, 259 (1984).

62. Furr, B.J.A. and Hutchinson, F.G. Biodegradable sustained release formulation of the LHRH analogue "Zoladex" for the treatment of hormone-responsive tumours. In "EORTC Genitourinary Group Monograph 2, Part A: Therapeutic Principles in Metastatic Prostatic Cancer", F.H. Schroeder, and B. Richards (Eds.), Alan R. Liss, Inc., 1985, p. 143.

63. Jacobi, G.H., Wenderoth, U.K. and Hohenfellner, R. Three-year follow-up of 58 patients with advanced prostatic carcinoma treated with the LHRH analogue buserelin under phase-II conditions. J. Urol., 133 153A (1985).

64. Klijn, J.G.M., deJong, F.H., Lamberts, S.W.J. and Blankenstein, M.A. LHRH-agonist treatment in metastatic prostate carcinoma. Eur. J. Cancer Clin. Oncol., 20, 483 (1984).

65. Koutsilieris, M. and Tolis, G. Long-term follow-up of patients with advanced prostatic carcinoma treated with either buserelin (Hoe 766) or orchiectomy: classification of variables associated with disease outcome. Prostate, 7, 31 (1985).

66. Waxman, J.H., Man, A., Hendry, W.F., Whitfield, H.N., Besser, G.M. and Tiptaft, R.C. Importance of early tumor exacerbation in patients treated with long-acting analogues of gonadotrophin releasing hormone for advanced prostatic cancer. Brit. Med. J., 291, 1387 (1985).

67. Labrie, F., Dupont, A., Belanger, A., Lachance, R. and Giguere, M. Long-term treatment with luteinizing hormone releasing hormone agonists and maintenance of serum testosterone to castration concentrations. Brit. Med. J., 291, 369 (1985).

68. Klijn, J.G.M., deVoogt, H.J., Schröder, F.H. and deJong, F.H. Combined treatment with buserelin and cyproterone acetate in metastatic prostatic carcinoma. Lancet, 493 (1985).

69. Klijn, J.G.M. and deJong, F.H. Treatment with a luteinizing-hormone-releasing-hormone analogue (buserelin) in premenopausal patients with metastatic breast cancer. Lancet, 1213 (1982).

70. Harland, S.J., Waxman, J.H., Rees, L., Ford, H.T., Gazet, J.C. and Nash, A. The treatment of premenopausal patients with breast cancer with buserelin nasal spray. Brit. J. Cancer, 52, 421 (1985).

71. Klijn, J.G.M., deJong, F.H., Lamberts, S.W.J. and Blankenstein, M.A. LHRH-agonist treatment in clinical and experimental human breast cancer. J. Steroid. Biochem., 23, 867 (1985).

72. Harvey, H.A., Lipton, A. and Max, D.T. LHRH analogs for human mammary carcinoma. In "LHRH and its Analogues", B.H. Vickery, J.J. Nestor, Jr., and E.S.E. Hafez (Eds.), MTP Press, Boston, 1984, p. 329.

73. Waxman, J.H., Harland, S.J., Coombes, R.C., Wrigley, P.F.M., Malpas, J.S., Powles, T. and Lister, T.A. The treatment of postmenopausal women with advanced breast cancer with buserelin. Cancer Chemother. Pharmacol., 15, 171 (1985).

74. Miller, W.R., Scott, W.N., Morris, R., Fraser, H.M. and Sharpe, R.M. Growth of human breast cancer cells inhibited by a luteinizing hormone-releasing hormone agonist. Nature, 313, 231 (1985).

75. Eidne, K.A., Flanagan, C.A. and Millar, R.P. Gonadotropin-releasing hormone binding sites in human breast carcinoma. Science, 229, 989 (1985).

76. Donaldson, M.D.C., Stanhope, R., Lee, T.J., Price, D.A., Brook, C.G.D. and Savage, D.C.L. Gonadotrophin responses to GnRH in precocious puberty treated with GnRH analogue. Clin. Endocrinol., 21, 499 (1984).

77. Ward, P.S., Ward, I., McNinch, A.W. and Savage, D.C.L. Reversible inhibition of central precocious puberty with a long-acting GnRH analogue. Arch. Dis. Child. 60, 872 (1985).

78. Comite, F., Cassorla, F., Barnes, K.M., Hench, K.D., Dwyer, A., Skerda, M.C., Loriaux, D.L., Cutler Jr., G.B. and Pescovitz, O.H. Luteinizing hormone releasing hormone analogue therapy for central precocious puberty. JAMA 255, 2613 (1986).

79. Fraser, H.M., Sandow, J. and Krauss, B. Antibody production against an agonist analogue of luteinizing hormone-releasing hormone: evaluation of immunochemical and physiological consequences. Acta Endocrinol. (Kbh.), 103, 151 (1983).

80. Michel, E., Bents, H., Akhtar, F., Hönigl, W., Knuth, U.A., Sandow, J. and Nieschlag, E. Failure of high-dose sustained release luteinizing hormone releasing hormone agonist (buserelin) plus oral testosterone to suppress male fertility. Clin. Endocrinol., 23, 663 (1985).

81. Vickery, B.H. Physiology and antifertility effects of LHRH and agonistic analogs in male animals. In "LHRH Peptides as Female and Male Contraceptives", G.I. Zatuchni, J.D. Shelton and J.J. Sciarra (Eds.), Harper & Row, Philadelphia, 1981, p. 275.

82. Sandow, J., Seidel, H.R., Krauss, B. and Jerabek-Sandow, G. Pharmacokinetics of LHRH agonists in different delivery systems and the relation to endocrine function. In International Symposium on "Hormonal manipulation of cancer: peptides, growth factors and new (anti)steroidal agents", June 4.-6., 1986, Rotterdam (in press).

83. Kitchell, J.P., Crooker, S.C., Wise, D.L. and Zaneveld, L.J.D. Preparation of biodegradable levonorgestrel rods. In "Long-Acting Contraceptive Delivery Systems", G.I. Zatuchni, A. Goldsmith, J.D. Shelton and J.J. Sciarra (Eds.), Harper & Row, Philadelphia, 1984, p. 164.

84. Healy, D.L., Lawson, S.R., Abbott, M., Baird, D.T. and Fraser, H.M. Toward removing uterine fibroids without surgery: subcutaneous infusion of a luteinizing hormone-releasing hormone agonist commencing in the luteal phase. J. Clin. Endocrinol. Metab., 63, 619 (1986).

25
Trials with Leuprolide

M.B. GARNICK[1], A. LIPTON[2], A. HARVEY[2],
D.T. MAX[3], J.A. SMITH[4] and L.M. GLODE[5]

[1]Dana-Farber Cancer Institute, Boston MA 02115; [2]Hershey Medical Center, Hershey, PA 17033; [3]Abbott Laboratories, North Chicago, IL 60064; [4]The University of Utah Medical Center, Salt Lake City, UT 84132; [5]University of Colorado Medical Center, Denver, CO 80262, USA

INTRODUCTION

Leuprolide ([D-Leu^6,Pro^9-NHEt]LHRH; leuprolide) is a potent analog of the hypothalamic human gonadotropin-releasing hormone (LHRH). It is available as Lupron®, Leuprolide Acetate Injection, TAP Pharmaceuticals. The function of the naturally occurring LHRH is to regulate the release of gonadotropins from the pituitary gland. Chronic administration of highly potent LHRH analogs such as leuprolide results in the inhibition of gonadotropin release, with the consequence that testicular and ovarian function are suppressed [1-4]. These observations led to trials of leuprolide in human prostate and breast cancer patients.

PROSTATE CANCER

The use of hormonal therapy constitutes the main stay of treatment for individuals with advanced, metastatic carcinoma of the prostate. The landmark observations by Huggins et al. [5-7] in the early 1940s demonstrated that prostate cancer was under the trophic influence of male hormones such as testosterone and dihydrotesto-sterone; indeed, one could achieve disease regression of metastatic deposits of prostate cancer with the ablation of androgens and one could cause disease progression and stimulation with the exogenous administration of androgens.

These cardinal observations lead to the widespread use of surgical or medical castration in the management of patients with metastatic prostate cancer. Up until recently, the two mainstays for systemic management of patients with prostate cancer have been surgical removal of the testicles (bilateral orchiectomy) or the exogenous administration of feminizing hormones such as diethyl-stilbestrol (DES). While both of these modalities have been extremely effective in controlling patients' symptoms from their disease, both are associated with side effects. The psychological impact of surgical castration, though difficult to assess, has certainly been seen commonly in clinical practice. Likewise, the studies from the Veterans Administration Cooperative Urologic Research Group (VACURG) clearly demonstrated the thromboembolic and cardiovascular complication risk rate associated with estrogens which was also found to be dose dependent [8,9]. In those studies, the daily administration of 5 mg DES was able to reduce the rate of death from prostate cancer which was, unfortunately, offset by an increased rate of death from cardiovascular complications. Subsequent VA studies demonstrated a lower cardiovascular complication rate from a 1 mg DES daily dose.

Clearly, the biochemical and pharmacological aspects of LHRH analogs opened up another, rational, and feasible modality of treating individuals with prostate cancer. The finding that chronic administration of LHRH analogs could induce and maintain castrate levels of circulating testicular androgens led to their evaluation for treatment of prostatic cancer.

Leuprolide studies

Two large, controlled, multi-institutional studies have been conducted evaluating the safety and efficacy of leuprolide in advanced prostate cancer patients [10-12].

Study 1 was an open, noncomparative study, initiated in 1980 to evaluate the safety, efficacy and endocrinological effects of leuprolide in patients with prostate cancer. Patients with Stage D_2 carcinoma of the prostate (prostate cancer which was no longer amenable to curative therapy with surgery and radiation therapy; disease which had spread to the lymph nodes above the aortic bifurcation; soft tissue or osseous metastases) were entered into the study. They had measurable or evaluable disease that met the following criteria.
1. measurable prostatic cancer
2. osteoblastic or osteolytic bone lesions
3. elevation of the serum acid phosphatase
4. objective evidence of ureteral obstruction
5. measurable soft tissue metastases.
Individuals with a history of adrenalectomy, hypophysectomy, or a concurrent cancer other than prostatic as well as medical illnesses predicting a life expectancy of less than two months were excluded from entry.

The criteria for objective response of those previously defined by the National Prostate Cancer project are outlined in Table 1.

One hundred eighteen patients entered the study between December 1980 and November 1981. Age ranged from 42 to 93 years with a mean age of 66 years. Varying doses of leuprolide were given with the majority of patients receiving 1 mg or 10 mg per day. Patients enrolled in the study belonged to one of three groups depending on previous treatment period. Fifty-nine patients received no prior hormonal therapy or chemotherapy. Twenty-eight patients had received previous hormonal therapy mainly in the form of diethylstilbestrol. Thirty-one patients had undergone a bilateral orchiectomy as their initial form of hormonal therapy. In addition, 21 of these 31 patients received additional therapy with DES. One hundred eleven patients had Stage D_2 disease, 4 patients had Stage D_1 and 3 patients had Stage C disease at the time of study entry. Eighty-four percent of the patients had abnormal elevations in serum acid phosphatase. The control groups

384

Table 1. National Prostatic Cancer Project Criteria for Evaluation of Clinical Responses to Treatment of Prostate Cancer.

	Tumor Masses	Elevated Acid Phosphatase	Osteoblastic Lesions	Osteolytic Lesions	Hepatomegaly /Abnormal LFTs[*]	Weight, Symptoms, Performance Status
Complete response (all, if present)	Complete disappearance No new lesions	Normalized	Disappeared	Recalcified	Normalized/ normalized	No deter- ioration
Partial response (all, if present)	>50% reduction of at least 1 mass	Normalized	No progres- sion	Recalcifica- tion of some	30% decrease/ 30% decrease	No deter- ioration
Objectively stable --no change (all, if present)	No increase in size by >25% No new lesions	Decreased in value	Stabilized	Not worse	No increase by >30%/ not worse	No deter- ioration
Progression (any of following)	Increase in size by >25% New lesions	Increase in acid and/or alkaline phosphatase with other evidence of progression				Deter- ioration

*LFTs denotes liver-function tests. From N. Engl. J. Med., 311, 1281 (1984).

for this study were composed of those individuals treated with 3 mg of diethylstilbestrol daily or orchiectomy in a concurrent study run by the National Prostate Cancer Project.

Hormonal assays. Long-term testosterone levels in previously untreated and orchiectomized patients in Study 1 are seen in Figure 1. The mean testosterone and dihydrotestosterone values continued at castrate levels, in patients treated with leuprolide for up to four years. FSH levels fell to significantly lower than baseline by Day 4 in all treated groups in Study 1 while LH levels declined but remained above baseline.

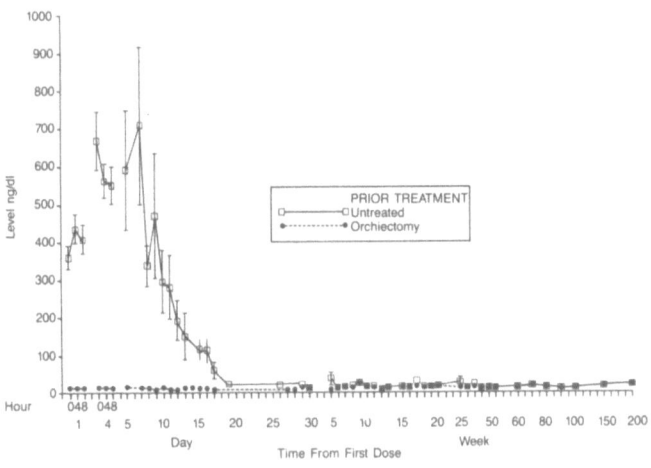

Figure 1. Testosterone levels (Mean ± S.E.M.) by prior treatment in prostatic cancer patients enrolled in Study 1.

385

In patients without previous hormonal treatment, leuprolide induced an objective disease response of 72% which was comparable to alternative endocrine therapy. There was minimal evidence of objective response (26% had stable disease for 3 months or longer) in patients who had become refractory to prior endocrine therapy with either orchiectomy or estrogens. There was no evidence of a dose response relationship with treatment of 1 or 10 mg/day.

Side effects. The most frequently reported adverse side effects were vasomotor hot flashes. The incidence in previously untreated patients was 61%. Characteristically, they varied in their intensity and frequency from occasional mild symptoms to hourly flushing and sweating. Hot flashes were not seen in the castrated patients.

Of great importance was the fact that there were no apparent drug-related cardiovascular or thromboembolic problems. Deep venous thrombosis did not occur in the leuprolide population. There was no drug induced gynecomastia. Though difficult to evaluate, there was a reduction in the libido and erectile potency in patients treated with leuprolide. There were no major drug-related adverse reactions.

The results of this study suggested that compounds such as leuprolide may prove to be the preferred initial endocrine therapy for patients with metastatic carcinoma of the prostate.

Beginning in October 1981, a second multi-institutional randomized prospective trial was undertaken in previously untreated patients with Stage D_2 metastatic prostate cancer. The study compared the safety and efficacy of leuprolide, given in a dose of 1 mg subcutaneously daily with DES given in a dose of 3 mg orally daily. A total of 199 patients were enrolled into the trial. They fulfilled the following entrance criteria: carcinoma of the prostate with bone metastases, lymph node metastases above the aortic bifurication, or metastases to other soft tissues; two measurable or evaluable manifestations of prostate cancer; performance status of 2 or less according to the Eastern Cooperative Oncology Group Scale; no previous systemic therapy or radiation therapy; recovery from other illnesses; informed voluntary consent. Patients were not to have received previous hormonal therapy of any form. Of the 199 patients enrolled, 186 were fully evaluable for response.

After several weeks of therapy, there was no difference in the levels of testosterone and dihydrotestosterone, between the DES or leuprolide treated groups. Castrate levels were maintained for the duration of the treatment period (Figures 2 and 3).

The objective response of all evaluable patients at the 12-week evaluation point demonstrated that 86% of the leuprolide population (complete response 1%; partial response 37%; stabilization of disease 48%) and 85% in the DES population (complete response 2%; partial response 44%; stable disease 39%) had favorable objective responses to treatment. There was no difference in survival between patients initially assigned to leuprolide and those initially assigned to DES treatment. Actual survival rates after one year were 87% for the leuprolide population and 78% for the DES population. When median duration of survival was reached

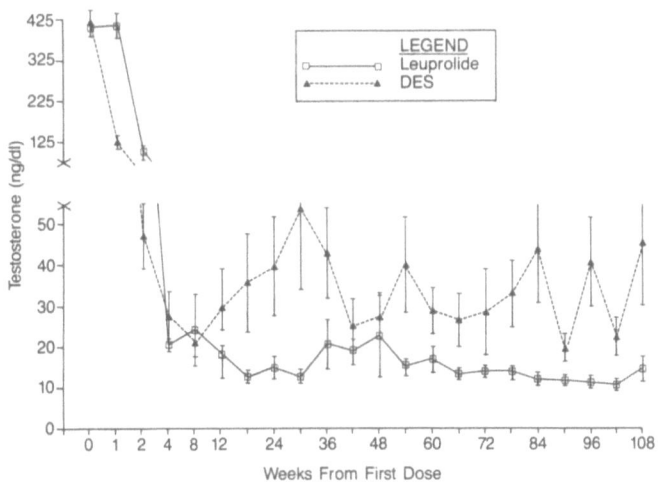

Figure 2. Testosterone levels (Mean ± S.E.M.) for patients
receiving leuprolide or DES in Study 2.

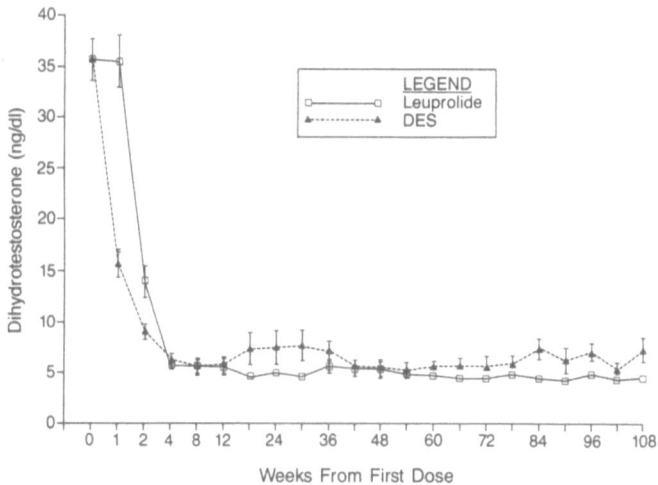

Figure 3. Dihydrotestosterone levels (Mean ± S.E.M.) for patients
receiving either leuprolide or DES in Study 2.

(Figure 4), the survival curves for the leuprolide and DES groups
were not statistically different (p = 0.90). The medians of the
distributions were 136 weeks for the leuprolide group and 149 weeks
for the DES group. However, due to the conditional crossover
design of the study, many patients crossed over to the alternative
therapy because of either disease progression or intolerable side
effects. Therefore, each group included patients receiving either
leuprolide or DES, as well as patients receiving both drugs
subsequently as first and second treatments.

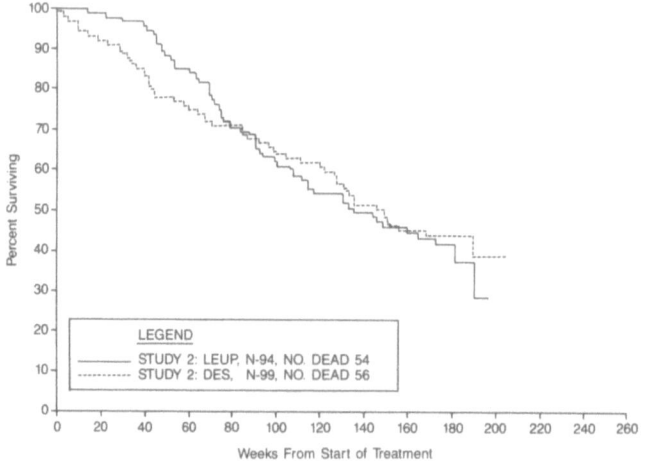

Figure 4. Time from study entry to death in previously untreated evaluable Stage D$_2$ patients, in patients treated with leuprolide or DES in Study 2.

Side effects. Table 2 details the significant side effects that were seen with either leuprolide or DES. There was a greater tendency toward the development of gynecomastia or breast tenderness, nausea and vomiting, peripheral edema, thrombosis, phlebitis and pulmonary embolism in the estrogen-treated population compared to the leuprolide population.

Table 2. Adverse side effects in patients receiving leuprolide or diethylstilbestrol (DES)

Side Effect	Leuprolide Group (N = 98)	DES Group (N = 101)	p VALUE
	no. of patients		
Hot flashes	51	11	<0.00001
Gynecomastia/breast tenderness	3	49	<0.00001
Nausea/vomiting	5	16	0.02
Edema	2	16	0.008
Thrombosis/phlebitis/ pulmonary embolus	1	7	0.065

Additionally, subjective parameters of improvement were seen in both the leuprolide and DES populations. Table 3 demonstrates the percentage of of patients who had improvement in pain in the early evaluation when treated with either leuprolide or DES. Both Tables 2 and 3 are reproduced, with permission, from The New England Journal of Medicine, 1984 [11].

388

Table 3. Evaluation of early changes in bone pain in patients treated with leuprolide or diethylstilbestrol (DES)

Week of Treatment	Leuprolide Group					DES Group				
	No. of Patients	% of patients				No. of Patients	% of patients			
		Better	Same	Worse	None*		Better	Same	Worse	None*
1	86	9	3	7†	48	81	17	40	1†	42
2	84	20	25	6	49	79	28	23	6	43
4	87	29	16	8	47	79	33	19	5	43
12	85	38	11	3	48	82	40	11	7	42

*Percentage of evaluable patients at each interval who had no bone pain throughout the study.
†$P = 0.118$, two-sided Fisher's exact test.

Results of both studies indicate that leuprolide is a new alternative treatment for metastatic prostate cancer, which may be preferable to current therapies for selected patients because of a lack of serious side effects.

BREAST CANCER

Surgical castration was first performed for the palliation of metastatic breast cancer by G. T. Beatson on July 15, 1895 [13].

Studies in animals have shown that LHRH analogs can produce regression of spontaneous or dimethylbenzanthracene-induced mammary tumors in female rats [14]. These observations led to trials of leuprolide in breast cancer patients.

Postmenopausal patients

The initial leuprolide studies in breast cancer were performed in postmenopausal patients with metastatic disease. The safety of the drug when administered by subcutaneous daily injection was demonstrated in these patients [15]. A total of 72 postmenopausal women received 1-10 mg of leuprolide daily in a pilot trial [16]. No suppression of estrogen production was observed in these women whose ovaries were no longer functional. Only 10% of women experienced objective tumor regression for a median duration of 20 weeks, and 22% had stabilization of their disease. Any effect of the analog must then have resulted from a direct action on the tumor.

Premenopausal patients

Clinical Results. We next turned our attention to premenopausal women with regular menses [17]. Twenty-six women with proven metastatic breast carcinoma and measurable disease were selected for the study. One patient received only one dose of leuprolide before it was discovered that she was ineligible for this study because she had preexisting severe thrombocytopenia. The remaining 25 patients were all evaluable for safety, efficacy, and hormonal analysis (Table 4).

389

Table 4. Characteristics of 25 Evaluable Premenopausal Women Treated with Leuprolide

Median Age:	43 yr. (range 23-52 yr.)
ECOG* performance status:	0-3 (capable of at least limited self-care)
Race:	12 Caucasians, 12 Mestizas (all living in Mexico) and 1 black
Estrogen receptors (ER):	14 ER(+), 10 ER(-), 1 ER unknown
Sites of matastases:	Soft tissue in 12, bone in 3, viscera in 3, and 2 or more sites in 7
Prior treatment:	None in 23, tamoxifen in 2

*Eastern Cooperative Oncology Group.

All patients had progressive disease at the time they were started on therapy. Each patient initially received 1 mg leuprolide sc once daily. Each investigator could elect to increase the dose to 5 or 10 mg daily at any time during the study based on the patient's clinical condition. Treatment was continued until there was renewed evidence of progressive disease. Criteria of response to therapy were as follows: Objective remission was classified as a decrease of 50% or greater in the sum of the products of the two largest perpendicular diameters in all measurable lesions, partial recalcification of osteolytic lesions for a least 3 months, or both. Stabilization of osteoblastic lesions with regression of other lesions was also considered an objective response. Stable disease was defined as a decrease of less than 50% or an increase of less than 25% in metastatic lesions with marked symptomatic improvement for at least 3 months. Progression required an increase of 25% or greater over original measurements or appearance of new metastatic lesions.

Eleven patients (44%) experienced a partial response with a median duration of benefit of 39 weeks. Five patients (20%) had a stabilization of disease with a median duration of benefit of 19 weeks. Thus, the overall response rate with leuprolide was 64% (Table 5). Nine patients (36%) had progression of the disease. Six of these patients had a rapid disease progression within two to nine weeks of initiating leuprolide treatment. Twenty patients had an increase in dosage of leuprolide during the study from 1 to 5 or 1 to 10 mg daily. In only two of these patients did an increased dosage lead to an improvement in objective response.

The following Tables 6, 7 and 9 are reproduced, with permission, from The Journal of Clinical Oncology, Harvey, et al., 1985 [17]. Table 6 shows the response rates for different individual sites of involvement in the 25 evaluable patients. Responses were primarily seen in soft-tissue and bony sites of involvement. Clinical outcome was also assessed with regard to the estrogen-receptor result (Table 7). Responses were noted in both estrogen-receptor-positive and estrogen-receptor-negative patients.

390

Table 5. Results of Leuprolide Therapy in 25 Premenopausal Patients With Advanced Breast Cancer

	Patients No.	%	Median duration in weeks[a]
Remissions	11	44	39 (12-141)
Stable disease	5	20	19 (16-93)
Failures	9	36	

[a]Numbers in parentheses are ranges.

This finding may be explained by a high incidence of false-negative estrogen receptor determinations. Several samples were shipped a great distance and no clinical laboratory quality control standards were prospectively included with each sample. Another explanation which has been suggested is that leuprolide and other LHRH super-agonist analogs could exert direct antitumor effects. Two laboratories recently demonstrated specific GnRH agonist binding sites in breast tumor tissues [18,19]. Miller et al. [19] detected inhibition of growth of MCF-7 human breast cancer cells in culture when exposed to concentrations of LHRH analogs in the range of 10^{-9} to 10^{-7} M. These effects were unrelated to nonspecific toxicity since coincubation with an LHRH antagonist prevented the inhibitory effects of the agonists.

Table 6. Response by Individual Site of Involvement

	Response			
Type of Tissue Involved	PR	Stable	Progression	Total
Soft-tissue only	7	3	2	12
Visceral only	0	1	2	3
Bone only	3	0	0	3
Multiple sites of involvement	1	1	5	7
Total	11	5	9	25

Table 7. Response by Estrogen-Receptor Status

	Response			
Estrogen-Receptor Status	PR	Stable	Progression	Total
Positive	6	3	5	14
Negative	4	2	4	10
Unknown	1	0	0	1
Total	11	5	9	25

391

Results similar to those mentioned above with leuprolide have been obtained by other investigators (Table 8) using two different analogs and dosage schedules [20-22]. Taken together, these pilot data suggest that LHRH analogs are a new class of agents that are useful in the treatment of premenopausal women with metastatic breast cancer.

Table 8. Premenopausal Women with Breast Cancer

Study	Number of Patients Entered	Number with Objective Response	Percent	Reference(s)
1	25	11	44%	17
2	22	9	41%	20,21
3	16	5	31%	22

Toxicity of Leuprolide. The side effects encountered by our 25 patients are listed in Table 9. As expected, hot flashes were among the most common as a result of cessation of ovarian function. The flare phenomenon characterized by increased bone pain was observed in two patients, probably as a result of the initial transient stimulation of the pituitary-gonadal axis by leuprolide before the paradoxic inhibitory effect takes place. The side effects did not appear to be dose dependent, and no patient discontinued treatment because of them. Patients appeared to welcome giving themselves daily injections as this gave them an active role in their own care.

Table 9. Side Effects from Leuprolide

Side Effect	Severity		
	Mild	Moderate	Severe
Hot flashes	2	3	
Nausea/vomiting	3	1	1
Headache	1	3	
Dizziness	2	1	
Taste in mouth	1	1	
Increase bone pain	0	1	1
Diarrhea	1	1	
Local reaction	1	1	
Nervous/irritable	0	1	
Hives	0	1	
Vaginal bleeding	1	0	
Polyuria and polydipsia	0	0	1

Endocrinologic effects of leuprolide

Effects on menses. Of the 25 evaluable patients, 11 had no menstrual cycles while receiving leuprolide and nine patients had only one menstrual cycle. The remaining five patients had two menstrual cycles within the first ten weeks of treatment. All of the 19 patients who received leuprolide for more than ten weeks had cessation of their menses by week 11, which continued as long as they remained on therapy.

Hormonal Effects. After an initial rise, both FSH and LH levels became suppressed after 1 week of therapy and remained so throughout the treatment period. Serum estradiol levels (Figure 5) were suppressed into the postmenopausal range after 4 weeks of therapy and remained so for as long as leuprolide was administered. Similarly, serum estrone and estrone sulfate were profoundly suppressed during treatment with this LHRH analog. Progesterone levels were likewise suppressed, whereas no consistent changes were observed in the serum levels of androstendione, prolactin and cortisol.

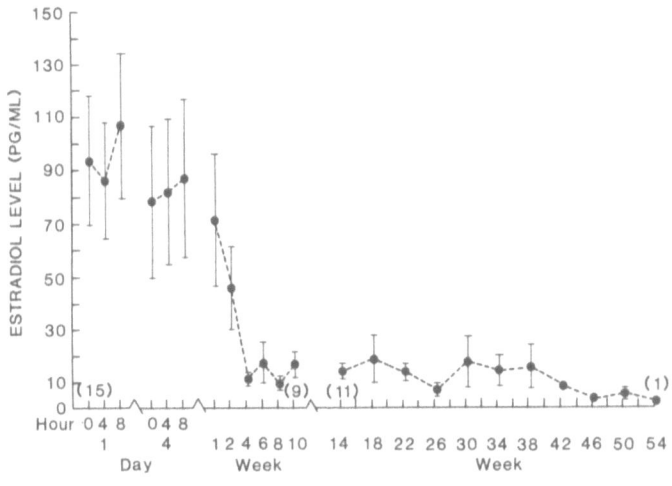

Figure 5. Chronologic evaluation of estradiol in 15 leuprolide-treated patients. Sample size is number in parentheses. The mean is presented ± S.E.M. Reproduced from Harvey, et al., J. Clin. Oncol., 3, 1068 (1985), with permission.

CONCLUDING REMARKS

Chronic parenteral administration of leuprolide is able to induce a medical castration in premenopausal patients with breast cancer as assessed by cessation of menses and hormonal measurements. In addition, this compound has an antitumor effect which is compatible to that observed with surgical ovariectomy.

These pilot trials with the LHRH superagonist analogs in women with breast cancer provide a basis for future investigations. Controlled trials of LHRH agonists vs. surgical oophorectomy are initially required. Later, these compounds could be studied as adjuvant endocrine treatment or as components of regimens of hormonal synchronization. A final potential clinical use of LHRH analogs in the treatment of breast cancer may be in association with antiestrogen therapy, the rationale for this combined approach would be to obtain a complete blockade of estrogen action. The administration of antiestrogens could, in fact, potentiate the antitumor effect of these compounds by blocking the action at the tumor level of the residual postmenopausal levels of estrogens observed during chronic therapy with LHRH analogs. Furthermore, coadministration of antiestrogens may prevent the flare phenomenon observed in some patients and may shorten the time required for tumor regression to occur, since it takes several weeks for the LHRH analogs to optimally suppress ovarian steroidogenesis. Such treatment strategy is currently being applied in the treatment of advanced prostate cancer where therapy with LHRH analogs is combined with antiandrogens [23].

REFERENCES

1. Schally, A.V. Aspects of hypothalamic regulation of the pituitary gland. Its implications for the control of reproductive processes. Science, 202, 18 (1978)
2. Maynard, P.V. and Nicholson, R.I. Effects of high doses of a series of new luteinizing hormone-releasing hormone analogues in intact female rats. Brit. J. Cancer, 39, 274 (1979)
3. Ying, S.Y. and Guillemin, R. (D-TRP)-Luteinizing-hormone-releasing factor inhibits follicular development in hypophysectomized rats. Nature, 180, 593 (1979)
4. Rabin, D. and McNeil, L.W. Pituitary and gonadal desensitazation after continuous luteinizing hormone-releasing hormone infusion in normal females. J. Clin. Endocrinol. Metab., 51, 873 (1980)
5. Huggins, C. and Hodges, C.V. Studies on prostatic cancer. I. The effect of castration, of estrogen and of androgen injection on serum phosphatases in metastatic carcinoma of the prostate. Cancer Res., 1, 293 (1941)
6. Huggins, C., Stevens, R.E., Jr. and Hodges, C.V. Studies on prostatic cancer. III. The effects of castration on advanced carcinoma of the prostate gland. Arch. Surg., 43, 209 (1941)
7. Huggins, C., Scott, W.W. and Hodges, C.V. Studies on prostatic cancer. III. The Effects of castration on advanced carcinoma of the prostate gland. Arch. Surg., 43, 209 (1941)
8. Byar, D.P. VACURG studies of conservative treatment. Scand. J. Urol. Nephrol. [Suppl], 55, 99 (1980)
9. Bailar, J.C., III and Byar, D.P., Veterans Administration Cooperative Urological Research Group. Estrogen treatment for cancer of the prostate: early results with 3 doses of diethlystilbestrol and placebo. Cancer, 26, 257 (1970)
10. Smith, J.A., Glode, L.M., Wettlaufer, J.M., Stein, B.S., Glass, A.G., Max, D.T., Anbar, D., Jagst, C.L., and Murphy, G.P. Clinical effects of a gonadotropin-releasing hormone analogue in patients with metastatic carcinoma of the prostate. Urol., 24, 106 (1985)

11. The Leuprolide Study Group. Leuprolide versus Diethystil-
    bestrol for Metastatic Prostate Cancer. N. Engl. J. Med., 311,
    1281 (1984)
12. Garnick, M.B. Leuprolide versus diethylstilbestrol for
    previously untreated stage D2 prostate cancer: Results of a
    prospectively randomized trial. Urol. [Suppl], 21 (1986)
13. Beatson, G.T. On the treatment on inoperable cases of
    carcinoma of the mamma: Suggestions for a new method of
    treatment, with illustrative cases. Lancet, 2, 104 (1896)
14. Johnson, E.S., Seely, J.A., White, W.F., and De Sombre, E.R.
    Endocrine-dependent rat mammary tumor regression: Use of a
    gonadotropin releasing hormone analog. Science, 194, 329
    (1976)
15. Harvey, H.A., Lipton, A., Santen, R.J., Escher, G.C., Hardy,
    M.A., Glode, L.M., Segaloff, A., Landau, R.L., Schneier, H.
    and Max, D.T. Phase II study of a gonadotropin-releasing
    hormone analogue (leuprolide) in postmenopausal advanced
    breast cancer patients. Proc. Am. Soc. Clin. Oncol., 22, 4444
    (1981) (Abstract C-436)
16. Harvey, H.A., Lipton, A., and Max, D.T. LHRH analogs for human
    mammary carcinoma. In "LHRH and its Analogs", Vickery, B.H.,
    Nestor, J.J., Jr., and E.S.E. Hafez (Eds.), MTP Press, Boston,
    1984, p. 329.
17. Harvey, H.A., Lipton, A., Max, D.T., Pearlman, H.G.,
    Diaz-Perches, R., and de la Garza, J. Medical castration
    produced by the GnRH analogue leuprolide to treat metastatic
    breast cancer, J. Clin. Oncol., 3, 1068 (1985)
18. Eidne, K.A., Flanagan, C.A. and Millar, R.P. Gonadotropin-
    releasing hormone binding sites in human breast carcinoma.
    Science, 229, 989 (1985)
19. Miller, W.R., Scott, W.N., Morris, R., Fruser, H.M., and
    Sharpe, R.M. Growth of human breast cancer cells inhibited by
    luteinizing hormone releasing hormone agonist. Nature, 313,
    231 (1985)
20. Klijn, J.G.M., deJong, F.H., Blankenstein, M.A., Doctar, R.,
    Alexieva-Figush, J., Blank, J., and Lambert, S.W. Antitumor
    and endocrine effects of chronic LHRH agonist treatment
    (Buserelin) with or without tamoxifen in premenopausal meta-
    static breast cancer. Breast Cancer Res. Treat., 4, 209 (1984)
21. Klijn, J.G.M. Long-term LHRH agonist treatment in metastatic
    breast cancer as a single treatment and in combination with
    other additive endocrine treatments. Med. Oncol. Tumor
    Pharmacother., 1, 123 (1984)
22. Walker, K.J., Nicholson, R.I., Turkes, A., Plowman, N., and
    Blamey, R. Therapeutic potential of the LHRH agonist, Zoladex
    ICI 118630, in the treatment of advanced breast cancer in pre-
    and postmenopausal women. J. Steroid Biochem., 20, 1409 (1984)
    (Abstract)
23. Labrie, F., Dupont, A., Belanger, A., and Members of the Laval
    University Prostate Cancer Program. Dramatic response to a new
    antihormonal treatment for prostate cancer. Proc. 7th Int.
    Congr. Endocrinol., Excerpta Medica, Int. Congr. Ses. 652,
    Elsevier Science Publishers, B.V., Amsterdam, 1984, p. 98
    (Abstract)

26
Zoladex Studies in Prostatic and Breast Cancer

R.J. DONNELLY and R.A.V. MILSTED

ICI Pharmaceuticals Division, Alderley Park, Macclesfield, SK10 4TG England

INTRODUCTION

'Zoladex'[†] ([D-Ser(Bu^t)^6, Azagly^{10}]-LHRH) is an LHRH analogue with a potency 50-100 times that of LHRH [1]. It entered clinical trials in 1982 as an aqueous formulation which was administered daily by subcutaneous injection. A depot formulation of the drug [2] became available for clinical study in early 1984. This depot consists of a cylindrical rod of a biodegradable and biocompatible d,1-lactide-glycolide co-polymer within which the drug is homogeneously dispersed. The depot is supplied in an applicator with a 16 gauge needle. Drug is released continuously for at least 28 days following subcutaneous injection.

The principal pharmacological effect of LHRH agonists in man occurs at the pituitary gland where, following an initial stimulatory phase, they inhibit the release of gonadotrophins. Consequently, with chronic therapy, sex hormone production in patients with functional gonads is reduced to levels found in the surgically gonadectomised state. This profile led to the evaluation of 'Zoladex' in the sex hormone dependent malignancies of advanced prostate and breast cancer.

ADVANCED PROSTATE CANCER - PREVIOUSLY UNTREATED PATIENTS

Prostate cancer is one of the most common causes of death from cancer in men in Western countries. Over 80% of patients present with advanced disease [3] and in these therapy can only be palliative. Huggins and Hodges [4] showed that reduction of serum testosterone by surgical castration or oestrogen therapy will provide temporary control of the disease in the approximately 70% of previously untreated patients who have androgen-dependent disease [5]. Non-comparative studies of 'Zoladex' were designed to define the long term suppressive effect of the drug on serum testosterone and to confirm that such an endocrine change would produce the

[†]'Zoladex' is a trade mark, the property of Imperial Chemical Industries PLC.

anticipated anti-tumour effects. A randomised comparison of 'Zoladex' and surgical orchidectomy was also initiated. Patients undergoing orchidectomy had the same assessments performed as those receiving 'Zoladex'.

Methods

Selection criteria. Previously untreated patients with histologically confirmed prostate cancer with metastases or locally advanced disease were selected if they had no other malignancy and gave informed consent.

Details of dosage. Patients entering studies of 'Zoladex' before 1984 received 'Zoladex' as daily subcutaneous injections of the aqueous formulation in doses ranging from 25 to 500 μg. The endocrine effects of these doses are presented elsewhere [6] and show that 250 μg daily suppresses serum testosterone. This dose was used for the majority of the patients who received the aqueous formulation. From 1984 patients received 'Zoladex' as subcutaneous injections of the depot formulation every four weeks. The initial studies examined the endocrine effects of 0.9, 1.8 and 3.6 mg of the drug [7], these giving an average daily release of 30, 60 and 120 μg respectively. The 3.6 mg depot dose was subsequently selected as optimum and further trials were conducted with this dose. The effect of extending the dosing interval of the 3.6 mg depot from four weeks to five or six weeks was studied in a sub-group of patients.

Endocrine assessments. Serum LH and testosterone concentrations were assessed at four weekly intervals up to 12 weeks and 12 weekly thereafter. Serum FSH, prolactin, oestradiol, sex hormone binding globulin and dehyroepiandrosterone sulphate concentrations were measured in a sub-set of patients.

Subjective assessments. The subjective response was determined by assessing performance status (scored 0-4), urological symptoms (scored 0-3), bone pain (scored 0-4) and analgesic use (scored 0-4). Patients were defined as symptomatic if they had a score of at least 2 for any assessment or had a total score of at least 4. A favourable subjective response in symptomatic patients was defined as a fall of at least 2 in any assessment or a fall in the total score of at least 4 (subjective response by protocol criteria) or a symptomatic improvement as judged by the clinician (subjective response by clinician's assessment).

Objective assessments. The objective response to therapy was monitored by frequent assessment of the primary tumour (by digital examination and, in some centres, ultrasonography), by serum total and prostatic acid phosphatases, by isotope bone scans and skeletal radiography and by assessment of extra-skeletal metastases.

The criteria for objective response were:

i)   Complete regression (CR)   - No evidence of residual tumour

ii) Partial regression (PR)   - No evidence of progression and
                                     any of the following:
     Primary tumour   - A decrease in (a) T-category
                                     (UICC) [8] or (b) product of
                                     length and width by 50% or
                                     (c) volume by 35%
     Bone metastases   - A decrease in radiological or
                                     bone scan evidence of
                                     metastases
     Extra-skeletal metastases   - Reduction in size by 35%
     Acid phosphatase   - Return to normal or reduction
                                     by 80%

iii) Stable disease (SD)   - Lack of progression and
                                     insufficient evidence for PR

iv) Progression (Prog)   - Any of the following:
     Primary tumour   - An increase in (a) T-category
                                     or (b) product of length and
                                     width by 50% or (c) volume by
                                     35%
     Bone   - Appearance of new metastases on
                                     X-ray or bone scan
     Extra-skeletal metastases   - Appearance of new metastases or
                                     increase by 35% of any existing
                                     measurable metastases

Tolerance. The safety of 'Zoladex' was assessed by specific enquiry
for the possible pharmacological side-effects of suppression of
libido, impairment of erections and the occurrence of hot flushes
and breast swelling or tenderness. In addition standard
haematological and biochemical tests were performed and patients
were monitored for possible adverse reactions. Local tolerance to
the subcutaneous injection of the depot was also assessed.

Results - Non-comparative studies

Patient details. Eight hundred and thirty patients were entered
into studies of 'Zoladex' in 12 European countries. All of these
patients are included in the tolerance analysis. The endocrine,
subjective and objective assessment analyses were performed on a
sub-set of 503 patients. These patients had a mean age of 71.0
years (SD 7.9, range 45-88), with 61% of them aged greater than 70.
The percentages of patients with well, moderately and poorly
differentiated prostate cancer were 15.9%, 43.5% and 34.8%,
respectively. Metastases were present in 83% of patients, the
remainder having locally advanced disease only.

Endocrine response. The mean serum testosterone concentrations of the patients are shown in Table 1.

Table 1. Mean serum testosterone values (nmol/1)

		Duration of therapy (weeks)								
	0	4	12	24	48	72	96	120	144
Mean	14.0	1.8	1.4	1.5	1.0	0.9	1.0	1.0	0.9
SD	7.7	3.0	2.4	3.1	0.6	0.5	0.5	0.6	0.5
n	476	431	322	143	110	49	15	9	7

These data show that the suppression of serum testosterone noted by week 4 is maintained for over two years, indicating that pharmacological tolerance does not develop on long term therapy. Mean serum LH also remained suppressed over this time period.

Mean serum FSH was suppressed by four weeks of therapy. After 12 weeks it slowly rose, but did not regain its pre-treatment value. Mean serum oestradiol was suppressed by four weeks of therapy and remained suppressed thereafter. Mean serum prolactin, dehyroepiandrosterone sulphate and sex hormone binding globulin were unaltered with chronic therapy.

Dosing frequency of the depot. The effect on serum testosterone of increasing the dosing interval of the 3.6 mg depot is shown in Table 2.

Table 2. Effect of increasing the 3.6 mg depot dosing interval

Dosing interval	No. of patients with rise in serum testosterone to above the surgically castrate range
5 weeks	2/24 (8%)
6 weeks	10/36 (28%)

Extension of the dosing interval of the 3.6 mg depot from four weeks to five or six weeks leads to failure of maintenance of suppression of serum testosterone in an appreciable proportion of patients. Conversely, a few days delay in the administration of the 3.6 mg depot beyond the standard 28 day dosing interval should not cause loss of control of suppression of serum testosterone.

Subjective response. Of the 503 patients assessable for subjective
response, 256 (51%) were symptomatic as defined above. Of these,
153 (60%) and 202 (79%) had favourable subjective responses by the
protocol criteria and by the clinician's assessment, respectively.
The median time to favourable subjective response by the life-table
method was eight weeks by the protocol criteria and five weeks by
the clinician's assessment.

Objective response. Of the 503 patients assessable for objective
response, 387 were evaluable. The main reason for the balance not
being evaluable was that the patients had not been on therapy for at
least 12 weeks. Table 3 shows the overall objective response status
for the 387 patients.

Table 3. Objective response status

	Overall objective response			
	CR	PR	SD	Prog
Percentage of patients	0%	51.2%	20.2%	28.6%

The mean serum testosterone of the patients who had disease
progression was 1.8 nmol/l (SD=2.7), indicating that lack of
endocrine control was not the reason for the objective progression
of these patients and that they had developed disease that was not
androgen dependent.

Tolerance. The effects of 'Zoladex' on possible pharmacological
side-effects are shown in Table 4.

Table 4. Possible pharmacological side-effects of 'Zoladex'

	Percentage of patients	Number of assessable patients
Suppression of libido	59%	376
Impairment of erections	61%	372
Occurrence of hot flushes	48%	772
Occurrence of breast swelling	3%	770
Occurrence of breast tenderness	2%	788

The incidence of hot flushes noted with 'Zoladex' therapy is
higher than the incidence spontaneously reported to clinicians
following surgical castration, but accords with the results of
trials where specific enquiry was made [9]. The hot flushes were
sufficiently severe in one patient to require withdrawal of therapy.
A low incidence of gynaecomastia is noted in surgically castrated
men (2 out of 106 [10]) and the similarly low incidence of mild

401

breast complaints noted with 'Zoladex' is, therefore, not surprising.

Examination of the results of standard haematological and biochemical parameters did not reveal any adverse effect of 'Zoladex'. Local tolerance to subcutaneous administration of the depot was assessed in 475 patients who received a total of approximately 2600 depots. On 19 occasions (0.8%) in 16 patients (3.4%) mild bruising or erythema at the site of injection of the depot was noted. These minor episodes related to the trauma of the subcutaneous injection and not to the presence of the depot. Specifically, no abscess was noted in any depot-treated patient.

The patients included in these studies were elderly men who had, apart from their prostate cancer, many concurrent illnesses for which they received concomitant medication. Not unexpectedly, serious medical events occurred in some patients during the study period. Apart from some dermatological, bone pain, neurological and renal events (presented later) all of the reported possible adverse reactions were explicable in terms of the natural history of patients with prostate cancer.

Fourteen (1.7%) of the 830 patients had mild or moderate skin eruptions, most commonly described as generalised maculo-papular rashes. These were noted from four days to five months after the initiation of therapy. No patient required hospitalisation. The eruptions in 12 of the 14 patients resolved despite continuation of 'Zoladex'. Therapy was withdrawn in two patients with complete resolution of their skin eruptions.

Worsening of signs and symptoms of prostate cancer during the first month of therapy. Increases in bone pain and the development of ureteric and spinal cord compression have been noted during the first month of LHRH agonist therapy for advanced prostatic cancer [11-13]. Consequently, the histories of the 830 patients were examined to identify patients with an early worsening of the disease. Fifty one (6.1%) patients were identified as shown in Table 5.

Table 5. Worsening of disease in first month

Bone pain		Urinary Tract Obstruction		Spinal Cord Compression		Total
Mild/ Moderate	Severe	Upper	Lower	Paraplegia	Paraparesis/ Paraesthesiae	
21 (2.5%)	14 (1.7%)	5 (0.6%)	4 (0.5%)	6 (0.7%)	4 (0.5%)	51† (6.1%)

†three patients had two signs or symptoms

Bone pain was managed symptomatically and no patient was withdrawn because of it. The urinary tract obstructions and spinal cord compressions were managed conventionally. Paraplegia resolved in five patients but not in the sixth whose endocrine data revealed that he did not receive 'Zoladex'. Examination of the objective and subjective response status of these patients by type of worsening of disease did not reveal any correlation. Specifically, there was no correlation between bone pain and objective regression.

The cause of the early disease worsening noted with LHRH agonists is not clear, although some workers consider that it is due to the rise in serum testosterone in the first week of therapy [14, 15]. They advocate the use of anti-androgens at the initiation of therapy even though there is no data from controlled clinical trials to show that such a manoeuvre prevents the early worsening of disease.

If the initial rise in serum testosterone does indeed lead to the development of ureteric obstruction or paraplegia, then there should be an increased frequency of such events in LHRH agonist-treated patients compared with those receiving standard therapy. The incidence of ureteric obstruction shortly after diagnosis is not well documented but Rubin et al [16] found that of 152 patients, 6.6% had paraplegia and 5.3% had increasing paraparesis at presentation which suggests that the incidence of spinal cord compression noted in the 'Zoladex' studies (1.2%) is not excessive. Also, two comparative studies of LHRH analogues versus standard therapies have not demonstrated an increased incidence of early paraplegia [17,18].

There are two other possible explanations for the early disease worsening: the disease in some patients could have been androgen-independent at presentation and the worsening could have simply represented disease progression; and the delay of two weeks before serum testosterone was suppressed below pre-treatment values may have allowed continued growth of androgen-sensitive neoplastic tissue to a critical size to cause the worsening.

Results - randomised comparative study

More than 350 patients have been entered into this on-going randomised comparison of 'Zoladex' and surgical orchidectomy. Preliminary results from this study [19] reveal that there was no difference between the two therapies in terms of subjective and objective response rates, suppression of serum testosterone and possible pharmacological side effects. The data are too premature to allow a valid analysis of survival differences between the two groups of patients.

ADVANCED PROSTATE CANCER - PREVIOUSLY TREATED PATIENTS

Patients whose advanced prostate cancer is controlled by hormone manipulation therapy will ultimately develop androgen-independent disease and will relapse. Such previously treated patients occasionally have a second remission induced by the institution of an alternative hormone manipulation therapy. Consequently, the value of 'Zoladex' was assessed in 42 patients whose disease had relapsed following earlier orchidectomy or oestrogen therapy. These patients were assessed as detailed in the previous section. Twenty eight patients were evaluable for subjective response and the favourable subjective response rate was 29% by the protocol criteria and 61% by the clinician's assessment. Of the 25 patients evaluable for objective response, one (4%) showed evidence of a partial regression, five (20%) showed stable disease and 19 (76%) showed progression. The patient achieving a partial regression had received oestrogen therapy previously but his serum testosterone was fully suppressed before the institution of 'Zoladex' therapy.

ADVANCED PRE-MENOPAUSAL BREAST CANCER

'Zoladex' has been evaluated in 53 pre-menopausal patients with advanced breast cancer [20]. Of these, 27 patients were treated initially with daily subcutaneous injections of 500 (n=5) or 1000 µg (n=22). The remaining 26 patients received 3.6 mg of the drug in the subcutaneous depot formulation every 28 days. All patients had histologically proven breast cancer and locally advanced (>5 cm) disease (n=14) or metastases (n=39).

Endocrinological response

After an initial rise, serum LH and FSH decreased below pre-treatment values. This fall was associated with a fall in circulating concentrations of oestradiol and progesterone to levels seen in surgically oophorectomised or post-menopausal patients. Administration of the depot formulation produced endocrine results at least as good as the administration of 1000 µg of the aqueous formulation daily. Two patients on the daily injection and three on the depot showed recurrent, though suppressed, peaks of oestradiol. These occurred despite basal levels of serum LH and FSH. The mechanism and clinical importance of these peaks is not clear since one of these patients showed sclerosis of lytic bone metastases during the first three months of treatment.

Clinical response

Forty five patients were assessable for response, eight having been excluded (two were lost to follow up and six were withdrawn because of disease progression before an adequate trial of the drug). Response was determined by UICC criteria with the added stipulation that any remission should be maintained for at least 6 months.

Fourteen patients (31%) had a partial remission and three (6%) had stable disease at six months. Oestrogen receptor status was known in 38 of the 45 assessable patients. Of the 14 responders only one was ER negative, 10 being ER positive and 3 unknown. Of the three patients with stable disease one was ER positive and two ER negative. Of the 28 patients with progressive disease 8 were ER positive, 16 ER negative and 4 unknown.

Twenty six patients underwent surgical oophorectomy on disease progression and four patients appeared to gain a response following this. Of these, one had recurrent peaks of serum oestradiol after therapy with the daily injection and three had possibly received an inadequate trial of therapy (2, 2 and 3 months).

Therapy was well tolerated. The pharmacological effects of oestradiol withdrawal included hot flushes in 20 patients (38%). All patients who had suppressed serum oestradiol concentrations ceased to have normal menstrual periods after two months of therapy. No patient had a transient increase of signs or symptoms of the disease at the initiation of therapy.

ADVANCED POST-MENOPAUSAL BREAST CANCER

Ten previously untreated post-menopausal patients have been studied in a trial to examine the endocrine [21] and clinical [22] effects of 'Zoladex'. Six patients received the drug by daily subcutaneous injection, of whom four only received one month of therapy, making them non-evaluable for clinical response. The remainding four all received the 3.6 mg depot formulation for at least three months.

Endocrine response

After 14 days of therapy serum concentrations of LH and FSH were suppressed below pre-treatment values. There appeared to be no change in levels of serum oestradiol, progesterone, testosterone, dehydroepiandrosterone sulphate and growth hormone.

Clinical response

Two of the six patients evaluable for clinical response achieved a partial remission. One patient had regression of spinal metastases documented on serial bone scans at three months. She subsequently maintained this remission for over a year on 'Nolvadex' before progressing at this site. She was six years post-menopausal with post-menopausal values of LH and FSH at the start of therapy and was both ER and progesterone receptor positive. The other responder was clinically and endocrinologically post-menopausal at the start of therapy and achieved a partial remission of lung metastases which is continuing after 12 months. Her receptor status is unknown.

'Zoladex' was well tolerated in all patients, both systemically and locally at the site of the depot injection. Other studies, still in progress, appear to confirm the lack of endocrine effects in most patients, other than suppression of gonadotrophins, and have yielded a further response in the primary tumour of a previously untreated patient (A Harris, personal communication).

CONCLUSIONS

In previously untreated patients with advanced prostate cancer, 'Zoladex' is effective in maintaining long term suppression of serum testosterone. The subjective response rates and objective response rate (CR + PR + SD = 71.4%) observed with 'Zoladex' in non-comparative studies are consistent with those expected following conventional hormone manipulation therapies and confirm the benefit to such patients of adequate suppression of serum testosterone. Disease progression was not associated with loss of suppression of serum testosterone. Preliminary results from a comparative study indicate that 'Zoladex' produces similar subjective and objective response rates to surgical orchidectomy but longer term follow up is required to determine whether there is any difference in survival between the two groups of patients. 'Zoladex' was well tolerated systemically and, with specific regard to the depot formulation, locally. Approximately half of the patients experienced the anticipated side effects due to suppression of serum testosterone of hot flushes, reduction of libido and impairment of erections. During the first month, bone pain increased in 4.2% with 1.1% experiencing urinary tract obstruction and 1.2% spinal cord compression. In view of the uncertainty surrounding the cause of these events, routine use of anti-androgens at the initiation of LHRH agonist therapy cannot be recommended until controlled clinical data are available to establish the value of this manoeuvre. The availability of the four weekly depot formulation of 'Zoladex' should aid patient compliance particularly when compared to the alternative of daily subcutaneous injections.

The findings of lower favourable subjective response rates and a low incidence of objective response in previously treated prostate cancer patients suggest that 'Zoladex' is unlikely to prove to be of substantial benefit to this patient group. However, the number of patients studied was low and this aspect of the use of 'Zoladex' is worthy of further study.

In women with advanced breast cancer, a 3.6 mg 'Zoladex' depot given every 28 days produced satisfactory suppression of serum gonadotrophins and reduced the serum oestradiol concentrations into the surgically castrate range in pre-menopausal women. The response rate in pre-menopausal women was similar to that produced by surgical or radiation oophorectomy and responses were more common in women with ER positive tumours. Subsequent response to oophorectomy was not seen in pre-menopausal patients progressing after adequate therapy with 'Zoladex'. The mechanism of the responses seen in post-menopausal patients is not clear and a larger number of

patients require to be studied to define fully the utility of
'Zoladex' in this patient group. 'Zoladex' was well tolerated
systemically and locally by the women with only the pharmacological
side effects of hot flushes being apparent in those who were premenopausal.

REFERENCES

1. Dutta,A.S., Furr,B.J.A., Giles,M.B. and Valcaccia,B. Synthesis
   and biological activity of highly active α-aza analogues of
   luliberin. J. Med. Chem., 21, 1018 (1978).

2. Furr,B.J.A. and Hutchinson,F.G. Biodegradable sustained
   release formulation of the LHRH analogue 'Zoladex' for the
   treatment of hormone responsive tumours. In EORTC
   Genitourinary Group Monograph 2, Part A:Therapeutic Principles
   in Metastatic Prostatic Cancer, 1985, p.143.

3. The Veterans Administration Co-operative Urological Research
   Group. Treatment and survival of patients with cancer of the
   prostate. Surg. Gynaecol. Obstet., 124, 1011 (1967).

4. Huggins,C. and Hodges,C.V. Studies on prostatic cancer : 1.
   The effect of castration, of oestrogen and on androgen
   injection on serum phosphatases in metastatic carcinoma of the
   prostate. Cancer Res., 1, 293 (1941).

5. Resnick,M.I. and Grayhack,J.T. Treatment of stage IV carcinoma
   of the prostate. Uro. Clin. N. Amer., 2, 141 (1975).

6. Donnelly,R.J., Cotton,R.C., Ellis,S.H. and Richards,D.
   Subcutaneous administration of 'Zoladex' (ICI 118,630), an LHRH
   analogue in advanced prostatic cancer. In "LHRH and Its
   Analogues", Labrie,F., Belanger,A. and Dupont,A. (Eds),
   Elsevier Science Publishers BV, 1984, p.305.

7. Walker,K.J., Turkes,A.O., Turkes,A., Zwink,R., Beacock,C.,
   Buck,A.C., Peeling,W.B. and Griffiths,K. Treatment of patients
   with advanced cancer of the prostate using a slow-release
   (depot) formulation of the LHRH agonist ICI 118,630
   ('Zoladex'). J. Endocrinol., 103, R1 (1984).

8. UICC. TNM classifiction of malignant tumours. Harmer,M.H.
   (Ed), Geneva, Union Internationale Contre le Cancer, 1978.

9. Frodin,T., Alund,G., and Varenhorst,E. Measurement of skin
   blood-flow and water evaporation as a means of objectively
   assessing hot flushes after orchidectomy in patients with
   prostatic cancer. The Prostate, 1, 203 (1985).

10. Gardner,A.M.N. and Setakis,N. Carcinoma of prostate. Increased mortality and cardiovascular complications associated with oestrogen therapy as compared with orchidectomy. Bristol Medico-Chirurg J., __98__, 117 (1983).

11. Faure,N., Lemay,A., Laroche,B., Robert,G., Plante,R., Jean,C., Thabet,M., Roy,R. and Fazekas,A.T.A. Preliminary results on the clinical efficacy and safety of androgen inhibition by an LHRH agonist alone or combined with an antiandrogen in the treatment of prostatic carcinoma. The Prostate, __4__, 601 (1983).

12. Kahan,A., Delrieu,F., Amor,B., Chiche,R. and Steg,A. Disease flare induced by D-Trp[6]-LHRH analogue in patients with metastatic prostatic cancer. The Lancet, __1__, 971 (1984).

13. Winfield,H. and Trachtenberg,J. A comparison of a powerful luteinising hormone releasing hormone analogue agonist and estrogen in the treatment of advanced prostatic cancer. J. Urol., __131__, 1108 (1984).

14. Labrie,F., Dupont,A., Belanger,A., Lacoursiere,Y., Raynaud,J.P., Husson,J.M., Gareau,J., Fazekas,A.T.A., Sandow,J., Monfette,G., Girard,J.G., Emond,J. and Houle,J.G. New approach in the treatment of prostatic cancer: Complete instead of partial withdrawal of androgens. The Prostate, __4__, 579 (1983).

15. Waxman,J. Early tumour exacerbation in patients treated with long acting analogues of gonadotrophin releasing hormone. Brit. Med. J., __292__, 58 (1986).

16. Rubin,H., Lowe,L.G. and Presman,D. Neurological manifestation of metastatic prostatic carcinoma. J. Urol., __111__, 799 (1974).

17. Leuprolide Study Group. Leuprolide versus diethylstilboestrol for metastatic prostate cancer. The New Eng. J. Med., __311__, 1281 (1984).

18. Parmar,H., Lightman,S.L., Allen,L., Phillips,R.H., Edwards,L. and Schally,A.V. Randomised controlled study of orchidectomy versus long-acting D-Trp[6]-LHRH microcapsules in advanced prostatic carcinoma. Lancet, __1__, 1201 (1985).

19. Peeling,W.B., Beacock,C., Kaisary,A.V., Turkes,A. and Tyrell,C.J. A comparison between surgical orchidectomy and the LHRH agonist 'Zoladex' (ICI 118,630) in the treatment of disseminated prostatic carcinoma. Abstracts of presentations at the British Association of Urological Surgeons meeting, London, 1986, p.88.

20. Williams,M.R., Walker,K.J., Turkes,A., Blamey,R.W. and Nicholson,R.I. The use of an LHRH agonist (ICI 118,630, 'Zoladex') in advanced pre-menopausal breast cancer. Br. J. Cancer, __53__, 629 (1986).

21. Nicholson,R.I., Walker,K.J., Turkes,A., Dyas,J., Plowman,P.N., Williams,M. and Blamey,R.W. Endocrinological and clinical aspects of LHRH action in hormone dependent breast cancer. J. Steroid Biochm., 23, 843 (1985).

22. Plowman,P.N., Nicholson,R.I. and Walker,K.J. Responses in post-menopausal breast cancer with an LHRH analogue (ICI 118,630). Eur. J. of Cancer and Clinical Oncology (In Press).

27
Intermittent LHRH Agonist Sequentially Combined with a Progestogen as Antiovulatory Contraception

A. LEMAY and N. FAURE

Endocrinologie de la Reproduction, Hôpital Saint-François d'Assise,
Québec, Canada, G1L 3L5

INTRODUCTION

Continuous LHRH infusion in normal women leads to pituitary and gonadal desensitization [1]. Once daily intranasal administration of potent LHRH agonists consistently blocks ovulation and prevents progesterone secretion [2-5]. However under repetitive administration of LHRH agonist and pituitary down-regulation the inhibition of follicular activity is variable and there is a high incidence of oligomenorrhea and amenorrhea [3-5]. Endometrial biopsies taken after several months of treatment indicated inactive endometrium or variable stages of proliferation [6,7]. Potential drawbacks of long term treatment could be related to the persistent state of decreased and unopposed estrogens.

Discontinuous peptide administration for 22 days together with an orally active progestogen during the last 3 days of the treatment cycle was first reported by Hardt [8]. Recently, we presented the results of a dose-range finding study on the endocrine and clinical effects of discontinuous intranasal buserelin for 2 periods of 3 weeks [9]. Ovulation was blocked while estradiol secretion was stimulated during the 2 consecutive treatment cycles. Withdrawal bleeding was obtained after 5 days of progestogen taken during the 3rd week of treatment.

INTERMITTENT TREATMENT REGIMENS

We have then evaluated the pituitary-ovarian activity during different discontinuous periods of treatment [10]. Fourteen day regimens were compared with 21 day regimens of [D-Ser(tBu)^6,Pro^9-NHEt] LHRH (buserelin). Since the frequency of administration is important in LHRH agonist action on the pituitary, 400µg of buserelin was administered intranasally once daily 400µg/24h) or in 2 dosings (200µg/12h). After 2 pretreatment cycles, 4 groups of 6 or 7 women were treated during 4 consecutive periods starting on day 3 of the regular cycle. The LHRH agonist was administered intranasally via a metered nasal spray delivering 100µg per insufflation (kindly provided by Hoechst Canada Inc., Montreal, Quebec, Canada). Five mg of medroxy-progesterone acetate (Provera) was taken orally twice daily on days 15 to 21 of the treatment periods as a progestogen complement to achieve a more adequate uterine bleeding. A pause of 7 days with no drug administration followed each treatment period. Volunteers were evaluated during 2 recovery cycles following the cessation of the medication.

Figure 1 illustrates the endocrine and clinical assessments during the 8 consecutive cycles of the study in a single subject protocol (ML). For radioimmunoassays of LH, FSH, estradiol (E_2) and progesterone (P), blood samples were drawn every other day at approximately the same time (generally at 8h00 am) and every day from day 10 to 16 of the pretreatment and post-treatment cycles. During the treatment periods blood was drawn every other day. The first 2 pretreatment cycles showed normal endocrine profiles of LH, FSH, E_2 and P.

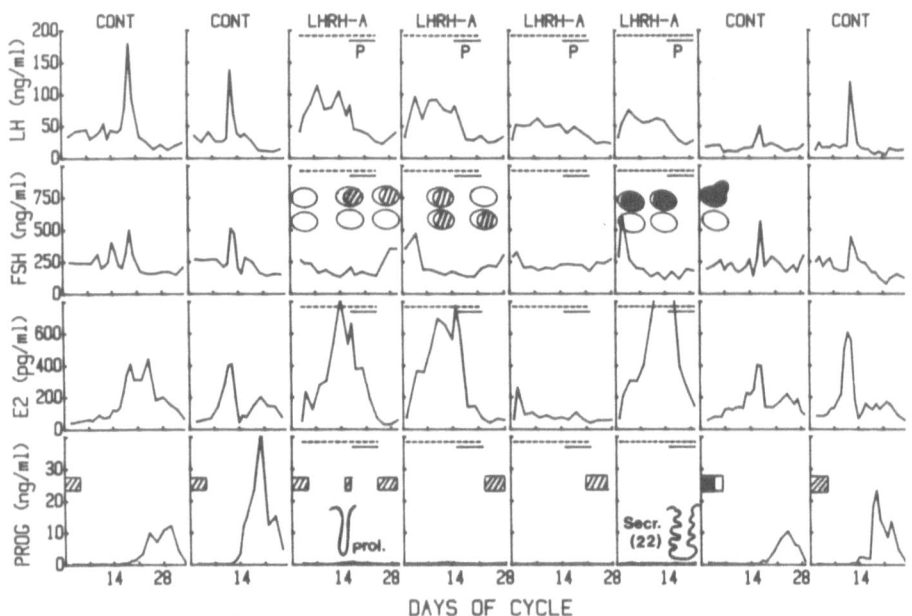

FIGURE 1 Serum LH, FSH, E_2 and P profiles in subject ML during 8 consecutive cycles. 200µg/12h of the LHRH agonist (LHRH-A) buserelin, was administered intranasally for 21 days starting on day 3 of the 3rd cycle. 5mg of medroxyprogesterone acetate (P) was taken by mouth twice daily from days 15 to 21. No medication was given between days 22 and 28 of each treatment cycle. Blood samples were drawn daily before dosing from day 10 to 16 of control cycles and otherwise every other day. ◘ light, ▨ moderate, ■ heavy uterine bleeding, ◯ quiescent ovary, ◑ large follicle, ● follicular cyst. The tubular proliferative and tortuous secretory glands are schematically drawn for endometrial biopsy illustration.

412

Intermittent administration of buserelin (200µg/12h) was started on day 3 of the third cycle. Ovarian ultrasound performed at the beginning of the treatment showed quiescent ovaries. Predosing levels of LH and FSH were elevated on days 2 and 4 of the treatment. Thereafter FSH returned to pretreatment levels whereas LH remained elevated. Serum E_2 rapidly increased following the FSH and LH stimulation at the beginning of the treatment and remained elevated during the LHRH agonist treatment. Repeated ovarian scan on treatment day 15 relealed a single large follicle in the right ovary. An endometrial biopsy performed the same day corresponded to a late proliferative phase. During the progestogen administration (week 3), LH and E_2 progressively decreased towards pretreatment levels of the early follicular phase although the large follicle was still present in the right ovary. During the pause (week 4), the hormones had returned to basal levels except for FSH which rose progressively. There was no significant elevation of progesterone during the entire treatment cycle. A 6-day uterine bleeding occurred during the pause.

A similar endocrine pattern was observed during the subsequent 3 other treatment cycles. Serum E_2 levels were lower in treatment cycle 3. Large follicles were seen in both ovaries of cycle 2. A large follicle was present at the beginning of the 4th treatment period. During that cycle, serum E_2 levels were markedly increased and a follicular cyst was observed in the right ovary at the end of the treatment. The endometrial biopsy taken on day 22 of the last treatment period showed secretory changes of an incompletely matured endometrium corresponding to day 21 of a normal 28 day cycle. The first recovery cycle was started on the first day of bleeding following the last medication period. The follicular phase was prolonged by a few days but the luteal phase was normal. The second posttreatment cycle was entirely comparable to pretreatment cycles.

SERUM LH AND FSH CHANGES

The mean predosing levels of serum LH of treatment cycles 1 and 4 are illustrated in Figure 2 and are compared with the normal range of control cycles. Following the stimulation at the beginning of the treatment cycle, serum LH levels were increased 1 to 3 fold above pretreatment levels. They remained significantly elevated above the normal range during the entire period of administration of buserelin. LH levels decreased to within control range after the medication was discontinued either after day 14 or day 21. During the pause, LH values were in the normal range as compared to the end of a normal cycle.

Serum FSH levels were significantly increased (0.5 to 2 fold) only on days 2 and 4 of each treatment cycle in all the groups (P < 0.01). Thereafter, serum FSH levels returned into the normal range for the entire period of buserelin administration. In the 200µg/12h groups, serum FSH levels were lower reaching the lower half of the normal range. Serum FSH levels could be seen to rise progressively when buserelin medication was discontinued either after day 14 or day 21. This spontaneous rise in FSH levels was statistically significant.

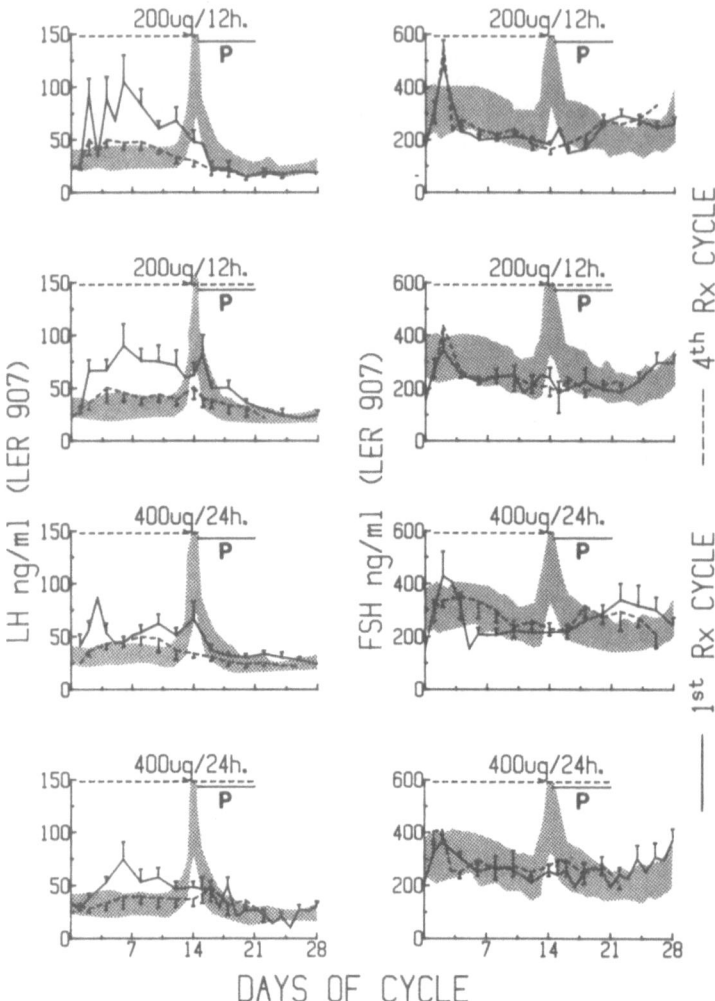

FIGURE 2 Means ± SEM of predosing serum LH and FSH measured every
other day during the 1st and 4th treatment cycles with the
LHRH agonist (----). Curves are presented according to the
frequency (200µg/12h vs 400µg/24h) and schedule (14 vs 21
days) of intranasal insufflation of buserelin. 5mg of (P)
medroxyprogesterone acetate (——) was taken by mouth on
days 15 to 21. The shaded area represents the range of
values of control cycles within ± 1 SD.

Thus intermittent LHRH agonist for 14 or 21 days caused an apparent different effect on LH and FSH. While serum LH was maintained
elevated during the duration of LHRH agonist administration, serum
FSH was only briefly increased during the beginning of each treatment cycle. We have previously reported that, during chronic LHRH
agonist treatment of endometriosis and leiomyoma, immunological LH

remained elevated above basal levels although ovarian function was suppressed to castration levels [11,12]. A loss of biological activity was associated with modified chromatographic behavior and secretion of LH fragments [13,14]. It is possible that during intermittent LHRH agonist administration, the biological activity would be decreasing after a few days of treatment. It is important to note that at cessation of LHRH agonist dosing, serum LH decreased to pretreatment levels whereas serum FSH spontaneously rose as at the beginning of normal cycle. These observations would indicate a short action of LHRH agonist and a rapid recovery of the pituitary. It is also important to note that serum LH was less stimulated in the 4th treatment cycle than in the first treatment cycle.

SERUM E_2 AND P CHANGES

The changes in gonadotropin secretion were reflected on serum E_2 levels illustrated in Figure 3. Early in the treatment cycles, serum E_2 was increased 2 to 4 fold over early follicular phase levels in all the groups. As for gonadotropin stimulation, serum E_2 remained elevated as long as the LHRH agonist was administered either for 14 or 21 days. Higher E_2 stimulations were observed in the group treated with 200μg/12h. On day 14 of the 14 day schedule, the mean E_2 level was comparable to the mean value of the preovulatory E_2 rise of control cycles. The mean serum E_2 value on day 14 of the 21 day schedule was lower. Similar but lower elevations of serum E_2 were obtained in the 400μg/24h groups.

An abrupt fall in serum E_2 was noted in the groups treated for 14 days whereas a more gradual fall was seen during the 3rd week of treatment in the 21 day treatment schedules (Figure 3). During the pause (week 4), serum E_2 returned in the early follicular phase range. It is to be noted that E_2 was already increasing at the end of the pause in the groups in which LHRH agonist has been used for only 14 days.

As also illustrated in Figure 3, higher E_2 levels were obtained at the 200μg/12h dosage. By comparison with the mean areas under the curves of control cycles, serum E_2 was significantly increased ($P < 0.05$) in the treatment cycles with 200μg/12h for 14 days. With the 400μg/24h dosage for 14 days, the total amount of E_2 secreted was within the range of the control cycles. Using this dosage once daily for 21 days, there was a significant ($P < 0.01$) decrease in total E_2.

In order to evaluate the possibility of ovulation, serum P has also been measured every other day during the 4 treatment cycles. As shown in Figure 3, there was no P elevation that could compare with a luteal phase. Starting early in the treatment cycle (day 4 to 9), elevations of serum P up to 10 to 20ng/ml could be detected in occasional cycles of the 14 day regimens. The rise in P was short-lived ending on day 16. In the 21 day regimens, serum P always remained in the early follicular phase range.

Thus the LHRH agonist administration caused a biphasic stimulation-inhibition of the ovary. The increase in serum E_2 would come from stimulated follicle(s) without ovulation. Inappropriate P secretion would also come from luteinized follicle(s).

415

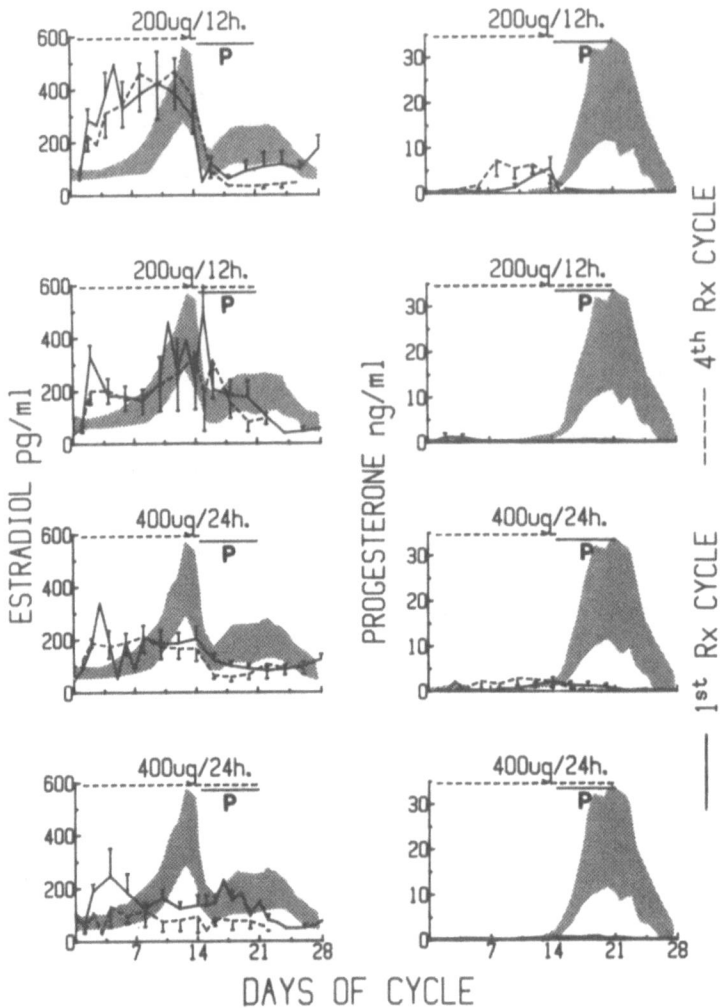

FIGURE 3 Means ± SEM of predosing serum E₂ and P measured every other day during the 1st and 4th treatment cycles with the LHRH agonist (----). Curves are presented according to the frequency (200μg/12h vs 400μg/24h) and schedule (14 vs 21 days) of intranasal insufflation of buserelin. 5mg of (P) medroxyprogesterone acetate (——) was taken by mouth from days 15 to 21. The shaded area represents the range of values of control cycles within ± 1 SD.

OVARIAN ULTRASONOGRAPHIC FINDINGS

In order to assess the incidence and evolution of follicular activity, ovarian scans were performed between days 1 to 6 and 12 to 15 of the first and fourth treatment cycles. The incidence and distribution of follicles are reported in Table 1. At the beginning of the first treatment cycle, occasional small follicles could be seen in 5 cases. At the end of the second week of the first treatment period, there was no measurable follicular structure (< 4mm) in 8 subjects (32%). Various degrees of follicular stimulation were observed in 17 women (68%). The predominant development in the 2 ovaries was numerous small follicles in 6 women (24%), developing follicle(s) in 6 volunteers (24%) and follicular cysts (>27mm) in the 5 other cases (20%). Figure 4 illustrates numerous small follicles in both ovaries in a subject on day 14 of the 1st treatment cycle with 200µg/12h.

Table 1. Predominant stage of ovarian follicular development between days 12 to 15 of treatment periods.

Intranasal buserelin dosage regimen	Follicular size									
	< 4mm		4–10mm		10–18mm		18–27mm		> 27mm	
	Rx1	Rx4	Rx1	Rx4	Rx1	Rx4	Rx1	Rx4	Rx1	Rx4
200µg/12hx14 days	1	2	1		1		1	1	2	3
200µg/12hx21 days	1	3	3	1	1		1	1		1
400µg/24hx14 days	3	3	2	1	1			2	1	1
400µg/24hx21 days	3	5			1		1		2	

At the beginning of the 4th period of treatment in the 14 day regimens, there were small follicles in 5 cases (38%) and large or cystic follicles in 5 subjects (38%) whereas in the 21 day schedules small follicles were seen in 5 cases (45%) and 1 large follicle in 1 case (11%). At week 2 of the 4th treatment cycle (Table 1), large follicle(s) was the predominant observation in the 14 day schedules (7 out 8 stimulated ovaries) whereas ovarian scans did not reveal follicular stimulation in 8 of 12 cases (66%) in the 21 day schedules.

Follicular development correlated with daily serum E_2 levels. Cumulated serum E_2 were above control cycles in cycles with induced large follicles mainly in 14 day schedules at the 200µg/12h dose. In 21 day schedules at 400µg/24h, absence of follicular follicles was frequently associated with serum E_2 in the early follicular phase range.

Although follicles reached the preovulatory size, there was no ultrasound evidence of ovulation. Occasional brief and low elevations of P were compatible with luteinized follicles. Ultrasonic evidence for luteinization of unruptured follicles has been documented in women requiring therapy for induction of ovulation [15] or having unexplained infertility [16]. The absence of significant elevation of progesterone and the presence of persistent high LH are good evidence for unruptured luteinized follicles.

In continuous daily intranasal buserelin administration at 400µg/24h for contraception, ultrasonic examination of ovarian follicles have been reported in 7 women [17]. Four of the women having

417

uterine bleedings had follicular development up to or above the preovulatory size of a normal cycle. No or only small ovarian follicles were visualized by ultrasound in the 3 other amenorrheic subjects.

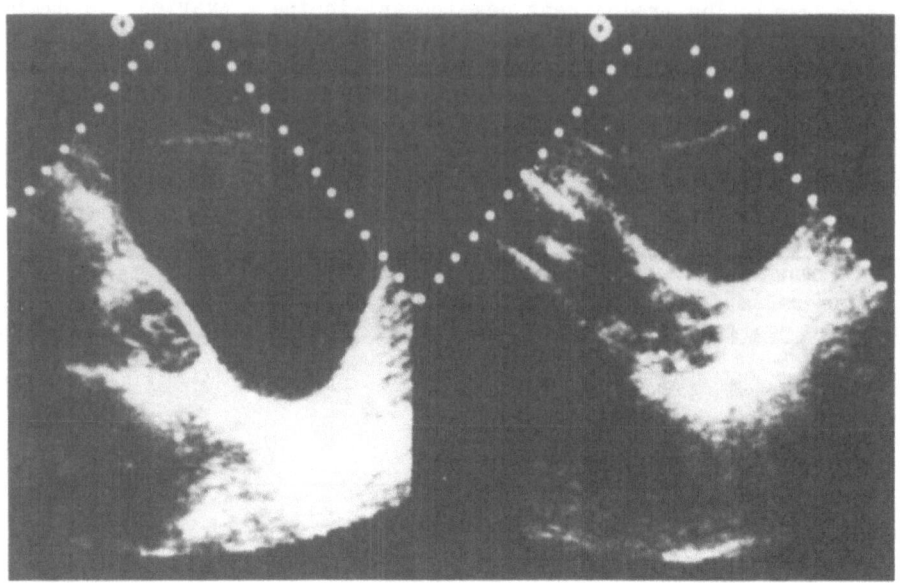

FIGURE 4 Transverse scans of right and left ovaries of subject SL on day 14 of the first treatment cycle with 200µg/12h of the LHRH agonist buserelin administered intranasally.

An intermittent 21 day regimen should be an appropriate contraceptive approach since the incidence of large follicles was small and decreased with repetitive treatment periods.

ENDOMETRIAL BIOPSIES

During the 1st treatment cycle, an endometrial biopsy was taken between days 12 to 15 before administration of the progestogen in 24 of the subjects. A normal proliferative endometrium was described in 16 cases. In 8 specimens, early secretory changes corresponded to day 16 or 17 of a normal menstrual cycle. This light degree of maturation of the endometrium was encountered in previously described cycles with precocious, low and short-lived rise in P (Figure 3).

Twenty biopsies were performed between days 18 and 24 of the 4th treatment cycle at the time of the progestogen administration (from days 15 to 21). Secretory transformation of the endometrium was found in 15 of 20 subjects: histological dating varied between day 16 to day 28. The histological appearance of a biopsy corresponding to day 23 of a normal cycle is illustrated in Figure 5.

At the end of the treatment, the endometrium remained proliferative in 5 cases. The histological examination did not reveal excessive proliferation or signs of hyperplasia. We have noticed that in
the 5 cases with proliferative endometrium, 4 subjects were in the
400µg/24h groups having lesser stimulation of E_2 in the early
follicular phase range. Two other women treated with 400µg/24h for
21 days and having weak stimulation of E_2 showed only early signs
of secretory maturation on their biopsy specimens.

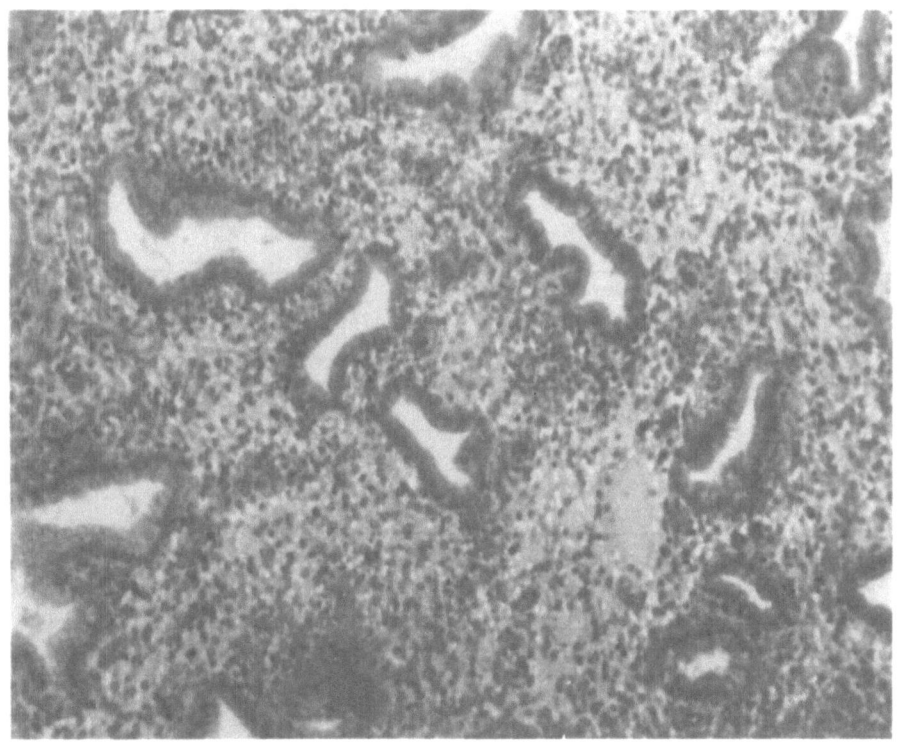

FIGURE 5 Histological picture of endometrial specimen of patient
FJ taken on day 22 of the 4th treatment cycle with
200µg/12h of intranasal LHRH agonist buserelin for 21 days
in combination with 5mg of medroxyprogesterone acetate
taken orally on days 15 to 21: secretory endometrium corresponding to day 24 of a normal menstrual cycle.

These results would indicate that at after 4 months of treatment
with a complement of progestogen during only 7 days, advanced but
yet incomplete maturation of the endometrium was obtained in the
presence of E_2 levels comparable to a normal cycle. Absence of
secretory transformation or poor maturation could be related to weak
estrogenisation of the endometrium. Inactive endometrium or variable
stages of proliferation were described in women using continuous
intranasal buserelin in contraceptive studies for several months

following variable and frequently low levels of E_2 [6,7]. An intermittent 21 day regimen should better preserve estrogen secretion for proliferation of the endometrium. The addition of an adequate amount of a progestogen should more completely mature the endometrium. In this study, the progestogen was given for only 7 days in order to best evaluate the LHRH agonist effect. In a definitive combination approach, an appropriate progestogen should be given for at least 10 days.

UTERINE BLEEDING

The effects of the different buserelin regimens on serum E_2 levels were reflected in the pattern of uterine bleeding. Uterine bleedings were related to the withdrawal of serum E_2 and to the administration of oral medroxyprogesterone acetate from days 15 to 21. The incidence and duration of bleedings are listed in Table 2.

Table 2. Incidence and duration of uterine bleeding.

Intranasal buserelin dosage regimen	Week 1 Total days	Days per cycle	Week 2 Total days	Days per cycle	Week 3 Total days	Days per cycle	Week 4 Total days	Days per cycle
200µg/12hx14 days	3	0.1	10	0.3	83	2.9	78	2.8
200µg/12hx21 days	2	0.1	2	0.1	6	0.2	86	3.6
400µg/24hx14 days	1	0.1	6	0.2	56	2.0	89	3.2
400µg/24hx21 days	1	0.1	2	0.1	7	0.3	105	4.4

There was no significant bleeding during the first 2 weeks of treatment. In the two 14 day schedules, breakthrough bleeding occurred for an average of 2.9 and 2.0 days/cycle. In these groups bleeding happened also frequently during the 4th week for an average of 2.8 and 3.2 days/cycle. A regular pattern of bleeding was obtained in the two 21 day schedules. Bleeding during the 3rd week happened in only 3 cycles for a total 6 and 7 days. In 91% and 96% of the cycles bleeding took place during the pause for an average of 3.6 to 4.4 days/cycle.

The breakthrough bleeding occurring in the 14 day schedules could be explained by the higher but shorter stimulation of serum E_2. The progestogen transformed the previously estrogenized endometrium but could not prevent the desquamation of the mucosa during the rapid decrease in serum E_2. In the 21 day schedules, the secretion of E_2 was moderate and did not decrease precipitously at mid-cycle. Although complete maturation of the endometrium was not achieved, withdrawal uterine bleeding normally occurred at the cessation of the medication. Appropriate uterine bleeding has also been shown by Hardt et al [8] in a similar 22 day schedule with adminis-

420

tration of norethisterone acetate during the last 3 days of the treatment period.

CLINICAL SYMPTOMS

Breast discomfort or congestion was present in 17% of the pretreatment cycles and was reported in 36% of the treatment cycles. There was no complaint of increased or decreased vaginal secretion. The incidence of premenstrual symptoms decreased from 77% in pretreatment cycles to 58% in treatment cycles. The incidence of dysmenorrhea was also reduced from 18% to 4% during the treatment cycles. There were no symptoms of lack of estrogen reported by the subjects during the treatment cycles. The incidence of symptoms such as headache and fatigue did not differ from those encountered in control cycles. No volunteer complained about nasal irritation following intranasal insufflation. There was no problem with nasal spraying during a few periods of nasal inflammation accompanying common cold.

RECOVERY CYCLES

The 2 immediate post-treatment cycles were ovulatory and showed normal hormonal profiles as illustrated in the example of Figure 1. The mean length of the follicular phase of the first recovery cycle was prolonged to 21.5 $\pm$ 1.8 days as compared to 14.8 $\pm$ 0.8 days (P < 0.01) in the pretreatment cycles. This delay in the follicular development was mainly encountered in the 21 day regimens. The duration of the luteal phase was normal in all the groups. The clinical events of the menstrual cycles were similar to those of the pretreatment cycles.

TESTOSTERONE AND PROLACTIN

Since the LHRH agonist effect was to block ovulation and temporarily increase serum E_2, we evaluated the effects of the different treatment regimens on parameters normally related to estrogen changes. Changes in serum testosterone and prolactin usually follow follicular development and increase at mid-cycle. We have compared the mean levels on day 14 of the treatment cycles with those on the day preceeding the preovulatory LH surge in the control cycles.

The histogram in Figure 6 demonstrates that there is an increase in the mean serum testosterone levels only in the group treated with 200µg/12h for 14 days. Although serum testosterone remained within the normal range, this increase was statistically significant (P < 0.01) when levels were compared with both pre and post-treatment control cycles. As described before, the largest follicles secreting E_2 above control cycles were mainly observed in the group treated with 200µg/12h for 14 days.

There was no significant changes in the mean prolactin levels in all the groups (Figure 7). In only the group treated with 400µg/24h for 21 days, serum prolactin was lower that in the pre- and

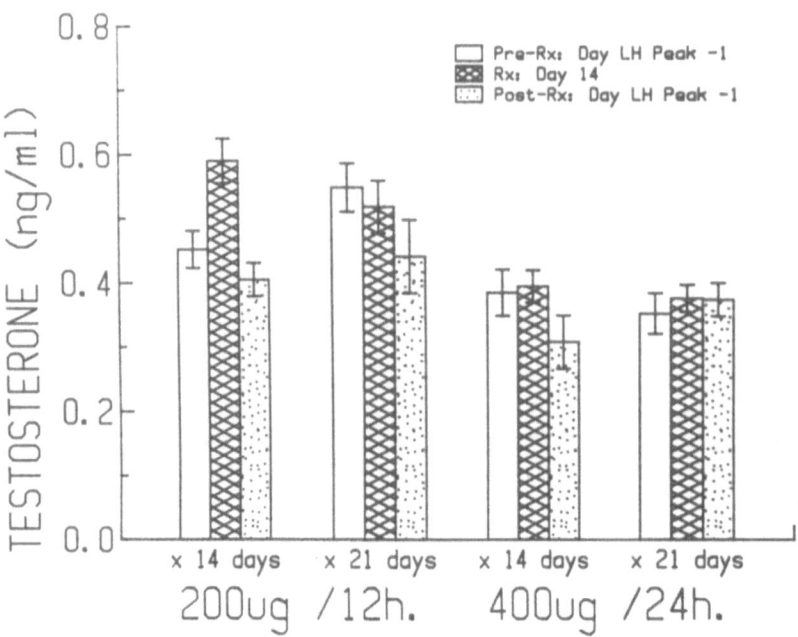

FIGURE 6 Means ± SEM of serum testosterone measured on the day preceeding the preovulatory LH surge in pre and post-treatment control cycles and on day 14 of the treatment cycles.

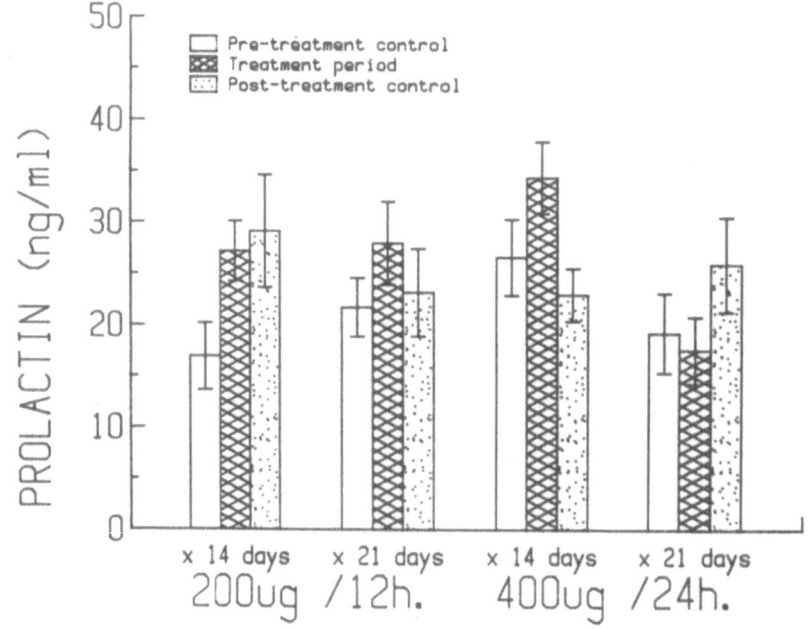

FIGURE 7 Means ± SEM of serum prolactin measured on the day preceeding the preovulatory LH surge in pre and post-treatment control cycles and on day 14 of the treatment cycles.

422

post-treatment cycles. As underlined before, lowest levels of E_2 were associated with frequent absence of follicular development in this group. In the other 3 groups, serum PRL was increased by comparison with pretreatment cycles.

LIPIDS AND SAFETY PARAMETERS

In this study, additional laboratory tests were performed at admission, at the end of the 1st and 4th treatment cycles and at the end of the study. There was no significant change or trend in total cholesterol and triglycerides. Total cholesterol and triglycerides of 188 ± 7 mg/dl and 81 ± 6 mg/dl at admission were 192 ± 6 mg/dl and 75 ± 4 mg/dl respectively at the end of treatment. The effect of a 6 month treatment with 300μg of intranasal buserelin given intermittently for 22 days in combination with 5mg norethisterone acetate from day 16 to 22 has been reported not to change total cholesterol but to increase HDL cholesterol [18]. The levels of HDL-cholesterol were more than 1/3 higher during the sixth cycle than those during the first cycle of medication. The increase in HDL-cholesterol is not explained but can be an important advantage in patients prone to arteriosclerosis.

The LHRH agonist did not alter metabolic parameters such as glucose, nitrogen, uric acid, creatinine, proteins, oxaloactic transaminase, glutamic pyruvic transaminase and alkaline phosphatase. Sodium, potassium, chloride, calcium and phosphorus remained in the normal range. There was also no change in T_3, T_4 or cortisol.

CONCLUDING REMARKS

The disordered follicular development during intermittent buserelin treatment results from inappropriate gonadotropin secretion in response to the biphasic stimulation/inhibition by repetitive LHRH agonist dosing. Although the 14 day schedule prevented ovulation, it was associated with development of large follicles, levels of estrogens above normal control cycles and breakthrough bleedings. When the LHRH agonist was discontinued after 14 days, the spontaneous rise of FSH initiated follicular development which was markedly stimulated at the beginning of the following period of treatment. At the beginning of the repeated 21 day schedule, the follicles had not been previously developed by FSH and in response to buserelin, only small follicles were developed secreting more physiological levels of E_2. Controlled withdrawal bleeding occurred during the pause.

In this study, medroxyprogesterone acetate was given for only 7 days in order to mainly evaluate the effect of the LHRH agonist. Although incomplete, a significant maturation of the endometrium was obtained at the endometrial biopsy. In the presence of stimulated estrogen levels a progestogen would be recommended on a longer period.

The 21 day regimen would satisfy the main objectives: inhibition of ovulation, preservation of E_2 secretion, controlled uterine bleeding and absence of side effects related to the medication. By comparison with the continuous administration of intranasal buserelin, discontinuous treatment should avoid or minimize the incidence of oligomenorrhea and amenorrhea secondary to continuous desensitization of the gonadotroph. The main advantage of intermittent LHRH agonist would be to avoid using a synthetic estrogen derivative and to use more physiological amounts of a progestogen, preferably natural progesterone, only in the second half of a contraceptive cycle. Although at this time such a contraceptive regimen would not compare on a practical basis with that of oral contraceptive, it could be useful in conditions where oral contraceptives are not satisfactory or are contraindicated. More work and development of new technologies should help in the validation of LHRH agonist as a contraceptive method.

ACKNOWLEDGEMENTS

This work was supported by a grant from NIH contraceptive branch to F. Labrie, A. Lemay and N. Faure. The authors are grateful to R. Dubois and R. Rehel for performing the radioimmunoassays, to N. Paquet and H. Brisson for doing the ultrasounds, to F. Labrecque for nursing assistance and to L. Mercier for typing the manuscript.

REFERENCES

1. Rabin, D. and McNeil, L.W. Pituitary and gonadal desensitization after continuous luteinizing hormone-releasing hormone infusion in normal females. J. Clin. Endocrinol. Metab., 51, 873 (1980).
2. Bergquist, C., Nillius, S.J. and Wide, L. Intranasal gonadotropin-releasing hormone agonist as a contraceptive agent. Lancet, 2, 215 (1979).
3. Hardt, W., Schmidt-Gollwitzer, M., von der Ohe, M. and Nevinny-Stickel, J. Der Einflu des dauer-medikation des LH-RH analogons Buserelin auf die zyklusregulation. Geburtsh. u. Frauenheilk, 41, 791 (1981).
4. Berquist, C., Nillius, S.J. and Wide, L. Long-term intranasal luteinizing hormone-releasing hormone agonist treatment for contraception in women. Fertil. Steril., 38, 190 (1982).
5. Gudmundsson, J.A., Nillius, S.J. and Bergquist, C. Inhibition of ovulation by intranasal nafarelin, a new superactive agonist of GnRH. Contraception, 30, 107 (1984).
6. Bergquist, C., Nillius, S.J., Wide, L. and Lindgren, A. Endometrial patterns in women on chronic luteinizing hormone-releasing hormone agonist treatment for contraception. Fertil. Steril., 36, 339 (1981).
7. Schmidt-Gollwitzer, M., Hardt, W., Schmidt-Gollwitzer, K., von der Ohe, M. and Nevinny-Stickel, J. Influence of the LH-RH analogue Buserelin on cyclic ovarian function and on endometrium. A new approach to fertility control? Contraception, 23, 187 (1981).
8. Hardt, W., Schmidt-Gollwitzer, K., Nevinny-Stickel, J. and Schmidt-Gollwitzer, M. Fortschritte in der kontrazeptiven anwendung des LH-RH agonisten Buserelin: diskontinuierliche

medikation mit gestagenin-duzierter abbruchblutung. Geburtsh. u. Frauenheilk, 42, 874 (1982).

9. Lemay, A., Faure, N., Labrie, F. and Fazekas, A. Inhibition of ovulation during discontinuous intranasal luteinizing hormone releasing hormone agonist dosing in combination with gestagen induced bleeding. Fertil. Steril., 43, 868 (1985).

10. Lemay, A. and Faure, N. Fourteen day versus twenty-one day regimens of intermittent intranasal LHRH agonist sequentially combined with an oral progestogen as antiovulatory contraceptive approach. J. Clin. Endocr. Metab. in press.

11. Lemay, A., Maheux, R., Faure, N., Jean, C., and Fazekas, A. Reversible hypogonadism induced by a luteinizing hormone-releasing hormone (LH-RH) agonist (Buserelin) as a new therapeutic approach for endometriosis. Fertil. Steril., 41, 863 (1984).

12. Maheux, R., Guilloteau, C., Lemay, A., Bastide, A. and Fazekas, A.T.A. Luteinizing hormone-releasing hormone agonist and uterine leiomyoma: a pilot study. Am J. Obstet. Gynecol., 152, 1034 (1985).

13. Evans, R.M., Doelle, G.C., Lindner, J., Bradley, V. and Rabin, D. A luteinizing hormone-releasing hormone agonist decreases biological activity and modifies chromatographic behavior of luteinizing hormone in man. J. Clin. Invest., 73, 262 (1984).

14. Meldrum, D.R., Tsao, Z., Monroe, S.E., Braunstein, G.D., Sladek, J., Lu, J.K.H., Vale, W., Rivier, J., Judd, H.L. and Chang, R.J. Stimulation of LH fragments with reduced bioactivity following GnRH agonist administration in women. J. Clin. Endocrinol. Metab., 58, 755 (1984).

15. Coulam, C.B., Hill, L.M. and Breckle, R. Ultrasonic evidence for luteinization of unruptured preovulatory follicles. Fertil. Steril, 37, 524 (1982).

16. Liukkonen, S., Koskimies, A.I., Tenhunen, A. and Ylöstalo, P. Diagnosis of luteinized unruptured follicle (LUF) syndrome by ultrasound. Fertil. Steril., 41, 26 (1984).

17. Bergquist, C. and Lindgren P.G. Ultrasonic measurement of ovarian follicles during chronic LRH agonist treatment for contraception. Contraception, 28, 125 (1983).

18. Schumacher, T., Zwirner, M., Unterberg, H., Pohl, C., Keller, E. and Schindler A.E. Effects of the LHRH-analogue buserelin given discontinuously as a contraceptive on ovarian cycle and lipometabolism. Neuroendocrinol., 5, 267 (1984).

28
LHRH Agonists and Male Contraception

S. BHASIN, B. S. STEINER and R. S. SWERDLOFF
Harbor-UCLA Medical Center, Torrance, CA 90509, USA

INTRODUCTION

Normal testicular function requires the stimulatory actions of the
pituitary gonadotropins LH and FSH [1,2]. Luteinizing hormone (LH)
stimulates Leydig cell steroidogenesis to generate and maintain high
intratesticular testosterone concentrations, which are essential for
initiating and maintaining spermatogenesis [1-4]. Most evidence
supports the concept that FSH in conjunction with LH is required for
the initiation of spermatogenesis which usually occurs during sexual
maturation. After puberty, however, the role of FSH in reproductive
function is less clear. Observations that hypophysectomy in man or
experimental animals predictably leads to azoospermia suggest that
complete suppression of LH and FSH by pharmacologic means could
provide effective suppression of spermatogenesis. Studies by Bremner
et al. have shown that in post-pubertal men, made hypogonadotropic
by testosterone enanthate, spermatogenesis can be reinitiated by LH
alone [3-6]. However, the quantitative level of sperm production in
the absence of FSH is not normal. Addition of FSH to hCG/LH
treatment regimen in this hypogonadotropic male model restores sperm
production to normal levels [5,6]. These results do not support the
concept that selective suppression of FSH will lead to an effective
male contraceptive [1,7].
    Agonist analogs of LHRH were originally developed as longer
acting therapeutic agents to treat GnRH deficient patients. After
early trials, it became apparent that chronic administration of
these LHRH agonists, after a brief initial period of stimulation,
leads to paradoxical inhibition of gonadal function in rodents [9-
10], primates [12-17] and humans [18-28]. Reports of these
paradoxical antigonadal effects raised hopes of their potential
application as male contraceptives.

RATIONALE FOR COMBINED THERAPY WITH LHRH AGONIST AND ANDROGEN

Inhibition of spermatogenesis by agents such as LHRH agonist that
act by inhibiting pituitary LH secretion is accompanied by a
predictable decline in serum testosterone (T) with attendant
decrease in libido and potency. In initial studies, Linde et al.

427

administered 50 ug of [D-Trp6,Pro9-NHET] LHRH daily to normal men
and observed a fall in serum T with a mean nadir of 2.1 nmol/L by
the fourth week of treatment [18]. Agonist treatment had to be
discontinued in 5 of 7 subjects because of impotence. Libido and
potency returned 2 weeks after stopping therapy. Occurrence of
these symptoms represented a significant drawback of the application
of LHRH agonist alone as a male contraceptive agent. In this
regard, our group proposed the use of combined LHRH agonist and
androgen therapy. We argued that their combined use is attractive
for two reasons. First, T treatment would prevent the undesirable
side effects of impotence and diminished libido; and second, since
androgens alone are potent inhibitors of spermatogenesis in man, the
addition of a second gonadotropin inhibitor might have additive
inhibitory effects on the testis. In this context, studies in the
rat by Heber et al. demonstrated a synergistic effect of combined
androgen and GnRH agonist therapy [29].

CLINICAL STUDIES WITH LHRH AGONISTS

Short term studies with LHRH agonists

Clinical studies in our laboratories have utilized the GnRH agonist
[D-Nal(2)6]LHRH (nafarelin, Syntex Research, Palo Alto, CA).
Preliminary studies assessed the effects of two doses (10 and 100
ug) of this potent agonist on LH, FSH and T secretion [20]. Daily
administration of this agonist resulted in an early phase of
stimulation followed by a progressive decline in serum LH, FSH and T
concentrations to serum levels below baseline by day 10 of
treatment. The higher dose was more potent in both the stimulatory
and downregulatory effects. Combined treatment with a single 200 mg
dose of testosterone enanthate (TE) on day 1 with daily
subcutaneous injections of 100 ug of LHRH agonist did not blunt the
peak LH and FSH responses on day 2, but resulted in lower LH and FSH
responses, as assessed by paired comparisons of the areas under the
curve from days 3-11 [30]. These studies suggested that the
addition of testosterone to LHRH analog had additive inhibitory
effects on LH and FSH secretion and encouraged us to test the
effects of combined treatment on spermatogenesis in long term
studies.

Long term studies with combined regimen of LHRH agonist and testosterone

In the long term studies, we treated seven normal men with daily
subcutaneous injections of 200 ug of [D-Nal(2)6]LHRH in combination
with 200 mg of TE every 2 weeks [19]. The mean sperm count declined
to a nadir of 17 million/cc. However, one subject did not show
significant suppression of sperm concentration as assessed by
regression analysis. While none of the 7 subjects became
azoospermic, one subject had sperm counts below 50,000 per ml of
semen. Thus, this combined regimen of intermittent LHRH agonist
administration with bimonthly injections of testosterone did not

induce azoospermia.

Basal serum LH concentrations, after an initial phase of stimulation, decined progressively to baseline by day 28, but were not significantly below baseline by the end of the 16 week treatment period. Twenty-four hour urinary immunoreactive LH excretion, (which represents a reasonable measure of 24 hour integrated LH secretion), after the initial rise on day 1 returned to baseline by day 10 but did not significantly decline below baseline at anytime during treatment. However, bioassayable LH concentrations declined by more than 70% below the pretreatment control level [19]. Basal FSH concentrations declined more rapidly than LH to 40-50% of baseline by the end of the second week and stayed decreased thereafter. Following discontinuation of treatment, both LH and FSH returned to baseline within 4-6 weeks without a significant rebound.

These data are quite similar to those of Doelle et al [22]. These investigators used 50 ug of [D-Trp[6],Pro[9]-NHEt]LHRH by daily subcutaneous injection along with bimonthly intramuscular injections of a lower dose (100 mg) of T.E. Azoospermia was not achieved in any of the 6 treated men.

Reasons for incomplete suppression of spermatogenesis by regimens employing single daily injections of LHRH agonist

The failure of combined regimens employing intermittent injections of LHRH agonist appears related, at least in part, to incomplete suppression of gonadotropins because complete hypophysectomy does lead to azoospermia. This may be due to several factors including: i) the human male may be biologically resistant to the inhibitory effects of the LHRH agonist; ii) the dose of the agonist may have been inadequate and/or iii) the regimen of intermittent daily injection may fail to provide constant and optimum blood levels.

Of these, the last appeared most likely since the serum concentrations of the LHRH agonist, measured by radioimmunoassay, decline to undetectable levels by 12h after the agonist injection (Bhasin, S. and Swerdloff, R.S., unpublished observations). Furthermore, studies in rhesus monkey, by Akhtar et al, have shown that constant infusion of LHRH agonist results in far greater suppression of gonadotropins and spermatogenesis than does intermittent injection [7,15].

Studies with constant infusion of LHRH agonist in the human male

Short term studies In order to assess if constant infusion of LHRH agonist will lead to greater suppression of gonadal function than will intermittent administration, we administered either 20 or 200 ug of nafarelin to two groups of normal volunteers for 28 days either by a single daily injection or by constant subcutaneous infusion from a portable infusion device (Autosyringe, Travenol Laboratories, Inc., Hookset, NH).
Basal or 24h. integrated LH, FSH and T responses were not

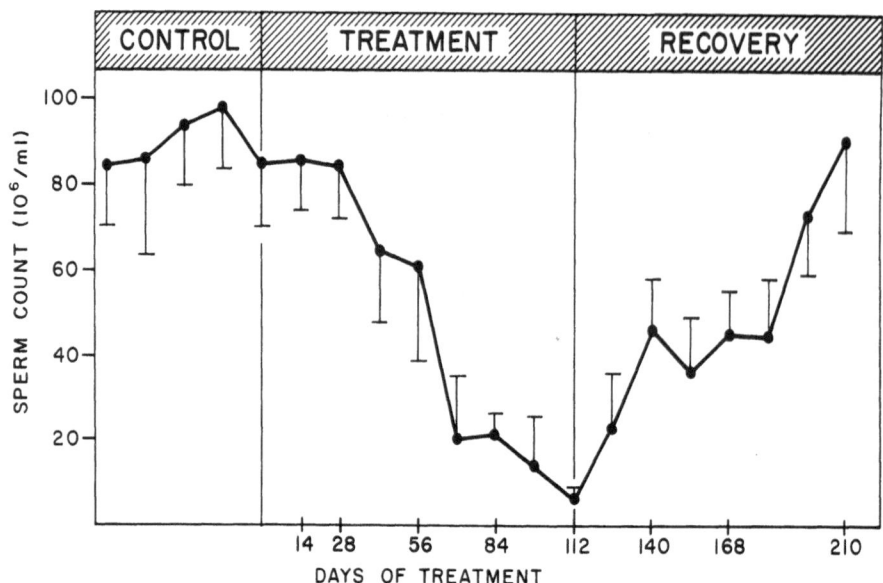

FIGURE 1:   Effect of long term constant infusion of LHRH agonist
               and bimonthly injections of testosterone enanthate
               on sperm concentrations. Data are mean ± SEM, n=7.

significantly different by the two modes of GnRH agonist delivery
either at 20 or the 200 mcg dose. Although both the mean basal and
24 hour integrated testosterone concentrations were lower in the
constant infusion group, these differences also did not approach
statistical significance.

     Thus, the effects of constant infusion of this LHRH agonist in
the human were not as striking as those reported for another agonist
in the rhesus monkey. Decline in serum testosterone in both the
groups occurred in the face of little or no change in serum LH
immunoreactivity suggesting that the antigonadal effects of
intermediate term LHRH agonist treatment in man cannot be fully
explained on the basis of downregulation of gonadotropin secretion
alone.

Long term studies with constant infusion of GnRH agonist In order
to determine if higher dose, constant infusion of LHRH agonist in
man would lead to azoospermia, we administered 400 ug of [D-Nal(2)6]
LHRH daily by constant subcutaneous infusion by a portable pump
along with bimonthly injections of 200 mg T.E. to 7 normal men for
16 weeks [27]. A higher dose of the LHRH agonist was used in these
studies because of data suggesting that plateau of the agonist dose
response curve had not been reached at the 200 mcg dose. Sperm
counts fell significantly in all 7 subjects during treatment, from
about 75 to a nadir of 6 million/ml between weeks 14-16 (Fig. 1
and Table 1). This represented a 92% mean suppression. Four

subjects had sperm counts less than 1.0 million/ml and 3 subjects became azoospermic. Sperm counts returned to normal within 6-12 weeks of discontinuation of drug therapy. No changes in sperm motility and morphology were noted during drug therapy.

Basal serum LH responses were qualitatively similar to those seen with the regimen employing single daily injections of the agonist. Serum LH concentrations rose quickly to a peak on day 1 and then progressively declined to baseline by day 28. However, basal serum LH concentrations did not decline below pretreatment level at anytime during the treatment phase.

Twenty-four hour integrated immunoreactive LH concentrations, computed by calculating areas under the curve above day 0 baseline showed marked increase on day 1 and declined to baseline by day 28, but did not significantly fall below baseline at anytime during treatment. Twenty-four hour urinary LH excretion rose significantly on day 1 and then returned to baseline by day 10. Urinary LH concentrations were modestly but significantly lower than pretreatment levels on days 28 and 112.

Serum FSH concentrations also showed a biphasic response with an early stimulatory phase and subsequent decline to baseline by day 10. However, neither the basal nor 24 hour integrated FSH concentrations fell below baseline at anytime during the treatment phase. After discontinuation of the LHRH agonist treatment, serum FSH concentrations showed a marked rebound rise peaking 4 weeks after termination of infusion and returning to pretreatment levels by day 210.

Serum testosterone concentrations rose after each injection of T.E. and then gradually declined to a nadir two weeks after the injection. Serum T concentrations remained essentially within the normal range during the entire treatment phase. This was consistent with the absence of any significant change in the subjects' sexual desire or activity. Serum estradiol (E_2) concentrations paralleled the serum T concentrations, rising after each injection of T.E. and gradually declining to a nadir 2 weeks after the injection.

Comparative effects of the two regimens of GnRH agonist administration

These data demonstrate that the regimen of combined treatment with constant infusion of LHRH agonist and testosterone led to greater suppression of spermatogenesis in men than the previous regimen employing single daily injections of a lower dose of the same agonist (Table 1). The combination of androgen and constant infusion of agonist consistently lowered sperm counts in all 7 subjects. The constant infusion regimen induced azoospermia in 3 subjects; the previous regimen had failed to induce azoospermia in any subject. The mean suppression of sperm counts after constant infusion of agonist was also greater than that seen with the previous regimen. Although basal LH and FSH concentrations were significantly lower on day 112 with the regimen employing single daily injections, 24 hour integrated LH and FSH concentrations were not significantly different by the two methods of GnRH agonist

431

administration. These differences in basal LH and FSH concentrations

Table 1. Comparative effects of two regimens of GnRH agonist administration

	Study I[a]	Study II
Method of Administration	Single Daily Injection	Constant Subcutaneous Infusion
Dose of Agonist	200 ug/d	400 ug/d
Mean Sperm Count on Day 112 (millions/ml)	28 ± 12^{b}	6 ± 3
Sperm Count Mean Percent Suppression	67 ± 22	93 ± 3
Azoospermic Men	0 of 7	3 of 7
Sperm Count Less than 1 million/ml	1 of 7	4 of 7
Sperm Count Less than 5 million/ml	3 of 7	5 of 7

a: Study I employed single daily subcutaneous injections of 200 ug. LHRH agonist and bimonthly intramuscular injection of 200 mg T.E. Study II employed constant subcutaneous infusion of 400 ug LHRH agonist per day in addition to bimonthly intramuscular injections of T.E. b: mean + SEM, n=7 in each group.

reflect different time courses of LHRH agonist action by the two methods of administration. Constant infusion of LHRH agonist leads to sustained (although modest) rise in serum LH concentrations throughout the 24 hour period. On the other hand, basal (pre-injection) LH concentrations on day 112 in subjects receiving single daily injections were lower, but rose significantly after LHRH agonist injection and then declined gradually to values below pretreatment levels by 24 hours after the injection.

These data are similar to those of Schurmeyer et al [23] and Pavlou et al [25]. Different dose regimens were used by these investigators. Furthermore, in vivo inhibitory potencies of different LHRH agonists used in these studies have never been rigorously compared so that the data from different laboratories are not directly comparable. However, it is notable that the dose of the LHRH agonist used by Schurmeyer et al in the human studies was significantly lower than that used by the same investigators in the monkey studies on a per kg basis. Data from studies in patients with prostate cancer suggest that at the doses of LHRH agonist currently being used in male contraceptive studies, the plateau of the agonist dose response curve has not been reached. It is unclear from our current studies whether the higher dose of the LHRH agonist or the mode of administration (constant infusion) was responsible for the greater suppression of spermatogenesis. These results are the most promising to-date and suggest that constant infusion of a still higher dose of the agonist might lead to azoospermia in all subjects.

DOES TESTOSTERONE ATTENTUATE ANTIFERTILITY EFFECTS OF LHRH ANALOGS IN MAN?

Akhtar et al recently reported that early addition of testosterone treatment attenuated the antifertility effects of LHRH agonist in the rhesus monkey [32]. However, it is notable that while exogenous testosterone can reinitiate and maintain spermatogenesis in the hypophysectomized male rat and stalk-sectioned monkey, testosterone has only been shown to inhibit rather than support spermatogenesis in man. The blood-testis barrier in man appears less permeable to exogenous testosterone. In fact, over a wide range of doses that can be practically administered to man, (up to 200 mg of testosterone enanthate per week) testosterone leads only to a dose dependent inhibition of spermatogenesis in man. The dose of testosterone used by our group (200 mg every two weeks) is higher than the doses used by other investigators, even though the results are not significantly different. Thus, the question of whether testosterone attenuates or delays the antifertility effects of GnRH agonist in man has not yet been adequately assessed. The issue is clearly of great importance to the formulation of contraceptive regimens employing GnRH agonist and androgen.

MECHANISMS OF LHRH AGONIST ACTION IN THE HUMAN MALE

In spite of the multiple uses proposed for LHRH agonists, the mechanisms of their antigonadal action in man remain poorly understood. Inhibitory effects of the agonists on LH and FSH secretion, assessed by measurement of serum LH and FSH concentrations, can only partially account for their antigonadal effects in man [33]. The confusion that exists in the literature with regard to their mechanism of action in man is due, at least in part, to the following factors:
    1. Significant differences exist between the data from the rat, mouse, monkey, and human studies. While a direct gonadal inhibitory effect of the GnRH agonist appears to predominate in the rat [34], similar effect have not been demonstrated in man [20,35,36].
    2. Significant cross-reactivity of human LH (alpha-) subunit exists in RIAs for hLH. The displacement curves obtained with serial dilutions of hLH (alpha) subunit tend to be nonparallel to those obtained with hLH reference preparations so that the relative contribution of serum hLH (alpha) to hLH immunoreactivity cannot be easily assessed.
    3. The effects of the LHRH agonist on pituitary and gonadal

Table 2: A Summary of Male Contraceptive Trials with LHRH Agonists

Reference	Number of Subjects	LHRH Agonist	Dose ug/day	Duration of Treatment (weeks)	Regimen of Androgen Replacement	Sperm Concentrations (10^6)	Azoospermia
Bergquist [41]	4	buserelin	5	17	None	No inhibition	
Linde et al. [18]	8	tryptorelin	50	6-10	None		1 of 8
Doelle et al.[22]	6	tryptorelin	50	20	[a]T.E. 100 mg every 2 weeks	12 ± 4[c]	0 of 6
Rabin et al. [24]	8	tryptorelin	100-500	20	T.E. 100 mg every 2 weeks	5.5	
Bhasin et al.[19]	7	nafarelin	200	16	T.E. 200 mg every 2 weeks	17 ± 6	0 of 7
Schurmeyer [23]	7	buserelin	118	12	[b]T.U. daily	18 ± 5	0 of 7
	4	buserelin	230	12	T.U. daily	10 ± 3	0 of 4
Pavlou et al.[25]	8	tryptorelin	500	16	T.E. 100 mg every 2 weeks		0 of 8
Michel et al.[26]	7	buserelin	440	12	T.U. daily	44 ± 14	
Swerdloff et al. [17]	7	naferelin	400	16	T.E. 200 mg every 2 weeks	8 ± 3	3 of 7

a   testosterone enanthate
b   testosterone undecanoate
c   million/ml, mean $\pm$ SEM

434

function vary with the duration of LHRH agonist treatment. For instance, in the male rat, direct inhibition of testicular steroidogenesis is the predominant mechanism in the early phases of treatment (1-3 weeks). But, after extended periods of LHRH agonist administration, down-regulation of pituitary LH secretion also contributes to inhibition of gonadal function. Thus, the data from short term studies cannot be extrapolated to fully explain the inhibition of spermatogenesis during long term LHRH agonist administration.

4. The status of gonadal function appears to influence the LH response to LHRH agonist [37]. This may partly explain why patients with prostate cancer, who tend to be hypogonadal as a group, show greater suppression of serum LH than normal adult men. Different subsets of patients (children with precocious puberty, normal adult men, and patients with prostate cancer) may differ in their responses to LHRH agonist.

Basal and integrated concentrations of immunoreactive LH after intermediate term (4-16 weeks) LHRH agonist treatment are only modestly decreased and cannot fully account for the far greater decline in serum T concentrations. Bioassayable LH concentrations, however, decrease markedly and parallel the fall in serum T, suggesting secretion of qualitatively different LH species with diminished biological activity [33,38]. While the circulating concentrations of beta-subunit parallel the measured bioassayable LH concentrations, free alpha-subunit secretion remains persistently and disproportionately elevated during chronic LHRH agonist treatment. Cross-reactivity of free alpha-subunits in the human LH RIA partly contributes to this disparity between the LH immuno- and bioactivity. Chromatography of serum LH during LHRH agonist treatment suggests secretion of a qualitatively different LH species. Unlike the rat, in which the antifertility effects of the agonist are mediated predominantly by direct inhibition of testicular steroidogenesis, significant direct gonadal effects have not been demonstrated in man. In fact, data from our laboratories have shown that the inhibition of steroidogenesis (steroid secretion as well as direct measurement of steroidogenic enzymes) in men treated with LHRH agonist is reversed by the administration of hCG [39]. Thus the bulk of evidence points to a predominant pituitary site of action in the human male. The molecular basis of the heterogeneity of LH during LHRH agonist treatment, however, remains to be elucidated. The hypothesis that co- or post-translational modification of glycosylation by the agonist may attenuate biologic activity of LH has not yet been directly tested.

CONCLUDING REMARKS

A perspective on the potential of LHRH agonists as male contraceptives

A summary of data from different investigators on the effects of LHRH agonist on spermatogenesis in man is outlined in Table 2. Although the regimens of LHRH agonist tested so far have failed to consistently induce azoospermia in man, achievement of azoospermia in the primate studies gives reason for hope.

Furthermore, absence of any significant systemic side effects

makes LHRH agonists extremely attractive as male contraceptive
agents. It is notable that the dose of LHRH agonist per kg used
in the primate studies was much higher than the dose used in any of
the human studies. Thus, a higher dose of LHRH agonist administered
by constant infusion might induce azoospermia in all the subjects.
The controversy regarding the optimum regimen for androgen
replacement also needs to be resolved. The issue of whether the
current regimens of T replacement attenuate the anti-fertility
effects of LHRH agonists is crucial to the successful application of
LHRH analogs for male contraception. Recent data suggest that 12-16
week treatment may not be sufficient to achieve maximal suppression
of spermatogenesis by the agonist analogs [40]. These provocative
data suggest the need for longer term studies (28 weeks) to assess
anti-fertility efficacy of LHRH analogs.

The above discussion has been predicated on the assumption that
azoospermia is required to assure contraceptive efficacy.
Unpublished data from trials with steroidal inhibitors of
spermatogenesis, however, have suggested that sperm function may be
impaired prior to the development of azoospermia. Field trials are
now being contemplated to determine if the partners of severely
oligospermic men are in fact, protected from pregnancy. The results
of such a study may result in modification of the absolute goal of
azoospermia to assure efficacy of LHRH agonists as male
contraceptives.

REFERENCES

1.   Bremner, W.J. and Matsumoto, A.M. Endocrine control of human
      spermatogenesis: Possible mechanisms for contraception. In
      "Male Contraception: Advances and Future Prospects", G.I.
      Zatuchni, A. Goldsmith, J.M. Spieler and J.J. Sciarra (Eds.),
      Harper and Row, Philadelphia, 1985, p. 81.
2.   DiZerega, G.S. and Sherins, R.J. Endocrine control of adult
      testicular function. In "The Testis", H. Burger, D. DeKretser
      (Eds.), Raven Press, New York, 1980, p. 127.
3.   Matsumoto, A.M. and Bremner, W.J. Stimulation of sperm
      production by human chorionic gonadotropin after prolonged
      gonadotropin suppression in normal men. J. Androl. 6, 137
      (1985).
4.   Matsumoto, A.M., Paulsen, C.A. and Bremner, W.J. Stimulation
      of sperm production by human luteinizing hormone in
      gonadotropin-suppressed normal men. J. Clin. Endocrinol.
      Metab., 59, 882 (1984).
5.   Bremner, W.J., Matsumoto, A.M., Sussman, A.M. and Paulsen, C.A.
      Follicle-stimulating hormone and human spermatogenesis. J.
      Clin. Invest., 68, 1044.(1981).
6.   Matsumoto, A.M., Karpas, A.E., Paulsen, C.A. and Bremner, W.J.
      Reinitiation of sperm production in gonadotropin-suppressed
      normal men by administration of FSH. J. Clin. Invest., 72,
      1005 (1983).
7.   Nieschlag, E. Reasons for abandoning immunization against FSH
      as an approach to male fertility regulation. In "Male
      Contraception: Advances and Future Prospects", G.I. Zatuchni,
      A. Goldsmith, J.M. Spieler and J.J. Sciarra (Eds.), Harper and

Row, Philadelphia, 1985, p. 395.

8. Pelletier, G., Cusan, L., Auclair, C., Kelly, P.A., Desy, L. and Labrie, F. Inhibition of spermatogenesis in the rat by treatment with D-Ala[6]desGly[10]-LHRH EA. Endocrinology 103, 641 (1978).

9. Labrie, F., Cusan, L., Seguin, C. and Belanger, A. Antifertility effects of LHRH agonists in the male rat and inhibition of testicular steroidogenesis in man. Int. J. Fertil., 25, 157 (1980).

10. Sandow, J., Von Rechenberg, W., Baeder, C. and Engelbart, K. Antifertility effects of an LHRH analog in male rats and dogs. Int. J. Fertil., 25, 313 (1980).

11. Tcholakian, R.K., DelaCruz, A., Chowdhury, M., Steinberger, A., Coy, D.H. and Schally, A.V. Unusual anti-reproductive properties of the analog [Dleu[6]-des-Gly-NH2[10]]-LHRH ethylamide in male rats. Fertil Steril., 30, 600 (1978).

12. Sundaram, K., Connell, K.G., Bardin, C.W., Samojlik, E., and Schally, A.V. Inhibition of pituitary-testicular function with D-Trp[6]-LHRH in rhesus monkey. Endocrinology 110, 1308 (1982).

13. Resko, J.A., Belanger, A. and Labrie, F. Effects of chronic treatment with a potent LHRH agonist on serum LH and steroid levels in the male rhesus monkey. Biol. Reprod., 26, 378 (1982).

14. Mann, D.R., Gould, K.G. and Collins, D.C. Influence of continuous GnRH agonist treatment on LH and testosterone secretion, the response to GnRH, and the testicular response to hCG in male rhesus monkeys, J. Clin. Endocrinol. Metab., 58, 262 (1984).

15. Akhtar, F.B., Marshall, G.R., Wickings, E.J. and Nieschlag, E. Reversible induction of azoospermia in rhesus monkeys by constant infusion of a GnRH agonist during osmotic minipumps. J. Clin. Endocrinol. Metab., 56, 534 (1983).

16. Vickery, B.H. and McRae, G.I. Effects of continuous treatment of male baboons with superagonists of LHRH. Int. J. Fertil., 25, 179 (1980).

17. Wickings, E.J., Zaidi, P. and Nieschlag, E. Do LHRH superagonists provide an approach to male fertility control? Pre-clinical trial in rhesus monkeys. Acta Endocrinol. (Copenh), 94, 79 (1980).

18. Linde, R., Doelle, G.C., Alexander, A.N., Kirchner, F. Vale, W., Rivier, J. and Rabin, D. Reversible inhibition of testicular steroidogenesis and spermatogenesis by a potent GnRH agonist in normal men. N. Engl. J. Med., 305, 663 (1981).

19. Bhasin, S., Heber, D., Steiner, B.S. and Swerdloff, R.S. Hormonal effects of GnRH agonist in the human male. III. Effects of long-term combined treatment with GnRH agonist and androgen. J. Clin. Endocrinol. Metab., 60, 998 (1985).

20. Heber, D., Bhasin, S., Steiner, B.S. and Swerdloff, R.S. Stimulatory and downregulatory effects of GnRH agonist in the human male. J. Clin. Endocrinol. Metab., 58, 1084 (1984).

21. Warner, B., Worgul, T.J., Drago, J., Demers, J., Dufau, M., Max, D., Santen, R.J., and members of the Abbott Study Group. Effects of very high dose D-leu[6]GnRH proethylamide on hypothalamic-pituitary-testicular axis as treatment of prostate

cancer. J. Clin. Invest., 71, 1842 (1983).

22. Doelle, G.C., Alexander, A.N., Evans, R.M., Linde, R., Rivier, J., Vale, W. and Rabin, D. Combined treatment with a LHRH agonist and testosterone in man: reversible oligospermia without impotence. J. Androl. 4, 298 (1983).

23. Schurmeyer, T.H., Knuth, U.A., Freischmen, C.W., Sandow, J., Akhtar, F.B. and Nieschlag, E. Suppression of pituitary and testicular function in normal men by constant GnRH agonist infusion. J. Clin. Endocrinol. Metab. 59, 19 (1984).

24. Rabin, D., Evans, R., Alexander, A.N., Doelle, G., Rivier, J., Vale, W. and Liddle, G. Heterogeneity of sperm density profiles following 20-week therapy with high dose LHRH analog plus testosterone. J. Androl. 5, 176 (1984).

25. Pavlou, S.N., Interlandi, J.W., Wakefield, G., Rivier, J., Vale, W. and Rabin, D. Heterogeneity of sperm density profiles following 16-week therapy with continuous infusion of high dose LHRH analogue plus testosterone. J. Androl. (In press), 1986.

26. Michel, E., Bents, H., Akhtar, F.B., Honigl, W., Sandow, J. and Nieschlag, E. Failure of high dose sustained release GnRH agonist plus testosterone to suppress male fertility. J. Androl. (Suppl.), 6, 37 (Abstract), (1985).

27. Swerdloff, R.S., Steiner, B.S. and Bhasin, S. Gonadotropin-releasing hormone (GnRH) agonists in male contraception. Med. Biol. 63, 218 (1985).

28. Swerdloff, R.S., Handelsman, D.J. and Bhasin, S. Hormonal effects of GnRH agonists in the human male: an approach to male contraception using combined agonist and androgen treatment. J. Steroid Biochem., 23, 855 (1985).

29. Heber, D. and Swerdloff, R.S. Male contraception: synergism between superactive GnRH analog and testosterone in suppressing gonadotropin secretion. Science, 209, 936 (1980).

30. Bhasin, S., Heber, D., Steiner, B.S., Peterson, M., Blaisch, B. Campbell, L.A. and Swerdloff, R.S. Hormonal effects of GnRH agonist in the human male. II. Testosterone enhances gonadotropin suppression induced by GnRH agonist. Clin. Endocrinol., 20, 119 (1984).

31. Bhasin, S., Steiner, B.S. and Swerdloff, R.S. Does constant infusion of GnRH agonist lead to greater suppression of gonadal function in man than its intermittent administration? Fertil. Steril., 44, 96 (1985).

32. Akhtar, F.B., Marshall, G.R. and Nieschlag, E. Testosterone supplementation attenuates the antifertility effects of an LHRH agonist in male monkeys. Int. J. Androl., 6, 461 (1983).

33. Bhasin, S. and Swerdloff, R.S. Mechanisms of GnRH agonist action in the human male. Endocr. Rev, 7, 106 (1986).

34. Hsueh, A.J.W. and Jones, P.C.B. Extrapituitary actions of GnRH. Endocr. Rev., 2, 437 (1981).

35. Schaison, G., Brailly, S., Vuagnat, P., Bouchard, P. and Milgrom, P. Absence of direct inhibitory effects of GnRH agonist D-Ser(TBU)^6-des-Gly-NH$_2$^{10} ethylamide (Buserelin) on testicular steroidogenesis in men. J. Clin. Endocrinol. Metab., 58, 885 (1984.

36. Evans, R.M., Doelle, G.C., Alexander, A.N., Uderman, H.D., and

Rabin, D. Gonadotropin and steroid secretory patterns during chronic treatment with an LHRH agonist analog in men. J. Clin. Endocrinol. Metab., 58, 862 (1984).

37. Bhasin, S., Fielder, T.J., Sod-Moriah, U.A. and Swerdloff, R.S. Testicular modulation of LH response to GnRH agonist. Biol. Reprod., (In press).

38. Evans, R.M., Doelle, G.C., Lindner, J., Bradley, V. and Rabin, D. An LHRH agonist decreases biologic activity and modifies chromatographic behavior of LH in man. J. Clin. Invest., 73, 262 (1984).

39. Rajfer, J., Sikka, S.S., Rivera, F. and Swerdloff, R.S. Lack of direct effect of gonadotropin-hormone releasing hormone agonist on human testicular steroidogenesis. J. Clin. Endocrinol. Metab., (In press).

40. Bouchard, P., Blondet, C., Spitz, I., Brailly, S., Jouannet, P. and Schaison, G. Sperm suppression by long acting GnRH agonist therapy in men: critical effect of testosterone substitution and duration of therapy. Endocrinology 118: 155A (Abstract), 1986.

41. Bergquist, C., Nillius, S.J., Bergh, T., Skarin, G. and Wide, L. Inhibitory effects on gonadotropin secretion and gonadal function in men during chronic treatment with a potent stimulatory luteinizing hormone-releasing hormone analog. Acta Endocrinol. 91: 601, 1979.

SECTION 7

GONADAL PROTECTIVE PROSPECTS WITH LHRH ANALOGS

29
Interactions between an LHRH Analogue and Cancer Chemotherapeutic Agents at the Testicular Level in Dogs

J. C. GOODPASTURE and B. H. VICKERY
Department of Physiology, Syntex Research, Palo Alto, CA 94304, USA

INTRODUCTION

Cytotoxic chemotherapy has advanced to a stage at which increased survivability or even complete remission from a variety of neoplasias such as Hodgkin's disease, or of nephrotic syndrome, is seen. However, such therapy often results in questionably reversible oligo- or azoospermia in men [1-3]. There is a known sensitivity of actively dividing tissue to these compounds [4,5]. It is also claimed that a better fertility prognosis follows chemotherapeutic treatment of prepubertal boys [6] in comparison to sexually mature men. These observations prompted studies by Glode et al. [7,8] who suggested that interruption of the hypothalamic-pituitary-gonadal axis prior to and during chemotherapy (thus returning the testis to a "prepubertal" state) might allow for a more rapid return of normal spermatogenesis after cessation of treatment while retaining the antineoplastic effects of the chemotherapy during treatment. Studies in rats had shown LHRH agonists to suppress gonadotropin secretion and reduce serum testosterone levels [9,10]. Glode et al. studied a combination treatment in mice using cyclophosphamide and [D-Leu^6,Pro^9-NHEt]LHRH. They reported a protective effect of the LHRH agonist against the antispermatogenic effects of cyclophosphamide therapy in this model. Subsequent studies have failed to confirm this [11], which is not surprising since, although LHRH agonists will release gonadotropins in the mouse, this species is particularly insensitive to the pituitary down-regulating effects of LHRH analogs. During agonist treatment, neither gonadotropin levels nor testicular steroids are decreased [12,13] and the mice are not rendered infertile [8], much less returned to a prepubertal state. Thus, if any protection occurs in the mouse model, it must be via some other mechanism, perhaps a stimulation of spermatogenesis along lines similar to methycobalamine [14]. The original hypothesis is nonetheless attractive and deserving of further evaluation, using an alternative species. The rat is not suitable for this purpose since LHRH agonists cause focal inhibition of spermatogenesis in this species [15] and are not fully suppressive of fertility [16]. For these reasons we chose to evaluate the hypothesis in the male beagle dog, in which LHRH agonists can induce complete azoospermia through aspermatogenesis [17,18].

EFFECTS OF CHEMOTHERAPY ON REPRODUCTIVE FUNCTION

Mature male beagle dogs were used for all the studies. They were housed in segregated quarters, quarantined from the remainder of the dog colony, but were otherwise kept under normal laboratory conditions in 12 hours light (06:00-18:00 h)/24 hours. They were fed commercial dog food and given water ad libitum. Blood was drawn weekly for creatinine and blood urea nitrogen (BUN) determination to monitor renal function, and for hematological work up to monitor bone marrow function. Weekly testicular volumes were determined and ejaculates were collected [17]. Duration and volume of ejaculation, sperm motility, count and morphology were determined and recorded.

Cyclophosphamide treatment

Two dogs were treated with cyclophosphamide (Cytoxan, Mead Johnson, Evansville, IN) orally (3.5-6.5 mg/kg 3 times weekly, with dose regulated according to the hematological profile) for 43 and 48 weeks for a total of 582 and 709 mg/kg cyclophosphamide, respectively. Nine and 5 weeks after cessation of treatment, respectively, the animals were hemicastrated for the study of testicular histology. Untreated contemporaneous control dogs housed in the same quarters were evaluated similarly.

Sperm numbers and motility were in the same range in all animals prior to treatment and continued in this range in control animals (Fig. 1). At the end of cyclophosphamide treatment, total sperm numbers per ejaculate for the two treated dogs had declined to 1.9×10^5 and 7.9×10^4, and the sperm were immotile. Total sperm numbers reached a nadir of approximately 2×10^4 at 7 weeks after stopping treatment. Sperm motility was not detectable for 22-24 weeks after cessation of treatment although sperm numbers slowly rose starting 11-13 weeks after the last drug dose (approximately 1¼ spermatogenic cycles in the dog [19]). A normal level of sperm motility was achieved by 45 weeks post-dosing and normal forward progression at about 48 weeks after the last drug dose for one animal. The second dog had approximately 50% sperm with forward progression by 62 weeks after stopping treatment, at which time the other testis was removed for histological study. Total sperm numbers were still 2 to 5 fold lower than pretreatment values, or values for the control animals, at 62 and 67 weeks after dosing was stopped.

Testicular volumes were significantly decreased by approximately 20 weeks of treatment (Fig. 2). They continued to decrease until, at cessation of treatment, they were approximately 50% of pretreatment values. Even at 62 to 67 weeks after cessation of dosing, testicular volume was still approximately 30% less than that of the control dogs.

Plasma testosterone levels did not change throughout the entire study and remained well within the normal range. Semen

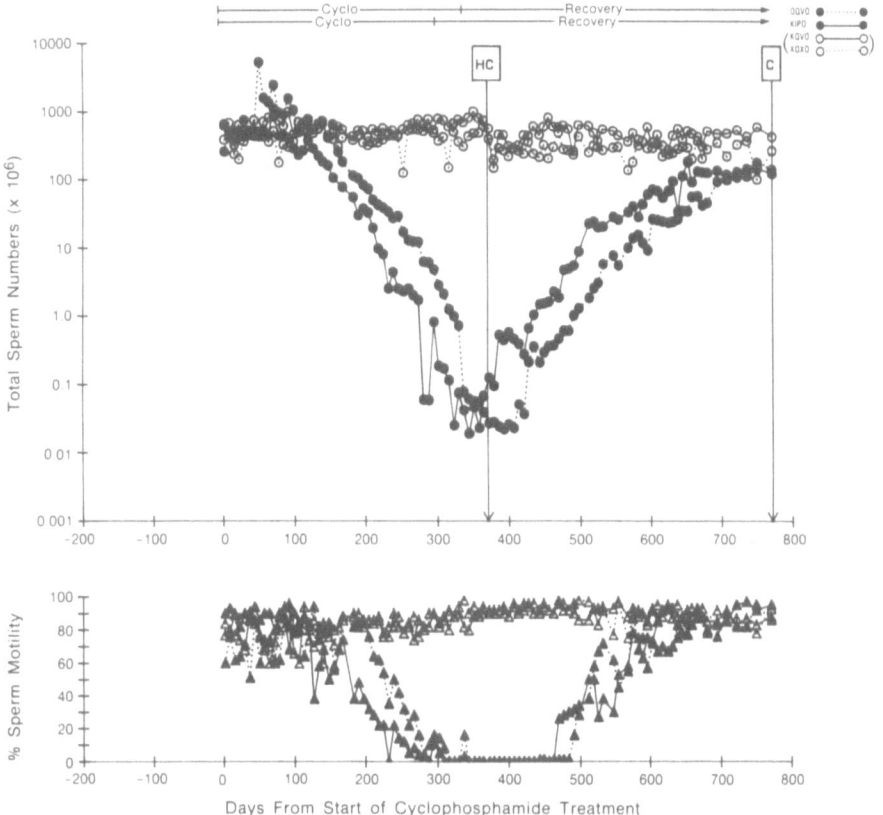

FIGURE 1.   Total sperm numbers and % sperm motility in ejaculates
of beagle dogs treated with cyclophosphamide as
indicated at top of figure. Animal tatoos are used in
key (control dogs in parenthesis). HC = hemicastration
and C = removal of remaining testis. Modified from
Goodpasture, J.C., Bergstrom, K., Waller, D.P. and
Vickery, B.H. In "LHRH and Its Analogues: Basic and
Clinical Aspects", Labrie, F., Belanger, A. and Dupont,
A. (Eds). Elsevier Science Publishers BV, Amsterdam,
1984, p. 156.

volume was also unchanged, reflecting these normal testosterone
levels.
    In the dog that was hemicastrated 5 weeks after the last drug
dose, the testis had atrophic seminiferous tubules containing only
Sertoli cells and occasional spermatogonia. In the other dog,
hemicastrated 9 weeks after the cessation of treatment, there was
also extensive seminiferous tubule atrophy, but in approximately
10% of the tubules there were germinal cells present at each stage
of spermatogenesis up to spermatid (Fig. 3,C). The Leydig cell
population appeared normal in both dogs, as expected. At 67 weeks

445

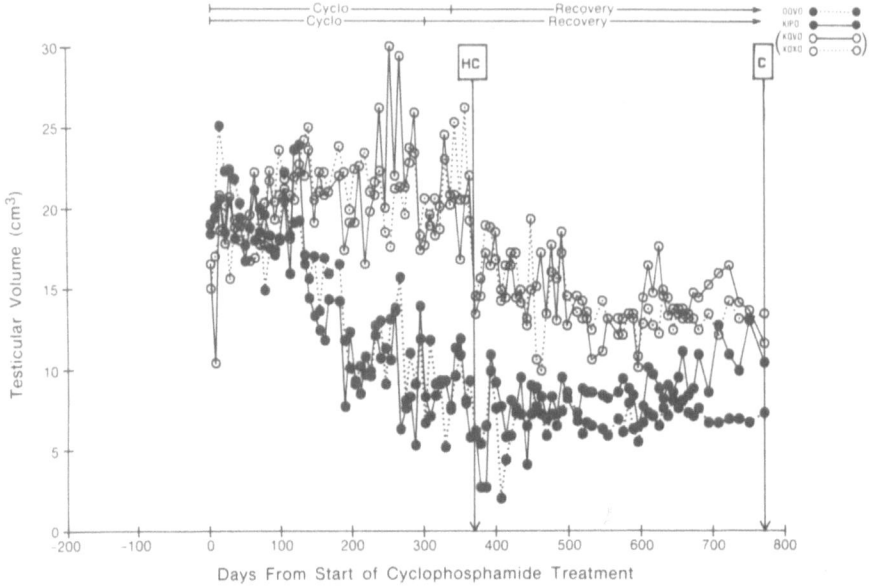

FIGURE 2.   Testicular   volumes   of   beagle   dogs   treated   with
            cyclophosphamide as indicated at top of figure.   Other
            details as in Figure 1.

after stopping treatment, more than 50% of tubules had complete
spermatogenesis (Fig. 3,D).

     BUN and creatinine remained normal, indicating no extensive
renal damage.   Bone marrow function was significantly affected.
White blood cell (WBC) counts were decreased after 2-3 weeks of
treatment   and   were   at   leukopenic   levels   (<6000 x 10^3/mm^3)
after approximately 5 weeks, and at severely leukopenic levels
(<2000 x 10^3/mm^3)   after   about   34 weeks.   WBC   counts   of
$\geq$6000 x 10^3/mm^3 were   regained   9 weeks   after   cessation   of
treatment.   Platelet counts decreased more slowly than WBC counts
and reached levels of <150 x 10^3/mm^3 at approximately 20 weeks
of treatment.

     Thus, long term therapy with cyclophosphamide in male beagles
causes severe oligozoospermia with total loss of sperm motility,
which   is   associated   with   virtually   complete   shutdown   of
spermatogenesis and a 50% reduction in testicular volume.   The few
spermatozoa in the ejaculate at the time of severe oligozoospermia
had   coiled   tails,   indicating   midpiece   defects.   Following
cessation of treatment, severe oligozoospermia with no sperm
motility persisted for 2-3 spermatogenic cycles, followed by a
slow, progressive return to sperm counts in the low normal range
and normal sperm motility.   The lack of sperm motility was not due
to androgen deprivation as the circulating testosterone levels
remained normal for the duration of treatment.   In addition, the
majority of sperm that were observed were of mature morphology

446

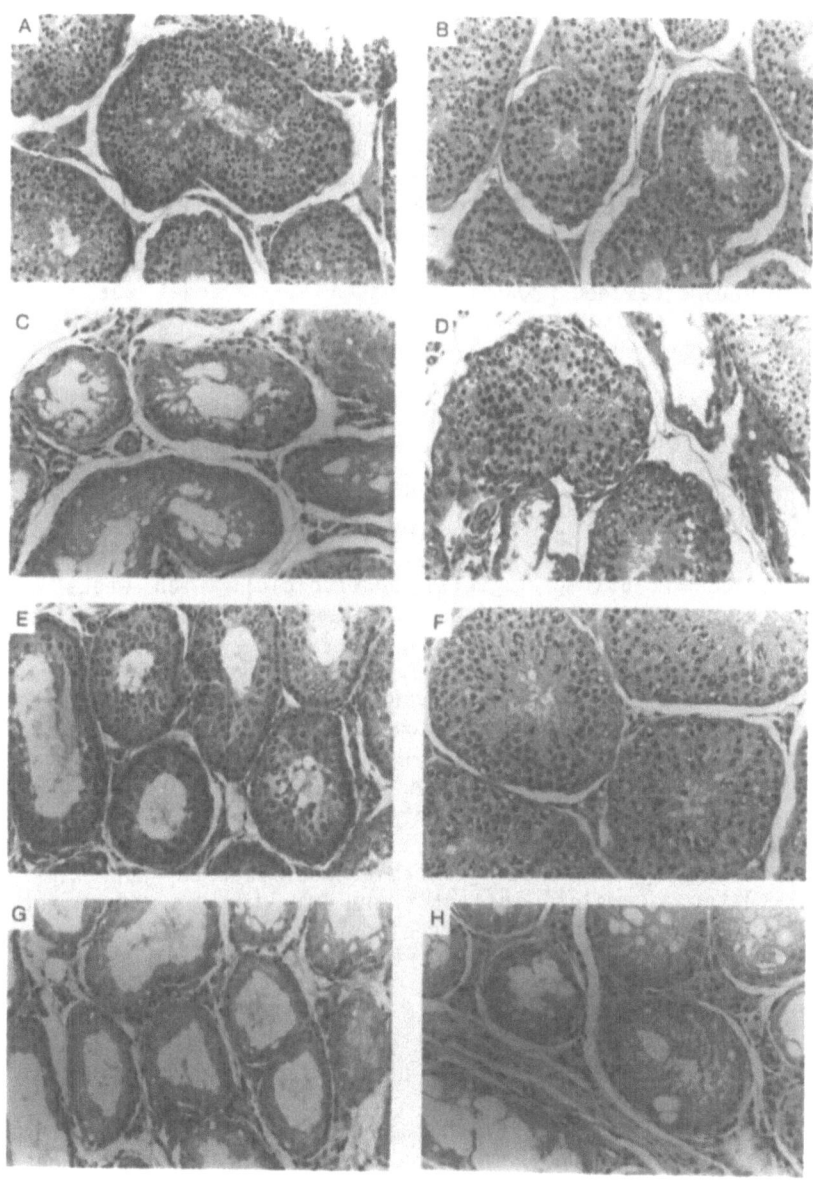

FIGURE 3. Photomicrographs of testes from animals at time of
hemicastration at 5 weeks after stopping treatment
(A,C,E,G), and at removal of the remaining testes at
approximately 67 weeks after stopping treatment
(B,D,F,H).   Animals   received   vehicle   (A,B),
cyclophosphamide only (C,D), nafarelin only (E,F) or
cyclophosphamide and nafarelin (G,H) as detailed in
text. Final magnification X 80.

(i.e., no residual cytoplasmic droplets) and ejaculate volumes remained in the normal range.

These findings are in keeping with those in young men. Although there are no prospective studies reported, clinically there appears to be decreased testicular volume, severe oligo- to azoospermia and infertility in response to treatment with cyclophosphamide [20]. Abnormal sperm morphology and motility have been noted [21], and there is depletion of the germinal epithelium lining the seminiferous tubules [21-24]. The degree of damage is associated in men with the total amount of cyclophosphamide administered. While decreased sperm count was reported after 3-6 g, azoospermia was rare, but became more common as doses of 6-10 g were reached [20].

Combination chemotherapy

Having established the effects of cyclophosphamide on male reproductive function in dogs, it was now possible to evaluate combination chemotherapy.

Three dogs were treated orally with both cyclophosphamide (as above) and doxorubicin (Adriamycin, Adria, Dublin, OH; 0.3 mg/kg once every 2 weeks) for 41 weeks (522-531 mg/kg total cyclophosphamide and 7.8-8.1 mg/kg total doxorubicin). Ten weeks after cessation of treatment the dogs were hemicastrated for evaluation of testicular histology.

The simultaneous administration of cyclophosphamide and doxorubicin for 24 weeks produced antireproductive effects equivalent to cyclophosphamide alone for 40 weeks (Fig. 4). Total sperm numbers were less than 6×10^4 in 2 dogs at the end of treatment. The third animal had less than 2×10^6 total sperm in the ejaculate when treatment was stopped. These numbers continued to decrease after cessation of treatment until azoospermia, or severe oligospermia was reached approximately 4 weeks later. Complete loss of sperm motility was seen after 19 to 48 weeks from initiation of treatment.

Fifty-seven weeks after cessation of treatment, total sperm numbers were still reduced by a factor of 2-2000 compared to pretreatment values, and ranged between 2.0×10^5 and 1.9×10^8 sperm per ejaculate. Sperm motility reached normal levels in two dogs at 31 and 44 weeks, and was up to 70% in the third animal at 57 weeks.

Decrease in testicular volume was more rapid in animals receiving both cyclophosphamide and doxorubicin (Fig. 5) than for those receiving cyclophosphamide alone. There was a continuous decrease to approximately 40% of the initial volume by the end of treatment, which did not increase up to 56 weeks after treatment cessation. Ejaculate volume was unchanged throughout treatment.

Testes histology at 8 weeks after cessation of treatment was similar to that observed in animals receiving cyclophosphamide alone. Seminiferous tubules were atrophic and contained only Sertoli cells and spermatogonia. The Leydig cell population appeared normal. At 57 weeks after stopping treatment, many tubules showed normal spermatogenesis.

448

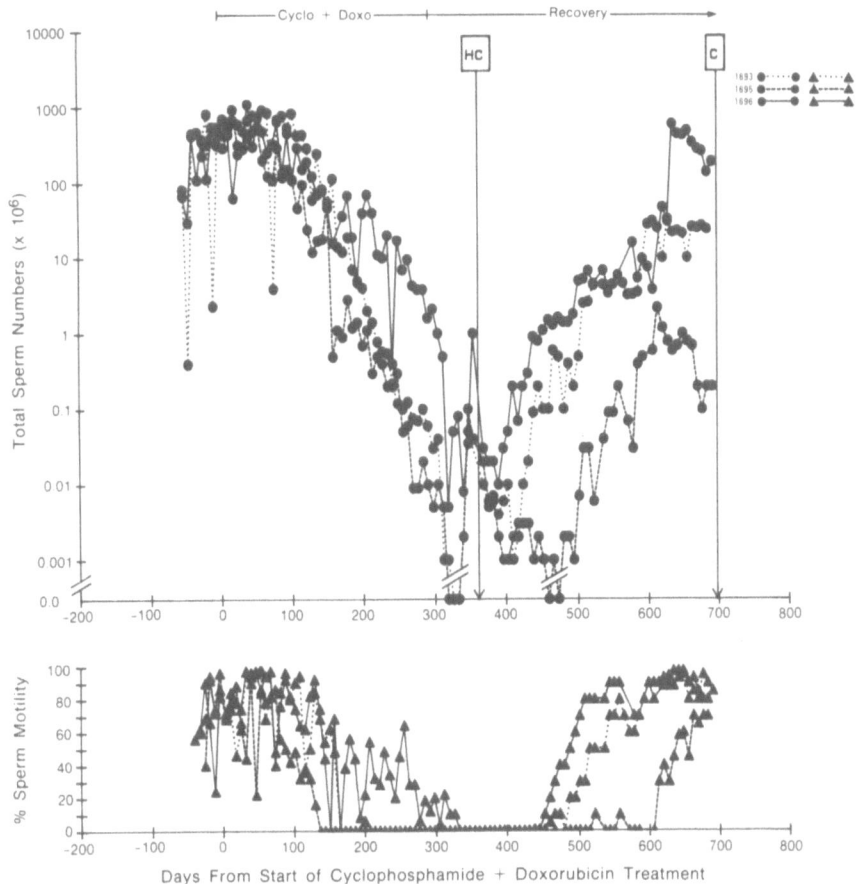

FIGURE 4. Total sperm numbers and % sperm motility in ejaculates
of beagle dogs treated with cyclophosphamide and
doxorubicin as indicated at top of figure. Other
details as in Figure 1.

BUN and creatinine levels remained unchanged throughout the
study. White blood cell counts were significantly decreased in
all animals during treatment. Rebound in white blood cell counts
occurred immediately after cessation of treatment. Platelet
counts were also depressed but did not reach levels as low as
those seen in animals receiving cyclophosphamide alone.

As expected, either therapy resulted in severe depression of
myeloid function in the dogs, with greatly reduced WBC and
platelet counts. In addition, there was evidence of
cyclophosphamide-induced cystitis. WBC and platelet counts
returned to normal more rapidly than did sperm counts and motility.

The addition of doxorubicin to cyclophosphamide therapy
resulted in a more rapid and more severe effect on testicular

449

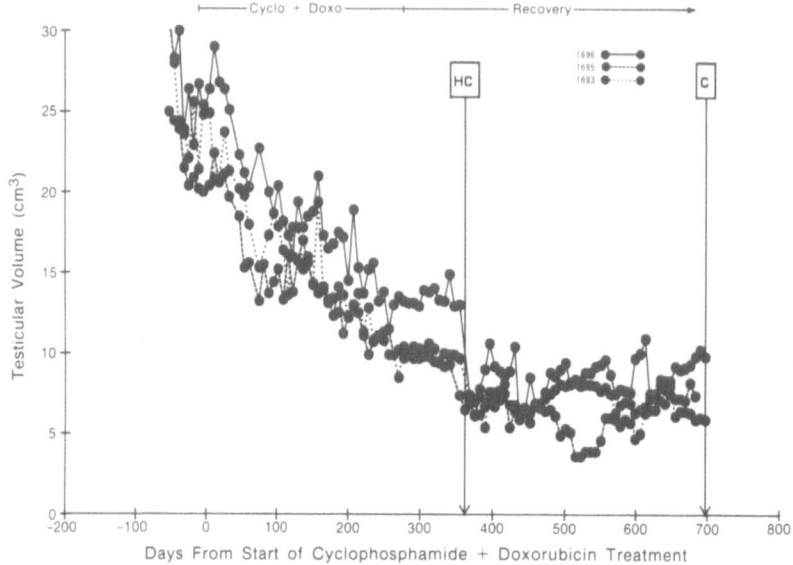

FIGURE 5. Testicular volume of beagle dogs treated with cyclophosphamide and doxorubicin as indicated at top of
figure. Other details as in Figure 1.

function in dogs, with ejaculates becoming azoospermic or so
severely oligozoospermic that centrifugation of the semen sample
was required in order to count the spermatozoa. Sperm motility
was absent for an extended period of time, although normal
motility levels were eventually reached in 2 out of 3 animals.
Similar results have been reported for men when doxorubicin was
used in chemotherapy [26].

In men it is believed that treatment with combination
chemotherapy is associated with a greater degree of testicular
toxicity and a more long lasting azoospermia than is therapy with
single agents [2].

These studies firmly established the suppressive effects of
cyclophosphamide and doxorubicin upon male reproductive function
in dogs and the protracted duration of the recovery phase. We
were now in a position to evaluate the ability of an LHRH agonist
to protect against these antireproductive effects.

EFFECTS OF CHEMOTHERAPY COMBINED WITH LHRH AGONIST TREATMENT

The LHRH agonist used in these studies was nafarelin
([D-Nal(2)6]LHRH). This analog is highly potent [27] and
completely suppresses spermatogenesis in dogs [17,18].

450

Effects of seven weeks pretreatment with LHRH agonist

Four dogs received nafarelin daily (2 µg/kg/day), two for 48 weeks and two for 52 weeks. Seven weeks after starting nafarelin treatment, two of the dogs (one from each group) also received cyclophosphamide treatment as described above for 41 and 45 weeks (570 mg/kg and 698 mg/kg total cyclophosphamide). Cyclophosphamide and nafarelin therapy stopped on the same day. Hemicastrations were performed 9 and 5 weeks after cessation of treatment, respectively.

After 4 weeks of nafarelin treatment none of the 4 dogs produced an ejaculate although erection was achieved and maintained, and anal contractions (normally associated with ejaculation) were evident.

All 4 animals produced ejaculates, which were azoospermic, by the 5th week after cessation of treatment (Fig. 6). The two

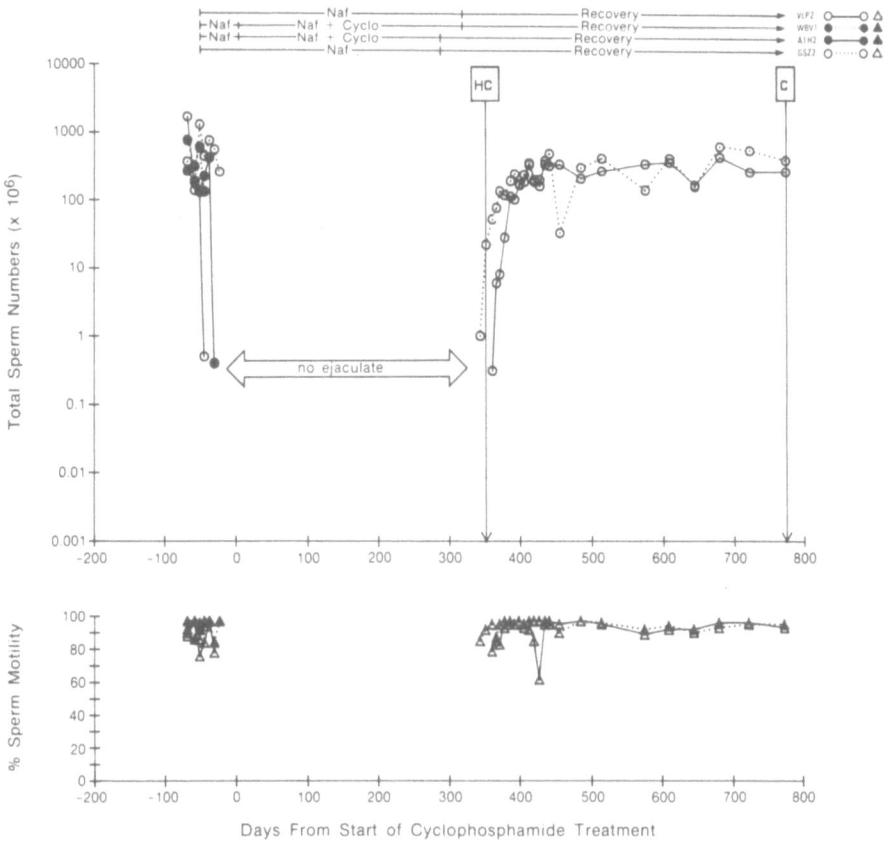

FIGURE 6.   Total sperm numbers and % sperm motility in ejaculates of beagle dogs treated with nafarelin or nafarelin plus cyclophosphamide as indicated at top of figure. Other details as in Figure 1.

animals receiving nafarelin alone had spermatozoa, which were
normally motile, in their ejaculates at 6-8 weeks after withdrawal
of therapy. No sperm were found in the ejaculates of animals
receiving cyclophosphamide in addition to nafarelin over the 65 to
69 week observation period after cessation of treatment.

Testes volumes declined over the first few weeks of nafarelin
treatment (Fig. 7) and reached a nadir after 8 weeks of dosing, at
approximately 30% of pretreatment values. Within 3 to 6 weeks
after cessation of treatment, testes volumes began to increase in
all animals, and at the time of hemicastration (5 and 9 weeks),
testes volume was 50-75% of pretreatment values. The remaining
testis of LHRH agonist only treated animals continued to increase
in size up to approximately 12 weeks after cessation of
treatment. Animals receiving combination treatment did not regain
pretreatment testicular volumes (single testis comparisons) and
never exceeded 60% of control values.

Plasma testosterone levels decreased to approximately
0.3 ng/ml by day 2 of nafarelin in 3 out of 4 animals. After some
variability during the following several weeks, testosterone
remained suppressed at castrate levels for the rest of the
treatment period in all 4 animals. Following cessation of
treatment, plasma testosterone rose to normal levels within
12 days (Fig. 8).

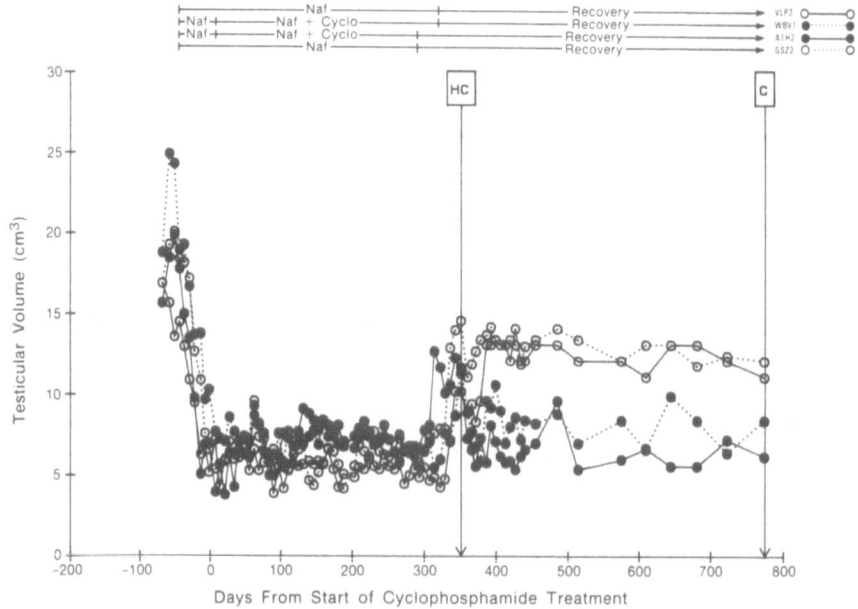

FIGURE 7.   Testicular volumes of beagle dogs treated with
             nafarelin or nafarelin plus cyclophosphamide as
             indicated at top of figure. Other details as in
             Figure 1.

452

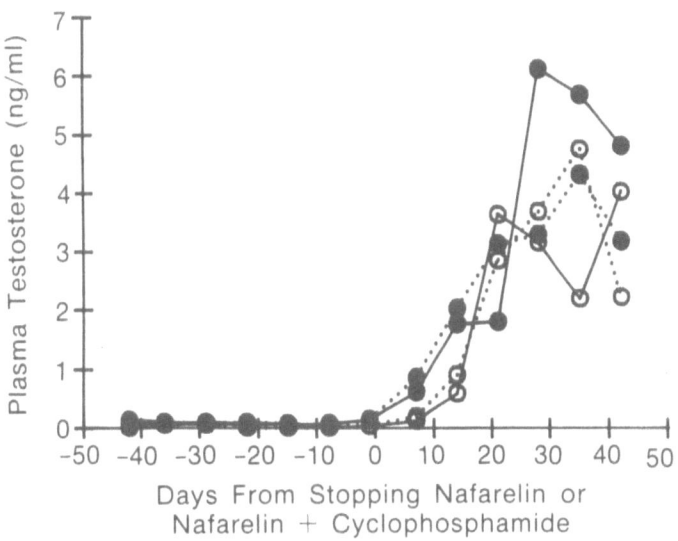

FIGURE 8.   Plasma testosterone levels of beagle dogs treated
            with nafarelin (open circles) or nafarelin plus
            cyclophosphamide (closed circles). Other details as
            in Figure 1.

Testicular histology at 5 and 9 weeks after cessation of
treatment in the two dogs which received cyclophosphamide together
with nafarelin, showed numerous seminiferous tubules with mitotic
activity and occasional tubules with virtually complete
spermatogenesis (Fig. 3,G). The two animals treated with
nafarelin alone had testes with complete spermatogenesis in most
tubules (Fig. 3,E). All 4 animals had normal Sertoli and Leydig
cells. At 65 weeks after stopping treatment, animals which had
received nafarelin only showed normal testicular histology
(Fig. 3,F). However, no germinal cells could be found in the
testes of animals which had received combination treatment,
although Sertoli and Leydig cells appeared normal (Fig. 3,H).

Effects of long term pretreatment with LHRH agonist

Five dogs were administered nafarelin for 58 weeks. After
14 weeks of nafarelin treatment, 3 of the dogs were started on
cyclophosphamide/doxorubicin therapy exactly as described
previously. Hemicastrations were performed 11 weeks after
cessation of treatment.
Animals responded to the nafarelin in this study in a similar
manner to the previous experiment. During the 10-12 week period
prior to azoospermia, ejaculates contained normally motile sperm
(Fig. 9). Ejaculate volume returned 6 weeks after cessation of
treatment. Spermatozoa were present in the ejaculates of
nafarelin-only treated animals by 8 weeks after stopping

453

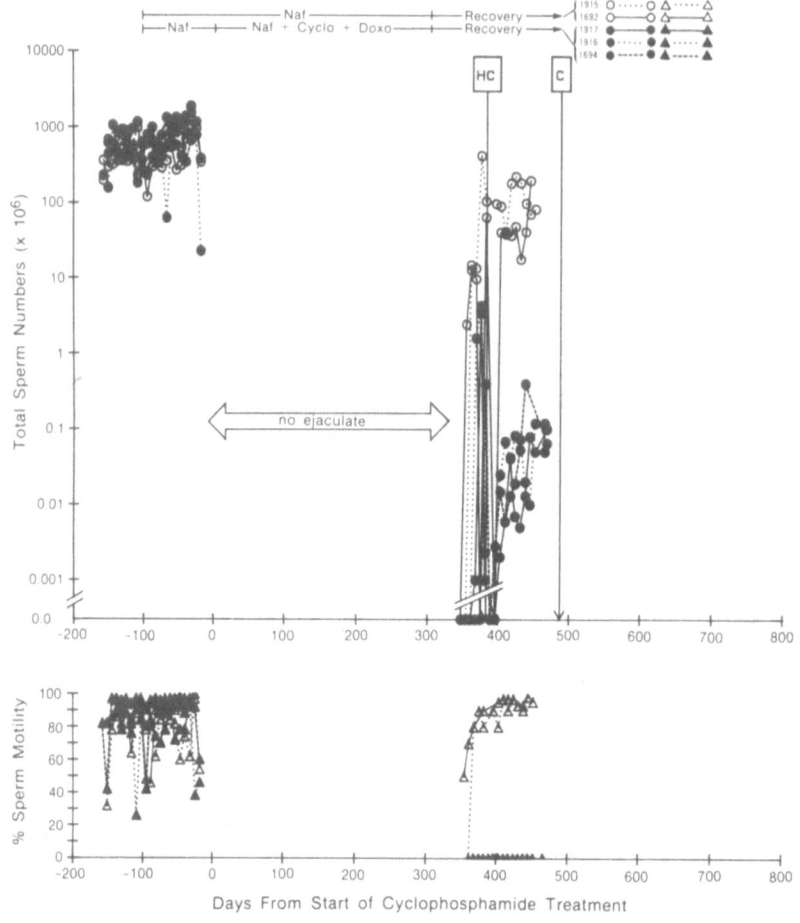

FIGURE 9. Total sperm numbers and % sperm motility in ejaculates of beagle dogs treated with nafarelin or nafarelin plus cyclophosphamide and doxorubicin as indicated at top of figure. Other details as in Figure 1.

treatment. Animals treated with nafarelin plus cyclophosphamide and doxorubicin had spermatozoa in their ejaculates by 9 to 11 weeks, unlike those animals receiving nafarelin plus cyclophosphamide, which did not ejaculate spermatozoa up to 69 weeks after stopping treatment. Eleven weeks after cessation of treatment, these 3 combination treatment animals had total sperm numbers between 1×10^3 and 4×10^5. Sperm motility was normal 9 weeks after stopping treatment in the animals receiving nafarelin alone. The animals that received nafarelin plus cyclophosphamide and doxorubicin did not have motile spermatozoa up to the time of removal of the remaining testis at 23 weeks after cessation of treatment.

454

Testicular volume decreased to a nadir of 25%-40% of pretreatment values (Fig. 10). The testes of animals receiving only nafarelin showed a rapid recrudescence starting approximately 4 weeks after stopping treatment, and reaching approximately 65% of pretreatment values by week 11. Animals receiving combination treatment had a lesser increase in testes size over the 11 week period to 35% of pretreatment values. At 24 weeks after stopping treatment, animals which had received the combined regimen still had testes volumes approximately 60% less than those which had been treated only with nafarelin.

Nafarelin treatment shut down both gametogenic and steroidogenic testicular function as previously published [17,18]. Since ejaculates were not obtainable from the dogs prior to start of chemotherapy (due to the nafarelin treatment), combination effects on sperm count could not be monitored. However, the decline in testicular volumes resembled that in the nafarelin only treated dogs rather than that in animals receiving

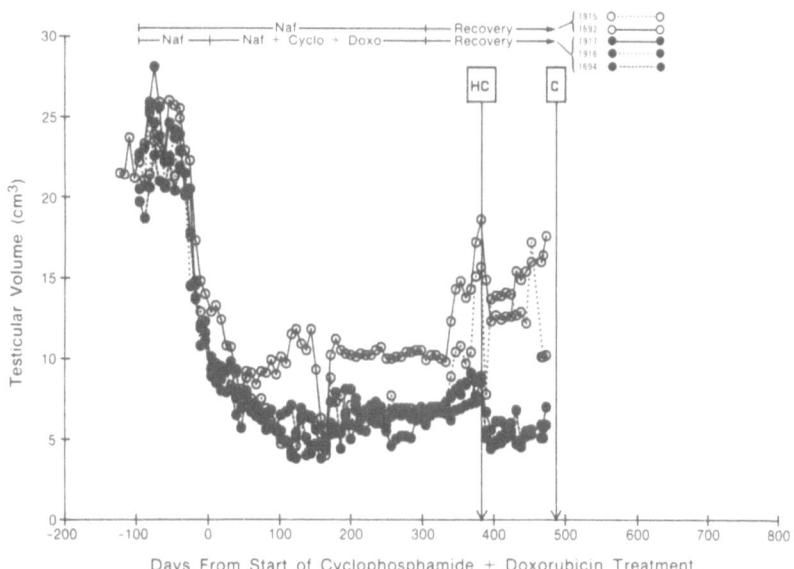

FIGURE 10. Testicular volumes of beagle dogs treated with nafarelin or nafarelin plus cyclophosphamide and doxorubicin as indicated at top of figure. Other details as in Figure 1.

chemotherapy alone. Nafarelin therapy did not alter the chemotherapy-induced effects on the blood parameters.

Return of testicular function following cessation of treatment with nafarelin was prompt. Circulating testosterone levels returned to the pretreatment range within 2 weeks, ejaculatory function was first evident 4 weeks later and the first sperm, already forwardly motile, were present at the 8th week after stopping treatment. Sperm motility was normal by 9 weeks after cessation of nafarelin administration. Testicular volume and consistency rapidly and progressively returned to the normal range over the course of 10 weeks, and testicular histology appeared normal at hemicastration. This confirms and extends a previous report which evaluated effects of 42 days of treatment [17] and underscores the reversibility and lack of toxicity of long term treatment with this LHRH agonist.

On the other hand, combined treatment with nafarelin and cyclophosphamide plus doxorubicin resulted in a situation similar to that observed in animals receiving cyclophosphamide and nafarelin. Testicular volume recovered to only approximately 40% of values for control animals. Although the nafarelin and cyclophosphamide plus doxorubicin treatment did not result in permanent azoospermia, sperm numbers never exceeded 1×10^5 and no motile sperm were observed through 24 weeks after cessation of treatment (time of removal of remaining testis). Based on the histological appearance of the testes at 24 weeks (no germ cells observed in any tubules), it is likely that these animals would have returned to an azoospermic state with a more extended period of observation. Animals receiving nafarelin and cyclophosphamide were azoospermic through approximately 65 weeks after stopping treatment, when they were castrated, at which time no germ cells could be found.

The gonadotoxic effects of both cyclophosphamide and cyclophosphamide plus doxorubicin were clearly potentiated in the presence of nafarelin. The testes remained at a reduced size, sperm numbers were very low or absent, and no germinal cells were found in the testes of any combination treatment animal at the time of removal of the second testis. All these parameters were either normal or near normal at the time of castration in animals receiving nafarelin or chemotherapy separately. Interestingly, at the time of hemicastration (5 to 11 weeks after stopping treatment), the combination-treated animals did have dividing spermatocytes in many tubules, and occasional tubules had complete spermatogenesis. This suggests that upon cessation of treatment germ cells were present in the testes and began to divide, but were then adversely affected to the extent that they were all subsequently destroyed.

OTHER STUDIES

Since the original report on protection in mice from the adverse testicular effects of cyclophosphamide treatment [7,8], several other reports have appeared.

In female rats, [D-Leu^6,Pro^9-NHEt]LHRH starting 2 days prior to and continuing for the 21 days of cyclophosphamide was concluded to inhibit the recruitment from small to large follicles [28]. As the latter are chemotherapy-sensitive, it was suggested that this effect might prevent chemotherapy-induced ovarian failure. In male rats treated with either buserelin or an LHRH antagonist ([Ac-D-Nal(2)^1,D-pCl-Phe^2,D-Trp^3,D-Arg^6,D-Ala^{10}]LHRH) together with cis-platinum, a potentiation of the damage to the germinal epithelium of the seminiferous tubule was noted [29].

In dogs, buserelin has been claimed to be protective against cyclophosphamide, cisplatinum and radiation therapy [30]. Protection was based upon shortened time to repopulation of the germinal epithelium in testicular biopsies. The timing and duration of therapies are not clear from the article so that it is difficult to compare that study with the present evaluation of nafarelin in dogs. Ejaculates were not obtained, so that the sperm immobilizing effect of cytotoxic therapy could not be addressed. In view of the interanimal variation in response to cytotoxic therapy noted in the present study, conclusions based on such small group sizes should be viewed with caution.

A further study in 3 baboons, 2 of whom were treated with [D-Trp^6]LHRH for 13 weeks prior to treating with cyclophosphamide, was also suggested to show decreased gonadal chemotherapy damage [31]. However, this was based upon one combined treatment animal recovering normal sperm count and motility in 8 months, and the other achieving a 7×10^6 sperm count with 40% motility at 10 months with a further increase in sperm count but a decrease in motility to 1% at 1 year. This was in contrast to the animal receiving cyclophosphamide alone, which had moderate oligospermia with no motile sperm.

Two clinical studies have been reported using patients with Hodgkins disease. In the first, preliminary report [D-Trp^6, Pro^9-NHEt]LHRH was started 3 to 10 days prior to chemotherapy plus, in some cases, radiation therapy [32]. Despite the achievement of azoospermia or oligospermia by the 8th week in all patients able to provide semen samples, 84 weeks following cessation of the 14 to 31 weeks of treatment only 1 patient had evidence of active spermatogenesis. It was concluded that no improvement in post treatment fertility due to the LHRH agonist was demonstrable.

In the second study, both men and women with Hodgkins disease received buserelin as adjuvant therapy to chemotherapy [33]. Again, no beneficial effect accrued from the LHRH agonist treatment.

CONCLUDING REMARKS

Five years after the original suggestion that LHRH agonists might be protective against the gonadotoxic effects of chemotherapy, no clear cut answer has been reached. Some animal studies have been interpreted as confirming the original suggestion but others have documented an increased sensitivity of the hypogonadal state.

Attempts to repeat the original finding in mice have failed. To date, experience in the clinic has not been able to show any helpful influence of the LHRH agonists; it is to be hoped that longer term follow-up does not show a detrimental influence.

The observation, in several studies, of an accelerated repopulation of the spermatogenic elements, followed in some cases by a redepletion of the germinal epithelium after cessation of treatment, suggests that the treatment regimen might be at fault. It seems possible that significant accumulation of the chemotherapeutic agents could take place in testicular or other tissues, to circulate and exert damaging cytotoxic effects at the gonad even after administration has ceased. If this were the case then continuation of the LHRH analog treatment until any tissue stores of the cytotoxins were depleted might be advantageous. In addition, the significant rebound of gonadotropins and testicular function noted in primates after cessation of long-term LHRH antagonist treatment [33] might also help in restoring gonadal function after cytotoxic therapy.

REFERENCES

1. Chapman, R.M. Gonadal injury resulting from chemotherapy. Am. J. Ind. Med., 4, 149 (1983).
2. Schilsky, R.L., Lewis, B.J., Sherins, R.J. and Young, R.C. Gonadal dysfunction in patients receiving chemotherapy for cancer. Ann. Intern. Med., 93, 109 (1980).
3. Thachil, J.V., Jewett, M.A.S. and Rider, W.D. The effects of cancer and cancer therapy on male fertility. J. Urol., 126, 141 (1981).
4. De Wys, W.D. and Kight, N. Kinetics of cyclophosphamide damage-sublethal damage repair and cell-cycle-related sensitivity. J. Natl. Cancer Inst., 42, 155 (1969).
5. Warwick, G.P. The mechanism of action of alkylating agents. Cancer Res., 23, 1315 (1963).
6. Trompeter, R.S., Evans, P.R. and Barratt, T.M. Gonadal function in boys with steroid-responsive nephrotic syndrome treated with cyclophosphamide for short periods. Lancet, 1, 1177 (1981).
7. Glode, L.M., Robinson, J. and Gould, S.F. Protection from cyclophosphamide-induced testicular damage with an analogue of gonadotropin-releasing hormone. Lancet, 1, 1132 (1981).
8. Glode, L.M., Robinson, J., Gould, S.F., Nett, T.M. and Merrill, D. Protection of spermatogenesis during chemotherapy. Drugs Exptl. Clin. Res., VIII, 367 (1982).
9. Rivier, C., Rivier, J. and Vale, W. Chronic effects of [D-Trp^6,Pro^9-NEt] luteinizing hormone-releasing factor on reproductive processes in the male rat. Endocrinology, 105, 1191 (1979).
10. Heber, D. and Swerdloff, R.S. Male contraception; synergism of gonadotropin-releasing hormone analog and testosterone in suppressing gonadotropin. Science, 209, 936 (1980).

11. Da Cunha, M.F., Meistrich, M.L., Nader, S. GnRH agonist treatment and cyclophosphamide-induced testicular toxicity. J. Androl., 6(Suppl.), 60P (1985).
12. Vickery, B.H. and McRae, G.I. Responses of the males of different laboratory species to continuous administration of an LHRH agonist. J. Androl., 1, 62 (1980).
13. Bex, F.J., Corbin, A. and France, E. Resistance of the mouse to the antifertility effects of LHRH agonists. Life Sci., 30, 1263 (1982).
14. Kimura, M., Ishikawa, H., Mitsukawa, S., Orikasa, S. and Kuamoto, Y. Effects of mecobalamin on spermatogenesis in rats treated with cancer chemotherapeutic drugs. J. Androl., 4, 36, J4 (1983).
15. Vickery, B.H. Physiology and antifertility effects of LHRH and agonistic analogs in male animals. In "LHRH Peptides as Female and Male Contraceptives", G.I. Zatuchni, J.D. Shelton, and J.J. Sciarra (Eds), Harper & Row, Philadelphia, 1981, p. 275.
16. Vickery, B.H., McRae, G.I., Bergstrom, K., Briones, W., Worden, A. and Seidenberg, R. Inability of continuous long-term administration of D-Nal(2)[6]-LHRH to abolish fertility in male rats. J. Androl., 4, 283 (1983).
17. Vickery, B.H., McRae, G.I., Briones, W., Worden, A., Seidenberg, R., Schanbacher, B.D. and Falvo, R. Effects of an LHRH agonist analog upon sexual function in male dogs. J. Androl., 5, 28 (1984).
18. Vickery, B.H., McRae, G.I., Briones, W.V., Roberts, B.B., Worden, A.C., Schanbacher, B.D. and Falvo, R.E. Dose response studies on male reproductive parameters in dogs with nafarelin acetate, a potent LHRH agonist. J. Androl., 6, 53 (1985).
19. Foote, R.H., Swierstra, E.E. and Hunt, W.L. Spermatogenesis in the dog. Anat. Rec., 173, 341 (1972).
20. Qureshi, M.S.A., Goldsmith, H.J., Pennington, J.H. and Cox, P.E. Cyclophosphamide therapy and sterility. Lancet, 2, 1290 (1972).
21. Fairley, K.F., Barrie, J.U. and Johnson, W. Sterility and testicular atrophy related to cyclophosphamide therapy. Lancet, 1, 1568 (1972).
22. Kumar, R., Biggart, J.D., McEvoy, J. and McGeown, M.G. Cyclophosphamide and reproductive function. Lancet, 1, 1212 (1972).
23. Miller, D.G. Alkylating agents and human spermatogenesis. JAMA, 217, 1662 (1971).
24. Buchanan, J.D., Fairley, K.F. and Barrie, J.U. Return of spermatogenesis after stopping cyclophosphamide therapy. Lancet, 2, 156 (1975).
25. Da Cunha, M.F., Meistrich, M.L., Reid, H.L., Gordon, L.A., Watchmaker, G. and Wyrobek, A.J. Active sperm production after cancer chemotherapy with doxorubicin. J. Urol., 130, 927 (1983).

26. Nestor, J.J. Jr., Ho, T.L., Simpson, R.A., Horner, B.L., Jones, G.H., McRae, G.I., Vickery, B.H. The synthesis and biological activity of some very hydrophobic analogs of luteinizing hormone-releasing hormone. J. Med. Chem., 25, 795 (1982).
27. Ataya, K.M., McKanna, J.A., Weintraub, A.M., Clark, M.R. and LeMaire, W.J. A luteinizing hormone-releasing hormone agonist for the prevention of chemotherapy-induced ovarian follicular loss in rats. Cancer Res., 45, 3651 (1985).
28. Handelsman, D.J., Peng, S., Sikka, S. and Raifer, J. Potentiation of cis-platinum induced testicular damage in rats by GnRH analogs. Endocrinology, 116, 1085A (1985).
29. Nseyo, U.O., Huben, R.P., Klioze, S.S. and Pontes, J.E. Protection of germinal epithelium with luteinizing hormone-releasing hormone analogue. J. Urol., 34, 187 (1985).
30. Lewis, R.W., Dowling, K.J. and Schally, A.V. D-Tryptophan-6 analog of luteinizing hormone-releasing hormone as a protective agent against testicular damage caused by cyclophosphamide in baboons. Proc. Natl. Acad. Sci. U.S.A., 82, 2975 (1985).
31. Johnson, D.H., Linde, R., Hainsworth, J.D., Vale, W., Rivier, J., Stein, R., Flexner, J., Van Welch, R. and Greco, F.A. Effect of a luteinizing hormone-releasing hormone agonist given during combination chemotherapy on post therapy fertility in male patients with lymphoma: preliminary observations. Blood, 65, 832 (1985).
32. Waxman, J. Is it possible to conserve the fertility of patients with Hodgkin's disease treated with cytotoxic chemotherapy? In "LHRH and Its Analogs: Contraceptive and Therapeutic Applications. Part 2". Vickery, B.H. and Nestor, J.J. Jr. (Eds.), MTP Press, Lancaster, 1987, in press.
33. Weinbauer, G.F., Surmann, F.J., Akhtar, F.B., Shah, G.V., Vickery, B.H. and Nieschlag, E. Reversible inhibition of testicular function by a gonadotropin hormone-releasing hormone antagonist in monkeys (Macaca fascicularis). Fertil. Steril., 42, 906 (1984).

30

Is it Possible to Conserve the Fertility of Patients with Hodgkin's Disease Treated with Cytotoxic Chemotherapy?

J. WAXMAN

Royal Postgraduate Medical School, Hammersmith Hospital,
Du Cane Road, London W12 0HS, England

INTRODUCTION

Changes in the treatment of malignant disease have led to the survival of previously incurable young people with lymphomas, leukemias, germ cell tumors and gestational trophoblastic tumors. As a result, the side-effects of treatment have become apparent, and include gonadal failure. Amongst this group of "curable" malignancies, gonadal failure is reported most frequently in Hodgkin's disease. This review describes the features of gonadal failure in patients with Hodgkin's disease and the attempts to circumvent this with a long-acting analogue of LHRH.

GONADAL FAILURE IN HODGKIN'S DISEASE

Prior to the development of combination chemotherapy programmes, the expectation for the majority of patients with advanced Hodgkin's disease was death within 18 months. The introduction of "MOPP" chemotherapy (mustine, vincristine, procarbazine and prednisone) and its variants has led to the cure of approximately 50 per cent of this group of patients, the majority of whom are young people [1]. As a result of this treatment, gonadal failure develops in a significant proportion of patients and this is of great importance in a young population.

The gonadal effects of cytotoxic chemotherapy were first described by Spitz in 1948 [2]. In a post-mortem study, 27 of 30 men treated with nitrogen mustard were shown to have testicular abnormalities. In patients who are sterilised by treatment, the testis is characteristically described as showing an absence both of mature sperm and spermatogenic precursors. Sertoli and Leydig cells are less affected by cytotoxic agents, and may be preserved [3]. Women are seen to have gross follicular destruction, and the ovary is replaced by fibrous tissue. Consequent to gonadal failure, women develop amenorrhoea with dyspareunia, hot flushes, sterility and may be liable to develop premature osteoporosis [4,5]. Women become deficient in ovarian steroids, and have high circulating levels of the gonadotropins [5]. Hormonal

461

replacement therapy may assuage the symptoms of the menopause, but germ cell destruction cannot be compensated for. Men, because of the comparative resistance of Leydig cells to the effects of treatment, have normal serum concentrations of testosterone, with normal basal luteinizing hormone but may have elevated basal follicle stimulating hormone concentrations [3,5]. Men become sterile, but usually retain normal potency.

LONG-TERM FOLLOW-UP IN HODGKIN'S DISEASE PATIENTS

The following study was conducted to investigate in detail the long-term gonadal sequelae of treatment for Hodgkin's disease. This investigation was performed in order to assess the exact incidence of gonadal failure in a carefully observed patient population and to investigate whether or not there was long-term recovery of gonadal function within this group of patients. Forty-six men and twenty-eight women were studied in whom complete remission of advanced Hodgkin's disease had been achieved between 1968 and 1978 and who had not relapsed by 1981 (Table 1). All women were premenopausal at the time of treatment.

Table 1. Patient details.

	Age (yrs) at treatment (mean).	Age (yrs) at follow-up (mean).	Years after chemotherapy (mean).
MEN	12-55 (27)	16-61 (34)	2-12.5 (6.5)
WOMEN	17-48 (30)	25-60 (39)	1-12.5 (7.2)

Cyclical combination chemotherapy with nitrogen mustard, vinblastine, prednisolone and procarbazine (MVPP) was given for either six or 16 cycles.

Seminal analysis was performed after a minimum of three days' abstinence. Forty-one men produced serial samples of semen over periods of two to 12.5 years after chemotherapy. Profound oligospermia was noted in 36 men, with total counts between 0 and 0.66 million. The remaining 5 men had total counts between 20 and 88.4 million. Three patients who initially had azoospermia, and 1 with a count of 10 million, showed recovery to between 20 and 88.4 million over 2 to 10 years after the end of chemotherapy; they had all been aged between 20 and 30 years when treatment was started, and one fathered a normal child.

Menstruating women were studied on days 3-5 of their cycle. After basal blood specimens had been obtained for estimating of concentration of prolactin (mean of three measurements), sex-hormone-binding globulin, testosterone, and 17β-oestradiol, a standard test was performed in which LHRH (100 µg) was given. Concentrations of progesterone were measured on days 20–22 of a cycle (if present).

Concentrations of testosterone and sex- hormone-binding globulin were normal in all patients (Table 2). Three patients had marginally raised concentrations of 17β-oestradiol; 34 raised basal concentrations of follicle- stimulating hormone and luteinizing hormone; two raised basal concentrations of luteinizing hormone alone; and six raised basal concentrations of follicle-stimulating hormone alone; four men had normal basal gonadotropin concentrations despite azoospermia in three. All 37 men tested had excessive responses of follicle- stimulating hormone, while 34 had excessive responses of luteinizing hormone. Four of the five patients with evidence of recovery of spermatogenesis had raised gonadotropin concentrations basally and after administration of LHRH. Prolactin concentrations were normal in all but eight patients.

Twenty-two of the 28 women with regular menses before chemotherapy became amenorrhoeic. There was no late return of menstruation if periods had failed to return within three months after completion of treatment. Five of the six patients whose menses remained normal had been aged under 30 at the time of treatment, and two of these subsequently had normal pregnancies and delivered normal children. There was a positive correlation between age at the time of chemotherapy and subsequent menstrual state. Normal menses were retained in five out of 17 women aged under 30 at the time of chemotherapy (one out of three aged 10–19 and four out of 14 aged 20–29) compared with only one out of 11 aged 30 or over at therapy (one out of six aged 20–29 and none of five aged 40 or over).

Gonadotropin concentrations corresponded to menstrual state: in the women with amenorrhoea both high-basal concentrations and an exaggerated response to administration of luteinizing hormone-releasing hormone were seen. As would be expected with ovarian failure, both oestradiol and progesterone concentrations were low. Testosterone concentrations were normal in all patients. The concentration of sex-hormone-binding globulin was raised in two women. All but seven women had normal prolactin concentrations.

This study with a mean duration of follow-up of over 6 years from chemotherapy has demonstrated irreversible gonadal failure in over 80 per cent of patients. In this context, the idea of applying an adjuvant therapy to circumvent infertility without altering a successful treatment programme is attractive.

ATTEMPTED PREVENTION OF TREATMENT-RELATED INFERTILITY IN PATIENTS TREATED WITH CYTOTOXIC CHEMOTHERAPY

This study investigated the hypothesis that decreased secretion of the pituitary gonadotropins might, by decreasing ovarian and testicular function, protect against the sterilizing effects of

463

Table 2. Hormone concentrations in 46 men and 28 women treated for Hodgkin's disease.

HORMONE	MEN			WOMEN		
	RANGE	MEAN	NORMAL RANGE	RANGE	MEAN	NORMAL RANGE
Prolactin (mU/l)	98 -1114	273	>360	163 - 562	289	>360
Sex-hormone-binding globulin (nmol/l)	16 - 42	27	17 - 50	20 ->120	56	38 -102
Testosterone (nmol/l)	13 - 33	21	10 - 38	1 - 3.2	1.85	0.5 - 3.0
17β-Oestradiol (pmol/l)	<30 - 205	101	<30 -128	<30 - 525	172	110-1290 premenopausal 37- 129 postmenopausal
Progesterone (nmol/l)				<1 - 42.4	7.33	>33
Luteinizing hormone (U/l): Baseline	2.9 - 28	12	1.4- 9.7	2.9 - >50	29	2.5 - 14.1
After 100 µg LHRH at 20 min at 60 min	34 ->50 29.8 ->50	48 37	13.1-57.6 11 -47.6	33 - >50 46 - >50	48 49	15 - 42 12 - 35
Follicle-stimulating hormone (U/l): Baseline	3.7 ->25	15	1 - 7	1.5 - >25	18	1 - 10
After 100 µg LHRH at 20 min at 60 min	6.6 ->25 7.6 ->25	23 24	1 - 7 0.8- 5.2	10.7 - >25 11.7 - >25	23 23	1.2 - 11.1 1.2 - 24.5

Conversion: SI to traditional units - Sex-hormone-binding globulin: 1 nmol/l = 5.2 µg/100 ml.
Testosterone: 1 nmol/l = 28.8 ng/100 ml.
17β-Oestradiol: 1 pmol/l = 26.5 pg/ml.
Progesterone: 1 nmol/l = 31.4 ng/100 ml.

464

treatment. The evidence that reduced secretion of the gonadotropins decreases germ cell activity comes from the finding of arrested spermatogenesis in patients proceeding to orchiectomy after treatment with buserelin [6], and the observation that both men and women with Kallmann's syndrome have hypogonadism. Although the findings are controversial, as children treated for malignancy are less vulnerable than adults to the sterilizing effects of chemotherapy [7,8] and prepubertal rats are less liable to radiation-induced testicular damage than adult rats [9], it may be that the repeated administration of an LHRH agonist analogue could protect against infertility. The animal studies supporting this hypothesis are described in detail in this volume [10].

Thirty-nine patients entered this study (Table 3). The following hormonal assessment was performed in all patients: basal blood samples were taken at 9:00 am for measurement of prolactin (mean of 3 readings), sex hormone binding globulin, testosterone, 17β-oestradiol, progesterone and a standard LHRH test was performed. After two days' abstinence from intercourse, seminal analysis was performed. This was repeated on at least two occasions to confirm oligospermia, and thrice if the analysis was normal to allow for cryopreservation of semen. In both sexes, if randomization was to "gonadal protection," treatment was started with buserelin at 200 μg thrice daily intranasally. Eleven men and 8 women were randomised to receive buserelin; ten men and ten women did not. In men six-weekly depot testosterone supplements were given to potentiate the effect of the agonist analogue and to prevent loss of libido [10]. After one week, the hormonal profile was repeated and cytotoxic chemotherapy given. Adjuvant treatment continued with buserelin for the duration of chemotherapy and for a further three days after its completion. Each patient was treated with up to six cycles of standard MVPP (mustine, vinblastine, prednisolone and procarbazine) chemotherapy. Subsequent to the early results of this study, the dosage regimen of buserelin was altered. An additional nine men received 1 mg of

Table 3. Patient details.

	Age Mean	Years Range	Follow-Up Mean	Years Range
MEN				
BUSERELIN TREATED	27.1	18-44	2.3	1-3
CONTROLS	27.1	18-43	1.9	1-2.5
WOMEN				
BUSERELIN TREATED	28.5	17-34	2.3	1.8-2.5
CONTROLS	25.9	17-46	2.0	1-2.5

buserelin subcutaneously for one week prior to chemotherapy, and then 200 μg thrice daily intranasally during treatment, which was increased to 200 μg five times daily for three days before day 1 of each treatment cycle. Five men of this group were treated with ChlVPP (chlorambucil, vinblastine, prednisolone and procarbazine) and four with MVPP. Patients were followed for up to three years after completing treatment. In men seminal analysis was repeated, and in women menstruation was assessed together with measurement of day 20-22 progesterone. The results of 2 males who were non-compliant, another who developed treatment-related hypersensitivity, 2 men who relapsed, and 1 women who died during treatment, are included until chemotherapy was altered or non-compliance demonstrated.

Women

Menstration. All women receiving buserelin, and three of ten who were not, developed amenorrhoea during treatment. Four of eight women treated with buserelin, and six of nine controls menstruated after treatment.

Serum hormone concentrations. In comparison to pretreatment levels there was persistent significant suppression of concentrations of LH (p <0.05: Student's t test) but not FSH measured at 20 and 60 minutes after injection of 100 μg LHRH (Figure 1A,B). Two patients who had received buserelin ovulated during the period of follow-up, as did control (progesterone day 20-22 of menstrual cycle >30 nmol/l). In patients who were treated with buserelin, low 17-β-oestradiol levels persisted throughout therapy and were consistently in the post-menopausal range in two of eight women. Serum testosterone, sex hormone binding globulin and prolactin levels did not significantly change during treatment with buserelin.

Men

Seminal analysis. Thirteen of 30 men had abnormal seminal analysis at presentation (total sperm counts $<20 \times 10^6$ or <50% sperm motile). All men were profoundly oligospermic with total counts $<0.6 \times 10^6$ during follow-up for three years following treatment.

Serum hormone concentrations. Basal FSH concentrations and levels of both gonadotropins at 20 and 60 minutes after 100 μg of LHRH were significantly suppressed (p<0.05: Students' t test) by buserelin after one week's treatment with both dosage regimens. After the institution of treatment, LH but not FSH responses to LHRH were suppressed throughout treatment. The results of sequential LHRH tests for both treatment regimens have been plotted in Figure 1C,D. An overall Chi square test compared their differences. LH alone was more significantly suppressed (p<0.002) by the higher dosage regimen. No significant change in the serum concentrations of testosterone, progesterone, prolactin, sex hormone binding globulin or 17ß oestradiol occurred comparing patients treated with buserelin and controls.

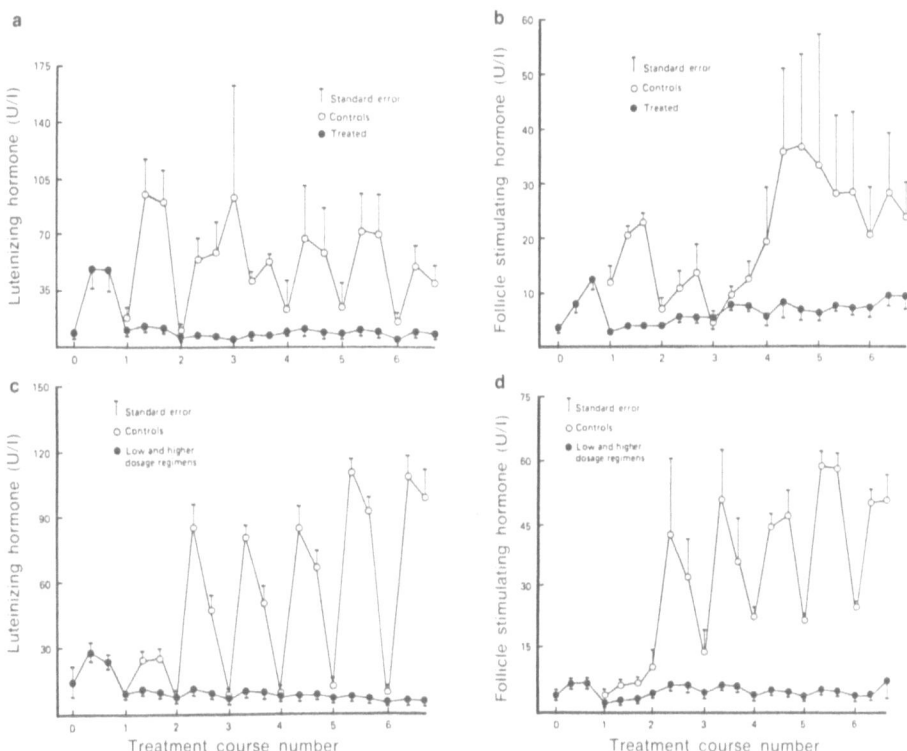

Figure 1. Results of sequential LHRH tests in treated and control patients. Values of LH and FSH are reported for female (A and B) and for male patients (C and D) following an injection of 100 µg of LHRH.

DISCUSSION

This study investigated whether or nor suppression of the pituitary gonadotropins in patients receiving sterilizing chemotherapy resulted in the preservation of fertility. In the dosages and schedules investigated, buserelin resulted in suppression of peak responses of luteinizing hormone to LHRH in both men and women throughout the receipt of cytotoxic chemotherapy. In men both high and low dosage buserelin regimens led to an initial suppression of folicle-stimulating hormone that ceased after one course of cytotoxic chemotherapy. At follow-up, all men were profoundly oligospermic, whilst four of eight women who received buserelin and six of nine controls continued to menstruate. Menstruation was ovulatory in two treated women and

467

two controls. One patient in the control group had a normal pregnancy.

CONCLUSIONS

The long-term gonadal sequelae of cytotoxic chemotherapy given to patients with Hodgkin's disease have been described. Infertility occurs in 80% of men and women. A long-acting agonist analogue of the gonadotropin-releasing hormone was given to patients prior to, and for the duration of chemotherapy in an attempt to prevent treatment-related sterility. This attempt failed. This may have been because the hypothesis investigated was incorrect or because the dosage regimen applied was suboptimal. The evidence from animal studies suggest that there may be a protective effect from these agents, when given for a prolonged period prior to the receipt of cytotoxic chemotherapy. Unfortunately, the opportunity for an adequate period in which to achieve gonadal "down-regulation" does not frequently present itself. There is generally an urgency to press on with treatment. It may be possible that the antagonist analogues of the gonadotropin-releasing hormone will offer an advantage. This is because of their lack of stimulatory effect. Their use may be associated with more rapid "down-regulation" of the pituitary-gonadal axis. A further more practical approach could be to alter therapy and apply a treatment regimen which is said to be less sterilizing and as effective as more commonly applied programmes [11].

REFERENCES

1.   De Vita, V.T., Serpick, A.A., Carbone, P.P. Combination chemotherapy in the treatment of advanced Hodgkin's disease. Ann. Intern. Med., 73, 881 (1970).
2.   Spitz, S. The histological effects of nitrogen mustard on human tumors and tissues. Cancer, 1, 383 (1948).
3.   Chapman, R.M., Sutcliffe, S.B., Rees, L.H., Edwards, C.R., Malpas, J.S. Cyclical combination chemotherapy and gonadal function. Lancet, 1, 285 (1979).
4.   Chapman, R.M., Sutcliffe, S.B., Malpas, J.S. Cytotoxic-induced ovarian failure in women with Hodgkin's disease. JAMA, 242, 1877 (1979).
5.   Waxman, J.H., Terry, Y.A., Wrigley, P.F. Gonadal function in Hodgkin's disease: long-term follow-up of chemotherapy. Brit. Med. J., 285, 1642 (1982).
6.   Waxman, J.H., Hendry, W.F., Whitfield, H.N., Wallace, D.M.A., Oliver, R.T.D. Response and relapse in patients with prostatic cancer treated with buserelin. In "LHRH and its analogues," F. Labrie, A. Belanger, A. Dupont (Eds) Elsevier, 1984, p. 359.
7.   Blatt, J., Poplack, D.G., Sherins, R.J. Testicular function in boys after chemotherapy for acute lymphoblastic leukaemia. N. Engl. J. Med., 304, 1121 (1981).

8. Whitehead, E., Shalet, S.M., Morris Jones, P.M., Beardwell, C.G., Deaking, D.P. Gonadal function after combination chemotherapy for Hodgkin's disease in choldhood. Arch. Dis. Child., 47, 287 (1982).

9. Delic, J.I., Shalet, S.M., Hendrix, J.H., Morris, I.D. Influence of age and pubertal status on radiation-induced testicular damage in the rat. Ped. Res., 19, 632 (1985) and Heber, D., Swerdloff, R.S. Male contraception: synergism of gonadotrophin-releasing hormone analog and testosterone in suppressing gonadotrophin. Science, 209, 936 (1980).

10. Santoro, A., Vivani, S., Zucali, R., et al. Comparative results and toxicity of MOPP vs ABVD combined with radiotherapy (TR) in PS 11B, 111(A,b) Hodgkin's disease. Proceedings ASCO and AACR Abstract C871 Oncol (1983).

11. Goodpasture, J.C. and Vickery, B.H. Interactions between an LHRH analogue and cancer chemotherapeutic agents at the testicular level in dogs. In "LHRH and its Analogs: Contraceptive and Therapeutic Applications, Part 2." Vickery, B.H. and Nestor, J.J. Jr. (Eds), MTP Press, Lancaster, 1987, in press.

SECTION 8

DIAGNOSTIC APPLICATIONS

31
Predicting Predisposition to Osteoporosis: GnRH Antagonist for Acute Estrogen Deficiency

G. D. HODGEN[1], D. KENIGSBERG[2] and R. ABBASI[3]
[1]The Jones Institute for Reproductive Medicine, Dept. of Ob/Gyn, Eastern Virginia Medical School, Norfolk, VA 23507: [2]Dept. Ob/Gyn, SUNY, Stony Brook, NY 11794; [3]Dept. Ob/Gyn, Brooke Army Medical Center, Fort Sam Houston, San Antonio, TX 78234 - 6200, USA.

INTRODUCTION

Few naturally occurring diseases adversely affect the quality and longevity of so many human lives as the sequelae to severe estrogen deficiency in the postmenopausal years. The scope of this health problem is reflected in both the more than 34 million American women over 50 years of age and the average lifespan of American women, which approaches 80 years [1]. Because the potential consequences with hormone replacement vs risks of non-treatment loom large for each individual, an early and accurate therapeutic decision can greatly extend an active and productive life.

The benefits of estrogen-replacement therapy for conserva tion of bone calcium, prevention of hot flushes and amelioration of urogenital tissue atrophy in most postmenopausal and ovariectomized women are well known [2-4]. Often, progestins are overlapped sequentially to shed proliferative endometrium, thereby reducing the risk of endometrial carcinoma [5]. Inherently, such regimens are controversial with regard to incidences of endometrial carcinoma and cardiovascular complications [6-11]. In addition, usually women would prefer to avoid menstruation beyond the natural menopause; some uterine bleeding is manifest by most of the women on current estrogen replacement therapy/progestin regimens [12].

Although most postmenopausal women gain obvious benefits from estrogen-replacement therapy, this is particularly true when a family history, skeletal type, habits, and genetic predisposition suggest that the individual is at significant risk [18].

Importantly, a smaller number of women do not require estrogen-replacement therapy in the postmenopausal years or can gain considerable symptomatic relief from progestins alone [19]. Evaluations by bone densitometry for discrimination of those women needing estrogens prophylactically may come too late to avert osteoporosis because such assessments are retrospective. Accordingly, a reliable predictive test to identify individually perimenopausal women who are highly vulnerable to the negative sequelae of severe estrogen deficiency may be useful to practitioners deciding for whom, when, and how to implement estrogen-

473

replacement therapy, or a combination regimen to prevent osteo-porosis.

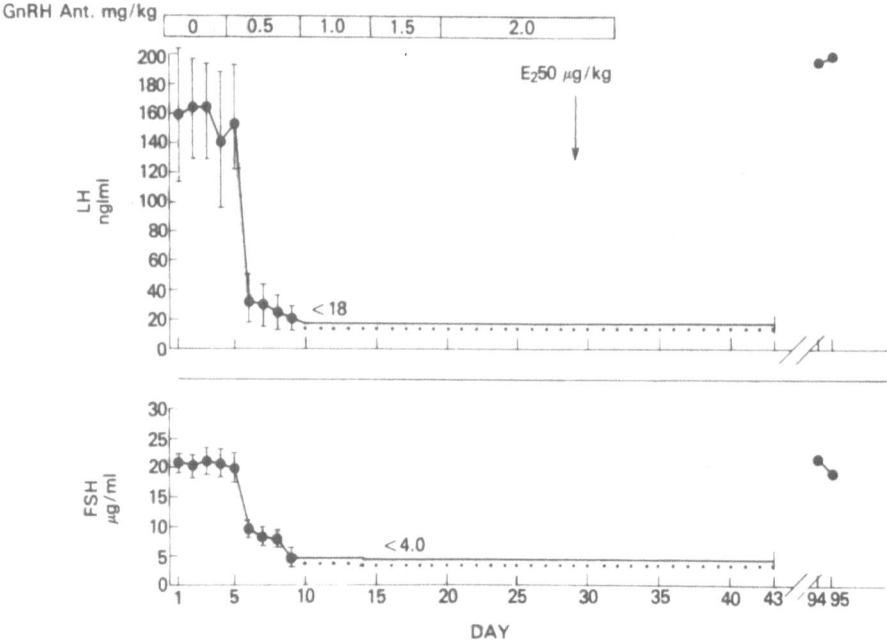

FIGURE 1 GnRH antagonist suppresses FSH and LH levels in serum to below limits of assay detection. Long-term ovariectomized monkeys did not respond to an estrogen challenge test. Note the full recovery of gonadotropin secretion by 2 months after cessation of treatment. Reproduced from Kenigsberg D, Littman BA and Hodgen GD. Fertil. Steril., 42, 112 (1984), with permission.

In earlier studies, we have demonstrated the potential utility of GnRH (LHRH) antagonists for (a) rapid achievement of a "medical hypophysectomy", with regard to reversible effects on pituitary gonadotropin secretion [15] (Fig 1); (b) adjunctive pituitary suppression during gonadotropin therapy for ovulation induction or in vitro fertilization [16]; and (c) contraception by once weekly ablation of the oncoming dominant follicle [17] (Fig 2). Here, we have incorporated our recent findings which suggest the means for a diagnostic test to predict predisposition to osteoporosis during severe estrogen deficiency [18, 19].

In the present study, primate models were employed to determine (1) whether short-term GnRH-antagonist treatment allows prospective identification of those individuals most acutely vulnerable to a negative calcium balance during overt estrogen deficiency; (2) whether daily treatment with high-dose clomiphene citrate is sufficiently estrogenic to abate urinary calcium loss and to sustain vaginal and perineal tissues after ovariectomy; and (3) whether clomiphene citrate will provide these beneficial effects, without inducing endometrial proliferation and menstruation after progestin withdrawal.

PRIMATE MODELS FOR PREDICTING PREDISPOSITION TO OSTEOPOROSIS

Adult female rhesus monkeys (4.2 to 8.6 kg) were housed and maintained in environmentally controlled laboratory conditions as described previously [20-21]. Urine collections were made between 6 AM and 9 AM, after overnight fasting and provision of distilled drinking water. As necessary, urine was taken from the bladder by suprapubic aspiration. Similar methods have proven reliable in both human and animal metabolic studies of calcium and creatinine excretion in urine [2,3,22,23]. Here, the ratio of calcium to creatinine was calculated on the final three days of a ten-day control vs treatment regimen.

The protocol for these studies is illustrated in Fig 3. In Phase 1 the objective was to achieve acute suppression of estrogens in circulation by GnRH-antagonist treatment (N=19) and to compare the urinary calcium/creatinine ratio to pretreatment controls. The dosage of the GnRH antagonist([N-Ac-D-pCl-Phe[1],D-p-Cl-Phe[2],D-Trp[3],D-Arg[6],D-Ala[10]]LHRH)employed was 2mg/kg/day, intramuscularly. This dose was sufficient to suppress serum gonadotropin levels below measureable limits in long-term castrate monkeys within 48 to 72 hours [14]; even 1 mg/kg/day intramuscularly greatly depleted circulating estradiol levels in intact females [16]. Gonadotropin releasing hormone-antagonist treatments were initiated on days 1 to 5 of the monkeys' menstrual cycles. Notice that the days illustrated in Fig 1 refer to the experimental course, not the menstrual cycle. Phase 2 was a nontreatment rest interval of 90 days, permitting resumption of the ovarian menstrual cycle. Lastly, Phase 3 achieved hypoestrogenic status by bilateral ovariectomy during the early follicular phase. Among these short-term castrates, the postcastration urinary calcium/creatinine ratio was compared to that observed under short-term GnRH antagonist therapy in Phase 1, as well as with that of intact controls. Arbitrarily, individuals were ranked in the high, middle, or low third according to their respective calcium/creatinine ratios in urine. Concurrently, 3.5 ml of femoral blood was taken on the final day of each control of treatment regimen for measurement of estradiol levels [24].

Urinary calcium/creatinine ratios were reassessed at 88 to 90 days and 178 to 180 days after ovariectomy. Thereafter, estrogen replacement-therapy was given to monkeys assigned randomly; the treatment interval was 30 days and in two forms--conjugated equine estrogens (N=8, 0.15 mg/day, orally) and clomiphene citrate (N=7, 48 mg/day, orally).

On days 21 to 30 of the estrogen replacement therapy, a Silastic[R] implant providing progesterone at midluteal phase levels (approximately 5 ng/ml of serum) was administered [25]. After eight to ten days of progesterone treatment, urinary calcium excretion was measured; then, progesterone treatment was discontinued to test for withdrawal bleeding.

To assess the peripheral estrogenicity of these estrogen-replacement therapy regimens, weekly vaginal epithelial smears

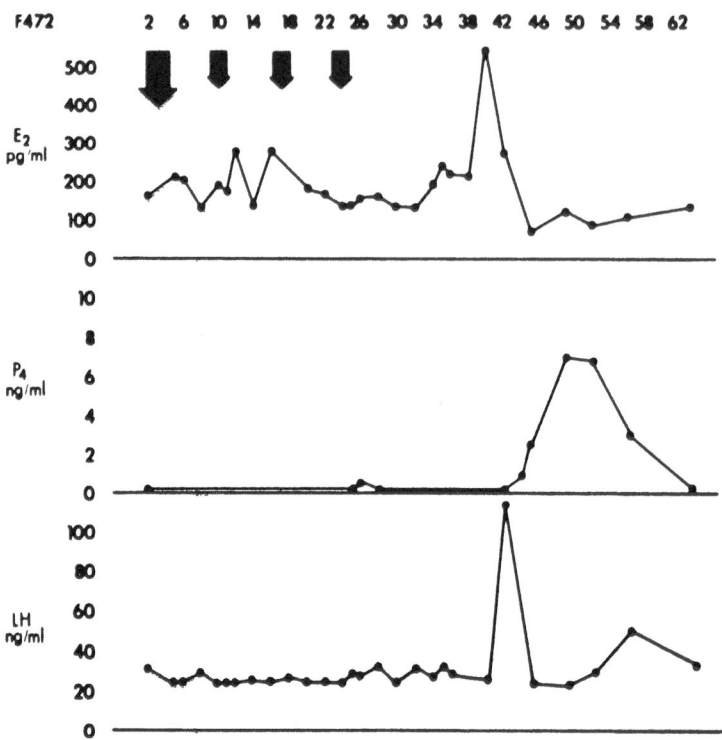

FIGURE 2 Peripheral serum E_2, P_4, and LH levels in a monkey (six of eight) during and after weekly administration of GnRH antagonist (arrows). Note that within about 15 days after the last GnRH antagonist treatment, high serum E_2 levels and a LH surge occurred, followed by an increase in serum P_4. Day 1 was the spontaneous onset of menstruation (top line). Compared to the normal interval from menstruation to ovulation (20), the delay of apparent ovulation and next menses associated with GnRH antagonist treatment was high significant ($P < 0.01$). Reproduced from Kenigsberg D and Hodgen GD.   J. Clin. Endocrinol. Metab., 62, 734 (1986), with permission.

were evaluated histologically; concurrently, coloration of perineum (red indicates estrogenization) was recorded photographically.

The dose of conjugated equine estrogens was chosen to approximate the high-dose range for women receiving estrogen-replacement therapy. For convenience, human conjugated equine

PROTOCOL

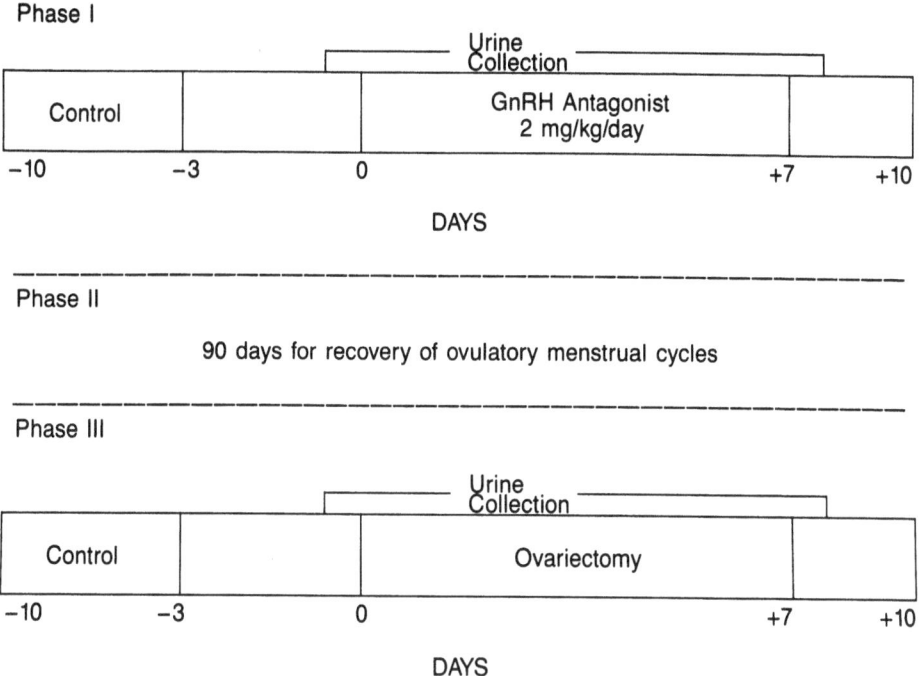

Phase I

Urine Collection

| Control | | GnRH Antagonist 2 mg/kg/day | |

-10   -3   0   +7   +10

DAYS

Phase II

90 days for recovery of ovulatory menstrual cycles

Phase III

Urine Collection

| Control | | Ovariectomy | |

-10   -3   0   +7   +10

DAYS

FIGURE 3   Protocol for studying effects of gonadotropin-releasing hormone (GnRH antagonist vs surgical ovariectomy on urinary calcium/creatinine ratio in rhesus monkeys. Gonadotropin-releasing hormone treatments were begun between first and fifth day of menstrual cycle. Phase 1 was designed to detect whether short-term administration of a GnRH antagonist increased calcium excretion. Phase 2 allowed reversal of GnRH-antagonist-induced suppression of ovarian cycle. Phase 3 was used to assess onset of negative calcium balance after ovariectomy. Reproduced from Abbasi R and Hodgen GD. J.A.M.A., 255, 1600 (1986), with permission.

estrogen pills of 0.3 mg were cut in half, making the monkey dose 0.15 mg. On a body-weight basis, this corresponds to a human dose of about 1.5 mg of conjugated equine estrogens daily. For clomiphene citrate, the 48-mg dose was selected on the basis of a previous study in long-term castrate monkeys. These ovariectomized monkeys (N=20) were divided into four groups of five each and given clomiphene citrate tablets for one month as follows: group

477

one, 12 mg/day; group two, 24 mg/day; group three, 48 mg/day; or
group four, daily placebo controls. Daily blood samples were
assayed for levels of gonadotropins, estradiol, and prolactin by
established methods [26]. Laparotomy and hysterotomy were
performed to assess endometrial proliferation on days 15 and 30.
Monkeys were checked daily for menstrual flow, vaginal
cornification and redness of the perineal skin.

Significant differences in numerical responses were detected
by use of the F statistic for groups of equal or unequal size
[28]. Tests were analyzed at P<.05 and P<.01 levels. Linear
regression analysis allowed comparison of the degree of negative
calcium balance during GnRH-antagonist treatment versus that after
ovariectomy. The coefficient of correlation was calculated as:

$$r=B([\textstyle\sum (x_i-X)^2]/[\textstyle\sum (y_i-y)^2])^{1/2}$$

ESTROGEN-CALCIUM METABOLISM RELATIONSHIPS

That severe acute depletion of ovarian estrogen secretion in these
primates by either GnRH-antagonist treatment or ovariectomy led to
increased (P<.05) calcium excretion is apparent in Fig 2. At the
end of Phase 1, after ten days of GnRH-antagonist treatment, serum
estradiol levels had declined to 24 ± 7 pg/ml, compared to 97 ± 36
pg/ml among intact controls (P<.01). Note that the calcium/creat-
inine ratio in urine rose from 0.11 ± 0.03 (controls) to 0.18 ± 0.05
(P<.05) after eight to ten days of GnRH-antagonist administration.
Following resumption of ovulation in 18 of 19 females during the
recovery interval of Phase 2, ovariectomy (Phase 3) caused an even
greater (P<.05) negative calcium balance than did the GnRH
antagonist 0.10 ± 0.02 vs 0.21 ± 0.04 among intact controls and
castrates, respectively. Concurrently, serum estradiol levels
declined from 86 ± 28 pg/ml (controls) to 13 ± 4 pg/ml at ten days
after ovariectomy (P<.01).

A significant decline (P<.05) in the urinary calcium/
creatinine ratio was observed during the initial six months after
ovariectomy. More importantly, administration of either conjugated equine estrogens or clomiphene citrate reversed (P<.01 and
P<.05, respectively) this status by reducing calcium loss in
urine. Note that conjugated equine estrogen therapy was more
effective than clomiphene citrate at the doses employed (P<.05).
None of the treatments had significant effects on creatinine
excretion in urine.

It was of interest to determine whether individual monkeys
who manifested the highest calcium/creatinine ratios during acute
suppression by the GnRH antagonist were among those expressing the
greatest negative calcium balance soon after ovariectomy. Figure
5 depicts three groups separated according to the degree of
elevation of the calcium/creatinine ratio during Phase 1 (short-
term GnRH-antagonist treatment). We asked whether they would rank
similarly after ovariectomy (Phase 3). There was a strong
correlation (r=.87, P<.01) between monkeys having high urinary
calcium/creatinine ratios during GnRH-antagonist suppression of

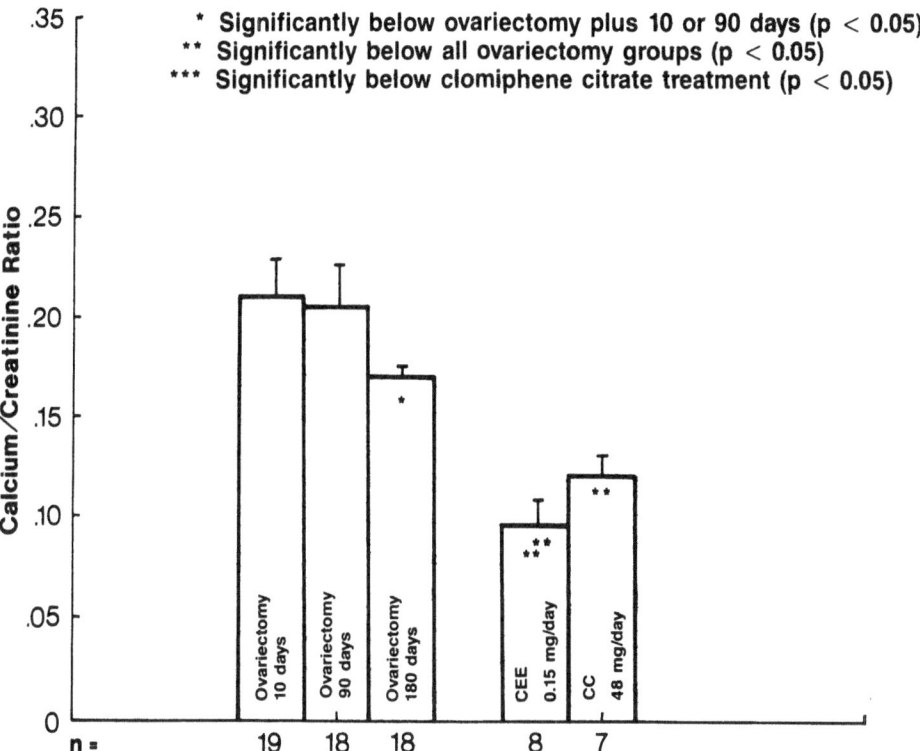

FIGURE 4   Urinary calcium/creatinine ratio in ovariectomized rhesus monkeys (X ± SEM).   Note calcium conservation effects of conjugated equine estrogens (CEE) or clomiphene citrate (CC) administrered for 30 days. Reproduced from Abbasi R and Hodgen GD.   J.A.M.A., 255, 1600 (1986), with permission.

ovarian estrogen secretion and after ovariectomy, less so in the middle (r=.42, P<.05) and low (r=.14, P>.05) ratio groups. Indeed, among the latter group five of seven individuals showed no effect of either the GnRH antagonist or ovariectomy on calcium excretion.

Both conjugated equine estrogens and clomiphene citrate had profound estrogenic effects on peripheral estrogen-dependent tissues.   Either estrogen-replacement therapy regimens induced cornified epithelial cells in the vagina and enhanced redness of the previously blanched perineum of long-term castrate monkeys. One   month   of   conjugated   equine   estrogen   administration proliferated endometrial tissues, as evidenced by withdrawal bleeding after progesterone treatment.   In contrast, clomiphene citrate did not cause endometrial proliferation; moreover, there was no menstrual flow following equivalent progesterone treatment.

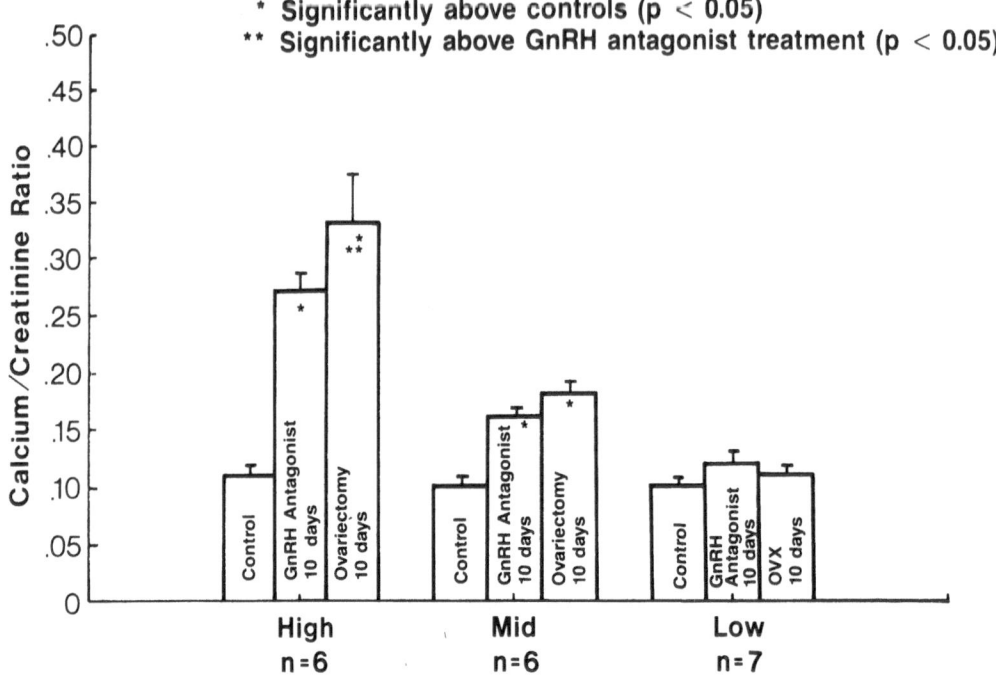

FIGURE 5 Comparison of calcium/creatinine ratio (X ± SEM) in urine of intact controls, gonadotropin-releasing hormone (GnRH)-antagonist treated, and ovariectomized monkeys according to rank by the GnRH-antagonist test (high third, middle third, low third). Note predictive value of GnRH-antagonist test for identification of those females most apt to manifest a large negative calcium balance after ovariectomy (r = .87). Reproduced from Abassi R and Hodgen GD. J.A.M.A., 255, 1600 (1986), with permission.

A negative-feedback suppression of follicle-stimulating hormone and luteinizing hormone secretion was observed in a long-term ovariectomized monkey receiving 48 mg of clomiphene citrate daily. This response manifested broad individual variation, with lower doses of clomiphene citrate inhibiting blood levels of follicle-stimulating hormone and luteinizing hormone less markedly. Serum estradiol remained less than 12 pg/ml; prolactin levels were not affected by clomiphene citrate treatments.

Table 1. Responses of estrogen dependent tissues to 30 days of estrogen replacement therapy, including a progesterone challenge test in rhesus monkeys ovariectomized 190 days previously.

Groups	Cornified Vaginal Epithelium	Perineal Coloration	Progesterone Withdrawal Bleeding
Conjugated Equine Estrogens (0.15 mg/day)	8/8	8/8	8/8
Clomiphene Citrate (48 mg/day)	7/7	7/7	0/7[a]

[a]Hysterotomy revealed absence of proliferative endometrium.

CONCLUDING REMARKS

The findings presented extend our earlier opinion that menopausal primate models may be useful paradigms for estrogen-calcium metabolism in women [29]. In particular, it is of some considerable significance that short-term (reversible) pituitary-ovarian suppression by the GnRH antagonist, with its attendant increases in calcium excretion, allowed identification of those individual monkeys most likely to have high urinary calcium/creatinine ratios after ovariectomy.

As demonstrated here, this discrimination was made after a seven-day regimen of the GnRH antagonist (beginning days 1 to 5 of the menstrual cycle), which achieves a "medical hypophysect-omy" status within 48 to 72 hours [15]. In contrast, GnRH agonists, which have an initial stimulatory effect before desensitization of the pituitary, would require a longer treatment interval, up to 21 days, to produce an equivalent hypogonadotropic and hypoestrogenic milieu, thereby reducing the practical value of the agonistic analogues of GnRH for this purpose.

Perhaps the greater degree of hypoestrogenic status after ovariectomy vs the GnRH antagonist accounts for more rapid calcium excretion after surgical castration. A similar phenomenon has been reported in women [30]. Moreover, despite achieving a state of GnRH-antagonist-induced medical hypophysectomy, the "quiescent" ovaries may secrete modest amounts of estrogens. Although not evaluated here, estrogens may derive from gonadotropin-independent peripheral aromatization [31].

It is noteworthy that the calcium loss rate in urine slowed marginally over six months, even without estrogen replacement therapy. Thereafter, administration of either conjugated equine estrogen or clomiphene citrate strikingly reduced urinary calcium loss. That clomiphene citrate was less effective than conjugated equine estrogen in deterring calcium excretion may be a matter of relative dose. Clomiphene citrate is known to be weakly estrogenic in some tissues, while it is antiestrogenic in others [32,33]; thus, even higher doses may be required to achieve the estrogenicity manifested by conjugated equine estrogens.

Clomiphene citrate did not induce mitogenic effects on the uterine endometrium, as observed in other animals [34]. In monkeys, whereas conjugated equine estrogen stimulated overt endometrial proliferation and withdrawal bleeding after progesterone, clomiphene citrate did neither. Similarly, among women given clomiphene citrate during conjugated equine estrogen therapy, proliferative endometrium became atrophic [35]. These findings offer some promise of developing effective estrogen replacement therapy without proliferation of endometrium by searching for a regimen that is desireably estrogenic at certain tropic sites (bone, central nervous system, and perineum), yet paradoxically antiestrogenic at the endometrial and cervical level. Theoretically, such a treatment mode might reduce the risk of endometrial carcinoma, while preserving skeletal calcium, suppressing hot flushes, and preventing vaginal atrophy.

The 48-mg/day dose of clomiphene citrate usually produced a significant decline in circulating levels of luteinizing hormone and follicle stimulating hormone within 30 days of treatment. While there was wide individual variation in this response, generally less suppression of pituitary gonadotropin secretion was achieved at clomiphene citrate doses of 12 or 24 mg/day. Note that red perineal coloration and vaginal cornification were achieved regularly at all doses of clomiphene citrate. Thus, the threshold for estrogenic effects of clomiphene citrate on urogenital tissues may be lower than that regulating gonadotropin secretion.

During the course of the study, one monkey was eliminated from the conjugated equine estrogen group and two were removed from the clomiphene citrate treatment because they lost body weight in association with anorexia; however, all three were without overt clinical symptoms. While we did not observe any specific indications of toxicity among monkeys receiving the GnRH antagonist or either estrogen replacement therapy regimen, this was not the focus of our attention. The remaining 16 primates were healthy throughout the study.

In summary, these primate models seem useful for the study of some hypoestrogenic sequelae that affect postmenopausal women [35-39]. While the present data are not offered as conclusive evidence, they indicate the potential utility of short-term GnRH-antagonist test to identify individuals likely to excrete calcium more rapidly after ovariectomy, during medical castration (such as GnRH agonist treatment for endometriosis or contraception) or spontaneous menopause. Much more research in both women and the primate model, including longitudinal studies

482

of bone densitometry, is required before our current interpretations can be held valid or rejected.

High-dose clomiphene citrate was nearly as effective as high-dose conjugated equine estrogens for conservation of urinary calcium, especially because clomiphene citrate did not cause endometrial proliferation and withdrawal bleeding after cessation of progesterone therapy. Moreover, we know little of the central nervous system effects of clomiphene citrate, specifically whether it can ameliorate hot flushes [40]. Indeed, clomiphene citrate at lower doses can cause hot flushes in women undergoing ovulation induction [41].

Overall, our findings indicate the worth of extending these primate studies, as well as considering related clinical investigations. Since the postmenopausal years make up an increasing part of womens' lives, improving the quality of this longevity through appropriately selective, safe, and effective estrogen-replacement therapy is among the most significant advances that reproductive medicine can offer to these growing millions of American women .

ACKNOWLEDGMENTS

We thank Ms. Barbara Murphy, Mr. Gregg Bloomquist, Mr. Charles Turner, Mr. Donald Barber and Mr. Adrian Coleman for superb primate husbandry and technical activities. Also, we express our sincere appreciation to Serono Laboratories, Inc., Randolph, MA for the gift of Serophene and to Dr. Marvin Karten of the Contraceptive Development Branch, NICHD, Bethesda, MD for the GnRH antagonist. Thanks, too, for the editorial assistance of Ms. Rose-Marie Bradley Jones.

REFERENCES

1. U.S. Bureau of the Census Current Population Reports, Series P-25, No. 965, Estimates of the Population of the United States, by Age, Sex, Race: 1980-1984, U.S. Government Printing Office, Washington, D.C., March 1985

2. Nordin, B.E.C., Horsman, A., Grilly, R.G., Marshall, D.H., and Simpson, M. Treatment of spinal osteoporosis in postmenopausal women. Brit. Med. J., 280, 5212 (1980)

3. Horsman, A., Nordin, B.E.C., Gallagher, J.C., Kirby, P.A., Milner, R.M., and Simpson, M. Observations of sequential changes in bone mass in postmenopausal women: a controlled trial of oestrogen and calcium therapy. Calcified Tissue Research, 22(supp), 217 (1977).

4. Campbell, S., Whitehead, M. Estrogen therapy and the postmenopausal syndrome. Clin. Obstet. Gynecol., 4, 31 (1977).

5. Geola, F.L., Frumar, A.M., Tataryn, I.V., Lu, K.H., Hershman, J.M., Eggena, P., Sambhi, M.P., Judd, H.L. Biological effects of various doses of conjugated equine estrogens in

postmenopausal women. J. Clin. Endocrinol. Metab., 51, 620 (1980).

6. Kenigsberg, D., Littman, B.A., and Hodgen, G. Medical hypophysectomy: I. Dose-response using a gonadotropin-releasing hormone antagonist. Fertil. Steril., 42, 112 (1984).

7. Kenigsberg, D., Littman, B.A., Williams, R.F., and Hodgen, G.D. Medical hypophysectomy: II. Variability of ovarian response to gonadotropin therapy. Fertil. Steril., 42, 116 (1984).

8. Kenigsberg, D. and Hodgen, G.D. Ovulation Inhibition by Administration of Weekly Gonadotropin-Releasing Hormone Antagonist. J. Clin. Endocrinol. Metab., 62, 734 (1986).

9. Abbasi, R. and Hodgen, G.D. Predicting the Predisposition to Osteoporosis: Gonadotropin-Releasing Hormone Antagonist for Acute Estrogen Deficiency Test. J.A.M.A., 255, 1600 (1986).

10. Yen, S.S.C. Estrogen withdrawal syndrome (editorial). J.A.M.A., 255, 1614 (1986).

11. Mandel, F.P., Geola, F.L., Lu, J.K.H., Eggena, P., Sambhi, M.P., Hershman, J., and Judd, H.L. Biologic effects of various doses of equine estradiol in postmenopausal women. Obstet. Gynecol., 59, 573 (1982).

12. Stern, M.P., Brown, B.W., Haskell, W.L., Farquhar, J.W., Wehrle, C.L., and Wood, P.D.S. Cardiovascular risk and use of estrogens or estrogen-progestagen combinations. J.A.M.A., 235, 811 (1976).

13. Bradley, D.D., Wingard, J., Petitti, D.B., Krauss, R.M., and Ramcharan, S. Serum high-density-lipoprotein cholesterol in women using oral contraceptives, estrogens and progestins. N. Engl. J. Med., 299, 17 (1978).

14. Nachtigall, L.E., Nachtigall, R.H., Nachtigall, R.D., and Beckman, M. Estrogen replacement therapy I: a 10-year prospective study in the relationship to osteoporosis. Obstet. Gynecol., 53, 277 (1979).

15. Hirvonen, E., Malkonen, and M., Manninen, V. Effects of different progestogens on lipoproteins during postmenopausal replacement therapy. N. Engl. J. Med., 304, 560 (1981).

16. Gordon, T., Castelli, W.P., Hjortland, M.C., Kannel, W.B. and Dawber, T.R. High density lipoprotein as a protective factor against coronary heart disease: The Framingham Study. Am. J. Med. 62, 707 (1977).

17. Sturdee, D.W., Wade-Evans, T., Peterson, M.E.L., Thom, M. and Studd, J.W.W. Relations between bleeding pattern, endometrial histology, and oestrogen treatment in menopausal women. Brit. Med. J. 1, 1575 (1978).

18. Gallagher, J.C., Melton, L.J. and Riggs, B.L. Epidemiology of fractures of the proximal femur in Rochester, Minnesota. Clin. Orthop., July-August 163 (1980).

19. Albrecht, B.H., Schiff, I. and Tulchinsky, D. Objective evidence that placebo and oral medroxyprogesterone acetate diminish menopausal vasomotor flushes. Am. J. Obstet. Gynecol., 139, 631 (1981).

20. Hodgen, G.D., Dufau, M.L., Catt, K.J., and Tullner, W.W. Estrogens, progesterone and chorionic gonadotropin in pregnant rhesus monkeys. Endocrinology, 91, 896 (1972).

21. Goodman, A.L., Nixon, W.E., Johnson, D.K., and Hodgen, G.D. Regulation of folliculogenesis in the rhesus monkey: selection of the dominant follicle. Endocrinology, 100, 155 (1977).

22. Hodgen, G.D., Erb, R.E., and Plotka, E.D. Estimating creatinine excretion in sheep. J. Anim. Sci., 26, 586 (1967).

23. Erb, R.E., Tillson, S.A., Hodgen, G.D., and Plotka, E.D. Urinary creatinine as an index compound for estimating rate of excretion of steroids in the domestic sow. J. Anim. Sci., 30, 79 (1970).

24. Goodman, A.L. and Hodgen GD. Post partum patterns of circulating FSH, LH, prolactin, estradiol and progesterone in nonsuckling cynomolgus monkeys. Steroids, 31, 731 (1978).

25. Hodgen, G.D. Surrogate embryo transfer combined with estrogen-progesterone therapy in monkeys. J.A.M.A., 250, 2167 (1983).

26. Freund, J.E., Livermore, P.E., and Miller, I. Manual of Experimental Statistics, A.A. Bennett (Ed.), Prentice-Hall, Inc, Englewood Cliffs, 1960.

27. Hodgen, G.D., Goodman, A.L., O'Connor, A., and Johnson, D.K. Menopause in rhesus monkeys: model for study of disorders in the human climacteric. Am. J. Obstet. Gynecol., 127, 581 (1977).

28. Nordin, B.E.C., Horsman, A. and Brook, R. The relationship between oestrogen status and bone loss in post-menopausal women. Clin. Endocrinol., 5, 353 (1976).

29. Siiteri, D.K., McDonald, P.C. Role of extraglandular estrogen in human endocrinology. In Handbook of Physiology, Section 7 - Endocrinology, RO Greep, E Astwood (Eds), American Physiological Society, Washington, D.C., Vol 2, Part 1, p 615, 1973.

30. Marut, E.L. and Hodgen, G.D. Antiestrogenic action of high-dose clomiphene in primates: pituitary augmentation but with ovarian attenuation. Fertil. Steril. 38, 100 (1982).

31. Clark, J.H. and Markaverich, B.M. The agonistic-antagonistic properties of clomiphene: A review. Pharmacol. Ther., 15, 467 (1982).

32. Clark, J.H. and Guthrie, S.C. Agonistic and antagonistic effects of clomiphene citrate and its isomers. Biol. Reprod., 25, 667 (1981).

33. Kokko, E., Janne, O., Kauppila, A., and Vihko, R. Cyclic clomiphene citrate treatment lowers cytosol estrogen and progestin receptor concentrations in the endometrium of postmenopausal women on estrogen replacement therapy. J. Clin. Endocrinol. Metab., 52, 345 (1981).

34. Mashchak, C.A., Lobo, R.A., Dozono-Takano, R., Eggena, P., Nakamura, R.M., Brenner, P.F., and Mishell, Jr. D.R. Comparison of pharmacodynamic properties of various estrogen formulations. Am. J. Obstet. Gynecol., 144, 511 (1982).

485

35. Lindsay, R., Hart, D.M., Purdie, D., Ferguson, M.M., Clark, A.S., and Kraszewski, A.   Comparative effects of oestrogen and a progestogen on bone loss in postmenopausal women. Clin. Sci. Mol. Med., 54, 193 (1978).

36. Lindsay, R., Aitken, J.M., Anderson, J.B., Hart, D.M., MacDonald, B., and Clarke, A.C.   Long-term prevention of postmenopausal osteoporosis by oestrogen.   Evidence of an increased bone mass after delayed onset of estrogen treatment.   Lancet, I(7968), 1038 (1976).

37. Yen, S.S.C., Martin, P.L., Burnier, A.M., Czekala, N.M., Greaney, Jr., M.O., and Callatine, M.R.   Circulating estradiol, estrone and gonadotropin levels following the administration of orally active 17b-estradiol in postmenopausal women.   J. Clin. Endocrinol. Metab., 40, 518 (1975).

38. Molnar, G.W.   Body temperatures during menopausal hot flashes.   J. Appl. Physiol., 38, 499 (1975).

39. Macgregor, A.H., Johnson, J.E., and Bunde, C.A.   Further clinical experience with clomiphene citrate.   Fertil. Steril., 19, 616 (1968).

SECTION 9

APPLICATIONS IN ANIMALS

32
The Use of LHRH Analogs in Aquaculture

L.W. CRIM[1], R.E. PETER[2] and G. VAN DER KRAAK[2]
[1]Marine Sciences Research Lab., Memorial University
of Newfoundland, St. John's, NFLD, Canada ALC5S7 and
[2]Department of Zoology, University of Alberta, Edmonton,
Alberta, Canada T6G2E9

INTRODUCTION

Our increased dependence on cultured as opposed to wild stocks of fish as a dietary source of protein has necessitated steps to control reproduction of fish as many species fail to ovulate under captive conditions. Some fish species exhibit a protracted breeding season and it is desirable to control the timing and synchrony of breeding to increase the efficiency of aquaculture operations. Historically, fish culturists have relied upon the administration of fish pituitary extracts, or in certain cases mammalian gonadotropin preparations to induce ovulation [1]. More recently, efforts have been made to substitute the use of LHRH peptide hormones for the more expensive pituitary hormone preparations. Since the first demonstration that LHRH stimulates gonadotropin (GtH) release from carp pituitaries in vitro [2], there have been numerous reports showing that LHRH and LHRH analogs stimulate GtH release in a variety of teleosts [3-5]. To date, the use of these compounds to regulate fish reproduction has met with varied success. In recent studies it has been demonstrated that distinct forms of LHRH are present in submammalian vertebrates [6] and these findings have opened new avenues of research investigating the use of fish, bird and mammalian LHRH analogs for the hormonal control of reproduction of fish in aquaculture [7-8].

The following sections review by fish family recent studies of various types of LHRH and LHRH analogs testing the effectiveness of these peptide hormones in promoting release of GtH and inducing spawning in laboratory fish or commercially valuable fish species of aquaculture interest.

LHRH STUDIES IN FISH

Family Cyprinidae

Ovulation in goldfish, Carassius auratus, and common carp, Cyprinus carpio, is normally induced by a surge in the blood levels of GtH in response to environmental factors including primarily the presence of floating vegetation, warm temperatures and the daily photoperiod

[9-11].

Farmed cyprinid fish generally have to be artificially induced to spawn because appropriate environmental cues to trigger ovulation are often absent. Although claims were made that injections of [D-Ala^6,Pro^9-NHEt]LHRH alone could induce a high rate of ovulation in grass carp, Ctenopharyngodon idellus, black carp, Mylopharyngodon piceus, silver carp, Hypophthalmichthys molitrix and spotted silver carp, (bighead carp) Aristichthys nobilis [12-14], this was not confirmed in more recent studies on goldfish [15-19], common carp [11,20-23], and mud carp, Cirrhinus molitorella [23]. However, injection of [D-Ala^6,Pro^9-NHEt]LHRH was found to be effective in inducing a high rate of ovulation in the Indian major carp Cirrhina mrigala (Ham) [24] and the bream, Parabramis pekinensis, although the ovulatory response was delayed to 24 hours post-injection [11]. Also, both [D-Ala^6,Pro^9-NHEt]LHRH and [D-Tle^6,Pro^9-NHEt]LHRH were found to be effective analogs for inducing ovulation in the Tench (Tinca tinca L.), although the ovulatory response was delayed 27-51 hours following injection [25].

Studies in goldfish indicate that dopamine acts in a dose dependent manner directly on pituitary gonadotropes as a GtH release-inhibitory factor to modulate both spontaneous secretion and [D-Ala^6,Pro^9-NHEt]LHRH induced release of GtH [15-19,26-29]. Combination treatment of preovulatory goldfish with the dopamine receptor antagonist, pimozide and [D-Ala^6,Pro^9-NHEt]LHRH is a highly effective method of inducing ovulation within 13-16 hours following injection [15-19, R. Peter, M. Sokolowska, C. Nahorniak, unpublished]. Similar findings on augmenting GtH release in the goldfish were found with other dopamine receptor antagonists including metaclopramid, haloperidol, spiperone and domperidone [16,29].

In a study of the structure-activity relationships of different types of gonadotropin releasing hormones applied to goldfish, [D-Arg^6,Trp^7,Leu^8,Pro^9-NHEt]LHRH (an analog of salmon LHRH), was found to be more potent in stimulating GtH release in vivo than [D-Ala^6,Pro^9-NHEt]LHRH [7]. Intraperitoneal injection of 10 ug/kg [D-Arg^6,Trp^7,Leu^8,Pro^9-NHEt]LHRH and 10 mg/kg pimozide was as effective in inducing ovulation as 100 ug/kg of [D-Ala^6,Pro^9-NHEt] LHRH combined with the pimozide treatment (R. Peter, M. Sokolowska, C. Nahorniak, unpublished). The LHRH analogs, [D-Ser(tBu)^6,Pro^9-NHEt]LHRH (buserelin), [D-Trp^6,Trp^7,Leu^8,Pro^9-NHEt]LHRH, and [His^3, D-Arg^6,Trp^7,Tyr^8]LHRH (an analog of chicken II LHRH) are also highly potent stimulators of GtH release in the goldfish (R. Peter et al., unpublished results cited in [30]) and may be useful for inducing ovulation in goldfish and other cyprinids. It is clear from these studies that the specificity of pituitary gonadotropin-releasing hormone receptors in the goldfish differs from that in mammals and further structure-activity studies on LHRH peptides in teleosts are warranted.

Treatment of common carp with 50 ug/kg [D-Trp^6,Pro^9-NHEt]LHRH increased circulating levels of GtH and oocyte maturation; this LHRH analog combined with 10 mg/kg pimozide induced ovulation in 57% of test females, the balance showing only oocyte maturation [21]. Studies by Lin et al. [11,23] showed that the combination of 10 mg/kg pimozide with 100 ug/kg [D-Ala^6,Pro^9-NHEt]LHRH also induces ovulation in common carp. Reserpine, a drug depleting brain cate-

cholamines, also potentiated the GtH-releasing action of [D-Ala[6],
Pro[9]-NHEt]LHRH; ovulation followed within 12-16 hours. The effectiveness of pimozide and [D-Ala[6],Pro[9]-NHEt]LHRH in stimulating GtH
release and ovulation was shown to be temperature dependent with no
ovulation obtained below 20°C in spite of apparent GtH release.
Simultaneous injection of [D-Ala[6],Pro[9]-NHEt]LHRH and pimozide was
as effective as giving the injections 3 or 6 hours apart thus allowing the fish to be handled only once for administration of drugs to
induce ovulation. The usefulness of pimozide and [D-Ala[6],Pro[9]-NHEt]
LHRH or [D-Arg[6],Trp[7],Leu[8],Pro[9]-NHEt]LHRH for inducing ovulation of
the common carp on Polish fish farms has been demonstrated (K.
Bieniarz, P. Epler, M. Sokolowska, R. Billard and R. Peter, unpublished results).

The combination of pimozide and [D-Ala[6],Pro[9]-NHEt]LHRH induced
ovulation of fertile and viable oocytes in bream and silver carp
within 8 and 12-16 hours, respectively [11,23]. Preliminary tests
with grass carp and bighead carp gave similar positive results. In
mud carp pimozide treatment plus a pair of [D-Ala[6],Pro[9]-NHEt]LHRH
injections were required to achieve a high rate of ovulation[23]; to
date this is the only cyprinid species where such extensive drug/
hormone therapy is needed for inducing spawning.

Family Salmonidae

Many varieties of salmon and trout have been shown to respond to
LHRH treatment. For example, coho salmon, Onchorhynchus kisutch,
were first primed with salmon gonadotropic hormone and then ovulation induced with either [D-Ala[6],Pro[9]-NHEt]LHRH or [D-Ser(tBu)[6],
Pro[9]-NHEt]LHRH [31]. Double injections of 20 ug/kg [D-Ala[6],Pro[9]-
NHEt]LHRH given on days 0 and 3 induced ovulation in female coho
salmon [32]. In landlocked Atlantic salmon, Salmo salar, ovulation
of females and increased milt collection from mature males was
achieved by intraperitoneal implantion of a single compacted cholesterol pellet containing [D-Trp[6],Pro[9]-NHEt]LHRH [33]. This study
also demonstrated that a prolonged stimulation of gonadotropic
hormone release (at least 4 wk) resulted from treatment with a
sustained-release type of formulation containing LHRH analog. The
successful induction of ovulation of trout, Salmo gairdneri [34] and
Atlantic salmon [33,35,36] using the pelleted LHRH analog was
perhaps expected since a relatively extended GtH release profile had
been noted in the ovulating female trout [37]. In a separate study
of the onset of spermiation in male landlocked salmon [38], it was
demonstrated that LHRH analogs were effective when administered
either by acute injection or by chronic implantation.

A practical application of LHRH analog treatment of salmonid
fish in aquaculture operations is to advance the spawning of coho
salmon broodstock, which reduces prespawning mortality and correspondingly increases egg take [39,40]. In a Newfoundland strain of
rainbow trout, implantation of [D-Trp[6],Pro[9]-NHEt]LHRH accelerated
ovulation under the cold-winter holding conditions [34]. An earlier
production of offspring in April has the advantage of allowing young
fish a longer growing season at increasing spring and summer temperatures. LHRH analogs also can be used to synchronize the normally

protracted breeding season of captive Atlantic salmon [35,36] and the rainbow trout [41] with consequent decreases in the costs of fish handling. Growth of the gonads in female Atlantic salmon may be stimulated with slow-release implants of [D-Nal(2)^6]LHRH [36], but the degree of long-term LHRH stimulation must be carefully controlled since the inadvertent induction of premature ovulation leads to spawning of eggs of extremely poor quality [35].

Optimizing the hormonal induction of spawning in the salmonid fishes will require additional work. For example, several LHRH analogs, including [D-Ala^6,Pro^9-NHEt]LHRH, [D-Nal(2)^6,Pro^9-NHEt]LHRH, [D-Nal(2)^6,Pro^9-Aza-Gly]LHRH and [D-Arg^6,Trp^7,Leu^8,Pro^9-NHEt]LHRH, have super agonist activity on release of GtH in the rainbow trout [8, L. Crim, J. Nestor, Jr., C. Wilson, unpublished]. The combination treatment of [D-Ala^6,Pro^9-NHEt]LHRH analog with pimozide was tested in the rainbow trout [41] and coho salmon [42] but a weak potentiation of LHRH analog mediated GtH release in these fish was obtained compared with the results (above) obtained with cyprinid fishes. The economical advantages of inducing spawning with LHRH analog would appear to be obvious since the cost per fish for LHRH analog induced ovulation in the coho salmon was reported to be $0.03 for [D-Ala^6,Pro^9-NHEt]LHRH compared with >$4.00 in the case of treatment with a commercial preparation of pituitary hormone (43).

Family Chanidae

The industry for milkfish, <u>Chanos</u> <u>chanos</u>, the most widely aquacultured foodfish in Southeast Asia, is completely dependent upon the inshore collection of young milkfish fry due to the scarcity of wild spawners. Spontaneous gonad maturation and spawning of pen-reared milkfish in the Philippines was reported [44] but egg collections from the brookstock held in sea cages is particularly difficult due to heavy predation of freshly spawned eggs or simply inefficient egg recovery. In an attempt to solve these problems a few mature milkfish have been captured from the sea and quickly transported to the laboratory for induced spawning with gonadotropic hormone treatment. A few cases of successful ovulation were recorded, but the fish are easily stressed and estimating the best time for egg stripping is difficult usually resulting in low egg fertility [45]. For more dependable supplies of milkfish, rearing of captive milkfish to the broodstock stage and artificial induction of spawning would be necessary.

In recent studies in Hawaii, milkfish broodstock were matured prior to the normal breeding season with monthly implantations of single cholesterol pellets containing 200 ug [D-Ala^6,Pro^9-NHEt]LHRH [46]. Previous studies had shown that testosterone treatment of juvenile rainbow trout increased pituitary gonadotropin levels [47] and the rate of maturation and repeat spawning of milkfish was improved when the LHRH analog administration was combined with 17α-methyl-testosterone supplied via silastic capsules [46]. Spawning took place in relatively small laboratory breeding tanks where eggs could be efficiently collected. Induction of spawning of sea-pen reared milkfish was also obtained recently in the Philippines [48]. Oocyte size in the broodstock was routinely checked by aspiration of eggs from the cannulated oviducts of anesthetized milkfish and once the eggs reached 0.6 mm, females were treated with [D-Ala^6,Pro^9-NHEt]LHRH or they received the fish LHRH analog, [D-Ala^6,Trp^7, Leu^8, Pro^9-NHEt]LHRH administered IP via osmotic pump, cholesterol pellet or as a single injection. Male milkfish were injected with LHRH analog and the ripe males and females were returned to their sea-cage for natural spawning and egg fertilization. In one such trial 700,000 eggs were collected with a fertilization rate of 25 percent.

In addition to promoting the maturation and spawning of milk-fish, LHRH analogs appeared to reduce oocyte atresia since heavy oocyte regression, commonly observed following the handling of maturing female milkfish during the breeding season, did not occur. Clearly, LHRH analog treatment is effective for inducing ovulation of fully ripe female milkfish and it also appears useful for priming the males for spawning.

Families Siganidae and Serranidae

The rabbitfish, Siganus guttatus, and the seabass, Lates calcarifer, are tropical fish species of commerical interest in Southeast Asia. Pituitary hormone preparations have been used in past attempts to induce these species to spawn and recently LHRH analog treatment was utilized [49]. In the rabbitfish, spawning, which usually occurs in relation to lunar rhythms, was accelerated by implantation of pelleted [D-Nal(2)^6]LHRH. The seabass ordinarily spawns spontan-eously in July or August but spawning in captivity was induced as early as May with implants of either [D-Trp^6,Pro^9-NHEt]LHRH or [D-hArg(Et$_2$)^6,Pro^9-NHEt]LHRH and up to 2.6 million hatchings were collected.

Family Cobitididae

Due to its commercial significance in the market place, the loach, Paramisgurnus dabryanus, is becoming a popular fish for aquaculture in China. A low ovulation rate (0-20%) usually occurs in response to injection of 10-50 ug/kg [D-Ala^6,Pro^9-NHEt]LHRH alone [50]. However, the ovulation rate in fish held at warm temperatures can approach 100% when this LHRH analog is combined with 0.5 or 1.0 mg/kg pimozide [50]. Reserpine, α-methyl-para-tyrosine or carbidopa (drugs which block synthesis of norepinephrine) potentiated GtH release induced by [D-Ala^6,Pro^9-NHEt]LHRH in the loach and this combination was highly effective in inducing ovulation [11,51].

Family Clariidae

The African catfish, Clarias gariepinus is popular in western Europe. This fish must be induced to ovulate under captive condi-tions and treatment with [D-Ala^6,Pro^9-NHEt]LHRH is effective [52, 53]. Again, pimozide potentiates the GtH releasing action of [D-Ala^6,Pro^9-NHEt]LHRH and the combination, at doses of 50 ug/kg and 5 mg/kg, respectively can induce ovulation rates of more than 80%

resulting in fertile and viable oocytes [52].

Family Percidae

The walleye, Stizostedion vitrium, is a sport fish of interest in North American temperate lakes and in some regions aquaculture and stocking of young fish has been undertaken to prevent depletion of the declining fish populations. It was found that treatment with human chorionic gonadotropin, [D-Ala^6,Pro^9-NHEt]LHRH, pimozide alone or pimozide plus [D-Ala ^{6},Pro ^{9}-NHEt]LHRH analog were all equally effective in inducing oocyte maturation and ovulation in this species [54].

CONCLUDING REMARKS

LHRH analogs are effective agents for regulating spawning of several species of fish of commercial interest. The discovery and synthesis of new forms of LHRHs (e.g., fish and bird types) and their analogs has increased the number of LHRH analogs potentially available for use in aquaculture. From the work to date it is clear that several types of LHRH analogs have superactive biological properties and can be used to induce the spawning of captive fishes. For some kinds of fish, LHRH analog combined with pimozide seems to be the most effective treatment regime. In other cases, however, simple injection(s) of LHRH analog alone is sufficient to induce spawning but slow-release formulations can also prove valuable where longer-term LHRH treatment (days or weeks) is required (e.g., stimulation of gonadal development). It is likely that as LHRH protocols are optimized and proven to be reliable, their cost effectiveness will be improved and LHRH analogs may replace pituitary hormone preparations for induction of spawning of farmed fish under aquaculture conditions.

ACKNOWLEDGEMENT

This research has been supported by grants from the Natural Sciences and Engineering Research Council of Canada and the International Development Research Centre to LWC and REP. MSRL Contribution No. 668.

REFERENCES

1. Donaldson, E.M. and Hunter, G.A. Induced final maturation, ovulation and spermiation in cultured fish. In "Fish Physiology", Vol. IXB, W.S. Hoar, D.J. Randall and E.M. Donaldson (Eds.), Academic Press, New York, 1983, p. 351.
2. Breton, B., Weil, C., Jalabert, B. and Billard, R. Activite reciproque des facteurs hypothalamiques de belier (Ovis aries) et de poissons teleosteen sur la secretion in vitro des hormones gonadotropes G-HG et LH respectivement par les

hypophyses de carpe et de belier. C.R. Acad. Sci. Ser. D., 274, 2530 (1972).

3. Crim, L.W. Actions of LHRH and its analogs in lower verte-brates. In "LHRH and Its Analogs: Contraceptive and Thera-peutic Applications", B.H. Vickery, J.J. Nestor Jr. and E.S.E. Hafez (Eds.), MTP Press Ltd., Lancaster, 1984, p. 377.

4. Peter, R.E. Evolution of neurohormonal regulation of repro-duction in lower vertebrates. Amer. Zool., 23, 685 (1983).

5. Peter, R.E. The brain and neurohormones in teleost reproduc-tion. In "Fish Physiology", Vol. IXA, W.S. Hoar, D.J. Randall and E.M. Donaldson (Eds.), Academic Press, New York, 1983, p. 97.

6. Sherwood, N.M. Evolution of a neuropeptide family: Gonado-tropin-releasing hormone. Amer. Zool. (In Press).

7. Peter, R.E., Nahorniak, C.S., Sokolowska, M., Chang, J.P., Rivier, J.E., Vale, W.W., King, J.A. and Millar, R.P. Structure-activity relationships of mammalian, chicken, and salmon gonadotropin releasing hormones in vivo in goldfish. Gen. Comp. Endocrinol., 58, 231 (1985).

8. Crim, L.W. A variety of synthetic LHRH peptides stimulate gonadotropic hormone secretion in rainbow trout and the land-locked Atlantic salmon. In "The Journal of Steroid Biochemistry 20, 1390. Abstract A51 (1984).

9. Stacey, N.E., Cook, A.F. and Peter, R.E. Ovulatory surge of gonadotropin in the goldfish, Carassius auratus. Gen. Comp. Endocrinol., 37, 246 (1979).

10. Stacey, N.E., Cook, A.F. and Peter, R.E. Spontaneous and gonadotropin-induced ovulation in the goldfish, Carassius auratus L.: Effects of external factors. J. Fish. Biol. 15, 349 (1979).

11. Lin, H.R., Van Der Kraak, G., Liang, J.Y., Peng, C., Li, G.Y., Lu, L.Z., Zhou, X.J., Chang, M.L. and Peter, R.E. The effects of LHRH analogue and drugs which block the effects of dopamine on gonadotropin secretion and ovulation in fish cultured in China. In "Proceedings of the International Symposium on the Aquaculture of Carp and Related Species", R. Billard (Ed.), I.N.R.A. Publications, Versailles, France, 1986 (in press).

12. Anon (Cooperative Team for Hormonal Application in Piscicul-ture). A new highly effective ovulating agent for fish repro-duction. Practical application of LH-RH analogue for the in-duction of spawning of farm fishes. Sci. Sinica., 20, 469 (1977).

13. Fukien-Kiangsu-Chekiang-Shanghai Cooperative Group. A further investigation on the stimulatory effect of a synthetic analogue of hypothalamic luteinizing hormone releasing hormone (LRH-A) on spawning in "domestic fishes". Acta Biochim. Biophys. Sin., 9, 15 (1977).

14. Jiang, R., Huang, S. and Zhao, W. Changes of serum gonado-tropin levels before and behind induced spawning in grass carp and silver carp. J. Fish. China, 4, 129 (1980).

15. Chang, J.P. and Peter, R.E. Effects of pimozide and des Gly[10], [D-Ala[6]] luteinizing hormone-releasing hormone ethylamide on serum gonadotropin concentrations, germinal vesicle migration, and ovulation in female goldfish, Carassius

auratus. Gen. Comp. Endocrinol., 52, 30 (1983).

16. Chang, J.P., Peter, R.E., Nahorniak, C.S. and Sokolowska, M. Effects of catecholaminergic agonists and antagonists on serum gonadotropin concentrations and ovulation in goldfish: Evidence for specificity of dopamine inhibition of gonadotropin secretion. Gen. Comp. Endocrinol., 55, 351 (1984).

17. Sokolowska, M., Peter, R.E., Nahorniak, C.S., Pan, C.H., Chang, J.P., Crim, L.W. and Weil, C. Induction of ovulation in goldfish, Carassius auratus, by pimozide and analogues of LH-RH. Aquaculture, 36, 71 (1984).

18. Sokolowska, M., Peter, R.E., Nahorniak, C.S. and Chang, J.P. Seasonal effects of pimozide and des Gly^{10} [D-Ala^6] LH-RH ethylamide on gonadotropin secretion in goldfish. Gen. Comp. Endocrinol., 57, 472 (1985).

19. Sokolowska, M., Peter, R.E. and Nahorniak, C.S. The effects of different doses of pimozide and [D-Ala^6,Pro^9-N ethylamide]-LHRH (LHRH-A) on gonadotropin release and ovulation in female goldfish. Can. J. Zool., 63, 1252 (1985).

20. Weil, C., Fostier, A., Horvath, L., Marlot, S. and Berscenyi, M. Profiles of plasma gonadotropin and 17β-estradiol in the common carp, Cyprinus carpio L., as related to spawning induced by hypophysation or LH-RH treatment. Reprod. Nutr. Dev., 20, 1041 (1980).

21. Billard, R., Alagarswami, K., Peter, R.E. and Breton, B. Potentialisation par le pimozide des effets du LHRH-A sur la secretion gonadotrope hypohysaire, l'ovulation et la spermiation chez la Carpe commune (Cyprinus carpio). C.R. Acad. Sci. Paris, Serie III, 296, 181 (1983).

22. Billard, R., Bieniarz, K., Peter, R.E., Sokolowska, M., Weil, C. and Crim, L.W. Effects of LHRH and LHRH-A on plasma GtH levels and maturation/ovulation in the common carp, Cyprinus carpio, kept under various environmental conditions. Aquaculture, 41, 245 (1984).

23. Lin, H.R., Liang, J.Y., Peng, C., Li, G.Y., Liu, L.Z., Zhou, X.J., Chang, M.L., Van Der Kraak, G. and Peter, R.E. Pimozide and reserpine potentiate the effects of LHRH-A on gonadotropin secretion and ovulation in cultivated fishes in China. In "Proceedings of the Asian Symposium on Freshwater Fish Culture", China Society of Fisheries. The Academic Publisher of China, Beijing, P.R. China (1986).

24. Kaul, M. and Rishi, K.K. Induced spawning of the indian major carp, Cirrhina mrigala (Ham.), with LHRH analogue or pimozide. Aquaculture 54, 45 (1986).

25. Kouril, J., Dart, T., Hamackova, J. and Flegel, M. Induced ovulation in tench (Tinca tinca L.) by various LHRH synthetic analogues: effect of site of administration and temperature. Aquaculture 54, 37 (1986).

26. Chang, J.P. and Peter, R.E. Effects of dopamine on gonadotropin release in female goldfish, Carassius auratus. Neuroendocrinology, 36, 351 (1983).

27. Chang, J.P., Peter, R.E. and Crim, L.W. Effects of dopamine and apomorphine on gonadotropin release from the transplanted pars distalis in goldfish. Gen. Comp. Endocrinol., 55, 347 (1984).

28. Chang, J.P., MacKenzie, D.S., Gould, D.R. and Peter, R.E. Effects of dopamine and norepinephrine on in vitro spontaneous and gonadotropin-releasing hormone-induced gonadotropin release by dispersed cells or fragments of the goldfish pituitary. Life Sci., 35, 2027 (1984).

29. Peter, R.E., Chang, J.P., Nahorniak, C.S., Omeljaniuk, R.J., Sokolowska, M., Shih, S.H. and Billard, R. Interactions of catecholamines and GnRH in regulation of gonadotropin secretion in teleost fish. Rec. Progr. Horm. Res., 42, 513 (1986).

30. Peter, R.E. Structure-activity studies on gonadotropin-releasing hormone in teleosts, amphibians, reptiles, birds and mammals. In "Comparative Endocrinology: Developments and Directions", C.L. Ralph (Ed.), Alan R. Liss, New York, 1986, p. 75.

31. Donaldson, E.M., Hunter, G.A., Van Der Kraak, G. and Dye, H.M. Application of LH-RH and LH-RH analogues to the induced final maturation and ovulation of coho salmon (Oncorhynchus kisutch). In "Proceedings of the International Symposium on Reproductive Physiology of Fish", C.J.J. Richter and H.J.Th. Goos (Eds.), Pudoc, Wageningen, The Netherlands, 1982, pp. 177-180.

32. Van Der Kraak, G., Dye, H.M., Donaldson, E.M. and Hunter, G.A. Plasma gonadotropin, 17β-estradiol and 17β 20α dihydroxy-4-pregnen-3-one levels during luteinizing hormone releasing hormone analogue and gonadotropin induced ovulation in coho salmon (Oncorhynchus kisutch). Can. J. Zool., 63, 824 (1985).

33. Crim, L.W., Evans, D.M. and Vickery, B.H. Manipulation of the seasonal reproductive cycle of the landlocked Atlantic salmon (Salmo salar) by LHRH analogues administered at various stages of gonadal development. Can. J. Fish. Aquat. Sci., 40, 61 (1983).

34. Crim, L.W., Sutterlin, A.M., Evans, D.M. and Weil, C. Accelerated ovulation by pelleted LHRH analogue treatment of spring-spawning rainbow trout (Salmo gairdneri) held at low temperature. Aquaculture, 35, 299 (1983).

35. Crim, L.W. and Glebe, B.D. Advancement and synchrony of ovulation in Atlantic salmon with pelleted LHRH analog. Aquaculture, 43, 47 (1984).

36. Crim, L.W., Glebe, B.D. and Scott, A.P. The influence of LHRH analog on oocyte development and spawning in female Atlantic salmon, Salmo salar. Aquaculture (in press).

37. Scott, A.P., Sumpter, J.P. and Hardiman, P.A. Hormone changes during ovulation in the rainbow trout (Salmo gairdneri Richardson). Gen. Comp. Endocrinol., 49, 128 (1983).

38. Weil, C. and Crim, L.W. Administration of LHRH analogues in various ways: effect on the advancement of spermiation in pre-spawning landlocked salmon, Salmo salar. Aquaculture, 35, 103 (1983).

39. Fitzpatrick, M.S., Suzumoto, B.K. and Schreck, C.B. Luteinizing hormone-releasing hormone analogue induces precocious ovulation in adult coho salmon (Oncorhynchus kisutch). Aquaculture, 43, 67 (1984).

40. Sower, S.A., Iwamoto, R.N., Dickhoff, W.W. and Gorbman, A. Ovulatory and steroidal responses in coho salmon and steelhead trout following administration of salmon gonadotropin and

D-Ala ^{6}, des Gly ^{10} gonadotropin-releasing hormone ethylamide (GnRHa). Aquaculture, 43, 35 (1984).

41. Billard, R., Reinaud, P., Hollenbecq, M.G. and Breton, B. Advancement and synchronisation of spawning in Salmo gairdneri and S. trutta following administration of LRH-A combined or not with pimozide. Aquaculture, 43, 57 (1984).

42. Van Der Kraak, G., Donaldson, E.M. and Chang, J.P. Dopamine involvement in the regulation of gonadotropin secretion in coho salmon. Can. J. Zool. 64, 1245 (1986).

43. Schreck, C.B. and Fitzpatrick, M. Induced maturation in salmon. In "Research Information Bulletin" No. 83-51, U.S. Fish & Wildlife Service.

44. Lacanilao, F. and Marte, C.L. Sexual maturation of milkfish in floating cages. Asian Aquaculture, 3, 4 (1980).

45. Kuo, C-M. A review of induced breeding of milkfish. In "Reproduction and Culture of Milkfish", C-S. Lee and I-C. Liao (Eds.), Published by The Oceanic Institute and Tungkang Marine Laboratory, Hawaii, 1985, p. 57.

46. Lee, C.-S., Tamaru, C.S., Banno, J.E., Kelley, C.D., Bocek, A. and Wyban, J.A. Induced maturation and spawning of milkfish, Chanos chanos Forsskal, by hormone implantation. Aquaculture, 52, 199 (1986).

47. Crim, L.W. and Evans, D.M. The influence of testosterone and/ or LHRH analogue on precocious sexual development in the juvenile rainbow trout. Biol. Reprod. 29, 137 (1983).

48. Marte, C.L., Sherwood, N.M., Crim, L.W. and Harvey, B. Induced spawning of maturing milkfish (Chanos chanos, Forskal) with gonadotropin-releasing hormone (GnRH) analogues administered in various ways. Aquaculture (in press).

49. Harvey, B., Nacario, J., Crim, L.W., Juario, J.V. and Marte, C.L. Induced spawning of sea bass, Lates calcarifer and rabbitfish, Siganus guttatus after implantation of pelleted LHRH analogue. Aquaculture, 47, 53 (1985).

50. Lin, H.R., Peng, C., Lu, L.Z., Zhou, X.J., Van Der Kraak, G. and Peter, R.E. Induction of ovulation in the loach (Paramisgurnus dabryanus) using pimozide and [D-Ala^6,Pro^9- N-ethylamide]-LHRH. Aquaculture, 46, 333 (1985).

51. Lin, H.R., Peng, C., Van Der Kraak, G., Peter, R.E. and Breton, B. Effects of [D-Ala^6,Pro^9-NHEt]LHRH and catecholaminergic drugs on gonadotropin secretion and ovulation in the Chinese loach (Paramisgurnus dabryanus). Gen. Comp. Endocrinol. (in press).

52. De Leeuw, R., Goos, H.J.Th., Richter, C.J.J. and Edig, E.H. Pimozide-LHRHa-induced breeding of the African catfish, Clarias gasiepinus (Burchell). Aquaculture, 44, 295 (1985).

53. De Leeuw, R., Resink, J.W., Rooyakkers, E.J.M. and Goos, H.J.Th. Pimozide modulates the luteinizing hormone-releasing hormone effect on gonadotropin release in the African catfish, Clarias lazera. Gen. Comp. Endocrinol., 58, 120 (1985).

54. Pankhurst, N.W., Van Der Kraak, G. and Peter, R.E. Effects of human chorionic gonadotropin, Des-Gly^{10} (D-Ala^6) LHRH- ethylamide and pimozide on oocyte final maturation, ovulation and levels of plasma sex steroids in the walleye (Stizostedion vitreum). Fish Physiol. Biochem., 1, 45 (1986).

33
Uses of LHRH and its Analogs in Cattle

H. A. GARVERICK* and J. S. STEVENSON**

*Department of Dairy Science, 111 Animal Sciences Center, University
of Missouri-Columbia, Columbia, MO 65211; ** Department of
Animal Sciences and Ind., Call Hall, Kansas State University,
Manhattan, KS 66506, USA

INTRODUCTION

Use of LHRH and its analogs in studies with human and laboratory
animals has encompassed antifertility (contraceptive) as well as
studies to increase fertility. In domestic farm species, however,
the overwhelming majority of studies have investigated regimens
designed to improve fertility and management of reproduction.
Reproductive failure and/or inefficiency result in significant
economic loss to livestock producers. The net result is fewer
animal products produced at increased cost to consumers.

In cattle, it is most economical for cows to calve every 12 to
13 months because more efficient production of milk is obtained
from dairy cows, and more meat from beef cows. In addition, calves
will be born at a similar time each year when environmental conditions might be favorable, and treatment regimens for improving
fertility can be concentrated into short segments of intensive
management during the year. Thus, use of therapeutic treatments
can be maximized while labor requirements are reduced. In other
livestock species, goals are to have swine farrow at least twice
annually and sheep produce three lamb crops in two years.

To achieve these goals in domestic farm species, cyclic
ovarian activity and pregnancy must be reestablished following a
variable postpartum period of anestrus. Cows must conceive within
90 days following parturition to achieve an annual calving interval. Often ovarian activity has not been reestablished by this
time, abnormal follicular growth has occurred, or fertility is not
optimal. Most of the studies in cattle with LHRH have addressed
these problems. Specific areas of interest have been: 1) inducing ovarian cycles in postpartum cows; 2) decreasing abnormal
ovarian cycles; 3)increasing fertility of subfertile cows, including therapeutic effects at breeding; and 4) treatment of abnormal
follicular structures (ovarian follicular cysts). These and other
areas are discussed later in this chapter. Possible applications
in other species include inducting follicular growth and ovulation
in lactational anestrous sows [1] and in seasonally anestrous ewes
[2,3]. Use of LHRH and its analogs in domestic farm animals for
profertility as well as antifertility therapy have been reviewed
recently [4]. However, neither LHRH nor its analogs have been
approved   for   therapeutic   use   in   pigs   or   sheep.

499

Most studies have investigated the effect of LHRH on pituitary release of gonadotropins during various reproductive states. In particular, LHRH-induced LH release is reduced following parturition and increases as the time postpartum increases [5,6]. Recently, LHRH-like compounds and receptors have been found in the ovaries of some species [7]. However, LHRH receptors do not appear to be present in ovine, bovine and porcine ovaries [8].

THERAPEUTIC APPLICATIONS

Ovarian follicular cysts

Ovarian cysts are anovulatory structures that occur spontaneously in a variety of mammalian species [9], and occur primarily in dairy cattle with an incidence of 6 to 30 percent [10]. Cows are generally infertile as long as the condition persists. In cattle, ovarian cysts are commonly defined as follicular structures of 2.5 cm in diameter or larger (normal Graafian follicle = 2 cm) that persist for at least 10 days in the absence of a corpus luteum. Whether the follicular cyst persists or is replaced by another has been questioned recently [11]. However, the condition usually persists for an extended period of time. Whereas ovarian follicular cysts in cattle and in women are anovulatory and have several similar characteristics, one major difference is that production of testosterone is not elevated in cattle [12] as observed in women [13,14]. Although there is voluminous literature concerning ovarian cysts in cattle, etiology of the condition remains obscure. Reviews addressing aspects of ovarian follicular cysts in cattle have been published [9,10,15,16].

If left untreated, approximately 20% of cows with ovarian cysts spontaneously resume cyclic ovarian function [17]. Many treatments have been attempted over the years, including bacteriostatic agents, different dietary regimens and various types of exercise. The earliest successful treatments for ovarian follicular cysts utilized crude pituitary extracts with high LH content. In later years, human chorionic gonadotropin was used with success rates of 65–80% [10].

Following elucidation of the structure for LHRH from porcine [18] and ovine [19] sources and its chemical synthesis [20], studies were initiated to determine: 1) if LHRH would elicit a surge of LH in cows with ovarian follicular cysts, and 2) if the ovaries of cows with ovarian follicular cysts responded to the LHRH-induced LH release. Subsequently, LHRH was shown to be an effective treatment for the condition [17,21-26] and an LH surge was induced by LHRH [21,22] (Fig. 1). Peak concentrations of LH in plasma were similar to those observed during the pre-ovulatory surge, although the duration was shorter. The ovary responded in approximately 80% of the cows when an optimal dose of LHRH was used [17,23,25] (Table 1). Estrus and ovulation occurred in most cases 18 to 23 days after treatment with LHRH. This interval can be reduced to 12 days by administering a luteolytic dose of prostaglandin $F_2\alpha$ ($PGF_2\alpha$) 9 days after LHRH [26]. Response to

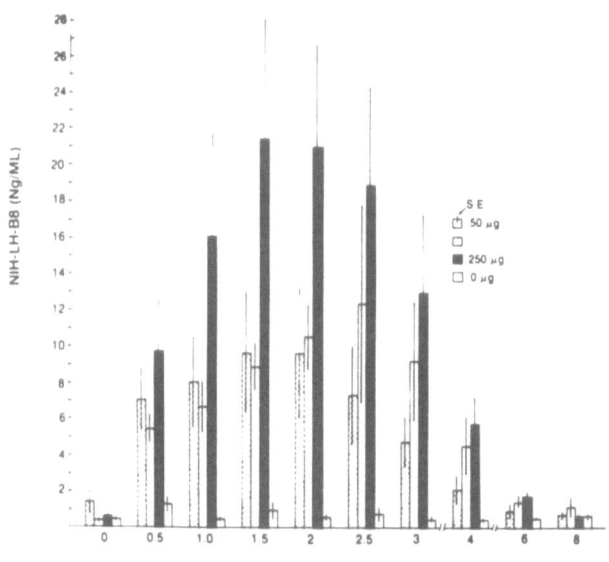

FIGURE 1.   Plasma LH concentrations in cows with ovarian cysts
following treatment (0 to 8 hr) with GnRH
[Reproduced from Cantley, T.C., Garverick, H.A.,
Bierschwal, C.J., Martin, C.E. and Youngquist, R.S.
J. Anim. Sci., 41, 1666 (1975), with permission].

treatment generally was characterized by the cyst decreasing in
size and becoming firmer over the subsequent 5 to 15-day period
[17,27].   In cows responding to treatment, concentrations of
progesterone in plasma increase and remain elevated until days 18
or 19 following treatment when luteolysis, follicular growth and
ovulation (day 21) occur.   However, ovulation of the ovarian
follicular cyst may occur when higher doses (0.5 to 1.5 mg) of LHRH
are administered [28,29].   Pituitary and ovarian responses of cows
with ovarian follicular cysts to analogs of LHRH appear to be
similar to those obtained with LHRH [30,31].

Use with artificial insemination

Conception rates for lactating dairy cows inseminated artificially
(AI) generally range from 40 to 60%.   With these levels of fertility, only 16 to 32% of cows will require more than two inseminations before conception occurs.   Administering LHRH immediately
following AI in dairy cattle has improved rates of conception at
first service in most [32-35], but not all studies [36] (Table 2).

Table 1. Subsequent fertility of cows with ovarian cysts responding to LHRH therapy [Reproduced from Bierschwal, C.J., Garverick, H.A., Martin, C.E., Youngquist, R.S., Cantley, T.C. and Brown, M.D. J. Anim. Sci., 41, 1660 (1975), with permission].

| Item | LHRH treatment group, μg | | | |
	0	50	100	250
No. of cows	28	28	28	30
No. of cows responding to treatment	6	18	23	23
Interval from treatment to first estrus, days[a]	24 ± 4	23 ± 4	22 ± 3	22 ± 3
Total no. conceived	4	13	20	17
Days treatment to conception[a]	45 ± 12	50 ± 7	43 ± 9	59 ± 9
No. conceiving first service	2	7	10	7
No. breedings/ conception[a]	1.5 ± .3	1.6 ± .3	1.6 ± .3	1.9 ± .3

[a]Mean ± SE.

Treating cows with LHRH at first service was most effective for cows in their first or third lactation, those who were treated 100 or more days postpartum, and those producing 26 to 30 kg milk per day [34]. An increase in first-service conception was not observed when LHRH was given at AI when first postpartum ovulations were induced by earlier LHRH treatment [35]. Success of second services was not improved by LHRH injections [36,37].

Apparently normal cows that have failed to conceive to at least two previous services are often referred to as repeat-breeders by dairy producers and veterinary clinicians. Causes for repeat breeding include a high incidence of fertilization failure and early embryonic mortality on days 6 to 7 after insemination [38]. Although the mechanism is not yet understood, administering LHRH to repeat-breeding dairy cows (third-service cows) improved conception rates by 21% [36] and 53% [35]. One field report suggested that LHRH given on day 12 of the cycle preceding insemination reduced the interval from treatment to conception compared with untreated control repeat-breeding dairy cows [39]. Whether the latter treatment influenced progesterone secretion significantly is not known, however, profiles of progesterone in milk indicated that persistent luteal activity, irregular-length estrous cycles, and periods of anestrus between normal estrous cycles are characteristic of repeat-breeders during the postpartum breeding period [40].

Table 2. Conception rates of dairy cows after LHRH administration at the time of artificial insemination.

Postpartum service	No. cows	% pregnant		Reference
		Control	LHRH	
First	133	32	48	37
	818	56	67	33
	118	49	59	32
	1,194	50	57	34
	328	46	47	36
Second	100	53	59	37
	204	46	55	36
Third	185	48	73	35
	97	51	66	36

APPLICATION TO REPRODUCTIVE MANAGEMENT

The postpartum period

Changes in reproductive hormones associated with reproductive function during the postpartum period [41,42] and estrous cycle [43] in domestic farm species have been reviewed recently. Following parturition, pituitary [44] and plasma [45,46] concentrations of LH are low and increase as the time postpartum increases. In addition, the pulsatile release of LH increases as time postpartum increases [45-47]. Increased pulsatile release of LH is associated with the first estrus and ovulation postpartum [47]. Pituitary responsiveness to LHRH also is low at parturition and increases as the time postpartum increases [5,6,48,49]. LHRH can induce a surge-like release of LH in cows postpartum well before the first spontaneous postpartum ovulation [41]. Pituitary responsiveness to LHRH is of great enough magnitude to release enough LH to induce ovulation by days 7 to 10 postpartum [5,6]. Pituitary release of LH in response to LHRH is probably delayed longer in suckled than in milked cows [50]. Concentrations of FSH in plasma and pituitary do not appear to change during the postpartum period [48,51,52]; however, responsiveness to LHRH may increase [48,51].

LHRH can release LH earlier postpartum than LH can induce ovulation. This phenomenon is probably related to ovarian follicular growth. Little follicular growth is present at parturition, but it increases markedly after the first week postpartum [42,44, 53,54]. After the second week postpartum in milked dairy and cows, later in suckled beef cows, follicles are probably large enough and contain sufficient LH receptors to respond to the LHRH-induced

LH surge. Ovulation can be induced in milked dairy cows by 2 weeks postpartum [5,55-57] and 3 to 4 weeks postpartum in beef cows [11]. In addition, repeated administration of LHRH to increase LH pulse frequency will initiate ovulation and ovarian cycles in acyclic cows during the postpartum period [58,59].

Thus, LHRH has been given during the early postpartum period to initiate cyclic ovarian activity. Of particular interest was the finding that inducing ovulation with LHRH-induced LH release 2 weeks postpartum reduced the incidence of ovarian cysts and improved subsequent fertility of dairy cows [57,60]. Zaied et al. [57] evaluated their results based on whether LHRH induced ovulation. None of the cows that ovulated following LHRH treatment developed ovarian cysts. Occurrence of ovarian cysts in cows not ovulating to LHRH treatment was similar to untreated cows. Thus, the observed decrease in abnormal ovarian function and the improved reproductive performance probably depends upon whether or not the LHRH-induced LH release stimulates ovulation. Follicular size at LHRH treatment determines the ovulatory response in most cases [56].

Improvment of reproductive function

Many of the effects on ovarian activity undoubtedly contribute to improved reproductive performance. Increased first-service conception rates, decreased number of services and reduced intervals to conception are observed in well-managed herds practicing early (beginning inseminations around 40 days postpartum) breeding [61,62]. Particular advantages were shown for cows classified as problem or abnormal breeders because of various periparturient problems including dystocia, retained placenta, metritis, endometritis, milk fever, or ketosis. Abnormal cows given LHRH had marked reduction in services per conception and intervals to conception than contemporary, untreated cows [61] (Table 3). Cows with retained placenta (retention of placenta for more than 12 hr) given LHRH around day 14 postpartum conceived earlier than controls if first inseminations occurred before 80 days postpartum, but not if delayed breeding was practiced [63]. In addition, involution of the uterus is advanced in response to early postpartum LHRH administration [55,57].

Contrasting results for the effects of LHRH on fertility were observed in one study [64]. Unless LHRH given on day 14 postpartum was followed 10 days later by $PGF_2\alpha$, LHRH-treated cows had longer postpartum intervals to estrus and conception because of increased incidence of pyometra and prebreeding anestrus. With the exception of the preceding study, all other studies provide evidence that early postpartum treatment of cows with LHRH will induce normal ovarian activity, reduce reproductive problems such as ovarian follicular cysts and involuntary culling [57,60], and enhance fertility of dairy cows. Prophylactic treatment of cows with LHRH seems warranted subject to further study of its economy to dairy producers.

Table 3. Fertility of dairy cows after LHRH treatment (200 µ g)
early postpartum (between days 10 and 14): Normal
versus abnormal puerperium [Reproduced from Benmard, M.
and Stevenson, J.S. J. Dairy Sci., 69, 800 (1986), with
permission].

Trait	Control	LHRH
Conception at first service, %	29	40
Normal	35	42
Abnormal	13	31
Days from calving to conception	115	88[a]
Normal	97	92
Abnormal	133	85[a]
Services per conception	2.3	1.7[a]
Normal	2.2	1.7[a]
Abnormal	2.4	1.7[a]

[a]Different from control (P<.05).

Synchronization of estrous cycles

Use of $PGF_2\alpha$ to regress the corpus luteum and thereby synchronize
estrus in cattle has been studied [65]. Its use is routinely
found in dairy and beef operations where AI is used. The various
protocols used allow for one injection of $PGF_2\alpha$ or its analogs,
followed by inseminations at estrus, or the use of two injections
given 10 to 12 days apart, followed by insemination at observed
estrus or AI at a predetermined time (timed AI) after the second
injection of $PGF_2\alpha$ [65]. Conception rates at observed estrus
generally are better than at timed AI.

Early work to determine if the timing of ovulation could be
made more precise to allow for improved conception rates after
timed AI by administering LHRH as part of a protocol for estrous
synchronization found little success. When LHRH was given at 48,
52, 60, 64, 68 or 72 hr after the second of two injections of
$PGF_2\alpha$ [65-69], conception rates were improved only in two studies
[65,70]. The magnitude of the LH peak was greater than that
normally observed at estrus, but its duration was attenuated
[70,71]. Precision of ovulation was increased when LHRH was given
52 hr after $PGF_2\alpha$ [72], but treatment of cattle in estrus with
LHRH has suppressed estrous behavior [46,75]. Although LHRH
treatment has improved the precision of preovulatory LH surges and
timing of ovulation, the conception rates after timed inseminations have not improved sufficiently to justify its use in practice.

505

Effect on luteal function

Secretion of LH that follows LHRH administration indicates that LHRH may have a luteotropic role in cattle. Treating cattle with natural LHRH [21,73,74] or with an LHRH analog [74] during the luteal phase of the estrous cycle resulted in transient increases of LH and progesterone in serum lasting 4 to 8 hr. Repetitive injections of the same LHRH analog also prolonged the cycle when given on days 9 to 12 of the estrous cycle [74]. Administering LHRH during the late luteal and early follicular phase of the cycle (days 16 to 18) did not alter duration of the cycle during which treatment occurred, nor duration of the subsequent cycle [75]. In addition, neither secretion of progesterone during the post-treatment cycle nor fertility were altered by previous LHRH treatment during the follicular phase. In contrast, when LHRH was given to heifers during metestrus (day 2), concentrations of progesterone in serum during the following luteal phase [76,77], as well as concentrations of unoccupied LH receptors in the plasma membranes of corpora lutea were reduced significantly [77]. Treatment of estrual cows with LHRH at the time of insemination also decreased subsequent concentrations of progesterone in serum of nonpregnant (luteal phase) and pregnant cows and heifers, whereas LHRH increased concentrations of estradiol-17β in serum of the same animals on days 4 to 6 after AI [70] (Figs. 2 and 3). A similar study, however, demonstrated increased progesterone in milk during the subsequent luteal phase of cows given LHRH treatment at estrus [78].

STUDIES WITH BULLS

Investigations in bulls have mostly been associated with attempts to hasten puberty or increase testosterone and sperm production after LHRH administration. At one week of age, bulls secrete LH in response to LHRH [79,80], and small increases in testosterone secretion also result [79]. However, without LHRH administration, pulsatile release of LH is infrequent and androgen secretion low the first few months of life [81]. Thereafter, pulsatile release of LH increases. However, pulsatile injections of LHRH to induce LH release and hasten puberty have been unsuccessful [82-84]. In general, the LHRH-induced LH release decreases over time during chronic LHRH administration, and testosterone production and sperm numbers are not increased [83].

In postpubertal bulls, LHRH elevates serum LH, FSH and testosterone concentrations [85,86]. However, repeated administration of LHRH also densensitized the pituitary to LHRH in postpubertal bulls [82,83,87] and no increase in testosterone and/or sperm numbers was observed [82,83]. Pulsatile administration of LHRH in bulls implanted with estradiol-17β to inhibit pulsatile LH secretion did override the inhibiting effects of estradiol-17β treatment [88]. Testicular size and sperm production were increased in the LHRH treated, estradiol-17β implanted bulls. More recently, a potent LHRH agonist (([D-Nal(2)[6]]LHRH) was injected

into bulls to decrease LH release and subsequent testosterone
production [87] because testosterone has been shown to decrease
carcass quality of bulls [89]. In that study [87], pulsatile
release of LH and FSH in serum and pituitary content of LH, FSH
and LHRH receptors were decreased. However, mean serum concentrations of testosterone were elevated as were testicular LH
receptors. Thus, treatment with a LHRH agonist did not appear to
be successful in this study as an agent to increase carcass
quality in bulls.

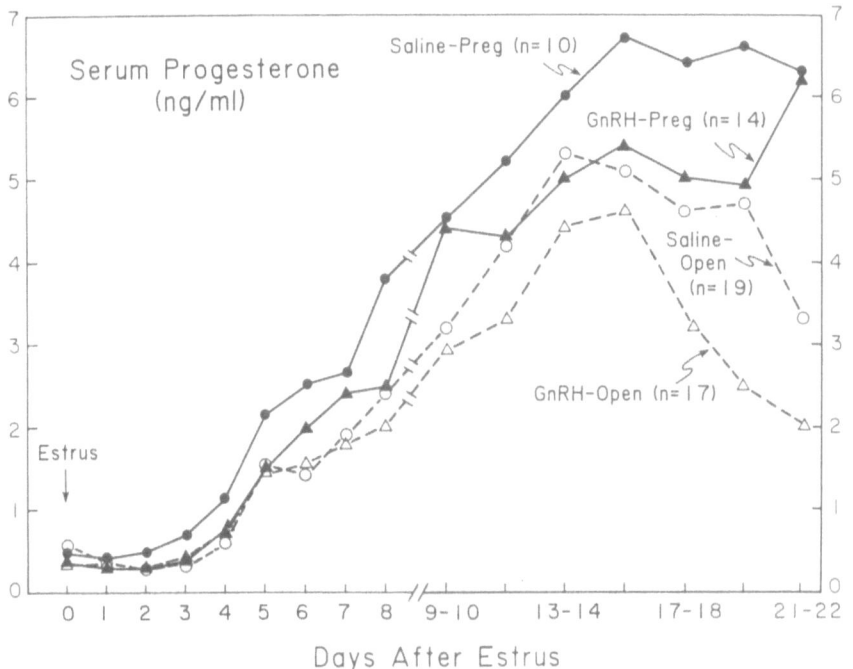

FIGURE 2. Average concentrations of progesterone in serum for cows
and heifers that either conceived (preg) or failed to
conceive (open) to a timed insemination (80 hr after a
luteolytic dose of prostaglandin $F_2\alpha$ or its analog,
cloprostenol). Gonadotropin-releasing hormone (GnRH) or
saline was given 8 hr before insemination. Day 0 desig-
nates the day of estrus or artificial insemination in the
absence of observed estrus [Reproduced from Lucy, M.C.
and Stevenson, J.S. Biol. Reprod., <u>35</u>, 300 (1986), with
permission].

507

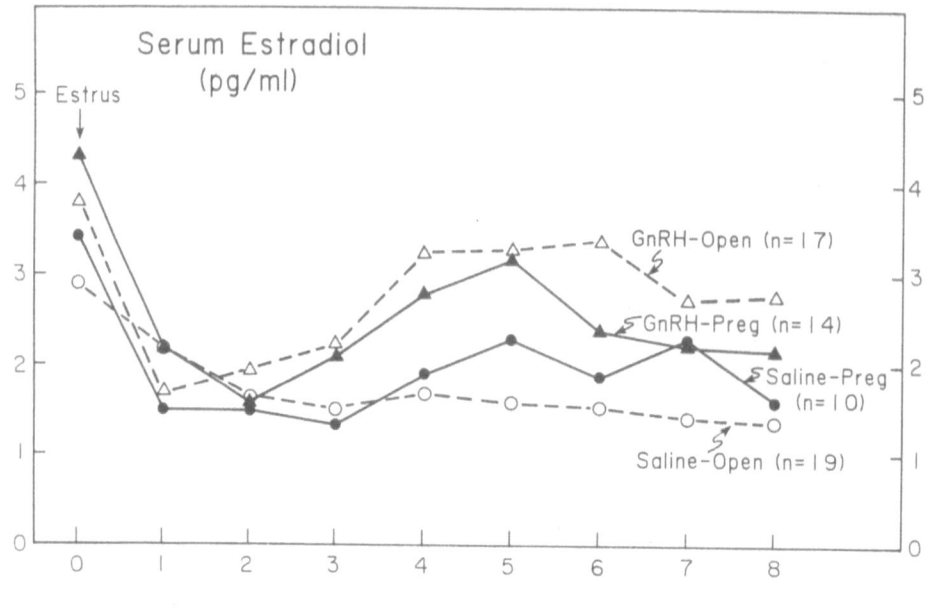

FIGURE 3. Average concentrations of estradiol in serum for cows
and heifers that either conceived (preg) or failed to
conceive (open) to a timed insemination (80 hr after a
luteolytic dose of prostaglandin $F_2\alpha$ or its analog,
cloprostenol). Gonadotropin-releasing hormone (GnRH) or
saline was given 8 hr before insemination. Day 0 desig-
nates the day of estrus or artificial insemination in
the absence of observed estrus [Reproduced from Lucy,
M.C. and Stevenson, J.S. Biol. Reprod., 35, 300
(1986), with permission].

CONCLUSIONS

LHRH has been used as a therapeutic agent in cattle for several
conditions. In particular, LHRH and its analogs have been shown
to be an effective treatment for cows with ovarian follicular
cysts, prevention of ovarian cysts, induction of cyclicity and
improved fertility in cows postpartum, and improvement of fertility in cows at insemination. Effectiveness of LHRH treatment in
those studies was related to the follicular activity present at
the time of treatment. Regimens for inducing follicular growth in
females without pituitary densensitization need to be developed.
Development of delivery systems also may allow LHRH and its
analogs to be used as antifertility agents in both cows and bulls.

REFERENCES

1. Armstrong, J.D. and Britt, J.H. Pulsatile administration of gonadotropin releasing hormone to anestrous sows: endocrine changes associated with GnRH-induced and spontaneous estrus. Biol. Reprod., 33, 375 (1985).

2. McNatty, K.P., Ball, K., Gibb, M., Hudson, N. and Thurley, D.C. Induction of cyclic ovarian activity in seasonally anoestrous ewes with exogenous GnRH. J. Reprod. Fert., 64, 93 (1982).

3. McLeod, B.J. and Haresign, W. Induction of fertile oestrus in seasonally anoestrous ewes with low doses of GnRH. Anim. Reprod. Sci., 7, 413 (1984).

4. Schanbacher, B.D. LHRH and analogs in relation to livestock. In "LHRH and Its Analogs: Contraceptive and Therapeutic Applications", B.H. Vickery, J.J. Nestor, Jr. and E.S.E. Hafez, (Eds.) MTP Press, Boston, MA, 1984, p.385.

5. Kesler, D.J., Garverick, Youngquist, R.S., Elmore, R.G. and Bierschwal, C.J. Effect of days postpartum and endogenous reproductive hormones on GnRH-induced LH release in dairy cows. J. Anim. Sci., 45, 797 (1977).

6. Fernandes, L.C., Thatcher, W.W., Wilcox, C.J. and Call, E.P. LH release in response to GnRH during the postpartum period of dairy cows. J. Anim. Sci., 46, 443 (1978).

7. Hsueh, A.J.W. and Jones, P.B.C. Extrapituitary actions of gonadotropin-releasing hormone. Endocr. Rev., 2, 437 (1981).

8. Brown, J.L. and Reeves, J.J. Absence of specific luteinizing hormone releasing hormone receptors in ovine, bovine and porcine ovaries. Biol. Reprod., 29, 1179 (1983).

9. Eyestone, W.H. and Ax, R.L. A review of ovarian follicular cysts in the cow with comparisons to the condition in women, rats and rabbits. Theriogenology, 22, 109 (1984).

10. Kesler, D.J. and Garverick, H.A. Ovarian cysts in dairy cattle: A review. J. Anim. Sci., 55, 1147 (1982).

11. Kesler, D.J., Garverick, H.A., Caudle, A.B., Elmore, R.G., Youngquist, R.S. and Bierschwal, C.J. Reproductive hormone and ovarian changes in cows with ovarian cysts. J. Dairy Sci., 63, 166 (1980).

12. Kesler, D.J., Garverick, H.A., Caudle, A.B., Bierschwal, C.J., Elmore, R.G. and Youngquist, R.S. Testosterone concentrations in plasma of dairy cows with ovarian cysts. J. Dairy Sci., 63, 1825 (1979).

13. Coney, P. Polycystic ovarian disease: Current concepts of pathophysiology and therapy. Fertil. Steril., 42, 667 (1984).

14. Goldzieher, J.W. Polycystic ovarian disease. Fertil. Steril., 14, 631 (1981).

15. Garm, O. A study of bovine nymphomania. Acta Endocrinol., 3(Suppl. 3), 1 (1949).

16. Garverick, H.A. and Bierschwal, C.J. Ovarian cysts in dairy cattle. In "Large Dairy Herd Management",

C.J. Wilcox and H.H. VanHorn (Eds.), Univ. Presses of Florida, Gainesville, 1979, p. 606.

17. Bierschwal, C.J., Garverick, H.A., Martin, C.E., Youngquist, R.S., Cantley, T.C. and Brown, M.D. Clinical response of dairy cows with ovarian cysts to GnRH. J. Anim. Sci., 41, 1660 (1975).

18. Matsuo, H., Baba, Y., Nair, R.M., Arimura, A. and Schally, A.V. Structure of the porcine LH- and FSH-releasing hormone. I. The proposed amino acid sequence. Biochem. Biophys. Res. Commun., 43, 1334 (1971).

19. Burgus, R., Butcher, M., Amoss, M., Ling, N., Monahan, M.W., Rivier, J., Fellows, R., Blackwell, R., Vale, W. and Guillemin, R. Primary structure of the ovine hypothalamic luteinizing hormone-releasing factor (LRF). Proc. Natl. Acad. Sci., USA, 69, 278 (1972).

20. Matsuo, H., Arimura, A. and Schally, A.V. Synthesis of the porcine LH- and FSH- releasing hormone by the solid phase method. Biochem. Biophys. Res. Commun., 45, 822 (1971).

21. Kittok, R.J., Britt, J.H. and Convey, E.M. Endocrine response after GnRH in luteal phase cows and cows with ovarian follicular cysts. J. Anim. Sci., 37, 985 (1973).

22. Cantley, T.C., Garverick, H.A., Bierschwal, C.J., Martin, C.E. and Youngquist, R.S. Hormonal response of dairy cows with ovarian cysts to GnRH. J. Anim. Sci., 41, 1666 (1975).

23. Elmore, R.G., Bierschwal, C.J., Youngquist, R.S., Cantley, T.C., Kesler, D.J. and Garverick, H.A. Clinical responses of dairy cows with ovarian cysts following treatment with 10,000 IU HCG or 100 mcg GnRH. Vet. Med./Sm. Anim. Clin., 70, 1346 (1975).

24. Garverick, H.A., Kesler, D.J., Cantley, T.C., Elmore, B.G., Youngquist, R.S. and C.J. Bierschwal. Hormone response of dairy cows with ovarian cysts after treatment with HCG or GnRH. Theriogenology, 6, 413 (1976).

25. Seguin, B.E., Convey, E.M. and W.D. Oxender. Effect of gonadotropin-releasing hormone and human chorionic gonadotropin in cows with ovarian follicular cysts. Amer. J. Vet. Res., 37, 153 (1976).

26. Kesler, D.J., Garverick, H.A., Caudle, A.B. Bierschwal, C.J., Elmore, R.G. and Youngquist, R.S. Clinical and endocrine responses of dairy cows with ovarian cysts to GnRH and PGF$_2\alpha$. J. Anim. Sci., 46, 719 (1978).

27. Kesler, D.J., Elmore, R.G., Brown, E.M. and Garverick, H.A. Gonadotropin releasing hormone treatment of dairy cows with ovarian cysts. I. Gross ovarian morphology and endocrinology. Theriogenology, 16, 219 (1981).

28. Berchtold, M., Rusch, P., Thun, R. and Kung, S. Wirkung oon HCG und GnRH auf die ovarien von kuhen mit zystos degenerietrten follikeln. Zuchthg, 15, 126 (1980).

29. Grunert, B., Hoffman, B. and Ahlers, D. Klinische und hormonanalytische untersuchungen bei kuhen mit ovarialzysten vor und nach gonadotropin-releasing-hormon (Gn-RH-)-verabreichung. Dtsch. Tierarztl. Wschr., 81, 373 (1981).

510

30.   Ax, R.L., Bellin, M.E., Schneider, D.K. and Haase-Hardie, J.A. Reproductive performance of dairy cows with cystic ovaries following administration of Procystin[TM]. J. Dairy Sci., 69, 542 (1986).

31.   Nakao, T., Kawata, K. and Numata, Y. Therapeutic effects of an analog of luteinizing hormone-releasing hormone (Des-Gly-LH-RH-ethylamide) on cows with cystic ovary. Jap. J. Vet. Sci., 42, 459 (1980).

32.   Schels, H.F. and Mostafawi, D. The effect of GnRH on the pregnancy rate of artificially inseminated cows. Vet. Rec., 103, 31 (1978).

33.   Leidl, W., Bostedt, H., Lamprecht, W., Prinzen, K., and Wendt, V. Zur ovulationssteuerung mit einem GnRH-Analogen und HCG bei der kunstlichen Besamung des Rindes. Tierarztl. Umschau, 34, 546 (1979).

34.   Nakao, T., Narita, S., Tanaka, K., Hara, H., Shirakawa, J., Nashiro, H., Saga, N., Tsunodo, N. and Kawata, K. Improvement of first-service pregnancy rate in cows with gonadotropin-releasing hormone analog. Theriogenology, 20, 111 (1983).

35.   Lee, C.N., Maurice, A., Ax, R.L., Pennington, J.A., Hoffman, W.F. and Brown, M.D. Efficacy of gonadotropin-releasing hormone administered at the time of artificial insemination of heifers and postpartum and repeater breeder dairy cows. Am. J. Vet. Res., 44, 2160 (1983).

36.   Stevenson, J.S., Schmidt, M.K. and Call, E.P. Gonadotropin-releasing hormone and conception in Holsteins. J. Dairy Sci., 67, 140 (1984).

37.   Bentele, W. and Humke, R. Versuch zur behandlung des verzogerten follikelsprungs beim rind mit dem synthetischen LH-FSH-releasinghormon. Tierarztl. Umschau, 31, 218 (1976).

38.   Ayalon, N. A review of embryonic mortality in cattle. J. Reprod. Fert., 54, 483 (1978).

39.   Humbolt, P. and Thibier, M. Effect of gonadotropin-releasing hormone and conception in Holsteins. Theriogenology, 16, 375 (1981).

40.   Bulman, D.C. and Lamming, G.E. Milk progesterone levels in relation to conception, repeat breeding and factors influencing acyclicity in dairy cows. J. Reprod. Fert., 54, 447 (1978).

41.   Wettemann, R.P. Postpartum endocrine function of cattle, sheep and swine, J. Anim. Sci., 51(Suppl.2), 2 (1980).

42.   Spicer, L.J. and Echternkamp, S.E. Ovarian follicular growth, function and turnover in cattle: A review. J. Anim. Sci., 62, 428 (1986).

43.   Hansel, W. and Convey, E.M. Physiology of the estrous cycle. J. Anim. Sci., 57(Suppl 2), 404 (1983).

44.   Saiduddin, S., Riesen, J.W., Tyler, W.J. and Casida, L.E. Relation of postpartum interval to pituitary gonadotropins, ovarian follicular development and fertility in dairy cows. Wisconsin Agr. Exp. Sta. Res. Bull., 270, 15 (1968).

45. Goodale, W.S., Garverick, H.A., Kesler, D.J., Bierschwal, C.J., Elmore, R.G. and Youngquist, R.S. Transitory changes of hormones in plasma of postpartum dairy cows. J. Dairy Sci., 61, 740 (1978).

46. Peters, A.R., Lamming, G.E. and Fisher, M.W. A comparison of plasma LH concentrations in milked and suckling postpartum cows. J. Reprod. Fert., 62, 567 (1981).

47. Stevenson, J.S. and Britt, J.H. Relationships among luteinizing hormone, estradiol, progesterone, glucocorticoids, milk yield, body weight and postpartum activity in Holstein cows. J. Anim. Sci., 48, 570 (1979).

48. Williams, G.L., Kotwica, J., Slanger, W.D., Olson, D.K., Tilton, J.E. and Johnson, L.J. Effect of suckling on pituitary responsiveness to gonadotropin-releasing hormone throughout the early postpartum period of beef cows. J. Anim. Sci., 54, 594 (1982).

49. Azzazi, F., Krause, G.F. and Garverick, H.A. Alteration of the GnRH-induced LH release by steroids in postpartum dairy cattle. J. Anim. Sci., 57, 1251 (1983).

50. Peters, A.R. and Lamming, G.E. Reproductive activity of the cow in the post-partum period. II. Endocrine patterns and induction of ovulation . Brit. Vet. J., 140, 269 (1984).

51. Schallenberger, E., Schams, D. and Zottmeier, K. Response of lutropin (LH) and follitropin (FSH) to the administration of gonadoliberin (GnRH) in pregnant and post-partum cattle including experiments with prolactin suppression. Theriogenology, 10, 36 (1978).

52. Moss, G.E., Parfet, J.R., Marvin, C.A., Allrich, R.D. and Diekman, M.A. Pituitary concentrations of gonadotropin and receptors for GnRH in suckled beef cows at various intervals after calving. J. Anim. Sci., 60, 285 (1985).

53. Kesler, D.J., Troxel, T.R. and D.L. Hixon. Effect of days postpartum and exogenous GnRH on reproductive hormone and ovarian changes in postpartum suckled beef cows. Theriogenology, 13, 287 (1980).

54. Dufour, J.J. and Roy, G.L. Distribution of ovarian follicular populations in the dairy cow within 35 days after parturition. J. Reprod. Fert., 73, 229 (1985).

55. Britt, J.H., Kittok, R.J. and Harrison, D.S. Ovulation, estrus and endocrine response after GnRH in early postpartum cows. J. Anim. Sci., 39, 915 (1974).

56. Garverick, H.A., Elmore, R.G., Vaillancourt, D.H. and Sharp, A.J. Ovarian response to GnRH in postpartum dairy cows. Am. J. Vet. Res., 41, 1582 (1980).

57. Zaied, A.A., Garverick, H.A., Bierschwal, C.J., Elmore, R.G., Youngquist, R.S. and Sharp, A.J. Effect of ovarian activity and endogenous reproductive hormones on GnRH-induced ovarian cycles in postpartum dairy cows. J. Anim. Sci., 50, 508 (1980).

58. Riley, G.M., Peters, A.R. and Lamming, G.E. Induction of pulsatile LH release, FSH release and ovulation in post-partum beef cows by repeated small doses of GnRH. J. Reprod. Fert., 63, 559 (1981).

59. Walters, D.L., Short, R.E., Convey, E.M., Staigmiller, R.B., Dunn, T.G. and Kaltenbach, C.C. Pituitary and ovarian function in post-partum beef cows. III. Induction of estrus, ovulation and luteal function with intermittent small-dose injections of Gn-RH. Biol. Reprod., 26, 655 (1982).

60. Britt, J.H., Harrison, D.S. and Morrow, D.A. Frequency of ovarian follicular cysts, reasons for culling, and fertility in Holstein-Friesian cows given gonadotropin-releasing hormone at two weeks after parturition. Amer. J. Vet. Res., 38, 749 (1977).

61. Benmrad, M. and Stevenson, J.S. Gonadotropin-releasing hormone and prostaglandin $F_2\alpha$ for postpartum dairy cows: Estrous, ovulation and fertility traits. J. Dairy Sci., 69, 800 (1986).

62. Nash, J.G., Ball, L. and Olson, J.D. Effects on reproductive performance of administration of GnRH to early postpartum dairy cows. J. Anim. Sci., 50, 1017 (1980).

63. Leslie, K.E., Doig, P.A., Bosu, W.T.K., Curtis, R.A. and Martin, S.W. Effects of gonadotropin-releasing hormone on reproductive performance of dairy cows with retained placenta. Can. J. Comp. Med., 48, 354 (1984).

64. Etherington, W.G., Bosu, W.T.K., Martin, S.W., Cote, J.F., Dory, P.A. and Leslie, K.E. Reproductive performance in dairy cows following postpartum treatment with gonadotropin-releasing hormone and/or prostaglandin: A field trial. Can. J. Comp. Med., 48, 245 (1984).

65. Hansel, W. and Fortune, J. The applications of ovulation control. In "Control of Ovulation", D.B. Crighton, G.R. Foxcroft, N.B. Haynes, and G.E. Lamming (Eds.), Butterworth, London, (1978) p. 237.

66. Rodriguez, T.R., Fields, M.J., Burns, W.C., Franke, D.E., Hentges, J.F., Thatcher, W.W. and Warnick, A.C. Breeding at a predetermined time in the bovine following $PGF_2\alpha$ and GnRH. J. Anim. Sci., 40, 188 (1975).

67. Burfening, P.J., Anderson, D.C., Friedrich, R.L. and Williams, J. Fertility of cows treated with $PGF_2\alpha$ and GnRH. J. Anim. Sci., 42, 1565 (1976).

68. Chipepa, J.A.S., Kinder, J.E. and Reeves, J.J. Synchronized breeding in cattle using $PGF_2\alpha$ and LHRH/FSHRH stimulatory analogs. Theriogenology, 8, 25 (1977).

69. Lucy, M.C., Stevenson, J.S. and Call, E.P. Controlling first service and calving interval by prostaglandin $F_2\alpha$, gonadotropin releasing hormone, and timed insemination. J. Dairy Sci., 69, 2186 (1986).

70. Lucy, M.C. and Stevenson, J.S. Gonadotropin-releasing hormone at estrus: Luteinizing hormone, estradiol, and progesterone during the periestrual and postinsemination periods in dairy cattle. Biol. Reprod., 35, 300 (1986).

71. Coulson, A., Noakes, D.E., Hamer, J. and Cockrill, T. Effect of gonadotropin-releasing hormone on levels of luteinizing hormone in cattle synchronized with dinoprost. Vet. Rec., 107, 108 (1980).

513

72. Cumming, I.A., Baxter, R.W., White, M.B., McPhee, S.R. and Sullin, A.P. Time of ovulation in cattle following treatment with a prostaglandin analogue (PG), PG with LHRH, or intravaginal silastic coils impregnated with progesterone (PRID). Theriogenology, 8, 184 (1977).

73. Thompson, F.N., Clekis, T., Kiser, T.E., Chen, H.J. and Smith, C.K. Serum progesterone concentrations in pregnant and nonpregnant heifers and after gonadotropin-releasing hormone in luteal phase heifers. Theriogenology, 13, 407 (1980).

74. Milvae, R.A., Murphy, B.D. and Hansel, W. Prolongation of the bovine estrous cycle with a gonadotropin-releasing hormone analog. Biol. Reprod., 31, 664 (1984).

75. Helmer, S.D. and Britt, J.H. Progesterone secretion and fertility in dairy cattle treated with gonadotropin-releasing hormone (GnRH) before ovulation or human chorionic gonadotropin (hCG) after ovulation. J. Dairy Sci., 66 (Suppl. 1), 228 (1983).

76. Ford, S.P. and Stormshak, F. Bovine ovarian and pituitary responses to PMS and GnRH administered during metestrus. J. Anim. Sci., 46, 1701 (1978).

77. Rodger, L.D. and Stormshak, F. Effects of GnRH on bovine luteal function. J. Anim. Sci., 59(Suppl. 1), 336 (1984).

78. Lee, C.N., Critser, J.K. and Ax, R.L. Changes of luteinizing hormone and progesterone for dairy cows after gonadotropin-releasing hormone at first postpartum breeding. J. Dairy Sci., 68, 1463 (1985).

79. Kesler, D.J. and Garverick, H.A. Luteinizing hormone and testosterone concentrations in plasma of bull calves treated with gonadotropin releasing hormone. J. Dairy Sci., 60, 632 (1977).

80. Bass, J.J., McNeily, A.S. and Moreton, H.E. Plasma concentraions of FSH and LH in entire and castrated prepubertal bull calves treated with GnRH. J. Reprod. Fert., 57, 219 (1979).

81. Amann, R.P. and Walker, O.A. Changes in the pituitary-gonadal axis associated with puberty in Holstein bulls. J. Anim. Sci., 57, 433 (1983).

82. Mongkunpunya, K., Hafs, H.D., Convey, E.M. and Tucker, H.A. Serum LH and testosterone and sperm numbers in pubertal bulls chronically treated wtih GnRH. J. Anim. Sci., 41, 160 (1975).

83. Haynes, N.B., Hafs, H.D. and Manns, J.G. Effect of chronic administration of gonadotropin releasing hormone and thyrotropin releasing hormone to pubertal bulls on plasma luteinizing hormone, prolactin and testosterone concentrations, the number of epididymal sperm and body weight. J. Endocrinol., 73, 227 (1977).

84. Miller, C.J. and R.P. Amann. Effects of pulsatile injection of GnRH into 6- to 14-wk-old Holstein bulls. J. Anim. Sci., 62, 1332 (1986).

85.   Schanbacher, B.D.   Testosterone secretion in cryptorchid
      and intact bulls injected with gonadotropin-releasing
      hormone and luteinizing hormone.   Endocrinology, <u>104</u>, 360
      (1979).
86.   Schanbacher, B.D. and Echternkamp, S.E.   Testicular steroid
      secretion in response to GnRH mediated LH and FSH release
      in bulls.   J. Anim. Sci., <u>47</u>, 514 (1978).
87.   Melson, B.E., Brown, J.L., Schoenemann, H.M., Tarnavsky,
      G.K. and Reeves, J.J.   Elevation of serum testosterone
      during chronic LHRH agonist treatment in the bull.   J.
      Anim. Sci., <u>62</u>, 199 (1986).
88.   Schanbacher, B.D., D'Occhio, M.J. and Kinder, J.E.   Initi-
      ation of spermatogenesis and testicular growth in oe-
      stradiol-17β-implanted bull calves with pulsatile infusion
      of luteinizing hormone releasing hormone.   J. Endocrinol.,
      <u>93</u>, 182 (1982).
89.   Gortsema, S.R., Jacobs, J.A., Sasser, R.G., Gregory, T.L.
      and Bull, R.C.   Effects of endogenous testosterone on
      production and carcass traits in beef cattle.   J. Anim.
      Sci., <u>39</u>, 680 (1977).

34
Clinical Uses of LHRH Analogs in Dogs

B. H. VICKERY, G. I. McRAE and J. C. GOODPASTURE
Department of Physiology, Institute of Biological Sciences, Syntex Research,
3401 Hillview Avenue, Palo Alto, CA 94304, USA

INTRODUCTION

LHRH agonist analogs have been extensively investigated in humans
for both contraceptive and therapeutic applications [1-3]. Much
of this work was based upon preliminary studies in animals [4-9].
In our laboratory, many of the preclinical studies were performed
in dogs, who constitute sensitive and relevant model subjects for
humans [10-12]. The results of the endocrine studies in dogs,
together with the successful use of these agents in humans,
encouraged us to evaluate the utility of the LHRH agonist analogs
as contraceptive and therapeutic agents for pets.

The LHRH analogs are essentially inactive orally. For human
use the alternative parenteral administration by once daily
injection, one or more nasal insufflations per day, or more
recently once monthly depot injectable or implantable systems have
proven acceptable. However, for dogs, therapy for all but
life-threatening disease should require low frequency visits to
the veterinarian, preferably to coincide with yearly immunization
or check-up visits. It was therefore an integral part of these
studies that we explore the development of long term (up to one
year) depot delivery systems for the LHRH analogs in dogs.

Agonist analogs of LHRH, by their nature, cause an initial
stimulatory effect on gonadotropin release and gonadal steroid
output before shutting down the pituitary-gonadal axis. With the
exception of a biochemical and sometimes symptomatic flare in
cancer patients [13-16] causing contraindication of use in a very
small subpopulation [17], this transitory effect is acceptable and
well tolerated. However, for contraception in female dogs, such a
stimulation can result in the very phenomenon that it is desired
to prevent i.e. expression of heat. A further integral part of
these studies has therefore been the development of stratagems to
avoid the symptomatic expression of the stimulatory effects of the
LHRH agonists.

The antagonistic analogs of LHRH were, logically, forecast to
be the more useful as contraceptive agents. However the early
analogs had low potency and it has required an increase of
10,000 fold in potency for clinically useful analogs to be

identified [18,19]. With LHRH antagonists now available which have receptor binding affinities equal to the best of the agonistic analogs, studies are being reported which explore the gamut of their effects, from suppression of reproductive function [20-23] to slowing of the growth of both gonadal hormone dependent [24-26] and independent tumors [27]. The availability to us of some of the most potent and long lived of these antagonist analogs yet reported [28,29] prompted an evaluation of their contraceptive potential in dogs.

SUPPRESSION OF SEXUAL FUNCTION IN FEMALES

Suppression of estrus with LHRH agonists

Cholesterol pellet implants. For an initial evaluation of estrus suppression by LHRH agonists we used the analog [D-Trp^6, Pro^{9}NHEt]LHRH (analog A). This analog was formulated, at a level of 0.5%, into compacted cholesterol pellets weighing 25 to 34 mg each. These pellets deliver the agonist for at least 30 days in rats, heifers and baboons [6-8,30].

Three, 10.5 to 11 month old, prepubertal beagle bitches were subcutaneously implanted with 10 to 13 pellets, each. The implantations were repeated at monthly intervals for a total treatment period of one year. This treatment amounted to 1.2-2.2 mg each (approximately 125 μg/kg agonist per month). In keeping with the initial stimulatory effects of treatment with these agents, within 4 to 6 days after initiation of treatment the three bitches exhibited proestrus, which was followed by ovulation, as diagnosed by elevated levels of plasma progesterone. However, none of the treated bitches had a further estrous episode during the remaining 1 year of treatment. Seven untreated bitches born in the colony at the same time as the treated animals served as controls, and had their first estrus at an average age of 12.4 months and a second estrus at an average of 6.7 months later. At the end of treatment all pellets were surgically removed, and the 3 bitches came into estrus 3, 3.5 and 8 months later, respectively. They all cycled regularly thereafter and were bred and conceived at either the first or second estrus following treatment.

This preliminary study, although performed with a formulation of uncharacterized release kinetics, demonstrated the potential for use of LHRH analogs in reversible, long term suppression of estrus. In addition it pointed out the potential disadvantages of the initial transitory stimulation of reproductive function to be expected from these agents.

Initiation of treatment at different stages of the cycle. Continuous subcutaneous infusion of two more potent [31] agonist analogs (analogs B and C) of LHRH (Table 1) was achieved through subcutaneous implantation of osmotic minipumps (Alzet®, Alza Corp., California). Depending on the model used, these minipumps were replaced at 14 day (model 2002) or 28 day (model 2ML4)

Table 1. Potencies of LHRH and agonist analogs

Analog	Structure	Potency[*]
–	LHRH	1
A	[D–Trp^6,Pro^{9}NHEt]LHRH	100
B	[D–Nal(2)^6]LHRH (nafarelin)	200
C	[D–Nal(2)^6,Aza-Gly^{10}]LHRH (aza–gly nafarelin)	230

[*]Based on the rat estrus–suppression assay [31].

intervals. The aim of these studies was to assess the effects of beginning treatment during different hormonal milieux and to establish chronic dose requirements.

a) Treatment during proestrus. A dose response study was conducted with analog B. Doses of 2, 8 or 32 µg per day were administered by osmotic pump to each of 3 mature regularly cycling beagle bitches, starting during the first week of a spontaneous proestrous vaginal discharge and continuing for 18 months. The impending ovulation was unaffected by treatment, as judged by a rise in plasma levels of progesterone (Fig. 1). The dose of 32 µg per day prevented further clinical or hormonal signs of heat or ovulation [32]. Two of the three bitches receiving this dose came into heat 3 and 18 weeks after cessation of treatment respectively, were mated and produced normal litters. The third bitch exhibited an anovulatory heat at 5 weeks after stopping treatment, followed by an ovulatory (based on plasma progesterone levels) heat eleven weeks later.

During the luteal phase immediately following start of treatment, integrated levels of progesterone for bitches receiving 8 or 32 µg per day were significantly ($p<0.01$) lower than in vehicle treated controls. This suggested that the treatment may have compromised luteal function, as previously noted for non-pregnant females in other species [33]. To examine fertility under treatment, a further two bitches were treated with 32 µg per day of analog B starting during the first week of a spontaneous proestrus. They were mated at the ensuing estrus and treatment was continued for 63 days or until whelping occurred. Both bitches were diagnosed as pregnant by abdominal palpation 28 days after mating. One bitch whelped a litter of nine normal pups at term. The second bitch did not deliver pups at term but had a sanguineous vaginal discharge at eight weeks of gestation and at laparotomy one week later one uterine implantation site was noted. In contrast to the non-pregnant animals, the progesterone levels in these treated pregnant animals were in the normal range. This finding again has its parallel in other species

519

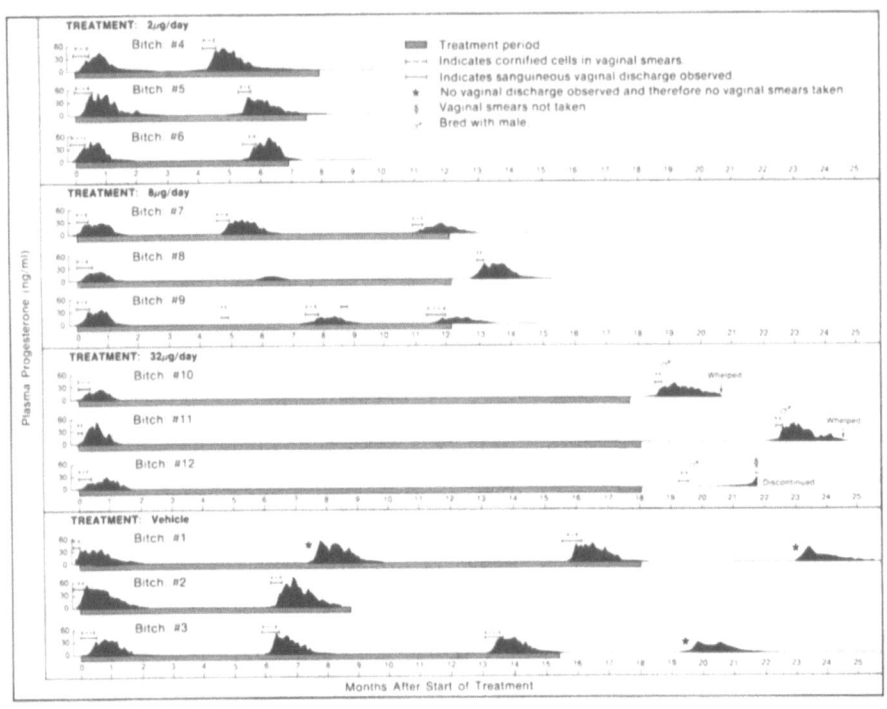

FIGURE 1.   Plasma progesterone and occurrence of vaginal discharge
             and vaginal cornification during and after continuous
             treatment with 2, 8 or 32 µg/day of analog B or
             vehicle alone. Reproduced from McRae, G.I. et al.
             J. Reprod. Fert., 74, 389 (1985), by permission.

[34,35]. In primates it appears that the luteal suppression is
overruled by a chorionic gonadotropin [34,36]. Whether a similar
principle lies behind the differing responses in the pregnant and
non-pregnant dog is unknown.

b) Treatment during diestrus. Three bitches were treated with
cholesterol pellets containing 0.5% analog A, at the same dose as
described for the preliminary study. Treatment started at 45 days
after their last proestrous discharge. As expected, at that time
the corpora lutea were functional, giving rise to plasma
progesterone concentrations of greater than 2 ng/ml. Starting
treatment at this time caused no sign of initial stimulation, i.e.
occurrence of proestrus or estrus. Repeated monthly implants of

520

the agonist pellets for one year prevented the occurrence of estrus in one of the three bitches. Four months after cessation of treatment, that bitch returned to estrus, mated and produced a normal litter.

c) Treatment during anestrus. A dose response study was conducted with analog C. Doses of 8 or 32 µg/day were administered, by osmotic pump, beginning 90 or more days after a spontaneous heat. As expected, approximately one week after start of treatment all the bitches exhibited signs of an induced heat, i.e. sanguineous vaginal discharge for 10 to 14 days. All but one bitch (one that was receiving 8 µg/day) ovulated at the induced heat, as diagnosed by a marked rise in plasma progesterone concentrations. Estrus was then suppressed throughout the 18 months of treatment in all 3 bitches receiving 32 µg/day and in 1 of 3 bitches receiving 8 µg/day (Fig. 2). The two bitches that expressed heat at 8 µg/day had their dosage increased to 16 µg/day and estrus did not occur during 18 months of treatment on that dose.

Measurement of the plasma concentrations of progesterone, which followed the induced heat and ovulation described above, indicated a lower than normal progesterone output [37] with shortened luteal phases, similar to the case in the study in which

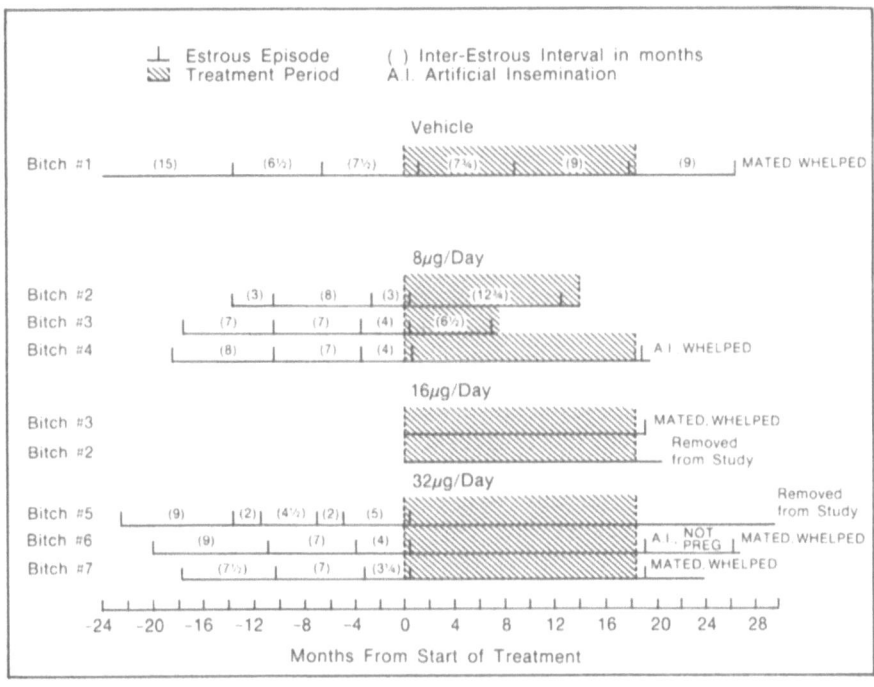

FIGURE 2.   Estrous episodes in beagle bitches before, during and after continuous treatment with 8, 16 or 32 µg/day of analog C or vehicle alone.

treatment started in proestrus. These findings suggested that fertility at the induced heat might be low. In order to evaluate this possibility, a further 3 bitches were treated continuously with 32 µg/day of analog B by subcutaneous osmotic pump starting between 92 and 100 days after a spontaneous heat. All three treated bitches exhibited an induced heat with sanguineous vaginal discharge and/or cornified cells in vaginal smears between 4 and 22 days after start of treatment. All three bitches were mated, at the induced heat, with a male beagle of proven fertility. Treatment was continued for at least 60 days. Uterine implantation sites were identified by abdominal palpation 3.5 to 4 weeks after mating in 1 of the 3 bitches. However, none of the bitches produced a litter or showed overt signs of pregnancy, abortion or parturition, indicating that fertility at the induced heat is low. This finding again has its parallel in other species. Although it must be stressed in the present instance that ovulation was inferred from a rise in progesterone levels and that follicular luteinization cannot be ruled out, induction of ovulation in anestrous sheep with LHRH was also followed by very low fertility [38].

Although the fertility at the induced heat has been demonstrated to be low, the induction of vaginal discharge and of behavioral estrus when treatment begins in anestrus is unwelcome. We therefore now evaluated alternative times to start treatment, which might not result in stimulation.

d) Treatment in the early prepubertal bitch. A convenient time to start treatment with a reversible estrus suppressant would be at the recommended time for routine vaccination, i.e. 3-4 months of age. This time in dogs is early prepubertal and studies in rats had demonstrated that starting LHRH agonist treatment at a very young age could delay puberty [39].

Accordingly, we began another study in which 32 µg per day of analog B was administered to each of 3 puppies. Treatment was started at 4 months of age and continued for 18 months. Estrus did not occur during treatment. Plasma progesterone concentrations remained below 0.3 ng/ml for the entire treatment period. Although body size and weight increased in a manner indistinguishable from controls, the vulvae remained immature in appearance for the duration of treatment. Estrus occurred within 4 months of cessation of treatment in all animals. All animals mated at that time but none conceived as judged by abdominal palpation. This is perhaps not surprising in view of the known low fertility at first estrus [40]. A second estrus occurred in these three bitches 6 to 6.7 months later and breeding at that time resulted in 2 pregnancies.

It thus appears that starting treatment prepuberally can reversibly postpone sexual development and puberty at least through 22 months of age, without overt signs of stimulation.

e) Treatment in the early post-partum bitch. In many species the lactational period following parturition is associated with suppressed ovarian function and responsivity, thought to be mediated through high levels of prolactin. We hypothesized that such a period in the bitch might be resistant to the initial

522

stimulatory effects of LHRH agonists. Accordingly, 7 bitches were treated with 32 µg per day of analog B starting either 1 day (4 bitches) or 7 days (3 bitches) postpartum and continuing for 56-60 days. None of these bitches showed overt signs of estrus in response to treatment, although in one animal (bitch B) progesterone levels were elevated between day 16 and day 64 postpartum with peak values between 6 and 7 ng/ml, consistent with incomplete luteinization (Fig. 3). Four other bitches (bitches C, D, E and G) showed transient elevation of plasma progesterone, to values between 1 and 2 ng/ml, immediately following initiation of treatment and lasting for 1 to 18 days. The timing of this response suggests that the luteal tissue of the recent pregnancy was re-activated by the LH released by the analog.

Reversibility. In the preceding sections, a variety of studies were presented showing that LHRH agonists can delay puberty or suppress estrus for periods of 12 to 18 months. Fourteen bitches

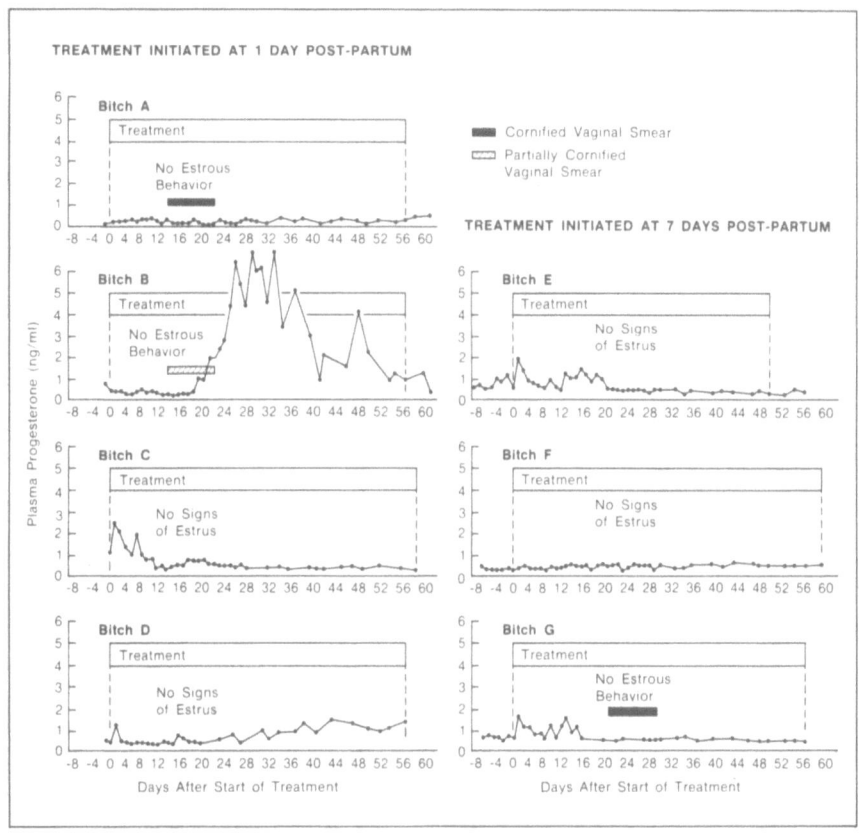

FIGURE 3. Plasma progesterone levels and signs of estrus in beagle bitches receiving continuous administration of 32 µg analog C/day starting at 1 or 7 days post-partum.

from studies described earlier, whose cycles were suppressed
during 12 to 18 months of treatment were followed until estrus
recurred to assess cyclicity and fertility following cessation of
treatment (Table 2). The first recovery estrus occurred at an
average of 3 months after the end of treatment. Ten bitches were
followed until a second estrus occurred and the average time
interval between the first and second estrus was 7 months.
Thirteen of 14 bitches were mated or artificially inseminated at
the first and/or second recovery estrus and 12 became pregnant and
whelped normal liters. These data show that estrus suppression
for up to 18 months with LHRH agonists is compatible with recovery
of normal cycling and fertility.

Table 2. Estrous cycle recovery and fertility following cessation of treatment in
bitches whose estrous cycles were suppressed during 12 or 18 months of continuous
treatment with analog A, B or C.

| | First Recovery Estrus | | Second Recovery Estrus | |
Start of Treatment	Months After End of Treatment	Result of Mating or Artificial Insemination	Months After 1st Recovery Estrus	Result of Mating or Artificial Insemination
Proestrus	0.7	PREGNANT	6.7	_a
	4.2	PREGNANT	6.3	_a
	3.8	_a	_b	_b
Diestrus	3.0	PREGNANT	6.5	_a
Anestrus	0.5	PREGNANT	_b	_b
	0.5	PREGNANT	_b	_b
	0.5	PREGNANT	_b	_b
	0.5	not pregnant	7.0	PREGNANT
Late Prepuberal (10-11 months old)	3.0	_c	6.0	PREGNANT
	8.0	PREGNANT	7.0	_a
	3.5	PREGNANT	7.0	_a
Early Prepuberal (4 months old)	4.0	not pregnant	6.7	not pregnant
	3.8	not pregnant	7.0	PREGNANT
	3.7	not pregnant	7.0	PREGNANT

[a]No mating was attempted. [b]Bitch was removed from study following first recovery
estrus. [c]Bitch refused male, no artificial insemination was performed.

Controlled release formulations. The studies described above
addressed the concept of reversible suppression of estrus by LHRH
agonists. However, daily injection or repetitive monthly
replacement of either cholesterol matrix pellets or osmotic
minipumps are not practical for widespread use. Radioimmunoassay
of blood samples obtained from animals receiving adequate estrus
suppressant doses of either analog B or C has established required
blood levels of these compounds (Table 3). This information is
now being used in the design of controlled release implantable or
injectable formulations. Injectable, biodegradable microsphere
formulations incorporating the analogs into copolymers of

524

Table 3. Plasma levels of analog B or analog C in beagle bitches during the first 6 weeks of continuous treatment by Alzet® pump

Dose	Bitch	Plasma Levels, mean ± S.E. (ng/ml)	
		Analog B (n=17 or 18)	Analog C (n=23)
8 µg/Day	1	0.21 ± 0.03	0.28 ± 0.02
	2	0.17 ± 0.02	0.14 ± 0.01
	3	0.16 ± 0.02	0.16 ± 0.02
16 µg/Day	1	–	0.28 ± 0.02
	2	–	0.25 ± 0.02
32 µg/Day	1	0.45 ± 0.08	0.66 ± 0.08
	2	0.50 ± 0.05	0.40 ± 0.04
	3	0.38 ± 0.04	0.59 ± 0.02

dl,polylactide-coglycolide have resulted in suppression of estrus for more than 1 year in rats [41]. A silicon elastomer matrix implant system delivered compound for more than 14 months in rats and was effective in suppressing male sexual function in monkeys over a 5.5 month observation period (E. Nieschlag, L. Sanders, B. Vickery, unpublished observations). The rapid advances in the technology of controlled release formulation, particularly as it applies to peptides, together with the low annual dose requirement of 12 or less mg of these LHRH agonists to suppress estrus, convince us that useful systems will be forthcoming shortly.

Interruption of heat with LHRH antagonists

The usual LHRH antagonist assay consists of administration of a range of doses of the compounds to rats at noon on the day of proestrus and establishment of an ED_{50} for prevention of ovulation [42]. On the basis of such an assay and by comparison with two literature standards (Table 4) we identified two promising compounds: analog F ([N-Ac-D-Nal(2)^1,D-pCl-Phe^2,D-Trp^3, D-hArg(Et$_2$)^6,D-Ala^{10}]LHRH; detirelix) and analog G ([N-Ac-D-Nal(2)^1,D-pCl-Phe^2,D-Pal(3)^3,D-hArg(Et$_2$)^6,D-Ala^{10}]LHRH). Further studies indicated analog G to be more potent in acute assays whereas analog F appeared to have a greater duration of action.

In a preliminary study analog F was administered to a mature beagle bitch starting at the first signs of proestrus (a sanguineous vaginal discharge). Seven consecutive daily doses of 300 µg/kg were administered subcutaneously. The proestrous vaginal cytology did not proceed in the normal fashion to a cornified appearance but rather regressed to an anestrous smear within 2 days of treatment. Estrous behaviour was prevented as the bitch would not accept the presence of a stud male (Table 5).

Table 4. Comparison of the ovulation inhibiting potency of various LHRH antagonistic analogs, when administered to rats at noon of proestrus

Analog	Structure	ED_{50}	Relative Potency
D	$[N-Ac-D-pCl-Phe^1,D-pCl-Phe^2,D-Trp^3,$ $D-Arg^6,D-Ala^{10}]LHRH$	1.8	100
E	$[N-Ac-D-Nal(2)^1,D-pF-Phe^2,D-Trp^3,$ $D-Arg^6]LHRH$	2.4	75
F	$[N-Ac-D-Nal(2)^1,D-pCl-Phe^2,D-Trp^3,$ $D-hArg(Et_2)^6,D-Ala^{10}]LHRH$ (detirelix)	0.7	257
G	$[N-Ac-D-Nal(2)^1,D-pCl-Phe^2,D-Pal(3)^3,$ $D-hArg(Et_2)^6,D-Ala^{10}]LHRH$	0.58	310

Circulating levels of estradiol declined, an LH surge was not detected and the animal did not ovulate as progesterone levels did not rise. This animal was detected in heat again 27 days after starting treatment.

We hypothesized that the treatment duration of 7 days might be causing the preovulatory follicles to suspend development and that a longer period of treatment might result in follicular atresia and regression and give a longer, more useful inter-estrus interval after treatment. A further 3 animals were therefore treated on a similar regimen but the treatment period was extended to 14 days. Although the average time to return of heat after

Table 5. Estrus interruption activity of subcutaneously injected analog F when given at onset of vaginal bleeding in beagle bitches

Dose	# Doses	# Showing Estrus Behavior	# Bitches Ovulating	Interval to Next Heat (Mean $\pm$ SEM)	# Pregnant Next Cycle
300 µg/kg	7	0/1	0/1	27 days	–
300 µg/kg	14	0/3	0/3	40 $\pm$ 6 days	1/1
2 mg/kg	1	2/9	0/13[a]	26 $\pm$ 1 days	6/6

[a]4 animals were treated again on the return heat.

start of treatment was prolonged slightly to 40 days, there was considerable variation.

A further group of nine animals was injected with a single i.m. dose approximating the sum of 7 days (2 mg/kg) of analog F on the first day of detected vaginal discharge. Four of these animals were reinjected at the first sign of heat returning after treatment. Other animals have been treated up to 4 times at the returning heats (data not shown). Although 2 animals did allow one day of breeding, other overt signs of heat were not present, no ovulations were detected. The return of heat was remarkably synchronous and suggests a useful management tool either for racing dogs or for commercial breeding purposes. All dogs bred at the first (in the case of 1 treatment) or subsequent return heat (in case of multiple treatments) have successfully conceived, attesting to the safety and utility of this approach.

Luteal suppression and termination of pregnancy

Previous studies had established 300 µg/kg of analog F to have luteal suppressive activity in rhesus (B. Vickery and G. McRae, unpublished) and stumptailed monkeys [43]. Accordingly, we administered 300 µg/kg/day of this analog by subcutaneous injection daily for seven days to two nonpregnant and one pregnant beagle bitchs during the mid-luteal/mid-gestational period. Plasma progesterone levels fell precipitously, were depressed to less than 2 ng/ml for the duration of treatment and resulted in abortion in the pregnant bitch (Fig. 4).

Luteal suppression in rhesus monkeys has been reported for another LHRH antagonist [44] and analog F has been noted to cause a precipitous decline in circulating levels and abortion in one of three pregnant baboons receiving approximately 200 µg/kg/day for seven days [45].

Analog G was administered by subcutaneous injection at 300 µg/kg/day for seven days to 3 pregnant beagle bitches during mid-gestation. Plasma progesterone levels declined in all 3 (Fig. 5); 1 bitch resorbed and 1 bitch aborted the pregnancy, progesterone levels subsequently rose to the normal range for the stage of pregnancy in the bitch that resorbed and a discharge was noted at term. The other two bitches continued through a normal pregnancy.

The same total dose (300 µg/kg/day) of analog G, when administered continuously for seven days by use of an osmotic minipump, maintained low levels of progesterone and terminated pregnancy in 2 of 2 treated bitches.

Studies in male dogs had indicated that remarkable duration of suppression of gonadal steroid output could be achieved from a single injection of higher doses of analog F (Fig. 6). Doubling of the dose from 1 mg/kg to 2 mg/kg extended the suppression from 4 to 12 days. We therefore evaluated the effect of 2 mg/kg of RS-68439 as a single injection given on different days of pregnancy. When this dose was given on day 20 or more of gestation pregnancy was routinely terminated. Treatment on day 15 was effective in 50% of treated animals but earlier treatment was

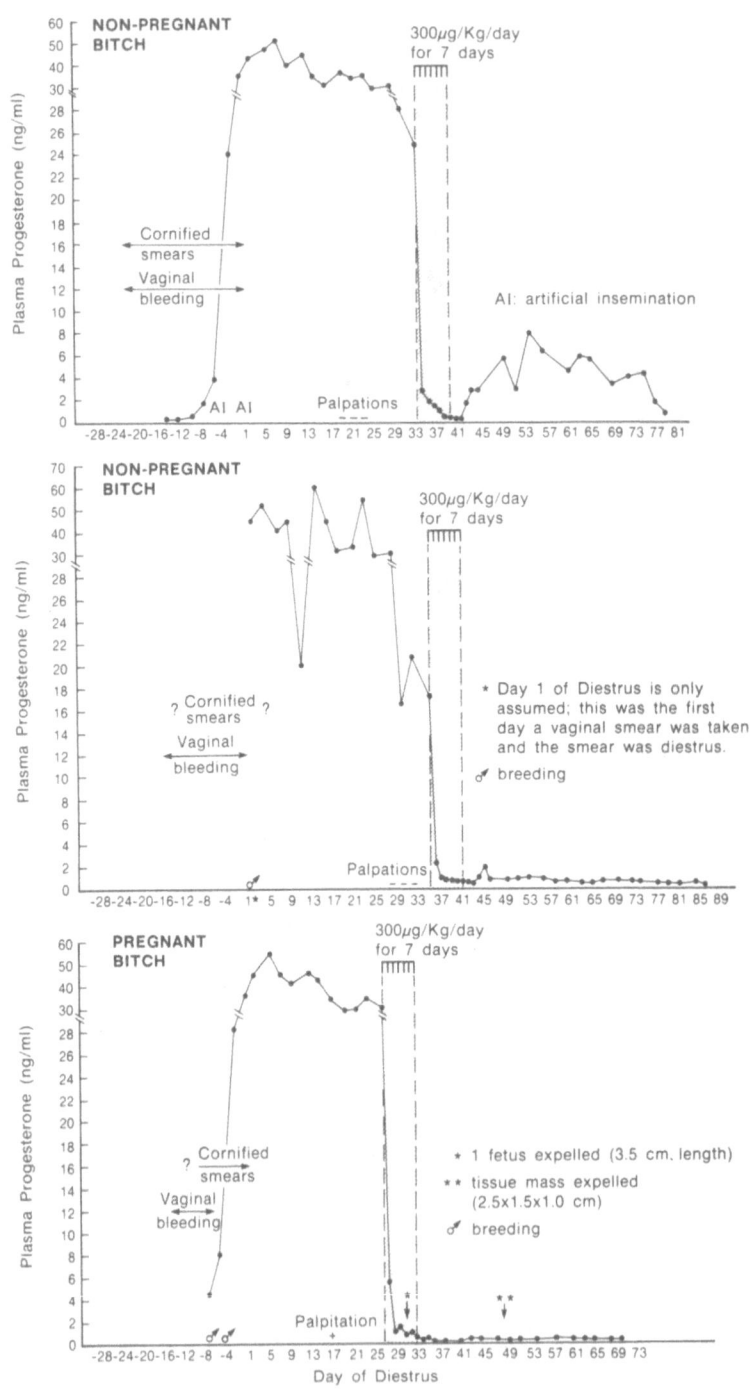

FIGURE 4. Plasma progesterone concentrations in nonpregnant and pregnant bitches receiving once daily subcutaneous injection of analog F during the mid-luteal phase.

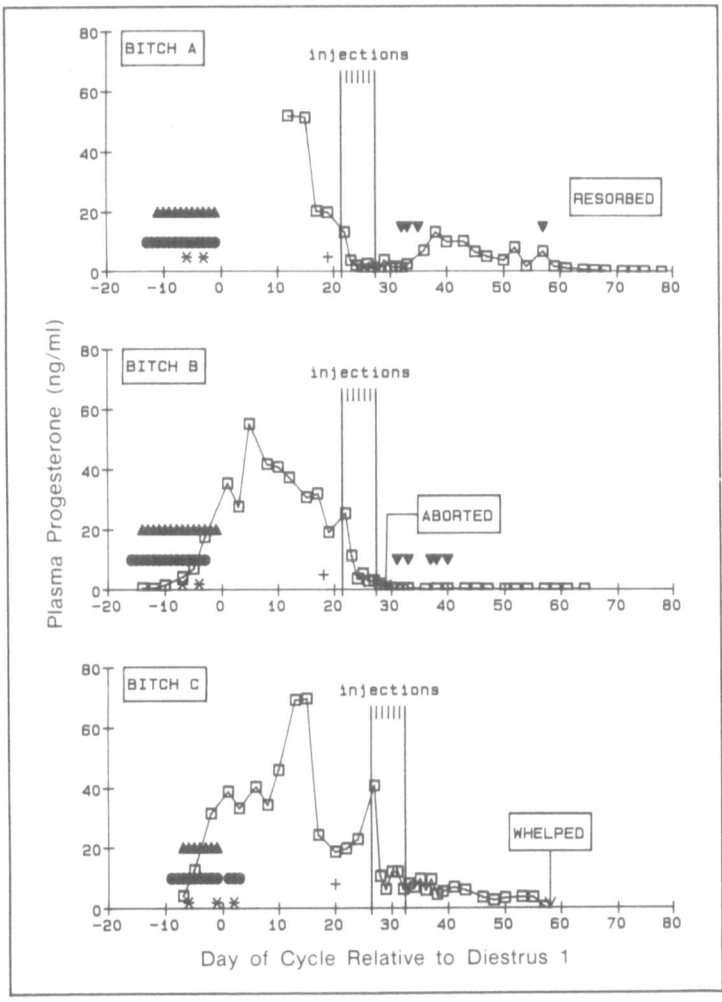

FIGURE 5. Plasma progesterone concentrations in pregnant bitches receiving once daily subcutaneous injections of 300 μg/kg/day of analog G during the mid-luteal phase (• vaginal bleeding; Δ cornified smear; * breeding or AI; ∇ vaginal discharge; + pregnancy diagnosis by abdominal palpation).

not successful. Analysis of circulating levels of progesterone revealed that early pregnancy treatment was associated with only a transient, incomplete fall in progesterone whereas later treatment caused a more complete, longer lasting suppression of gonadal steroid output (Fig. 7). This suggests a relative autonomy of the corpus luteum from pituitary gonadotropin requirement during early gestation. Most recently we have shown that injection of a

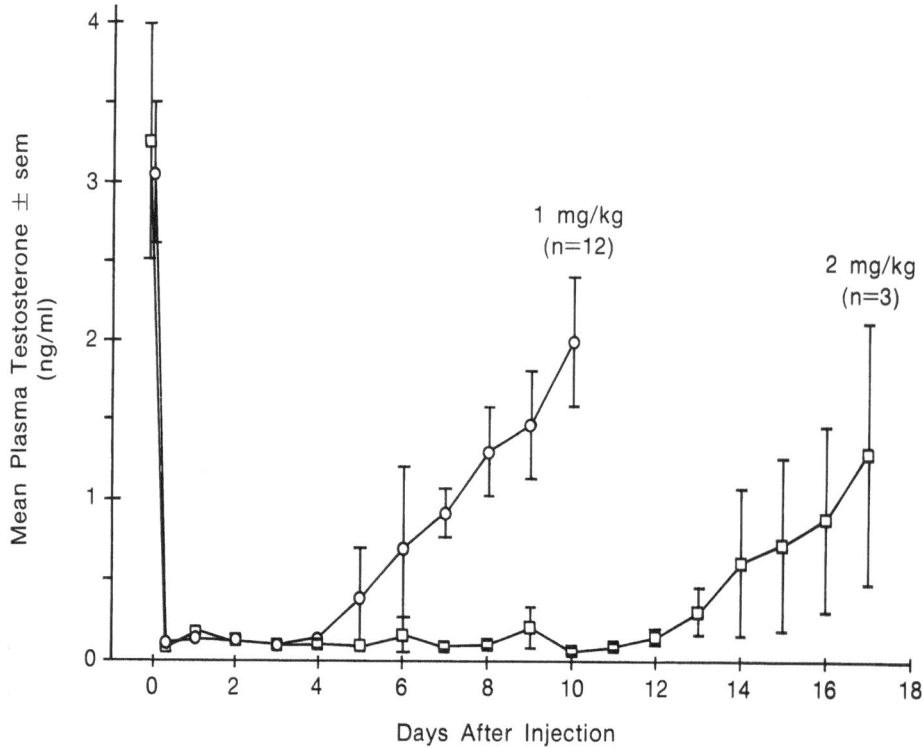

FIGURE 6. Plasma testosterone concentrations in male beagles following a single subcutaneous injection of analog F. Reproduced from Vickery, B.H. and Nestor, J.J. Jr. Sem. Reprod. Endocrinol., in press, by permission.

massive dose of analog F even as early as day 1 or 2 of gestation will terminate pregnancy. However, this results from progesterone withdrawal beginning 1-2 weeks after the treatment, i.e. the analog is present and gonadotropin suppression is prolonged until the time of luteal sensitivity is reached.

OTHER BENEFITS

As in other species, chronic treatment with LHRH analogs in the female dog may be likened to a reversible chemical ovariectomy. Thus, any disease or syndrome dependent on ovarian hormones should respond to treatment with LHRH analogs. The favorable responses to these agents in women with breast cancer [46,47] may also be

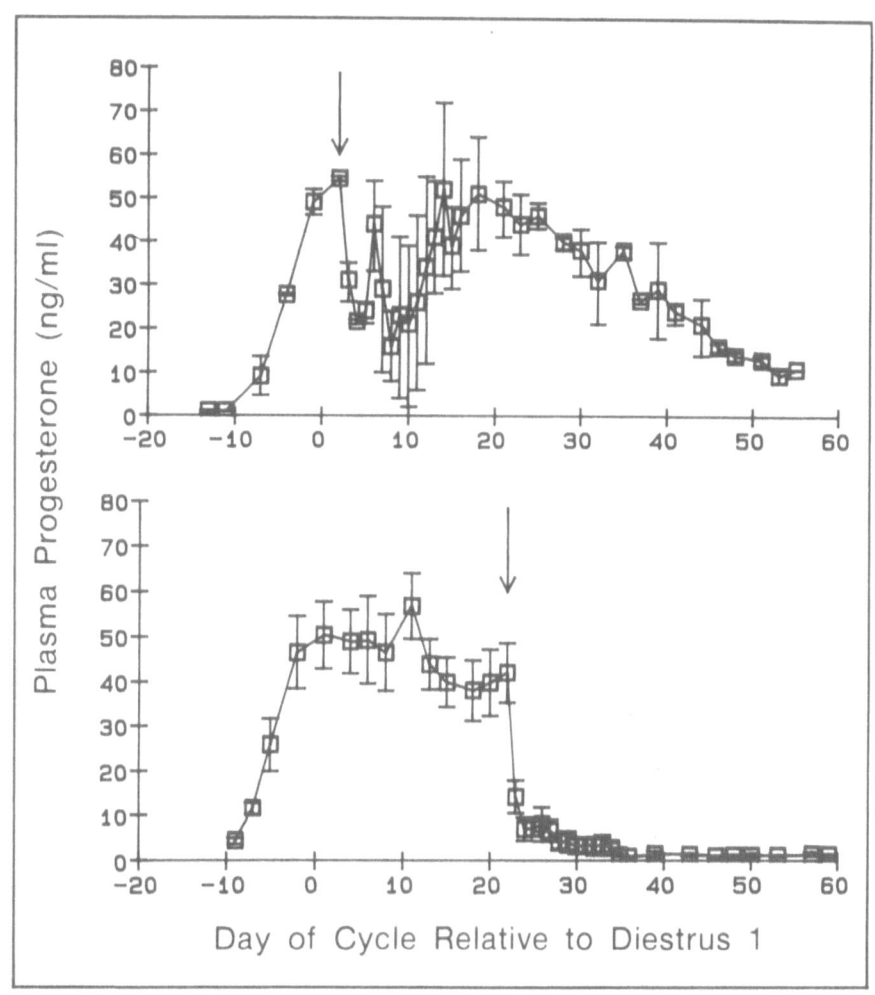

FIGURE 7. Plasma progesterone concentrations in pregnant beagle bitches receiving a single subcutaneous injection (arrow) of 2 mg/kg of analog F in the early luteal phase (upper panel, n=2, bars represent range) and mid-luteal phase (lower panel, n=5, mean ± SEM).

forecast for either benign or malignant mammary tumors in bitches. In addition, the progesterone-dependency of pyometra makes this condition likely to respond to LHRH analog treatment.

SUPPRESSION OF MALE SEXUAL FUNCTION

LHRH agonists

Early studies investigated the effect of daily s.c. administration of 10 µg/kg nafarelin in mature beagles [11]. The treatment caused a transient rise in plasma levels of testosterone followed by a marked decline to castrate levels by about 1 week of treatment. The testosterone withdrawal led to dry ejaculation by two to three weeks of daily treatment. Prior to the complete disappearance of ejaculatory volume there was a reduction in the numbers of normal, motile sperm and a corresponding increase in poorly motile sperm and immature cell stages in the ejaculate.

In the testis, by ten days of treatment, there was already a disruption of the cytoarchitecture of the seminiferous tubules with exfoliation of germ cells into the lumen and passage through the reproductive tract. By 6 weeks of treatment only spermatogonia and Sertoli cells remained in the tubules. These changes were reflected by decrease in testicular volume to a nadir of 30-40% of the value prior to treatment.

Dose response studies. Decreasing the daily dose of nafarelin to 2 µg/kg gave results which were superimposable on those at 10 µg/kg/day [12]. A further reduction of dose to 0.5 µg/kg/day prolonged the time required to achieve castrate levels of testosterone (3 weeks) and to inhibit ejaculation (6 weeks) (Fig. 8). This is probably a reflection of the more gradual evolution of desensitization at the pituitary level (Fig. 9). Complete inhibition of spermatogenesis was again evident histologically at 6 weeks of treatment even at the dose of 0.5 µg/kg/day. Lower doses have not been evaluated.

Time course of reversibility. Following the cessation of very short periods of analog B treatment e.g. 10 days in male beagles, plasma testosterone levels are within the normal range after only 4 days and ejaculate volume is normal after one week (Fig. 10). Sperm counts, however, continue to decline, reach their nadir 2-3 weeks later, and require a further 3 weeks to re-enter the normal range.

After more extended periods of treatment, such as 6 weeks, return to normal plasma levels of testosterone is more gradual and takes 2-3 weeks. Detectable ejaculate volume is not achieved until 6 weeks after stopping treatment and these ejaculates, which progressively increase in volume, are azoospermic for a further two weeks. Following appearance of sperm in the ejaculate at 8-9 weeks after cessation of treatment sperm numbers increase rapidly and are in the normal range 3 weeks later. The high degree of correlation of appearance of sperm in the ejaculate with the 8 week duration of the spermatogenic cycle in dogs [48] indicates the very rapid resumption of spermatogenesis when treatment is stopped.

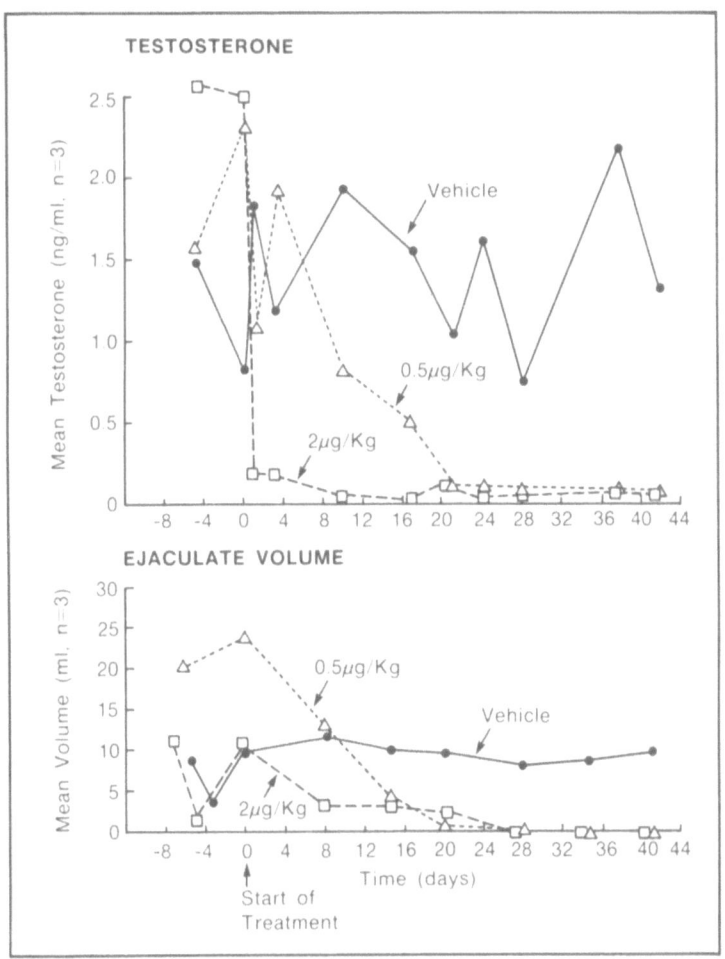

FIGURE 8.   Plasma concentrations of testosterone (upper panel) and ejaculate volume (lower panel) in male beagles injected subcutaneously once daily with analog B for 42 days.

With the exception of a rather more extended time to recovery of normal circulating testosterone values, a very similar pattern was observed following cessation of long-term treatment of 1 year duration [49].   Again, normal sperm numbers in the ejaculate were rapidly regained.   The only adverse effect noted for this long-term treatment was that the animals showed some discomfort for the first 2-3 ejaculations after cessation of treatment.   This observation did not persist and probably reflects some slower reversal of atrophic changes in the reproductive tract, because of the very extended period of time in which only castrate circulatory levels of testosterone were present.

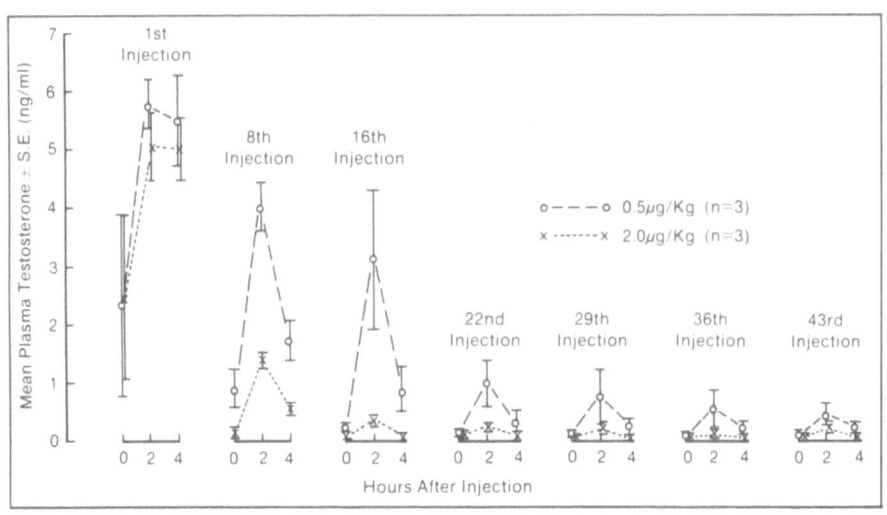

FIGURE 9. Acute LH response to daily injections of analog B in the male dog

Sustained release formulations. With the exception of some early work using a cholesterol matrix implant [30] all of the reported studies on the effects of LHRH agonist analogues in male dogs have been conducted using daily injection. The exponential decay in release rate from the cholesterol matrices and their short duration of action (30-60 days) make such implants uneconomic. However, it is clear that for long-term suppression of male sexual function in dogs with these peptides to be a viable proposition, a long-term sustained release formulation will be required. A good deal of effort is being extended toward this goal [50,51]. Perhaps the most promising are silastic matrix implants which can have a duration of release of 14 months or more and have been shown to suppress male sexual function in rhesus monkeys [52]. Alternative possibilities include implants of poly(dl,lactide-coglycolide) of relatively high lactide content [50,53] and the less extensively evaluated poly-ortho esters [54].

LHRH antagonists

In preliminary studies, analog F was evaluated for duration of action on pituitary gonadotropin release indirectly through effect on plasma levels of testosterone. Single subcutaneous injection of various doses of analog F was given to male beagles [55]. Plasma levels of testosterone were maximally suppressed for 8 hours after injection of 4 µg/kg. However, for suppression through 24 hours a dose of 100 µg/kg was required.

Accordingly, we elected to assess the effect on sexual function of 20 and 100 µg/kg administered by daily injection for

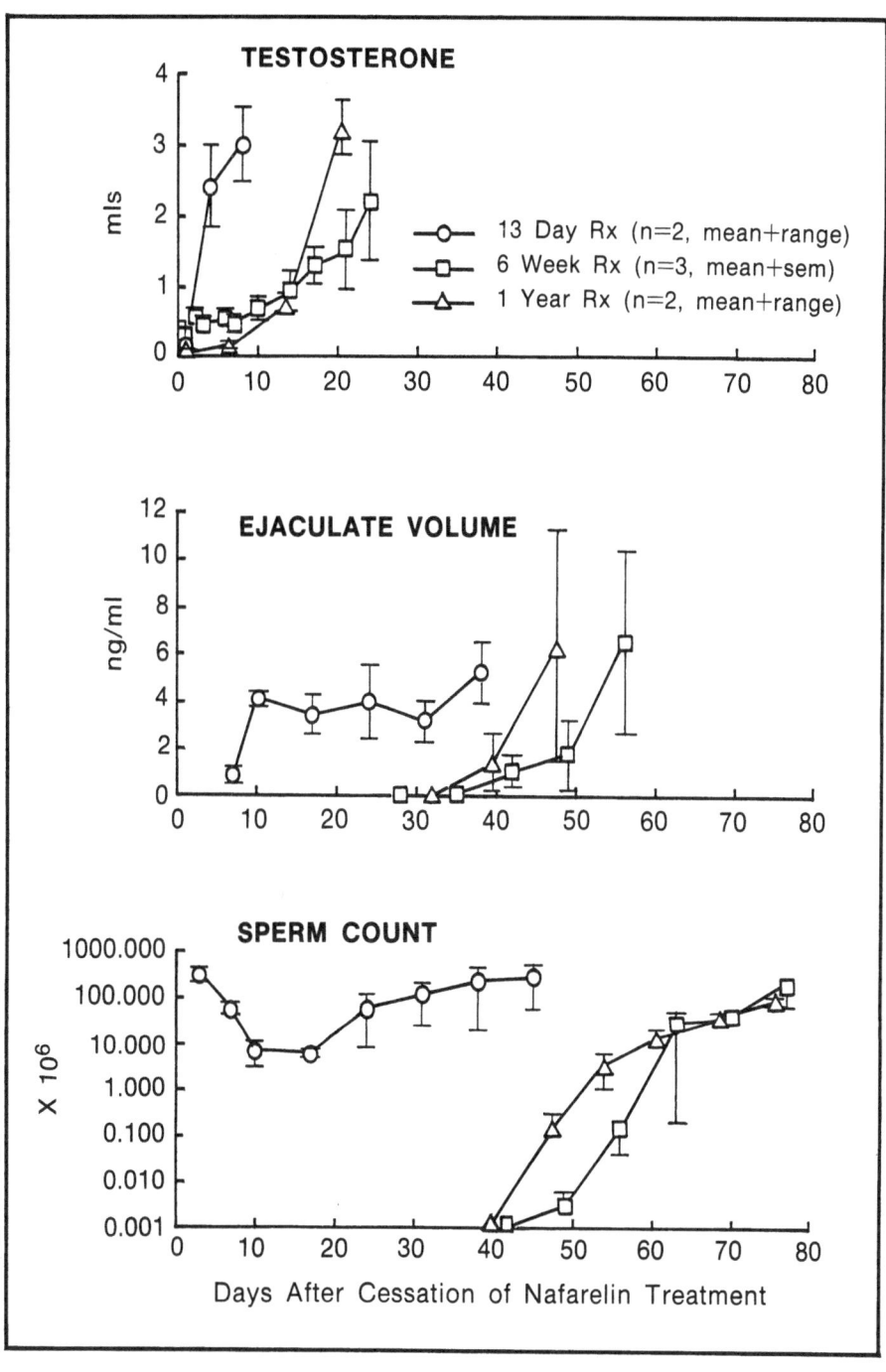

FIGURE 10. Reversibility of effects of analog B on plasma testosterone, ejaculate volume and sperm numbers after dosing for different periods of time.

63 days.   Plasma levels of testosterone in blood samples drawn
prior to the daily injection were consistently suppressed by the
dose   of   100 µg/kg   but   not   by   20 µg/kg (Fig. 11).   The

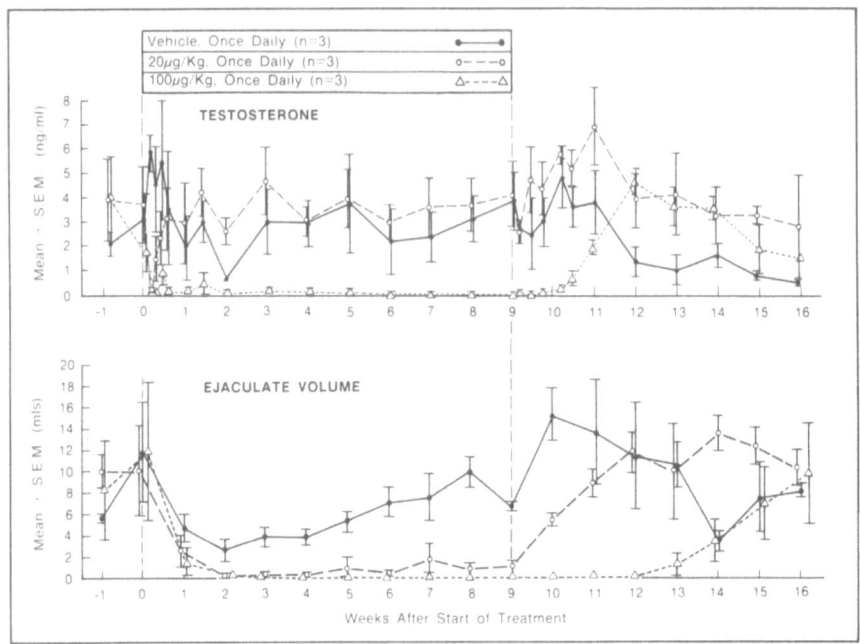

Figure 11. Plasma   testosterone   concentrations   (upper   panel)   and
           ejaculate   volumes   (lower   panel)   in   male   beagles
           receiving   once   daily   subcutaneous   injections   of
           analog F.

testosterone   withdrawal   in   dogs   receiving   100 µg/kg/day   of
analog F resulted in dry ejaculation by 3 weeks of treatment.
Interestingly, the withdrawal of testosterone each day, for less
than   24 hours,   in   the   animals   receiving   20 µg/kg/day   also
profoundly affected accessory organ secretion, as ejaculate
volumes declined to less than 1 ml in these dogs.   The lesser
degree of suppression was also reflected by the greater rapidity
of return to normal ejaculate volume after cessation of treatment
with 20 µg/kg/day than of 100 µg/kg/day.
     Following   cessation   of   treatment   with   100 µg/kg/day   of
analog F circulating levels of testosterone returned to the normal
range in 2 weeks; ejaculate volumes were measurable at 4 weeks and
were in the normal ranges two weeks later.   These early ejaculates
were azoospermic;   first   sperm   were   detected   7-10 weeks   after
stopping treatment.   Total sperm numbers then rose rapidly to the
normal 10^9 - 10^{10} in the following 3 weeks.   The timing of

appearance of sperm correlates well with the duration of the spermatogenic cycle in dogs [48] and this, plus the rapidity with which normal numbers are regained, suggests no carry-over effect.

Effects in cystic hyperplasia of the prostate and other androgen dependent syndromes

The rapid and sustained suppression of circulating levels of testosterone caused by administration of LHRH analogs to male dogs in addition to suppressing sexual function may have other therapeutic benefits. Cystic hyperplasia of the prostate regresses in response to LHRH analog treatment [10,56]. Prostatic cancer is alleviated in men with remission for extended periods of time; disappearance of bone and pleural metastases also occurs in some instances [57,58]. There is no reason why this malignant condition should not respond also in dogs. Other possible benefits may include regression of perianal tumors and alleviation of aggressive behavior, both of which are thought to be androgen dependent.

CONCLUDING REMARKS

It is clear that chronic administration of very low doses of the highly potent agonistic analogs of LHRH can reversibly inhibit the occurrence of estrus in bitches. Starting treatment during a spontaneous heat will likely not prevent fertility at that heat so that for such timing of treatment to be contraceptive, segregation would be needed initially. Treatment begun during anestrus allows expression of a transitory, stimulatory action of the LHRH agonist and although the fertility of the induced estrus appears to be low the inconvenience of the proestrous discharge and the estrous behavior would probably make this timing undesirable. However, starting treatment during diestrus (within 45 days of spontaneous heat), or up to 7 days postpartum, or at 4 months of age appears to effectively and indefinitely postpone the next heat episode without initial stimulation. These latter timings for starting treatment would probably be those of choice for eventual utilization of LHRH agonists for contraception. For the practical application of these materials further development of controlled release technology is required and such further development is viewed as promising. The nonsteroidal nature of these agents makes it unlikely that the problems associated in the past with the contraceptive use of steroids will impact on this treatment. On the contrary, the chemical equivalence to surgical castration makes it likely that therapeutic benefits in addition to contraception may result from treatment of bitches with these LHRH agonists.

Nafarelin (analog B) is a potent and effective agent to suppress sexual function in male dogs. Daily or continuous administration will rapidly inhibit libido, sperm motility, ejaculation and spermatogenesis, each of which would be expected to be contraceptive. Long-term dosage is compatible with rapid reversion of circulating testosterone levels to normal values after cessation of treatment; reappearance of sperm in the ejaculate is more protracted and dependent upon the length of the spermatogenic cycle. Use of the peptide is expected to carry the additional benefits of alleviation of androgen-dependent syndromes, in particular both benign and malignant prostatic hyperplasia. With regard to the antagonistic analogs of LHRH, long term suppressive effects on gonadal function in both sexes can again be achieved. However this clearly requires a higher dose and therefore a higher cost than with the agonistic analogs. It appears therefore that the preferred use of the antagonistic analogs will be in the female in situations such as interruption of heat and termination of pregnancy, for which the agonists are ineffective and in which the antagonists can act by a single administration.

Thus we visualize nonduplicative clinical utilities in dogs for both agonistic and antagonistic analogs of LHRH which, particularly in the field of fertility control, could be complementary and exert a major impact on control of the pet population.

REFERENCES

1. Zatuchni, G.I., Shelton, J.D. and Sciarra, J.J. (Eds.) "LHRH Peptides as Female and Male Contraceptives, Harper & Row, Philadelphia, 1981.
2. Vickery, B.H., Nestor, J.J. Jr. and Hafez, E.S.E. (Eds.) "LHRH and Its Analogs: Contraceptive and Therapeutic Applications", MTP Press, Boston, 1984.
3. Labrie, F., Belanger, A. and Dupont, A. (Eds.) "LHRH and Its Analogues: Basic and Clinical Aspects", Elsevier Science Publishers, New York, 1984.
4. Labrie, F., Belanger, A., Seguin, C., Cusan, L., Pelletier, G., Lefebvre, F-A., Kelly, P.A., Ferland, L., Reeves, J.J., Lemay, A. and Raynaud, J-P. Inhibition of testicular and ovarian functions by LHRH agonists. In "Bioregulators of Reproduction" Jagiello, G. and Vogel, H.J. (Eds.). Academic Press, New York, 1981, p. 305.
5. Corbin, A. and Beattie, C.W. Post-coital contraceptive and uterotrophic effects of luteinizing hormone-releasing hormone. Endocr. Res. Commun., $\underline{2}$, 445 (1975).
6. Herschler, R.C. and Vickery, B.H. The effects of [D-Trp[6], DesGly[10],ProNH$_2$ [9]]LHRH ethylamide on the estrous cycle, weight gain and feed efficiency in feedlot heifers. Am. J. Vet. Res. $\underline{42}$, 1405 (1981).
7. Vickery, B.H. Female contraceptive potential of "super" agonists of LHRH as assessed in infrahuman primates. In "LHRH Peptides as Female and Male Contraceptives", G.I. Zatuchni, J.D. Shelton, and J.J. Sciarra (Eds), Harper & Row, Philadelphia, 1981, p. 109.

8. Vickery, B.H. and McRae, G.I. Effects of continuous treatment with superagonists of LHRH when initiated at different times of the menstrual cycle in female baboons. Int. J. Fertil., 25, 171 (1980).

9. Fraser, H.M., Laird, N.C. and Blakeley, D.M Decreased pituitary responsiveness and inhibition of luteinizing hormone surge and ovulation in the stumptailed monkey (Macaca arctoides) by chronic treatment with an agonist of luteinizing hormone-releasing hormone. Endocrinology, 106, 452 (1980).

10. Vickery, B.H., McRae, G.I. and Bonasch, H. Effect of chronic administration of a highly potent LHRH agonist on prostate size and secretory function in geriatric dogs. The Prostate, 3, 123 (1982).

11. Vickery, B.H., McRae, G.I., Briones, W., Worden, A., Seidenberg, R., Schanbacher, B.D. and Falvo, R. Effect of an LHRH agonist analog upon sexual function in male dogs: suppression, reversibility and effect of testosterone replacement. J. Androl. 5, 28 (1984).

12. Vickery, B.H., McRae, G.I., Briones, W.V., Roberts, B.B., Worden, A.C., Schanbacher, B.D. and Falvo, R.E. Dose response studies on male reproductive parameters in dogs with nafarelin acetate, a potent LHRH agonist. J. Androl., 6, 53 (1985).

13. Waxman, J., Man, A., Hendry, W.F., Whitfield, H.N., Besser, G.M., Tiptaft, R.C., Paris, A.M. and Oliver, R.T. Importance of early tumor exacerbation in patients treated with long-acting analogues of gonadotrophin-releasing hormone for advanced prostatic cancer. Brit. Med. J. 291, 1387 (1985).

14. Kahan, A., Delrieu, F., Amor, B., Chiche, R. and Steg, A. Disease flare induced by D-Trp[6]-LHRH analogue in patients with metastatic prostate cancer. Lancet 1, 971 (1984).

15. Kerbrat, P., Toussaint, C., Gedjuin, D. and Lobel, B. Aggravation of obstructive renal insufficiency by prostate cancer under treatment with a gonadorelin agonist. Presse Med. 15, 165 (1986).

16. Deghenghi, R. and Misset, J.L. Disease flare induced by luteinizing hormone-releasing hormone analogues in cancer patients. Lancet 2, 1302 (1984).

17. Vickery, B.H., McRae, G.I., Sanders, L.M., Hoffman, P. and Parlou, S. Studies with nafarelin and a long-acting LHRH antagonist. In "Hormonal Manipulation of Cancer", Klijn, J. (Ed.) Raven Press, New York, 1986.

18. Rees, R.W.A., Foell, T.J., Chai, S-Y. and Grant, N. Synthesis and biological activities of LHRH modified in position 2. J. Med. Chem., 17, 1016 (1974).

19. Vickery, B.H. Pharmacology of LHRH Antagonists. Furr, B.J.A. and Wakeling, A. (Eds.) "Pharmacology and Clinical Uses of Inhibitors of Hormone Secretion and Action". Praeger Scientific, Eastbourne, 1986, in press.

20. Rivier, C., Rivier, J. and Vale, W. Antireproductive effects of a potent GnRH antagonist in the female rat. Endocrinology, 108, 1425 (1981).

21. Asch, R.H., Balmaceda, J.P. and Borghi, M. LHRH antagonists in rhesus and cynomolgus monkeys. In "LHRH and Its Analogs: Contraceptive and Therapeutic Applications", B.H. Vickery, J.J. Nestor, Jr. and E.S.E. Hafez (Eds), MTP Press, Lancaster, 1984, p. 107.

22. Weinbauer, G.F., Surmann, F.J., Akhtar, F.B., Shah, G.F., Vickery, B.H. and Nieschlag, E. Reversible inhibition of testicular function by a gonadotropin hormone-releasing hormone antagonist in monkeys (Macaca fascicularis). Fertil. Steril., 42, 1985, in press.

23. McRae, G.I., Vickery, B.H., Nestor, J.J. Jr., Bremner, W.J. and Badger, T.M. Biological evaluation of a highly potent LHRH antagonist. In "LHRH and Its Analogs: Contraceptive and Therapeutic Applications", B.H. Vickery, J.J. Nestor Jr., and E.S.E. Hafez (Eds), MTP Press, Lancaster, 1984, p. 137.

24. Corbin, A. From contraception to cancer: a review of the therapeutic applications of LHRH analogues an antitumor agents. Yale J. Biol. Med., 55, 27 (1982).

25. Redding, T.W., Coy, D.H. and Schally, A.V. Prostate carcinoma tumor size in rats decreases after administration of antagonists of luteinizing hormone-releasing hormone. Proc. Natl. Acad. Sci. U.S.A., 79, 1273 (1982).

26. Schally, A.V., Comaru-Schally, A.M. and Redding, T.W. Antitumor effects of analogs of hypothalamic hormones in endocrine- dependent cancers. Proc. Soc. Exp. Biol. Med., 175, 259 (1984).

27. Gonzalez-Barcena, D., Rangel-Garcia, N.E., Perez-Sanchez, P.L., Gutierrez-Dampenio, C., Garcia-Carrasco, F., Comaru-Schally, A.M. and Schally, A.V. Response to D-Trp[6]-LH-RH in advanced adenocarcinoma of pancreas. Lancet, July 10, 154 (1986).

28. Nestor, J.J. Jr., Tahilramani, R., Ho, T.L., McRae, G.I. and Vickery, B.H. New luteinizing hormone-releasing factor antagonists. In "Peptides-Structure and Function. Proceedings of the Eight American Peptide Symposium" V.J. Hruby, and D.H. Rich, D.H. (Eds), Pierce Chem. Co., Rockford, Illinois, 1983, p. 861.

29. Nestor, J.J. Jr., Ho., T.L., Tahilramani, R., McRae, G.I. and Vickery, B.H. Long acting LHRH agonists and antagonists. J. Steroid Biochem., 20, 1366 (A3) (1984).

30. Kent, J.S., Vickery, B.H. and McRae, G.I. The use of cholesterol matrix pellet implants for early studies on the prolonged release in animals of agonist analogues of luteinizing hormone-releasing hormone. Proc. 7th Int. Symp. on Controlled Release of Bioactive Materials. Fort Lauderdale, Florida, 1980.

31. Nestor, J.J. Jr., Ho, T.L., Simpson, R.A., Horner, B.L., Jones, G.H., McRae, G.I. and Vickery, B.H. The synthesis and biological activity of some very hydrophobic analogs of luteinizing hormone releasing hormone. J. Med. Chem., 25, 795 (1982).

32. McRae, G.I., Roberts, B.B., Worden, A.C., Bajka, A. and Vickery, B.H. Longterm, reversible suppression of oestrus in bitches with nafarelin acetate, a potent LHRH agonist. J. Reprod. Fert., 74, 389 (1985).

33. Lemay, A., Faure, N. and Labrie, F. Induction of luteolysis by postovulatory intranasal administration of [D-Ser(TBU)^6-des-Gly-NH$_2$ ^{10}]LHRH ethylamide (buserelin): a postcoital contraceptive approach. In "LHRH Peptides as Female and Male Contraceptives", G.I. Zatuchni, J.D. Shelton, and J.J. Sciarra (Eds), Harper & Row, Philadelphia, 1981, p. 184.

34. Casper, R.F., Sheehan, K.L. and Yen, S.S.C. Chorionic gonadotropin prevents LRH-agonist-induced luteolysis in the human. Contraception, 21, 471 (1980).

35. Skarin, G., Nillius, S.J. and Wide, L. Failure to induce abortion of early human pregnancy by high doses of a superactive LRH agonist. Contraception, 26, 457 (1982).

36. Vickery, B.H. and McRae, G. Antagonism by an LHRH agonist of the steroidogenic effects of exogenous human chorionic gonadotrophin in the female primate. Life Sci., 27, 1409 (1980).

37. Concannon, J.W., Hansel, W. and Visek, W.J. The ovarian cycle of the bitch: plasma estrogen, LH and progesterone. Biol. Reprod., 13, 112 (1975).

38. McLeod, B.J., Haresign, W. and Lamming, G.E. Response of seasonally anoestrous ewes to small-dose multiple injections of Gn-RH with and without progesterone pretreatment. J. Reprod. Fert., 65, 223 (1982).

39. Johnson, E.S., Gendrich, R.L. and White, W.F. Delay of puberty and inhibition of reproductive processes in the rat by a gonadotrophin releasing hormone agonist analog. Fertil. Steril., 27, 852 (1976).

40. Olson, P.N., Husted, P.W., Allen, T.A. and Nett, T.M. Reproductive endocrinology and physiology of the bitch and queen. Vet. Clin. North Am.: Small Anim. Pract. 14, 927 (1984).

41. Sanders, L.M., Kell, B.A., McRae, G.I. and Whitehead, G.W. Poly(lactic-co-glycolic)acid: properties and performance in controlled release delivery systems of LHRH analogues. Proceedings of 12th International Symposium on Controlled Release of Bioactive Materials, Geneva, Switzerland, 1985.

42. Corbin, A. and Beattie, C.W. Inhibition of the preovulatory proestrous gonadotropin surge, ovulation and pregnancy with a peptide analogue of LH-RH. Endocr. Res. Commun., 2, 1 (1975).

43. Fraser, H.M., Abbott, M., Laird, N.C., McNeilly, A.S. Nestor, J.J. Jr. and Vickery, B.H. Effects of an LH-releasing hormone antagonist on the secretion of LH, FSH, prolactin and ovarian steroids at different stages of the luteal phase in the stumptailed macaque. J. Endocrinol., 1986, in press.

44. Collins, R.L., Sopelak, V.M., Williams, R.F. and Hodgen, G.D. Induction of luteolysis and menstruation by a GnRH antagonist in primates. Prog. 31st Ann. Meet. Soc. Gynec. Invest., Washington D.C., p. 72 (1984).

45. Siler-Khodr, T.M., Kuehl, T. and Vickery, B. Action of a GnRH antagonist on the pregnant baboon. Program of the Annula Meeting of the Society for Gynecologic Investigation. Phoenix, Arizona, 1985.

46. Klijn, J.G.M. and DeJong, F.H. Treatment with a luteinizing hormone-releasing hormone analogue (buserelin) in premenopausal patients with metastatic breast cancer. Lancet, ii, 1213 (1982).

47. Harvey, H.A., Lipton, A. and Max, D.T. LHRH analogs for human mammary carcinoma. In "LHRH and Its Analogs: Contraceptive and Therapeutic Applications" B.H. Vickery, J.J. Nestor, Jr. and E.S.E. Hafez (Eds), MTP Press, Lancaster, 1984, p. 329.

48. Foote, R.H., Swierstra, E.E. and Hunt, W.L. Spermato-genesis in the dog. Anat. Rec., 173, 341 (1972).

49. Goodpasture, J.C., Bergstrom, K., Waller, D.P. and Vickery, B.H. (1985). Interactions between an LHRH analogue and cancer chemotherapeutic agents at the testicular level. In "LHRH Analogs: Basic and Clinical Aspects" Labrie, F., Belanger, A. and Dupont, A. (Eds). Elsevier, N. Holland, 1984, p. 156.

50. Vickery, B.H., McRae, G.I., Nestor, J.J. Jr., Sanders, L.M. and Kent, J. In vivo assessment of long acting formulations of LHRH analogs. In "Long Acting Contraceptive Delivery Systems" G.I. Zatuchni, A. Goldsmith, J.D. Shelton, and J.J. Sciarra (Eds), Harper & Row, Philadelphia, 1984, p. 180.

51. Sanders, L.M., McRae, G.I., Vitale, K.M., Vickery, B.H. and Kent, J.S. An injectable biodegradable controlled release delivery system for nafarelin acetate. In "LHRH Analogs: Basic and Clinical Aspects" Labrie, F., Belanger, A. and Dupont, A. (Eds.). Elsevier, N. Holland, 1984, p. 53.

52. Akhtar, F.B., Weinbauer, G.F., Vickery, B.H., Sanders, L.M. and Nieschlag, E. Pituitary and testicular function in rhesus monkeys under long-term sustained release of [D-Nal(2)^6]LHRH. Prog. 3rd Joint Meet. Brit. Endocr. Soc., Edinburgh, 1985.

53. Kent, J.S., Sanders, L.M., Tice, T.R. and Lewis, D.H. Microencapsulation of the peptide nafarelin acetate for controlled release. In "Long Acting Contraceptive Delivery Systems", G.I. Zatuchni, A. Goldsmith, J.D. Shelton, and J.J. Sciarra (Eds), Harper & Row, Philadelphia, 1984, p. 113.

54. Heller, J., Penhale, D.W.H., Fritzinger, B.K. and Ng, S.Y. Controlled release of contraceptive agents from poly(ortho) esters. In "Long Acting Contraceptive Delivery Systems", G.I. Zatuchni, A. Goldsmith, J.D. Shelton, and J.J. Sciarra (Eds), Harper & Row, Philadelphia, 1984, p. 113.

55. Vickery, B.H., McRae, G.I., Donahue, D.J., Roberts, B.B. and Worden, A.C. Suppression of testicular function in dogs with a highly potent LHRH antagonist. Program of IIIrd Int. Congress of Androl., Boston, Massachusetts, 1985.

56. Dube´, J.Y., Frenette, G., Tremblay, R.R., Tremblay, Y. and Belanger, A. Involution of spontaneous benign prostatic hyperplasia in the dog under the influence of chronic treatment with a LHRH agonist. The Prostate, 5, 417 (1984).
57. Faure, N., Lemay, A., Tolis, G., Labrie, F., Belanger, A. and Fazekas, A.T.A. Buserelin therapy for prostatic carcinoma. In "LHRH and Its Analogs: Contraceptive and Therapeutic Applications, B.H. Vickery, J.J. Nestor, Jr. and E.S.E. Hafez (Eds), MTP Press, Lancaster, 1984, p. 337.
58. Santen, R.J., Warner, B., Demers, L.M., Dufau, M. and Smith, J.A. Jr. Leuprolide therapy for prostatic cancer. In "LHRH and Its Analogs: Contraceptive and Therapeutic Applications", B.H. Vickery, J.J. Nestor, Jr. and E.S.E. Hafez (Eds), MTP Press, Lancaster, 1984, p. 351.

SECTION 10

FORMULATION AND METABOLISM

35

Intra-nasal Administration of LHRH and its Analogs

B. H. VICKERY

Department of Physiology, Institute of Biological Sciences, Syntex Research,
Palo Alto, CA 94304, USA

INTRODUCTION

The high peptidase activity present in the gastrointestinal tract
would be expected to result in rapid degradation of LHRH. In
addition, it is known that peptides of more than 3 amino acids,
even if resistant to proteolysis, are extremely poorly absorbed
across the intestinal mucosa. Together, these factors account for
the vanishingly small (0.01-0.1%) bioavailability of LHRH and its
agonist analogues by the oral versus parenteral routes. Even the
multiply substituted, metabolically blocked, LHRH antagonists
still only have oral bioavailabilities in the range of 0.1-1%.

Daily administration by injection is tolerable to patients
with life threatening disease, for example insulin for diabetics
and, LHRH agonists for prostatic cancer patients. It is not
preferred in these instances and is probably unacceptable for
non-life threatening disease such as endometriosis or hirsutism.

Attempts to increase acceptability and compliance for the
parenteral route with LHRH analogs have included the development
of injectable or inplantable sustained/controlled release
formulations, which continually administer drug for a month or
more after placement [1].

While these formulations will clearly be useful in certain
circumstances, the need to individualize the dose of agonist to
lessen side effects, and concerns about the therapeutic ratio for
the antagonists, leave the need open for a daily, noninvasive form
of therapy. This need seems to be satisfied by the intranasal
route of delivery. Bioavailability of the LHRH analogs lies in
the range of 2-5% from simple aqueous solutions. However, a
number of absorption enhancers have been described which enable
several fold increases in bioavailability. In addition,
considerable progress has been made in the development of metered
spray devices, enabling extremely accurate dispensing of dose.
Some of these developments have been recently reviewed [2].

547

EARLY STUDIES WITH LHRH

Early studies of intranasally administered LHRH evaluated absorption by reference to changes in circulating levels of LH and/or FSH. These responses are sensitive to very small amounts of absorbed LHRH. Dose levels of 2-5 mg of LHRH administered in 0.5 ml of saline or distilled water elevated blood levels of LH in a similar manner to 100 µg administered i.v. [3,4]. Changes in FSH were less marked.

A much higher dose was required by intranasal administration than by injection [5,6]. Transport across all mucous membranes is not equal. High doses of LHRH [4] or a potent analog, nafarelin [M. Henzl, personal communication] administered sublingually or buccally are without effect. Absorption from the vagina is detectable but much less than from the nasal chamber [7].

When the dose volume was controlled and reduced to 100 µl, minimizing losses due to drainage, a linear dose response for integrated values of LH was obtained in men over a range of 0.5-2.0 mg of LHRH [8]. Responses in women were less clear cut.

A bioavailability of 1% was found for intranasal versus i.v. administration of LHRH, with the peak LH response occurring somewhat later by nasal administration [9]. Pharmacokinetic measurements have confirmed a 1% bioavailability [10].

The elevations of gonadotropins resulting from intranasal administration of LHRH have direct application to the treatment of idiopathic hypogonadotropic hypogonadism [11,12] and cryptorchidism [13,14]. The latter indication in particular has been extensively researched [15]. Other direct applications include treatment of delayed puberty [16] and ovulation induction using prior clomiphene or gonadotropin treatment to induce follicular development [17-20].

STUDIES WITH AGONIST ANALOGS

Availability of long acting agonist analogs of LHRH and the emerging knowledge of their antireproductive activities stimulated the nasal evaluation of these agents also.

Animal studies

Comparative studies in rats showed the bioavailabilities of [D-Leu[6],Pro-NHEt[9]]LHRH (leuprorelin), [D-Trp[6],Pro[9]-NHEt]LHRH (tryptorelin) and [D-Ser(tBu)[6],Pro[9]-NHEt]LHRH (buserelin) to be quite similar when administered either by single or multiple daily dosing [21]. Further study with leuprorelin administered nasally as a saline solution in rats or dogs showed bioavailabilities of 19-35% compared to i.v. administration. In the rats a marked suppression of testicular steroid output and sex accessory organ weights was noted [22]. However, subsequent human studies did not show these high transmucosal fluxes, the 1-2% figure historically seen for LHRH being found.

Early studies by daily intranasal insufflation of the potent agonist [D-Nal(2)[6]]LHRH (nafarelin) evaluated the dose-dependent inhibition of ovulation in female rhesus monkeys [23]. Using a constant 2X 100 µl dose volume and varying dose concentration, 250 µg per day per animal was completely effective in blocking ovulation, i.e. a relative bioefficacy of 2% compared to i.m. administration. For further work on the optimization of nasal absorption, a highly sensitive and specific RIA method was developed which, measured only intact nafarelin as verified by radiometric HPLC [24]. Use of this assay established that final blood levels of nafarelin were dependent upon both total dose and concentration administered [23,25]. Keeping dosage volume constant and varying delivered dose by changing concentration showed that a 2.2-fold increase in dose from 125 µg to 270 µg gave a 6.5 increase in 8 hour integrated area under curve (AUC) values; increasing the dose to 430 µg resulted in a further 4-fold increase in AUC (Fig. 1). Similar results were obtained in human studies [23]. However when concentration was kept constant at 1.25 mg/ml and dose volume was varied, an increase in dose from 140 µg to 275 µg gave a 2-fold change in AUC [25]. The solubility of nafarelin in aqueous buffer (2.5 mg/ml), together with the maximum feasible dose volume effectively restricts the highest bioavailability and dose to 400 µg.

The noted low bioavailability from these simple aqueous solutions may be due in part to enzymatic degradation in the nasal mucosa [26] or poor flux due to the charged nature of the molecules, in which case absorption enhancers such as the bile salts [27] may be of use. However, at least in the case of nafarelin administered to monkeys, addition of the enzyme inhibitor Trasylol (0.5 U/ml) to the formulation did not increase absorption (S.T. Anik and J-Y. Hwang, personal communication). Better results have been noted using a variety of absorption enhancers. Thus, incorporation of 5% α-cyclodextrin to the leuprorelin formulation increased AUC over a saline formulation 2.5-3.7X in rats and dogs and 2X in humans [22].

In a series of experiments with nafarelin, EDTA, sodium glycocholate (NaGly), Brij 56® and Azone™ were all shown to significantly enhance absorption, while addition of Tween 60 or encapsulation in liposomes did not [28]. In all cases there was an interaction between concentration of drug, enhancer and degree of absorption enhancement (Table 1). However, the greatest blood levels for lowest dose of nafarelin were achieved in the presence of 1% NaGly and this formed the basis of an "enhanced" formulation which is in clinical trial in prostatic cancer patients [29].

Human trials

The only comparative study reported for normal men is that of Happ, et al. [30]. These workers found that an equivalent elevation in circulating levels of LH was induced by 25 µg LHRH i.v., 100 µg LHRH s.c., 5 µg buserelin or leuprorelin i.v., or 50 µg tryptorelin i.n. (given as 100 µl of saline solution by micropipette). The same 50 µg dose of leuprorelin applied

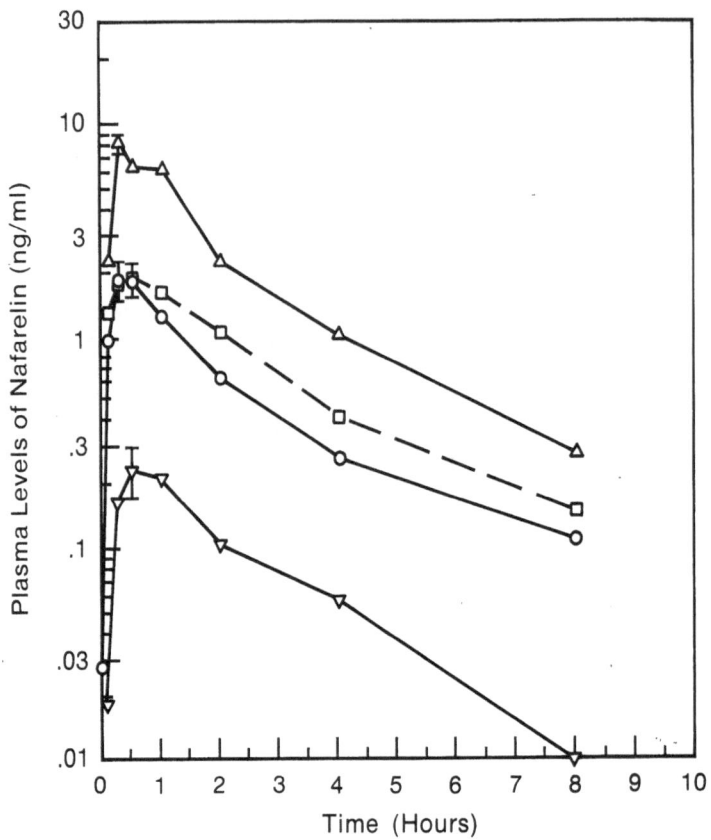

FIGURE 1. Mean concentrations of nafarelin in plasma of female
monkeys after a single subcutaneous or intranasal
dose. Subcutaneous □ 5 µg (10 ng/ml); intranasal
∇ 133 µg (0.625 mg/ml), 0.272 µg (1.25 mg/ml),
∆ 431 µg (2.5 mg/ml). From Anik, S.T. et al.
J. Pharm. Sci., 73, 684 (1984) with permission.

intranasally via "nasioles" (flexible LD-polyethylene ampoules,
25 µg/100 µl) was only half as effective [30]. The latter
preparation was used in the treatment of cryptorchidism where it
caused testicular descent in 4 of 11 patients [31].
    After development of a metered dose nebulizer (reviewed in
[32] detailed pharmacokinetic studies on intranasal application of
buserelin were performed in humans [33]. A nasal bioavailability
of about 1% was calculated from analysis of urinary excretion.
Using an experimental model of rhinitis induced by histamine, no

Table 1. Effect of various enhancers on the plasma levels of nafarelin resulting from intranasal administration to female rhesus monkeys.

Nafarelin Conc. (mg/ml)	Enhancer	Average Dose Per Monkey (µg)	$AUC_{8\ hr}$ ng/ml·hr	Enhancement[*]
0.3125	none	–	–	–
	0.1% NaGly	54	0.70	>2.0[**]
	0.1% Brij 56®	65	2.72	>4.3[**]
0.625	none	133	0.63	–
	1% NaGly	120	14.1	22.4
	1% Brij 56®	137	9.1	14.4
1.250	none	272	4.1	–
	0.1% EDTA	226	7.7	1.9
	1% Brij 56®	229	19.4	4.7
	1% Azone™	256	17.4	4.2
	1% NaGly†	252	27.6	6.5

[*]Fold enhancement over same dose (concentration of nafarelin alone).
[**]By extrapolation from 0.625 mg/ml nafarelin alone.
†Plus 0.5% Tween 20 in order to solubilize the nafarelin.

difference in absorption of buserelin was found versus non-histamine treated controls, as judged by serum LH levels [21]. However, it should be noted that a dose response study would be more properly required to reach this conclusion when such an indirect, saturable-response measure is used.

Determination of blood levels of nafarelin following intranasal administration to both men and women essentially confirmed earlier studies in monkeys. Bioavailability of this hydrophobic analog from simple buffered solution was about 5% for intranasal versus subcutaneous application [23]. Addition of 1% NaGly to the formulation ("enhanced" formulation) results in a doubling of absorption of nafarelin in man. These relatively high bioavailabilities together with the high plasma protein binding (~80%) of nafarelin [34], combine to make this analog highly potent and convenient in clinical use by nasal administration. Thus for the simple aqueous formulation daily administration of as little as 125 µg to normal women completely blocks ovulation and causes hot flashes [35]. Equivalent efficacy for buserelin appears to require 200-400 µg daily [36,37]. Similarly for treatment of endometriosis and precocious puberty, nafarelin is administered twice daily intranasally at total doses of

400-800 µg and 800-1200 µg, respectively [36-40]. For the former indication buserelin has been used in an intranasal total dose of 1200 µg in a thrice daily regimen following a five day induction period of 400 µg/day by injection [41]. Buserelin is also used for treatment of precocious puberty. However, in spite of a six month induction period with subcutaneous injection and a thrice daily intranasal dosage regimen, gonadal steroid output was not returned to prepubertal values [42]. The intranasal dose used (200 µg 3 times daily) was recently concluded to be suboptimal for initial management of patients with precocious puberty and only effective after induction of pituitary desensitization with injected high doses [43]. The recommended dosage regimen with buserelin in prostatic cancer patients is 500 µg subcutaneously every 8 hours for 7 days, followed by 400 µg intranasally thrice daily (total 1200 µg per day) [44]. Again, in contrast, nafarelin administered intranasally as the enhanced formulation appears fully effective by twice daily insufflation of a total dose of 700 µg, without need of any induction period [29].

CONCLUDING REMARKS

Great strides have been made since the early feasibility studies using LHRH and micropipettes or flexible tubing as delivery devices for the intranasal administration of LHRH analogs. Metered spray pumps have been optimized and with at least one analog (nafarelin) bioavailabilities on the order of 10% have been achieved clinically. The even higher absorption rates seen in animal studies, when the reasons are understood, may lead to further increases in bioavailability. In addition, the correlation between dose, concentration and absorption noted for nafarelin suggests that the LHRH antagonists, some of which are more soluble and require a higher dose, may have an intrinsically higher bioavailability. Indeed one of the LHRH antagonists, formulated in a propylene glycol vehicle has an intranasal bioavailability, relative to injection, in monkeys of 40% (R. Asch, personal communication).

In any event, the present state of the art is such that analogs such as buserelin may be applied intranasally as maintenance therapy following pituitary desensitization with injectable therapy. In the case of nafarelin, the high bioavailability (up to 10%) and the high potency combine to make intranasal administration feasible and economically viable for both initiation and maintenance of therapy in a range of indications. The increase in convenience and compliance with this non-invasive route to drug therapy will no doubt further broaden the applications and general efficacy of these peptidic LHRH analogs.

REFERENCES

1. Pitt, C.G. The controlled delivery of polypeptides including LHRH analogs. In "LHRH and Its Analogs: Contraceptive and Therapeutic Applications. Part 2", B.H. Vickery and J.J. Nestor Jr. (Eds), MTP Press, Lancaster, 1987, in press
2. Chien, Y.W. (Ed) Transnasal Biomedical Medications. Fundamental Developmental Concepts Biomedical Assessments. Elsevier Science Publishers B.V., Amsterdam (1985)
3. London, D.R., Butt, W.R., Lynch, S.S., Marshall, J.C., Owusu, S., Robinson, W.R. and Stephenson, J.M. Hormonal responses to intranasal luteinizing hormone-releasing hormone. J. Clin. Endocrinol. Metab., 37, 829 (1973)
4. Solbach, H.G. and Wiegelmann. Intranasal application of luteinizing-hormone releasing hormone. Lancet, 1, 1259 (1973)
5. Jeppson, S., Kullander, S., Rannevik, G. and Thorell, J. Intranasal administration of synthetic gonadotrophin-releasing hormone. Brit. Med. J., 4, 231 (1973)
6. Mortimer, C.H., Besser, G.M., Hook, J. and McNeilly, A.S. Intravenous, intramuscular, subcutaneous and intranasal administration of LH/FSH-RH: the duration of effect and occurrence of asynchronous pulsatile release of LH and FSH. Clin. Endocrinol., 3, 19 (1974)
7. Saito, M., Kumasaki, T., Yaoi, Y., Nishi, N., Arimura, A., Coy, D. and Schally, A.V. Stimulation of luteinizing hormone (LH) and follicle-stimulating hormone by [D-Leu^6,desGly^{10}-NH$_2$] LH-releasing hormone ethylamide after subcutaneous, intravaginal and intrarectal administration to women. Fertil. Steril., 28, 240 (1977)
8. Dahlen, H.G., Keller, E. and Schneider, H.P.G. Linear dose dependent LH release following intranasally sprayed LHRH. Horm. Metab. Res., 6, 510 (1974)
9. Fink, G., Gennser, G., Liedholm, P., Thorell, J. and Mulder, J. Comparison of plasma levels of luteinizing hormone-releasing hormone in men after intravenous or intranasal administration. J. Endocrinol., 63, 351 (1974)
10. Bourguignon, J.P., Burger, H.G. and Franchimont, P. Radioimmunoassay of serum luteinizing-hormone-releasing hormone (LHRH) after intranasal administration and evaluation of the pituitary gonadotrophic response. Clin. Endocrinol., 3, 437 (1974)
11. Happ, J., Neubauer, M., Egri, A., Demisch, K., Schoffing, K. and Beyer, J. GnRH therapy in males with hypogonadotropic hypogonadism. Horm. Metab. Res., 7, 526 (1975)
12. Klingmüller, D., Meschi, M. and Schweikert, H.U. Successful intranasal administration of LHRH in men with hypogonadotropic hypogonadism. J. Steroid. Biochem., 20, A62 (1984)
13. Happ, J., Kollman, F., Krawehl, C., Neubauer, M. and Beyer, J. Intranasal GnRH therapy of maldescended testes. Horm. Metab. Res., 7, 440 (1975)

14. Illig, R., Kollman, F., Borkenstein, M., Kuber, W., Exner, G.U., Kellerer, K., Lunglmayr, L. and Prader, A. Treatment of cryptorchidism by intranasal synthetic luteinizing-hormone releasing hormone. Lancet, 2, 518 (1977)

15. Happ, J. Correction of infertility with LHRH agonists in the male. In "LHRH and Its Analogs: Contraception and Therapeutic Applications", B.H. Vickery, J.J. Nestor Jr., and E.S.E. Hafez (Eds), MTP Press, Lancaster, 1984, p. 299

16. Happ, J., Schmitr, V., Cordes, U., Krause, U., Atzpodien, W. and Beyer, J. Treatment of delayed puberty by intranasal application of gonadotrophin-releasing hormone (GnRH). Int. J. Fertil., 25, 247 (1980)

17. Potashnik, G., Homberg, R., Eshkol, A., Insler, V. and Lunenfeld, B. Hormonal and clinical responses in amenorrheic patients treated with gonadotropins and a nasal form of synthetic gonadotropin-releasing hormone. Fertil. Steril., 29, 148 (1978)

18. Potashnik, G., Homberg, R., Eshkol, A., Insler, V. and Lemenfeld, B. Hormonal responses to nasal application of synthetic gonadotrophin-releasing hormone in amenorrheic patients treated with gonadotrophins. Int. J. Fertil., 25, 234 (1980)

19. Zarate, A., Canales, E.S., Schally, A.V., Ayala-Valdes, L. and Kastin, A.J. Successful induction of ovulation with synthetic luteinizing hormone-releasing hormone in anovulatory infertility. Fertil. Steril., 22, 188 (1971)

20. Phansey, S.A., Barnes, M.A., Willaimson, H.O., Sagel, J. and Nair, R.M.G. Combined use of cloniphene and intranasal luteinizing hormone-releasing hormone for induction of ovulation in chronically anovulatory women. Fertil. Steril., 34, 448 (1980)

21. Sandow, J. and Petri, W. Intranasal administration of peptides: biological activity and therapeutic efficacy. In "Transnasal Systemic Medications", Y.W. Chien (Ed), Elsevier Science Publishers B.V., Amsterdam, 1985, p. 183.

22. Shimamoto, T. Pharmaceutical aspects: nasal and depot formulations of leuprotide. J. Androl., 8(Suppl.), S-14 (1987)

23. Vickery, B.H., Anik, S., Chaplin, M. and Henzl, M. Intranasal administration of nafarelin acetate: contraception and therapeutic applications. In "Transnasal Systemic Medications", Y.W. Chien (Ed), Elsevier Science Publishers B.V., Amsterdam, 1985, p. 201

24. Nerenberg, C., Foreman, J., Chu, N., Chaplin, M.D. and Kushinsky, S. Radioimmunoassay of nafarelin ([6-(3-(2-naphthyl)D-alanine)]LHRH) in plasma or serum. Anal. Biochem., 141, 10 (1984)

25. Anik, S.T., McRae, G., Nerenberg, C., Worden, A., Foreman, J., Hwang, J., Kushinsky, S., Jones, R.E. and Vickery, B. Nasal absorption of nafarelin acetate, the decapeptide [D-Nal(2)^6]LHRH, in rhesus monkeys. I. J. Pharm. Sci., 73, 684 (1984)

26. Hirai, S., Yashiki, T. and Mima, H. Mechanism for the enhancement of the nasal absorption of insulin by surfactants. Int. J. Pharm., 9, 173 (1981)

27. Flier, J.S., Moses, A.C., Gordon, G.S. and Silver, R.S. Intranasal administration of insulin: efficacy and mechanism. In "Transnasal Systemic Medications", Y.W. Chien (Ed), Elsevier Science Publishers B.V., Amsterdam, 1985, p. 217

28. Anik, S.T., Benjamin, E., Maskiewicz, R., McRae, G., Nerenberg, C., Hwang-Felgner, J., Schneider, J., Worden, A. and Foreman, J. Nasal absorption of nafarelin acetate in rhesus monkeys. II. Effect of formulation variables. Submitted for publication.

29. Hoffman, P.G., Henzl, M.R., Chaplin, M.D. and Nerenberg, C.A. Clinical development of nafarelin acetate: Phase I and Phase II studies. J. Androl., 8(Suppl), S-17 (1987)

30. Happ, J., Hartmann, U., Weber, T., Cordes, U. and Beyer, J. Gonadotropin and testosterone secretion in normal human males after stimulation with gonadotropin-releasing hormone (GnRH) or potent GnRH analogs using different modes of application. Fertil. Steril., 30, 666 (1978)

31. Happ, J., Weber, T., Callensee, W., Ermert, J.A., Eshkol, A. and Beyer, J. Treatment of cryptorchidism with a potent analog of gonadotropin-releasing hormone. Fertil. Steril., 29, 552 (1978)

32. Petri, W., Schmeidel, R. and Sandow, J. Development of a metered-dose nebulizer for intranasal peptide administration. In "Transnasal Systemic Medications", Y.W. Chien (Ed), Elsevier Science Publishers B.V., Amsterdam, 1985, p. 161

33. Sandow, J., Jerabek-Sandow, G., Krauss, B. and Schmidt-Gollwitzer, M. Pharmacokinetics and metabolism of LHRH agonists, clinical aspects. In "LHRH and Its Analogues: Basic and Clinical Applications", F. Labrie, A. Dupont, A. Belanger (Eds), Elsevier Science Publishers B.V., Amsterdam, 1984, p. 123

34. Chan, R.L. and Chaplin, M. Plasma binding of LHRH and nafarelin acetate, a highly potent LHRH agonist. Biochem. Biophys. Res. Commun., 127, 673 (1985)

35. Gudmundsson, J.A., Nillius, S.J. and Bergquist, C. Inhibition of ovulation by intranasal nafarelin: a new super-active agonist of GnRH. Contraception, 30, 107 (1984)

36. Bergquist, C., Nillius, S.J. and Wide, L. Inhibition of ovulation in women by intranasal treatment with a luteinizing hormone-releasing hormone agonist. Contraception, 19, 497 (1979)

37. Schmidt-Gollwitzer, M., Hardt, W., Schmidt-Gollwitzer, K. and von der Ohe, M. The contraceptive use of buserelin, a potent LHRH agonist: clinical and hormonal findings. In "LHRH Peptides as Female and Male Contraceptives", G.I. Zatuchni, J.D. Shelton, and J.J. Sciarra (Eds), Harper & Row, Philadelphia, 1981, p. 199

38. Shriock, E., Monroe, S.E., Henzl, M. and Jaffe, R.B. Treatment of endometriosis with a potent agonist of gonadotropin-releasing hormone (nafarelin). Fertil. Steril., 44, 583 (1985)

39. Henzl, M.R., Monroe, S.E., Carson, S.L. and Moghissi, K.S. Treatment of endometriosis by nasal administration of nafarelin. In "LHRH and Its Analogs: Contraceptive and Therapeutic Applications. Part 2", B.H. Vickery and J.J. Nestor Jr. (Eds), MTP Press, Lancaster, 1987, in press

40. Lin, T-H., LePage, M.E., Henzl, M. and Kirkland, J.L. Intranasal nafarelin: An LHRH analogue treatment of gonadotropin-dependent precocious puberty. J. Pediatr., 109, 954 (1968)

41. Lemay, A., Maheux, R., Faure, N., Jean, C. and Fazekas, A.T.A. Reversible hypogonadism induced by a luteinizing hormone-releasing hormone (LH-RH) agonist (buserelin) as a new therapeutic approach for endometriosis. Fertil. Steril., 41, 863 (1984)

42. Luder, A.S., Holland, F.J., Costigan, D.C., Jenner, M.R., Wielgosz, G. and Fazekas, A.T.A. Intranasal and subcutaneous treatment of central precocious puberty in both sexes with a long-acting analog of luteinizing hormone-releasing hormone. J. Clin. Endocrinol. Metab., 58, 966 (1984)

43. Holland, F.J., Fishman, L., Costigan, D.C., Luna, L. and Leeder, S. Pharmacokinetic characteristics of the gonadotropin-releasing hormone analog $D-Ser(TBU)^{6}-EA-^{10}$ luteinizing hormone-releasing hormone (buserelin) after subcutaneous and intranasal administration in children with central precocious puberty. J. Clin. Endocrinol. Metab., 63, 1065 (1986)

44. Present, C.A., Soloway, M.S., Klioze, S.S., Kosola, J.W., Yakabow, A.L., Mendez, R.G., Kennedy, P.S., Wyres, M.R., Naessig, V.L., Ford, K.S., Wiseman, C.L., Bouzaglou, A., Tannenbaum, B. and Eventov, D. Buserelin as primary therapy in advanced prostatic carcinoma. Cancer, 56, 2416 (1985)

36
The Controlled Delivery of Polypeptides including LHRH Analogs

C. G. PITT
Research Triangle, PO Box 12194, Research Triangle Park, NC 27709, USA

INTRODUCTION

Controlled drug delivery received its impetus from studies in the 1960's that demonstrated the feasibility of using drug diffusion from subdermal silicone rubber implants as a mechanism of achieving sustained, constant blood levels [1]. These early studies focussed almost exclusively on delivery of steroids and other relatively lipophilic drugs in the molecular weight range 100-400 daltons. Once the merits of controlled drug delivery were recognized, it was a logical step to expand the classes of drugs to include both hydrophilic and higher molecular weight compounds. These properties posed new problems to the designer of delivery systems. The rate of diffusion in any polymer is the product of two drug dependent terms, the diffusion coefficient (D) and the solubility in the polymer. The value of D decreases inversely with the molecular weight of the drug, typically exhibiting a log-log relationship, eq. 1 [2]. As a result, diffusion of a drug with a molecular weight in excess of 1000 can be impractically slow in a convention-

$$\log D = a - b \log MW \tag{1}$$

al polymer such as silicone rubber. This problem is compounded by the fact that peptides and biological macromolecules are relatively hydrophilic compared to most polymers, and their solubility in the polymer bulk is vanishingly small.

Because of these limitations of conventional polymeric delivery systems, new approaches to the delivery of peptides are necessary. There is not enough published information on LHRH and its analogs to present a complete picture of the different approaches that have been implemented. Therefore, this chapter will review methods of drug delivery that are applicable to LHRH-like peptides by expanding the scope to include all macromolecules. The different approaches to the controlled delivery of macromolecules that have been employed are conveniently divided into five material types, (a) hydrogels, (b) monolithic systems, (c) microparticles, (d) biodegradable polymers, and (e) porous membranes.

557

Hydrogels are hydrophilic polymers that absorb and swell in water without dissolving. The insolubility of the hydrogel may be associated with some residual lipophilicity but, more typically, is achieved by crosslinking the polymer. The uptake of water can be controlled from a minor amount to several hundred percent by varying the degree of crosslinking. Simplistically, the hydrogel provides an restricted aqueous environment for diffusional migration of the macromolecular drug; in fact, experimental studies [3-5] suggest a distinction be made between transport through a domain composed of bulk water (pore mechanism) and a domain composed of polymer segments, interfacial water, and bound water (partition mechanism).

The first application of hydrogels to macromolecular delivery appears to be due to Davis, who used polyacrylamide as a matrix for the delivery of insulin [6]. He subsequently showed that polyacrylamide and polyvinylpyrrolidone gels crosslinked with 20 w/w-% N,N'-methylenebisacrylamide could be used for controlled delivery of immunoglobulin, luteinizing hormone (LH), bovine serum albumin (BSA), prostaglandin $F_{2\alpha}$ and sodium iodide [7] (Fig. 1).

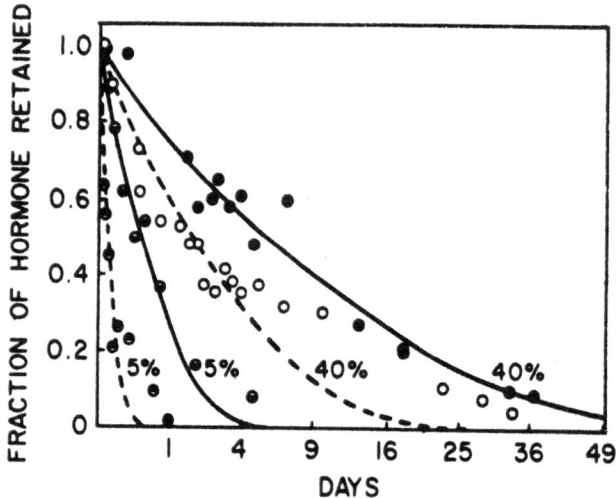

FIGURE 1   Depletion of ^{125}I-labeled LH from 5% and 40% polyacrylamide gels (20% crosslinked) in 10 mM phosphate-buffered saline, pH 7.2, at 37°, and in mature female hamsters. The curves were calculated using the average apparent diffusion coefficients obtained from the amount of solute retained by the gels at indicated times. **Continuous lines** denote implants, and **broken lines** are for depletion in vitro. Reproduced from Davis, B. K. in Proc. Nat. Acad. Sci. USA, 71, 3120 (1974) (with permission).

Implants were prepared as cylinders, 2 cm x 1.5 mm (od), by photo-initiated polymerization of the vinyl monomers and the drug in phosphate buffered saline (PBS) in glass capillaries. The rates of diffusion of the various drugs from the hydrogel matrix in vitro exhibited an inverse logarithmic dependence on the polymer concentration of the gel (C_p) and the drug molecular weight (M). This dependence was expressed mathematically by equation 2, where D and D_0 are the diffusion coefficients of the solute in the hydrogel and solvent, respectively.

$$D = D_0 \exp[- (0.05 + 10^{-6} M) C_p] \qquad (2)$$

The duration of release of LH in hamster could be varied between 1 and 36 days by increasing the polyacrylamide concentration in the gel from 5 to 40%. The rate of release of LH was approximately proportional to the square root of time, in accord with the kinetics expected for diffusion from a monolithic cylindrical device.

Sefton and Nishimura [8] also demonstrated the importance of the degree of hydration of the hydrogel. These authors determined the permeability of insulin in hydrogel membranes of polyhydroxyethyl methacrylate (37% water), polyhydroxyethyl acrylate (52% water), polymethacrylic acid (67.5% water), and cuprophane PT-150 (Fig. 2). The permeabilities (P) of the series correlated directly with the aqueous diffusion coefficient of insulin in water (D_w) and

$$P = \alpha H D_w \qquad (3)$$

the degree of hydration (H) of the hydrogel (equation 3) , in accordance with the free volume model of Yasuda, et al. [9].

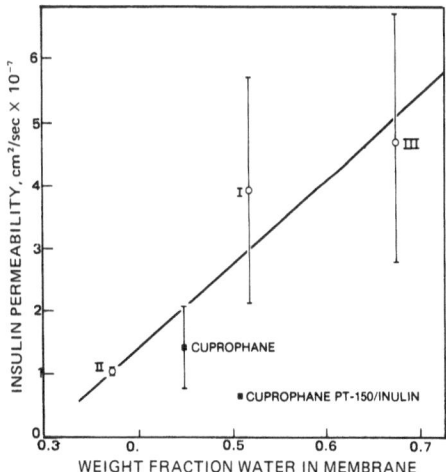

FIGURE 2 Relationship between the weight fraction of water and the insulin permeability of highly swollen polyacrylate membranes. Reproduced from Sefton, M.V. and Nishimura, E. in J. Pharm. Sci., 69, 208 (1980) (with permission)

Sato and Kim [10] described the use of hydrogels of hydroxyethyl methacrylate (HEMA), methoxyethyl methacrylate (MEMA), and

methoxyethoxyethyl methacrylate (MEEMA) as membranes for the dif-
fusion-controlled delivery of the following water-soluble solutes
with a wide range of molecular weights: sodium acetate, glucose,
maltose, insulin, cytochrome C and albumin. Both dense and porous
membranes were studied. The diffusivity was dependent on the solute size (Fig. 3) and the membrane hydration, and was consistent
with the model of permeation involving both "pore" and "partition"
mechanisms.

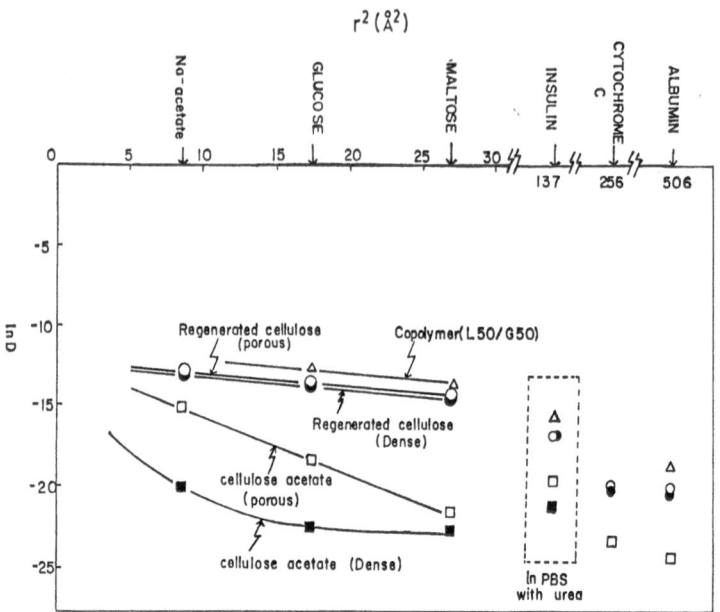

FIGURE 3 Dependence of cellulosic membrane diffusion coefficients
on the solute molecular size. Reproduced from Sata, S.
and Kim, S. W. in Int. J. Pharm., _22_, 229 (1984) (with
permission)

The use of biodegradable polymers for drug delivery is advantageous, eliminating the need to remove polymer residues from the
implant site after the drug is exhausted, as well as providing an
alternative mechanism of drug release from the polymer matrix.
Torchilin, et al. [11] showed that polyvinylpyrrolidone hydrogels
crosslinked with N,N'-methylenebisacrylamide are degradable if the
crosslinks are reduced to less than 1%. The methylene group of the
crosslinker is subject to slow hydrolytic cleavage at pH 7, and
gradual loss of crosslinks results in the controlled dissolution of
the hydrogel. This approach was demonstrated by incorporation of
chymotrypsin into the gel by mechanical trapping during emulsion
polymerization of N-vinylpyrrolidone. Chymotrypsin was released
from the gel under in vitro conditions over a period of one week or
longer, the rate depending on the crosslink density of the gel.
  This formulation suffered from the fact that the crosslink
density controlled the rates of both the hydrogel dissolution and
the diffusional release of the chymotrypsin. Only gels with a very

low crosslink density dissolved within a reasonable time period; such gels, by virtue of their highly porous structure, were unable to retain the entangled macromolecule, and rapid diffusional release occurred. Heller, et al. [12] sought to simplify this design problem by limiting the release mechanism to biodegradation. To this end, a more tightly crosslinked system was prepared to reduce diffusional release, while at the same time the hydrolytic instability was increased by introduction of fumaric or malonic ester linkages. Water soluble polyester prepolymers were first prepared from polyethylene glycol and fumaric acid, and then crosslinked by copolymerization with N-vinylpyrrolidone (Fig. 4). Structurally analogous hydrogels were prepared from combinations of fumaric acid with ketomalonic acid, 1:1-ketoglutaric acid and 1:1-diglycolic acid. The rate of release of BSA from these gels was constant (Fig. 5) and the duration of release could be varied between 10 days and greater than 7 weeks by the choice of chemical structure and amount of vinylpyrrolidone (20-150%).

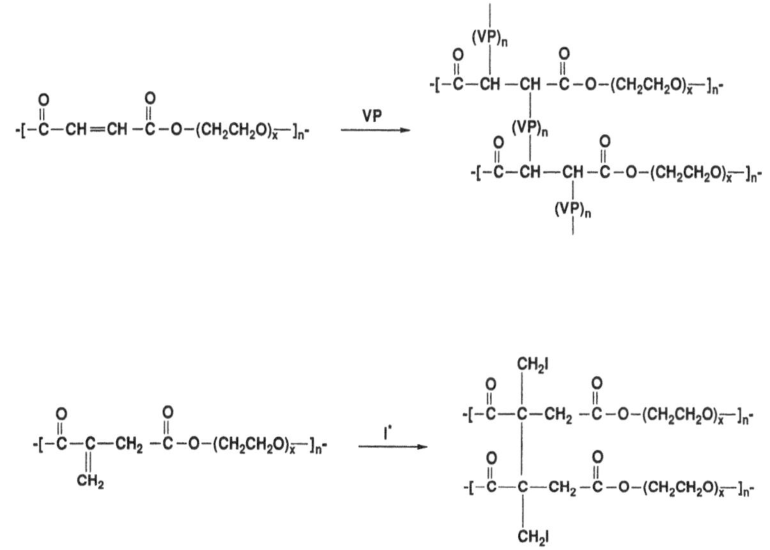

FIGURE 4   Preparation of biodegradable hydrogels from (a) fumarate polyesters crosslinked with N-vinylpyrrolidone and (b) crosslinked itaconate polyesters.

Because erosion of these hydrogels produces the non-degradable polymer polyvinylpyrrolidone as a by-product, a new group of hydrogels were prepared by vinyl polymerization of the polyesters of itaconic and allylmalonic acid [12]. These polymers were totally degraded to low molecular weight fragments. The rate of release of BSA from these hydrogels was controlled by the degree of crosslinking and the chemical structure (Fig. 6).

An example of a biodegradable but non-crosslinked hydrogel system, where the initial insolubility is the result of partial hydrophobic character, is provided by a patent to Churchill and

561

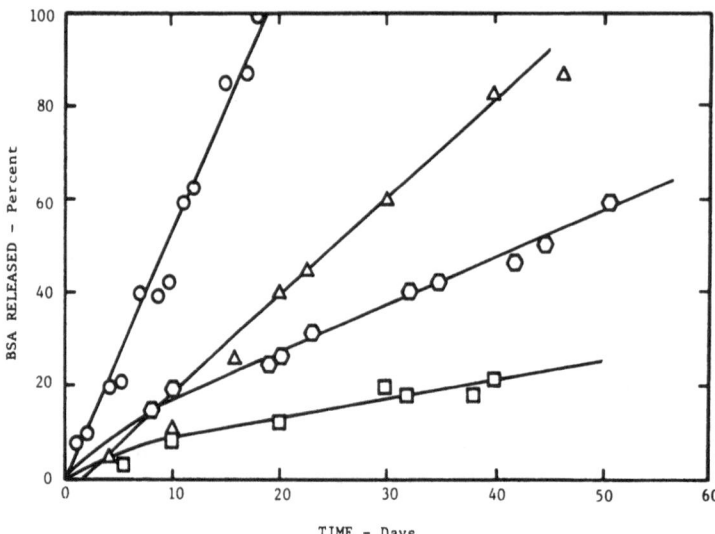

FIGURE 5 Release of bovine serum albumin at pH 7.4 and 37°C from microparticles prepared from various water-soluble unsaturated polyesters crosslinked with 60 wt-% N-vinyl pyrrolidone. Reproduced from Heller, J., et al. in Biomaterials, 4, 262 (1983) (with permission).

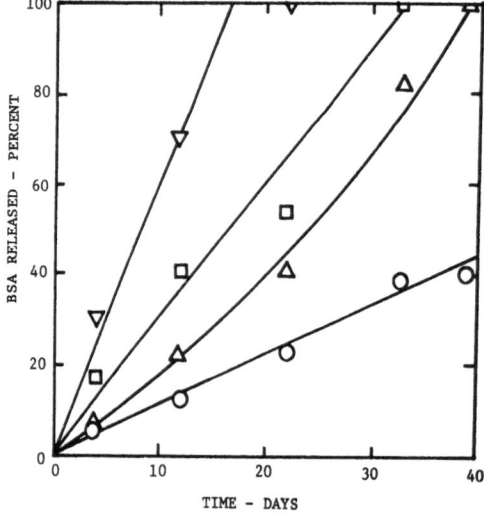

FIGURE 6 Release of bovine serum albumin at pH 7.4 and 37°C from microparticles prepared from water-soluble allylmalonic or itaconic polyesters crosslinked by free radical initiation. (O) itaconic acid, 18% concentration; (▽) allylmalonic acid, 18% concentration; (□) allylmalonic acid, 36% concentration, (△) allylmalonic acid, 53% concentration. Reproduced from Heller, J., et al. in Biomaterials, 4, 262 (1983) (with permission).

Hutchinson [13]. The authors described the preparation of block
copolymers consisting of a hydrophilic component and a degradable
hydrophobic component, and their use for the delivery of polypeptides such as LHRH, growth hormone releasing factor, EGF, ACTH, and
somatostatin. Examples of the hydrophilic component are polyvinyl
alcohol, polyethylene glycol, and polyvinylpyrrolidone, while the
degradable block may be polyesters such as polylactic acid, polyglycolic acid, or polyamides. Release proceeds by diffusion, further promoted by the degradation process.

MONOLITHIC SYSTEMS

While classical Fickian diffusion of macromolecules through the
polymeric bulk of semipermeable membranes is impractically slow,
Langer and his group [14-17] have shown that many different macromolecules are released from the hydrophobic polymer polyethylene-
co-vinyl acetate (EVA). Initially, difficulties in obtaining reproducible release rates were experienced. However, procedures for
fabrication by mixing the dry, powdered macromolecule with the
polymer solution at -80°C, then solvent evaporation at incremental-
ly higher temperatures, minimized drug settling and provided the
necessary reproducibility [18]. The list of drugs that have been
combined with the monolithic EVA system includes BSA, β-lactoglobu-
lin A, lysozyme, soybean trypsin inhibitor, alkaline phosphatase,
catalase, insulin, heparin, and DNA. Three examples are shown in
Fig. 7.

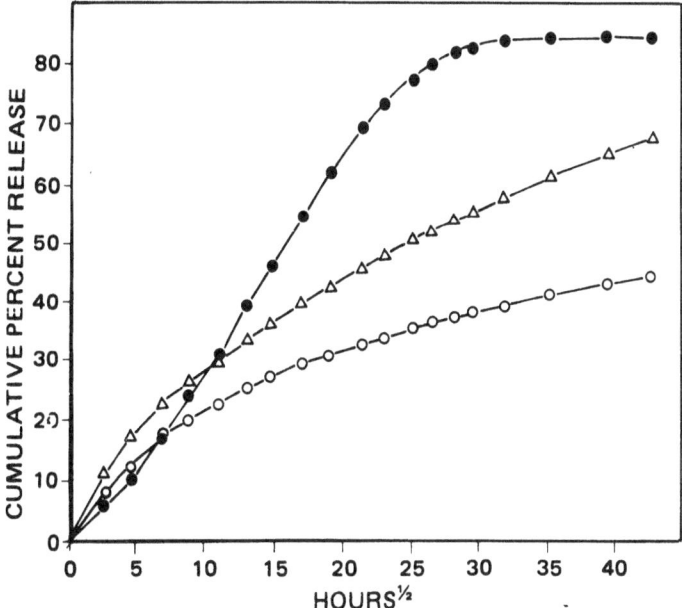

FIGURE 7   Cumulative release from EVA versus time$^{1/2}$ for three
           proteins. Key: ($\bullet$), β-lactoglobulin; ($\triangle$) BSA; and ($\circ$)
           lysozyme. Reproduced from Rhine, W.D., et al. in J.
           Pharm. Sci., 69, 265 (1980). (with permission)

563

A potential limitation of the use of a monolithic system a-
rises from the fact that the kinetics of drug release are not zero
order. For example, drug release from a monolithic slab is proportional to the square root of time. This shortcoming has been addressed [19-21] by changing the design of the monolith, and several
different geometries which provide nearly zero order release have
been identified. Hsieh, et al. [21] showed that the inward releasing hemisphere is one such geometry, illustrating its use with the
in vitro release of BSA (Fig. 8).

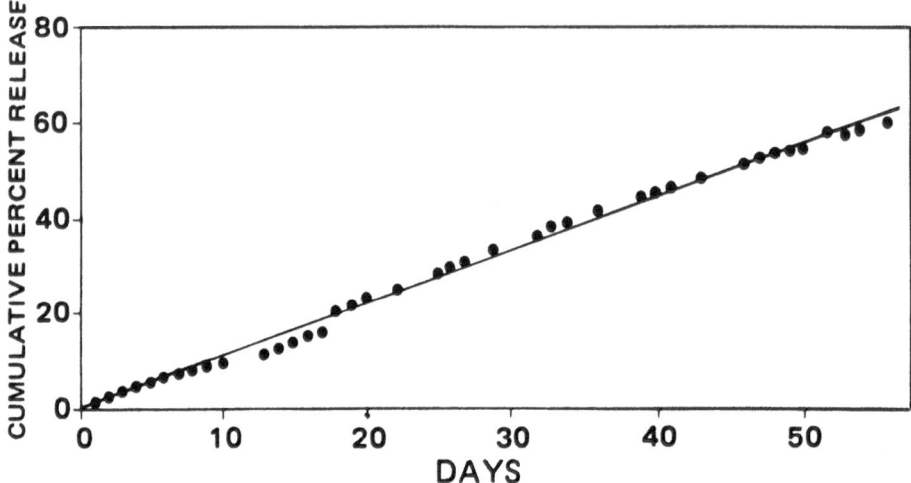

FIGURE 8   Cumulative release of BSA versus time from an inward
            releasing hemisphere. The matrix was made of EVA and
            BSA. Reproduced from Hsieh, D.S.T., et al. in J. Pharm.
            Sci., 72, 17 (1983) (with permission)

The versatility of the monolithic EVA system was significantly
enhanced by the discovery that the rate of release of the drug may
be reversibly increased by ultrasound [22]. Release rates up to 20
times the baseline rate can be achieved, depending on the intensity of the source. Mechanistic experiments suggest that the enhancement of the release rate is due to cavitation; local temperature increases and improved mixing (i.e. removal of any boundary
layer effects) are inconsequential. These findings provide a mechanism by which the recipient may control the rate of drug delivery,
a considerable advantage in therapy such as insulin administration
to diabetics, where pulsed rather than zero order release is
desirable. The application of a pulsed magnetic field to monolithic EVA-macromolecule delivery systems containing steel particles has been used to achieve a similar effect.
        Several studies have been devoted to the elucidation of the
mechanism of release of macromolecules from EVA [23-25]. The mechanism does not involve dissolution of the drug in EVA and classical
Fickian diffusion, or swelling of the polymer bulk as in the case
of a hydrogel. Rather it appears to involve diffusion though aqueous channels created by the protein itself. This is consistent

with the finding that a minimum drug loading is necessary before release of the drug from the EVA matrix is observed. Microscopy identified pores and connecting channels occupied by the drug (Fig. 9) [23]. A morphological study demonstrated that there is considerable swelling of the pores due to water uptake by the protein, and collapse of some pores occurs after loss of the protein [25].

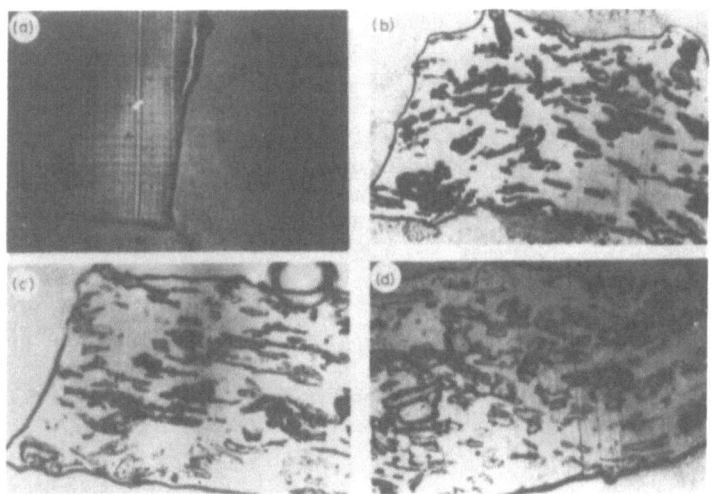

FIGURE 9   Optical microscopy (OM) micrographs of (a) pure EVA cast without drug (lines represent knife marks); (b) with 25% by weight BSA, (particle size 63-149 μm) prior to release; (c) slab similar to (b) after 16 hours release; (d) slab similar to (b) after 40 hours release. Slabs released to exhaustion have same appearance as (d). Reproduced from Bawa, R., et al. in J. Controlled Release, 1, 259 (1985). (with permission).

In a series of papers, Korsmeyer, et al. [26], discussed the mechanism of release of BSA and low molecular weight drugs from porous hydrophilic polymers, using poly(vinyl alcohol) discs as experimental models. The initial drug diffusion was attributed to dissolution into and diffusion through water filled pores near the surface of the polymer matrix. Subsequent polymer swelling leads to structural changes in the polymer and its porosity. Finally, as the swelling progresses, diffusion of the drug occurs through the polymer matrix as well as the water-filled pores. The rate and kinetic law, i.e., zero vs first order, depend on the relative contributions of these processes.

MICROCAPSULES AND MICROSPHERES

The first application of microcapsules to the delivery of macromolecules is due to Chang [27], who in 1976 described the release of insulin from polylactic acid microcapsules. It was

stated that the release rate could be varied from 50% in 5 hours to
2.5% in 24 hours.   Similarly, asparaginase was incorporated in
nylon 610 and polylactic acid microcapsules with retention of enzymatic activity [27,28]; however, in these cases activity was
achieved by diffusion of asparagine into the microcapsules and not
release of the enzyme into the environment.

    A number of publications [29-34] from the Syntex group have
described the use of biodegradable polyglycolic acid-co-DL-lactic
acid microcapsules for the delivery of the LHRH agonist Nafarelin.
The release of the peptide was shown to be polyphasic. The first
phase is diffusional, and is associated with loss of superficial
drug. The second phase, with a lower of release rate, is then
followed by one or more phases of higher release. The latter does
not occur until bulk hydrolysis of the polymer has caused erosion
and break up of the polymer-drug matrix to begin. The rate of the
hydrolysis and the duration of the secondary phase may be controlled by the initial polymer molecular weight. The glycolic acid:
lactic acid ratio also influences the duration of the second phase,
as well as the overall duration of Nafarelin delivery. By judi-
cious choice of these polymer properties, it was possible to sufficiently reduce the second phase to provide essentially continuous
efficacy in rat for greater than 8 months, with partially effective
levels of release continuing beyond 15 months (Fig. 10).

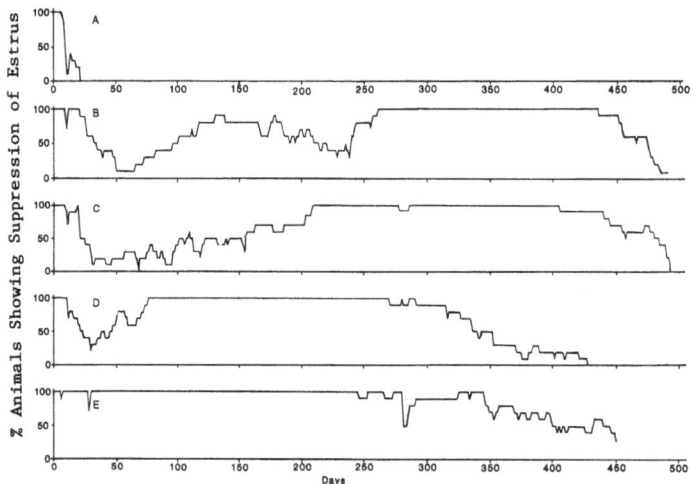

FIGURE 10   Influence of molecular weight of poly(DL-lactic acid)
            microcapsules on kinetics of Nafarelin release, measured
            by estrus suppression. Key: Polymer intrinsic viscosity
            (A) 1.75 dl/g, (B) 1.02 dl/g, (C) 0.72 dl/g, (D) 0.47
            dl/g, (E) 0.36 dl/g

    As part of a series of studies of protein immobilization,
Artursson, et al. [35] described the use of biodegradable microparticles prepared from crosslinked polysaccharides.   The method of
preparation involved chemical derivatization of the polysaccharide,
either maltodextrin or hydroxyethylstarch, with acrylic acid gly-
cidyl ester. This derivative, the protein to be encapsulated, a

566

surfactant and ammonium peroxodisulfate were dissolved in buffer, and homogenized in chloroform-toluene in the presence of a surfactant to produce a water-in-oil emulsion. Polymerization of the acrylate residues, initiated by addition of an amine, served to stabilize the suspended microspheres. The size range achieved was of the order of 1-10 microns and up to 40% (dry weight) of proteins such as human serum albumin, lysozyme, immunoglobulin, and carbonic anhydrase could be incorporated.

Very rapid biodegradation of these microspheres in serum, and in the target organelle, the lysosyme, was demonstrated. Release of the protein was sustained over a 12 week period but was not zero order (Fig. 11). The mechanism of release was thought to be diffusion through pores in the microspheres. The inclusion of the crosslinking agent N,N'-methylenebisacrylamide in the formulation increased the release rate, consistent with previous findings that the microsphere pore size is increased by addition of a crosslinking agent. The future use of these microspheres for controlled delivery will depend on the ability to control the relative contributions of diffusion and biodegradation to the release rate.

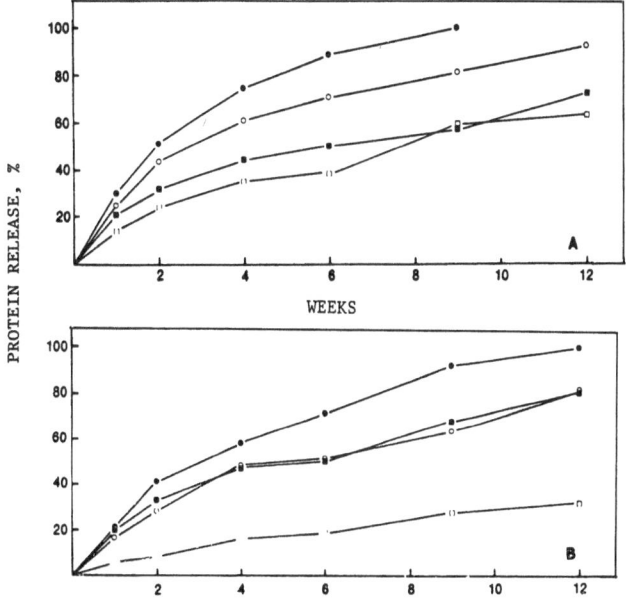

FIGURE 11 Release of immoblized proteins at room temperature from microparticles of (A) maltodextrin and (B) hydroxyethyl starch. The immobilized proteins were lysozyme (●), human serum albumin (O), carbonic anhydrase (■), and immunoglobulin G (☐). Reproduced from Artursson, P., et al. in J. Pharm. Sci., 73, 1507 (1984) (with permission).

Lee, et al. [36] described the development of serum albumin microbeads as an injectable, biodegradable system for the delivery of progesterone. This formulation was subsequently adapted to the delivery of insulin by Goosen, et al. [37]. Insulin crystals were

suspended in phosphate buffer containing BSA, and crosslinking was
initiated by addition of glutaraldehyde (2.5 or 5%). The suspension was stirred rapidly in a mixture of corn oil and petroleum
ether until the water in oil emulsion was fixed. The activity of
the resulting microcapsules, which ranged in size from 50-1000 µg,
was measured in diabetic rats. Blood insulin levels (RIA) decreased from 67 µU to 10 µU over a 60 day period (Fig. 12), while resorption of the BSA microbeads required about 5 months.

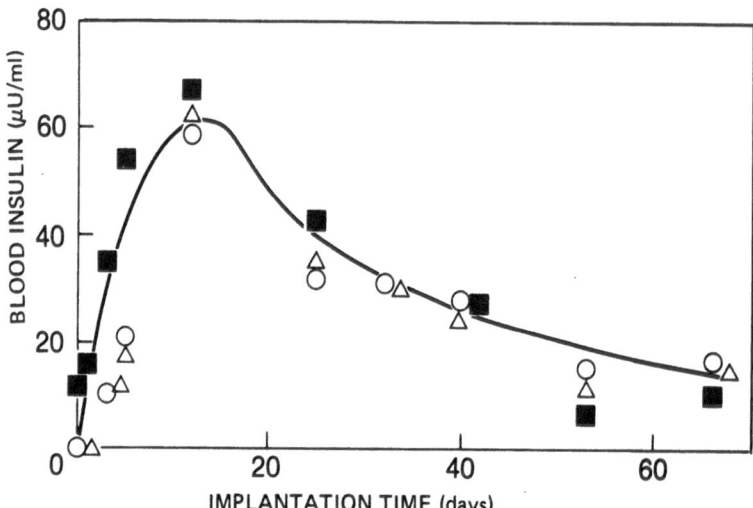

FIGURE 12 Blood-insulin levels of diabetic rats implanted with
varying doses of insulin-albumin microbeads (200 mg in-
sulin/gm microbeads). Symbols: (○) 10 mg dose, (△) 20
mg dose and (■) 40 mg dose. Reproduced from Goosen,
M.F.A., et al. in Biomat. Med. Dev. Art. Org., 10, 205
(1982) (with permission).

There are numerous examples of the encapsulation of macromolecules in liposomes, with the object of improved cell uptake and
tissue targeting. This subject has been reviewed recently [38] and
so need not be considered here. A variation of the standard formulation of liposomes is microencapsulation of proteins entrapped in
liposomes. Wheatley, et al., [39] described the coating of liposomes with alginate, followed by poly-L-lysine and polyvinylamine.
The kinetics of release of myoglobin from such capsules was bimodal, giving rise to the possibility of either pulsed or delayed
drug release [39].

BIODEGRADABLE POLYMER SYSTEMS

Some examples of the use of biodegradable hydrogels and microspheres for the controlled delivery of macromolecules have been
described in preceding sections. Other examples of biodegradable
systems may be mentioned. Mathiowitz, et al. [40] reported the use

568

of polyanhydride spheres (50-1000 μm) to deliver insulin and myo-globin, as well as lower molecular weight dyes. Spheres were pre-pared by mixing the drug and melted polymer, suspending in a hot non-miscible solvent, and cooling until solid. After screening a number of polyanhydrides, the copolymer of sebacic anhydride and bis(p-carboxyphenoxy)propane anhydride was identified as having the requisite material properties and rate of hydrolytic degradation. Incorporation of the drug affected the rate of surface erosion of the polymer. The rate of insulin release was not constant in vitro, but suppression of glucose levels in diabetic rats was demonstrated over a several day period.

Asano, et al. [41] prepared a hot-pressed rod (1 cm x 2 mm od) from powdered low molecular weight poly(DL-lactic acid) and the agonist [D-Leu[6],Pro[9],NHEt]LHRH. The two components were mixed at 70°C, and then compressed within a Teflon tube. After implantation in the dorsal region of rats, the release of the peptide and the extent of polymer weight loss were determined by recovery of samples at prescribed time intervals. Both the rates of polymer erosion and the peptide release decreased with time over a 15 week period, at which point no polymer was recoverable (Fig. 13).

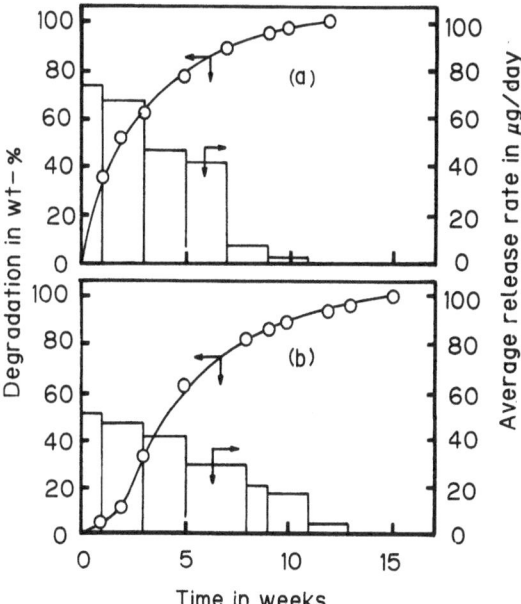

FIGURE 13 In vivo degradation of hot-pressed pure PLA and the aver-age daily dose of LHRH agonist released in vivo from hot-pressed PLA formulation. (a): PLA $\bar{M}_n$ = 1850, (b): PLA $\bar{M}_n$ = 2200. Reproduced from Asano, M., et al. in Makromol. Chem. Rapid Commun., 6, 509 (1985) (with permission).

Furr and Hutchinson [42] described the biological effects of sustained delivery of [D-Ser(tBu)[6],AzaGly[10]]LHRH (Zoladex, ICI) compounded with a 1:1 copolymer of DL-lactic acid and glycolic acid and implanted subdermally as a rod (1 mm x 3-6 mm). This formula-tion, which was totally biodegradable, was designed to deliver the peptide for at least 28 days.   Both polymer erosion and drug diffusion through drug-created pores in the polymer matrix contributed to the release rate. The rate could be controlled by the choice of copolymer composition and molecular weight and, because of the duality of the release mechanism, could be made biomodal [43].

Recently, Heller et al. [44] have demonstrated that polyorthoesters may be used to deliver LHRH analogs. This polymer system functions by surface erosion of the polymer-drug blend at physiological pH, and has been used previously for the delivery of a variety of lower molecular weight drugs. The rate of surface erosion is controlled by the specific polymer composition, the lipophilicity being one of several factors that determine the kinetics.

POROUS MEMBRANE SYSTEMS

Porous membranes are distinct from other polymeric membranes described in this article by having stable pores, the size and distribution of which do not depend on the presence of hydrophilic polymer sequences (hydrogels) or hydrophilic drugs (monoliths).

Porous cellulosic membranes have a long history of use as dialysis membranes. In 1971 Colton, et al. [45] characterized the permeabilities of commercial, modified, and laboratory-cast porous cellulose membranes, using fifteen water soluble solutes with molecular weights ranging from 58 to 68,000 daltons.   The rates of diffusion of the solutes decreased as their size increased. A log-log plot (cf eq. 1) of the membrane resistance (reciprocal of permeability) versus the drug molecular weight was linear for 7 of 9 solutes, with only heparin and polyethyleneglycol failing to conform. A semilog plot of the ratio, D_m/D_{water}, of the diffusion coefficients in the membrane and water versus the molecular radius of the solute was also linear (Fig. 14), these correlations permitting prediction of the permeabilities of other solutes.

Sato and Kim [10] showed that it was possible to obtain porous films of a 1:1 copolymer of DL-lactic acid and glycolic acid by casting from a methanol-chloroform solution.   Membranes of this biodegradable polymer were more permeable to glucose and insulin than several porous cellulosic and hydrogel membranes evaluated during the same study.   These biodegradable membranes are being used as part of an autoregulated insulin delivery system now under development [46].

The reproducible preparation of porous membranes for controlled delivery in geometries other than films is difficult. Eenink, et al. [47] have described the preparation of porous tubing (1 mm od) by coagulation spinning of polymer solutions. The polymers employed were poly-L-lactic acid and a copolymer of ℓ-ethyl-L-glutamate and ℓ-piperonyl-L-glutamate, both of which are biodegradable. The porosity of the tube walls was controlled by the choice of solvents for dissolution and coagulation of the tubing, and by inclusion of additives such as monomeric L-lactide and polyvinylpyrrolidone in the polymer solution.   The porosity of the tubing was determined by measurement of the rate of release of the dye cresyl violet acetate (MW 321) from capsules prepared using the

570

tubing. The application to higher molecular weight species has not been described, but may be feasible.

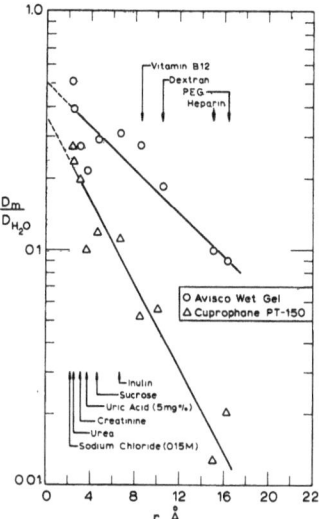

FIGURE 14 Diffusion coefficient reduction in porous cellulosic membranes as a function of characteristic molecular radius of solute. Reproduced from Colton, C.K., et al. in J. Biomed. Mater. Res., 5, 459 (1971) (with permission).

This wet spinning procedure is related to a method developed in the author's laboratory and now being applied to the preparation of LHRH analog delivery systems [48,49]. In this method, a biodegradable polyester such as polylactic acid or poly(ϵ-caprolactone) is melt extruded as a blend with an inert additive. The resulting tubing, typically 1-2 mm outer diameter, is extracted with a solvent to remove the additive and, in the process, to create a porous wall (Fig. 15). The porosity of the wall is controlled by such experimental variables as the choice and amount of additive, the temperature, and the solvent used for extraction. The tubing is suitable for preparation of reservoir (capsule) delivery systems that may be implanted subdermally. The rate of release of macromolecules is dependent on the porosity of the tube wall, and values ranging between 20 μg and 400 μg per day for [D-Trp^6,des-Gly^{10}]-LHRH ethyl amide have been achieved (Fig. 16). These capsules are equally useful for the delivery of higher molecular weight proteins.

A porous alumino-calcium-phosphorus oxide ceramic (ALCAP) is reported [50] to be capable of controlled release of a variety of drugs, including testosterone, gossypol, GRH, BSA, bovine gamma globulin, insulin, and chymotrypsinogen. The ceramic can be compounded with polylactic acid and formulated as a hollow cylinder. The release from such cylinders in vitro is determined by the size of the calcined particles.

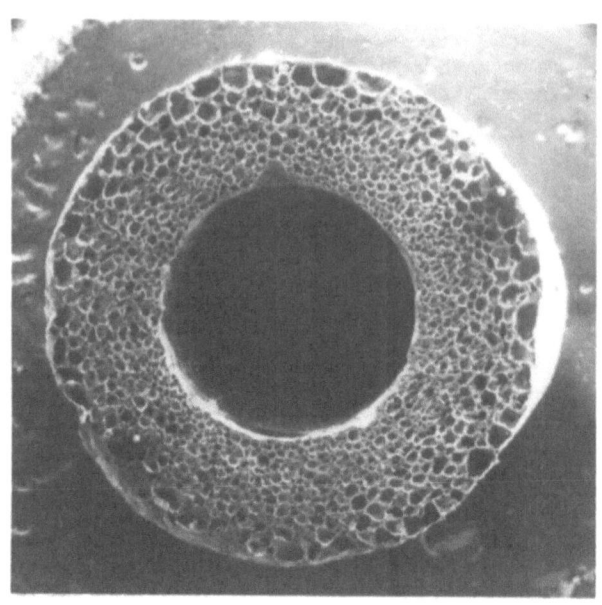

FIGURE 15 Scanning electron micrograph of cross-section of a porous
capsule of poly(ε-caprolactone) prepared by solvent extraction of an inert additive, magnification X15. (micrograph courtesy of P. Ingram).

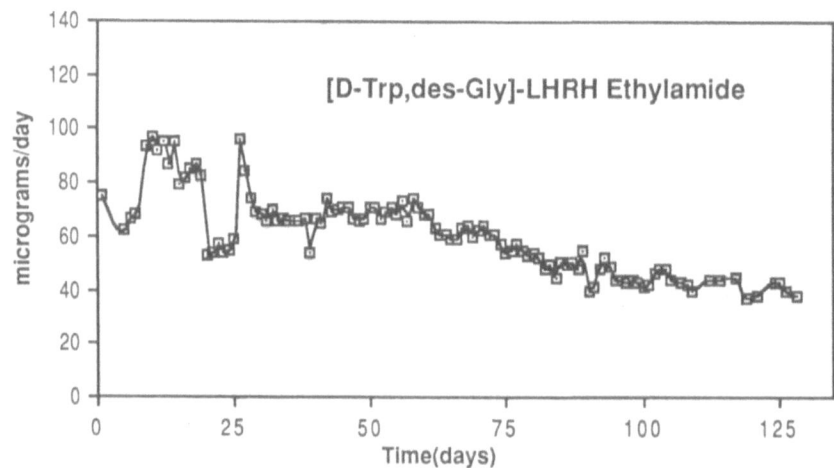

FIGURE 16 In vitro rate of release of [D-Trp⁶,des-Gly¹⁰]-LHRH ethyl
amide from a porous capsule of the type shown in Figure
15 [48].

CONCLUSIONS

This review of the literature has described a number of approaches
to the controlled subdermal administration of LHRH analogs and
higher molecular weight peptides. Very few, if any, of the methods can be considered to be reduced to practice; at this stage in
the development of the methodology, the focus has been on demonstrating feasibility rather than the achieving a specific dose rate
and duration of action. Significant practical problems remain.
For example, it is well known that some polypeptides, e.g. bovine
growth hormone, are unstable when formulated in a synthetic polymer
matrix. Mention has already been made of the advantages of delivering some drugs on an as-needed basis, and it is probable that
others will be much more effective when administered cyclically,
rather than at a constant rate. Presently, there are no simple
methods of self-regulated or pulsed subdermal drug delivery [51].
    Some peptides may require too large a daily dose for subdermal
implantation to be practical. Given the limitations of nasal delivery, the best approach in such cases may be to devise methods of
oral delivery which avoid proteolysis in the stomach and upper
intestine, permitting absorption in the colon. An ingenuous example of this strategy applied to the targeted delivery of insulin
was described very recently [52].

REFERENCES

1. Chien, Y.W. Novel Drug Delivery Systems, M. Dekker, New
    York, 1982, p. 312.
2. Pitt, C.G., Andrady, A.L., Bao, Y.T. and Samuel, N.K.P. The
    estimation of rates of drug diffusion in polymers. W.R. Good
    and P.I. Lee (Eds.), ACS Symposium Series, In Press.
3. Wisniewski, S. and Kim, S.W. Permeation of water-soluble
    solutes through poly(2-hydroxyethyl methacrylate) and poly(2-
    hydroxyethyl methacrylate) crosslinked with ethylene glycol
    dimethacrylate. J. Membrane Sci., 6, 299 (1980).
4. Zentner, G.M., Cardinal, J.R., Feijen, J. and Song, S. Pro-
    gestin permeation through polymer membranes IV: Mechanism of
    steroid permeation and functional group contributions to
    diffusion through hydrogel films. J. Pharm. Sci., 68, 970
    (1979).
5. Jhon, M.S. and Andrade, J.D. Water and hydrogels. J. Bio-
    med. Mater. Res., 7, 509 (1973).
6. Davis, B.K. Control of diabetes with polyacrylamide implants
    containing insulin. Experientia, 28, 348 (1972).
7. Davis, B.K. Diffusion in polymer gel implants. Proc. Nat.
    Acad. Sci. USA, 71, 3120 (1974).
8. Sefton, M.V. and Nishimura, E. Insulin permeability of hy-
    drophilic polyacrylate membranes. J. Pharm. Sci., 69, 208
    (1980).
9. Yasuda, H., Peterlin, A., Colton, C.K., Smith, K.A. and
    Merrill, E.W. Permeability of solutes through hydrated poly-
    mer membranes. Part III: Theoretical background for the

selectivity of dialysis machines. Makromol. Chem., 126, 177 (1969).

10. Sata, S. and Kim. S. W. Macromolecular diffusion through polymer implants. Int. J. Pharm., 22, 229 (1984).

11. Torchilin, V.P., Tischenko, E. G., Smirnov, V. N. and Chazov, E. I. Immobilization of enzymes on slowly soluble carriers. J. Biomed. Res., 11, 223 (1977).

12. Heller, J., Helwing, R.F., Baker, R.W. and Tuttle, M.E. Controlled release of water-soluble macromolecules from bio-erodible hydrogels. Biomaterials, 4, 262 (1983).

13. Churchill, J.R. and Hutchinson, F.G., Continuous Release Formulations, US Patent 4,526,938.

14. Langer, R.S. and Folkman, J. Polymers for the sustained release of proteins and other macromolecules. Nature (Lond.), 263, 797 (1976).

15. Langer, R.S. and Folkman, J. Sustained release of macromolecules from polymers. In "Polymeric Delivery Systems," R.J. Kostelnik (Ed.), Midland Macromolecular Monograph, Vol. 5, Gordon and Breach Science Publishers, New York, 1978, p. 175.

16. Langer, R.S., Rhine, W.D., Hsieh, D.S.T. and Bawa, R.S. Polymers for the sustained release of macromolecules: applications and control of release kinetics. In "Controlled Release of Bioactive Materials," R. Baker (Ed.), Academic Press, 1980, p. 83.

17. Langer, R., Lund, D., Leong, K. and Folkman, J. Controlled release of macromolecules: Biological studies. J. Controlled Release, 2, 331 (1985).

18. Rhine, W.D., Hsieh, D.S.T. and Langer, R. Polymers for sustained macromolecular release: Procedures to fabricate reproducible delivery systems and control release kinetics. J. Pharm. Sci., 69, 265 (1980).

19. Brooke, D. and Washkuhn, R.J. Zero-order drug delivery system: Theory and preliminary testing. J. Pharm. Sci., 66, 159 (1977).

20. Yalkowsky, S.H. and Kuu, W-Y. Multiple hole approach to zero-order release. J. Pharm. Sci., 74, 927 (1985).

21. Hsieh, D.S.T., Rhine, W.D. and Langer, R., Zero-order controlled release polymer matrices for micro- and macromolecules. J. Pharm. Sci., 72, 17 (1983).

22. Kost, J., Leong, K. and Langer, R. Ultrasonically controlled delivery systems. Proc. Int. Symp. Control. Rel. Bioact. Mater., 12, 73 (1985).

23. Bawa, R., Seigal, R.A., Karel, M. and Langer, R. An explanation for the controlled release of macromolecules from polymers. J. Controlled Release, 1, 259 (1985).

24. Siegel, R.A. and Langer, R. Effects of Pore Morphology and Topology on Macromolecular Drug Release from Macroporous Polymers. Abstr. 191st ACS National Meeting, American Chemical Society, New York, April 1986, INDE 182.

25. Miller, E.S., Peppas, N.A. and Winslow, D.N. Morphological changes of ethylene/vinyl acetate-based on controlled delivery systems during release of water-soluble solutes. J. Membrane Sci., 14, 79 (1983).

26. Korsmeyer, R.W., Gurny, R., Doelker, E., Buri, P. and Peppas, N.A. Mechanisms of solute release from porous hydrophilic polymers. Int. J. Pharm., 15, 25 (1983).

27. Chang, T.M.S. Biodegradable semipermeable microcapsules containing enzymes, hormones, vaccines, and other biologicals. J. Bioeng., 1, 25 (1976).

28. Chong, D.S.C. and Chang, T.M.S. In vivo effects of intraperitoneally injected L-asparaginase solution and L-asparaginase immobilized within semipermeable nylon microcapsules with emphasis on blood L-asparaginase, "Body" L-asparaginase, and plasma L-asparaginase levels. Enzyme, 18, 218 (1974).

29. Sanders, L.M., McRae G.I., Vitale, K.M., Vickery, B.H., and Kent J.S. An injectable biodegradable controlled release delivery system for Nafarelin acetate. In "LHRH and its Analogs," F. Labrie, A. Belanger, and A. Dupont (Eds.), Elsevier Science Publishers B.V., 1984, p. 53.

30. Sanders L.M., Kent J.S., McRae G.I., Vickery, B.H., Tice T.R., and Lewis, D.H. Controlled release of luteinizing hormone-releasing analogue from poly(DL-lactide-co-glycolide) microspheres. J. Pharm. Sci., 73, 1294 (1984).

31. Sanders, L.M., McRae, G.I., Vitale, K.M., and Kell, B.A. Controlled delivery of an LHRH analogue from biodegradable injectable microspheres. J. Controlled Release, 2, 187 (1985).

32. Sanders, L.M., Kell, B.A., McRae, G.I., and Whitehead, G.W. Prolonged controlled-release of Nafarelin, a luteinizing hormone-releasing hormone analogue, from biodegradable polymeric implants: Influence of composition and molecular weight of polymer. J. Pharm. Sci., 75, 356 (1986).

33. Sanders, L.M., Kell, B.A., McRae, G.I., and Mishky, P.B. Controlled delivery of Nafarelin, an agonistic analogue of LHRH, from microspheres of poly(DL-lactic-co-glycolic acid). In "Proceedings of NATO Advanced Research Workshop on Advanced Drug Delivery Systems for Peptides and Proteins". Copenhagen, 1986, in press.

34. Anik, S.T., Sanders, L.M., Chaplin, M.D., Kushinsky, S., and Nurenberg., C. Delivery systems for LHRH and analogs. In "LHRH and its Analogs. Contraceptive and Therapeutic Applications". B.H. Vickery, J.J. Nestor, Jr., and E.S.E. Hafez (Eds.), MTP Press Ltd. Boston, 1984, 421.

35. Artursson, P., Edman, P., Laakso, T. and Sjoholm, I. Characterization of polyacryl starch microparticles as Carriers for proteins and drugs. J. Pharm. Sci., 73, 1507 (1984).

36. Lee, T.K., Sokoloski, T.D. and Royer, G.P. Serum albumin beads: An injectable, biodegradable system for the sustained release of drugs. Science, 213, 233 (1981).

37. Goosen, M.F.A., Leung, Y. F., Chou, S. and Sun, A. M. Insulin-albumin microbeads: An implantable, biodegradable system. Biomat. Med. Dev. Art. Org., 10, 205 (1982).

38. Gregoriadis, G. (Ed.) Liposome Technology. Volume II; Incorporation of Drugs, Proteins and Genetic Material, CRC Press Inc., Boca Raton, Florida, 1985.

39. Wheatley, M.A., Eisen, H. and Langer, R. Alginate/poly-L-lysine microcapsules as a vehicle for controlled release of

macromolecules. Proc. Int. Symp. Control. Rel. Bioact. Mater., 12, 245 (1985).

40. Mathiowitz, E., Leong, K. and Langer, R. Macromolecular drug release from biodegradable polyanhydride microspheres. Proc. Int. Symp. Control. Rel. Bioact. Mater., 12, 183 (1985).

41. Asano, M., Yoshida, M., Kaetsu, I., Imai, K., Mashimo, T., Yuasa, H., Yamanaka, H., Suzuki, K. and Yamazaki, I. Biodegradability of hot-pressed poly(lactic acid) formulation with controlled release of LHRH agonist and its pharmacological influence on rat prostate. Makromol. Chem. Rapid Commun., 6, 509 (1985).

42. Furr, B.J.A. and Hutchinson, F.G. Biodegradable sustained release formulation of the LHRH analogue "Zoladex" for the treatment of hormone-responsive tumours. "EORTC Genitourinary Group Monograph 2, Part A: Therapeutic Principles in Metastatic Prostatic Cancer", 143 (1985).

43. Hutchinson, F.G. and Furr, B.J.A. Biodegradable polymers for sustained release of peptides. Trans. 609th Biochem. Soc. Meeting, Leeds, U.K., 13, 520 (1985).

44. Heller, J., Sanders, L.M., Mishky, P., and Ng, S.Y. Release of an LHRH Analog from Crosslinked Poly(ortho ester), Proc. 13th Int. Symp. Controlled Release Bioactive Materials, Norfolk, Virginia, 1986, p. 69.

45. Colton, C.K., Smith, K.A., Merrill, E.W. and Farrell, P.C. Permeability studies with cellulosic membranes. J. Biomed. Mater. Res., 5, 459 (1971).

46. Kim, S.W., Jeong, S.Y., Sato, S., McRae, J.C. and Fiejen, J. Self-regulating insulin delivery system - A chemical approach. In "Recent Advances in Drug Delivery Systems," J. M. Anderson and S. W. Kim (Eds.), Plenum, New York, N.Y., 1984, p. 123.

47. Eenink, M.J.D., Albers, H.J.M., Rieke, J.C., Olijslager, J., Greidanus, P.J. and Feijen, J. Biodegradable hollow fibers for the controlled release of drugs. Proc. Int. Symp. Control Rel. Bioact. Mater., 12, 49 (1985).

48. Schindler, A., Patents pending.

49. Schindler, A., Hendren, R.W. and Pitt, C.G. Unpublished studies.

50. Bajpai, P.K., Alcap ceramics in drug delivery, Polymer Preprints, 26, 2, 203 (1985).

51. Pitt, C.G. Self-regulated and triggered drug delivery systems. Pharm. Int., 7, 88 (1986).

52. Saffran, M., Kumar, G.S., Savariar, C., Burnham, J., Williams, F., and Neckers, D.C. Science, 233, 1081 (1986).

37
Pharmacokinetics and Metabolism
of LHRH Analogs

R.L. CHAN and C.A. NERENBERG

Bioanalytical and Metabolic Research, Syntex Research, Palo Alto,
CA 94304, USA

INTRODUCTION

The distribution, clearance and metabolism of LHRH have been extensively studied. The reported biological half-life (T 1/2) of
LHRH (2-8 min) in early studies [1-7] represented only the distribution phase of the compound after iv administration. In subsequent studies using radioimmunoassay specific for LHRH, plasma
T 1/2 were reported to be 13-27 min for the elimination phase in
man [8-10]. Plasma elimination T 1/2 of LHRH in rats, rhesus
monkeys and sheep were 6.7, 21 and 33 min, respectively [11,12].
The longer T 1/2 of LHRH in man compared to the T 1/2 in monkeys
and rats is reflected in its lower metabolic clearance rate
(MCR). Thus MCR were 1 to 1.8 ℓ/min, 31 ml/min/kg and 58 ml/
min/kg in man [5,6,8-10,13], monkeys and rats [12], respectively.
Volumes of distribution (Vd) of LHRH were 11-12ℓ, 0.56 ℓ/kg
and 1.5 ℓ/kg, respectively, in man [6,8], rats and monkeys
[12]. These Vd values in man are much larger than normal blood
volumes, indicating extensive distribution of LHRH into body
tissues. Values of Vd, T 1/2 and MCR in man were affected by
age, sex [9, 14] and various pathological conditions [5, 6]. In
organ distribution studies of ^{3}H-LHRH [3, 4] and ^{125}I-LHRH
[15, 16] in rats, significant accumulation of radioactivity was
found in the pituitary, pineal gland, liver and kidney.

In vitro metabolism of LHRH by tissue extracts involved the
action of cytosolic [17-19] as well as membrane-bound enzymes
[20-26]. Although intact hypothalamus and pituitary cells do not
degrade LHRH in vitro [27, 28], there is evidence that intracellular LHRH-metabolizing enzymes may play a physiological role in
regulating LHRH levels. Thus internalization of LHRH into pituitary [29-31] and ovarian cells [32, 33] occurs, and the activity
of these enzymes is dependent on sexual status [34-38] and on the
level of sex steroids [38-42].

Data on the metabolism of LHRH analogs are mostly restricted
to a few compounds under clinical development, such as buserelin
[43, [D-Ser(tBu)[6],Pro[9]-NHEt]LHRH], leuprolide [44, [D-Leu[6],
Pro[9]-NHEt]LHRH], nafarelin [45, [D-Nal(2)[6]]LHRH], tryptorelin
[46, [D-Trp[6]]LHRH], and a potent LHRH antagonist, detirelix
[47,[N-Ac-D-Nal-(2)[1],D-pCl-Phe[2],D-Trp[3],D-hArg(Et$_2$)[6], D-Ala[10]]LHRH].

Metabolic studies on these analogs, in particular those related to nafarelin and detirelix, form the focus of this chapter.

ANALYTICAL METHODOLOGY

A prerequisite for obtaining reliable pharmacokinetic data in metabolic studies of LHRH and its analogs is the development of specific assay procedures for these compounds. Bioassay, based on LH-releasing activity of LHRH or its analogs, has been used in monitoring concentrations of LHRH or its analogs in both in vivo [48,49] and in vitro [50] studies. However, sensitivity of bioassays is often low [16]. To quantitate low levels of LHRH or its analogs in biological samples, sensitive radioimmunoassays (RIA) are needed. Radioimmunoassays have been described for buserelin [16], leuprolide [51], tryptorelin [52,53] and nafarelin [54].

For pharmacokinetic and metabolic studies of nafarelin and detirelix, we used RIA or an HPLC-radiometric method. To produce the nafarelin antiserum, the hapten was modified by replacing pyroglutamic acid at the N-terminus with glutaric acid. This provided a free carboxyl group for conjugation to keyhole limpet hemocyanin using a water-soluble carbodiimide coupling procedure. The resulting antiserum from New Zealand White rabbits [54] showed little or no cross-reactivity with LHRH or peptide fragments of nafarelin (Table 1). The radioactive tracer for the assay was prepared by labeling nafarelin with ^{125}I and separating the labeled from unlabeled material to assure maximum specific activity. Sample purification prior to RIA was not required. The sensitivity of the assay is 50 pg/ml. For the nafarelin and detirelix HPLC-radiometric method, we used either ^{14}C or ^3H labels [55]. A C-18 reversed-phase extraction column was used for preliminary purification of plasma samples prior to separation by HPLC [13].

TABLE I. Cross reactivity data in radioimmunoassay of nafarelin

Compound	% Cross-Reactivity
Nafarelin	100.00
Nafarelin-free acid	80.00
[Glutaric acid^1] nafarelin	31.5
(1-5) pentapeptide of nafarelin	<< 0.001
(6-10) pentapeptide amide of nafarelin	0.052
(4-10) heptapeptide of nafarelin	0.70
[des-Gly-NH$_2^{10}$]nafarelin	0.46
[Aza-Gly-NH$_2^{10}$]nafarelin	100.0
[D-Tyr^5]nafarelin	1.8
[Trimethoxy-Phe^6]nafarelin	<< 0.1
LHRH	<< 0.001
(5-10) hexapeptide amide of nafarelin	0.27
(1-7) heptapeptide of nafarelin	<< 0.008
(6-7) dipeptide of nafarelin	<< 0.008
D-Nal(2)	<< 0.008
2-Naphthylacetic acid	<< 0.008
(5-7) tripeptide of nafarelin	<< 0.008

Antiserum for the antagonist detirelix was produced by coupling the hapten to BSA via a free carboxylic acid (C-terminal) or amino functional group (N-terminus). Antiserum produced by the N-terminal coupling was superior to that obtained with the C-terminal conjugation. Sensitivity of the assays was 0.15 and 0.70 ng/ml, respectively, for the N and C-terminal conjugates. Radioactive tracer was prepared by labeling with ^{125}I. For both nafarelin and detirelix, RIA showed good agreement with HPLC-radiometric analyses.

IN VITRO DEGRADATION

Preferential hydrolysis of LHRH at Tyr^5-Gly^6 by a non-chymotrypsin-like endopeptidase from pituitary homogenates [56,57] can be blocked by substitutions of Gly^6 with D-amino acids. Thus, analogs with D-Ala [58,59], D-Leu [59], D-Trp [59,60] or D-Nal(2) [N.I. Chu and M.D. Chaplin, unpublished] at position 6 were degraded by tissue homogenates more slowly than LHRH. Inactivation at the C-terminus by post-proline cleaving enzyme [61-66] can be deterred by replacement of $Gly^{10}NH_2$ with ethylamide [11,58, 67]. Modifications at positions remote from the scissile peptide bond can also influence the degradation by post-proline cleaving enzyme [67]. Analogs containing modifications at both position 6 and the C-terminus, such as [D-Ala^6, Pro^9-NHEt]LHRH [58,68], buserelin [11,67-73], [D-Phe^6, Pro^9-NHEt]LHRH [69], leuprolide[71-73], [D-Lys^6, Pro^9-NHEt] LHRH and [D-Gln^6,Pro^9-NHEt] LHRH [71], were more resistant to enzymatic degradation than LHRH. Modifications at other positions, for example, [D-Leu^6, (N$^\alpha$-Me)Leu^7] LHRH and [D-Ala^6,(N$^\alpha$-Me)Leu^7]LHRH [59], also increased the stability towards degrading enzymes. Another major soluble enzyme hydrolyzing LHRH in vitro is the pyroglutamate aminopeptidase [66, 67,74]. Antagonistic analogs containing position 2 modifications such as [des-His^2]LHRH, [D-Phe^2] LHRH, [D-Phe^2, D-Trp^{3,6}] LHRH, [D-pGlu^1,D-Phe^2,D-Trp^{3,6}] LHRH, were not degraded by this enzyme [67].

Resistance of LHRH analogs to enzymatic degradation may result in increased concentrations at target sites and peripheral sites. This has been used to rationalize the prolonged and increased LH/FSH releasing activity of many analogs [11,58,69,70, 73], though some workers reported lack of strict colinearity between biological activity and stability towards degradation [67, 75]. Other factors, such as protein and receptor binding, undoubtedly also contribute to the superactivity of LHRH analogs.

BINDING STUDIES

Receptor binding

Binding of LHRH analogs to LHRH receptors is important for biological activity [76]. Studies on LHRH-receptor binding are often complicated by membrane-associated degrading enzymes [21]. Superagonists and antagonists, however, are not hydrolyzed to any significant extent by pituitary membrane preparations [68]. Structure-activity studies indicate that biological potencies of many LHRH analogs closely parallel their receptor binding affinities [77-82], although the correlation is not necessarily linear [60].

Plasma protein binding

Protein binding is a physiochemical property that may affect the pharmacologic and therapeutic effects of a drug [83]. The _in vitro_ plasma binding of a strongly hydrophobic LHRH agonist, nafarelin, was very different from that of LHRH [84]. At 4°C, nafarelin was 78-84% bound, whereas LHRH was only 22-25% bound to plasma proteins from several species (Figure 1). Another agonist, leuprolide, was bound to plasma proteins [85] to the same extent (7-19%) as LHRH. The greater extent of plasma protein binding of nafarelin may be due to the hydrophobic nature of D-Nal(2) at position 6 and might contribute to its prolonged duration of action and enhanced potency compared with other LHRH agonists. An antagonist, [N-acetyl-D-pCl-Phe[1,2], D-Trp[3], D-Lys[6], D-Ala[10]]LHRH has recently been shown [86] to bind to human albumin also. The extent of binding, however, was not reported.

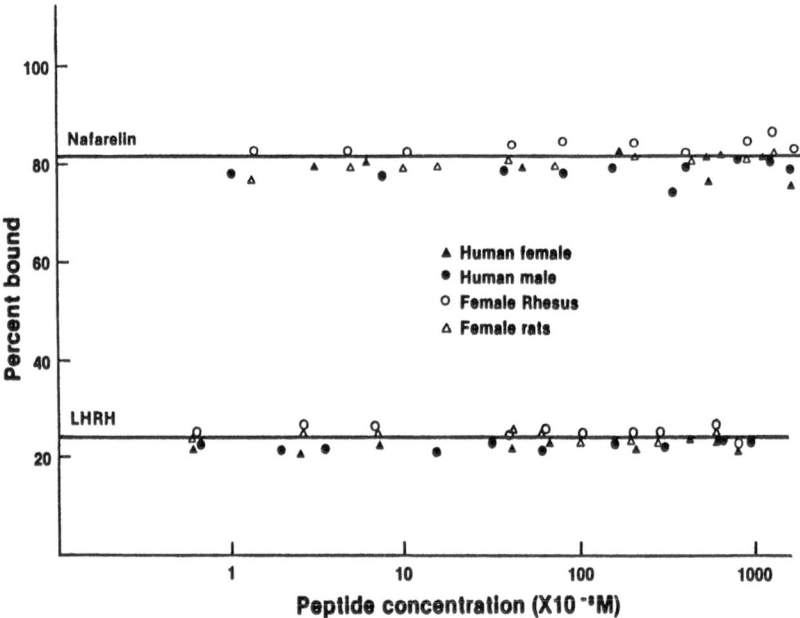

Figure 1 Binding of ^{3}H-nafarelin and ^{3}H-LHRH to plasma from the human, rat and rhesus monkey (Reproduced from Chan, R.L. and Chaplin, M.D., Biochem. Biophys. Res. Common, 127, 673 (1985) with permission).

580

PHARMACOKINETIC STUDIES

Studies in Animals

Agonists. Pharmacokinetic data of LHRH agonists are very limited and are mostly restricted to plasma T 1/2 values. Plasma profiles of LHRH and its analogs following an intravenous bolus dose generally consist of two phases. The first (α) phase is due to mixing throughout the vascular and extracellular fluid volumes. The second (β) is a slower metabolism and elimination phase. Comparison of plasma elimination T 1/2 between various agonists is often complicated by the different methods used in their estimations by different authors. Thus, based on plasma concentrations measured between 6 and 30 minutes postdose only, Swift and Crighton [11] reported no significant difference of plasma T 1/2 values between LHRH and three agonists: [Pro^9-NHEt]LHRH, buserelin and [D-Ser^6]LHRH. These values were 3-4 and 21-25 minutes, for the α and β phases, respectively. Other authors [87] reported similar plasma elimination T 1/2 for iodinated LHRH, [D-Ala^6,Pro^9-NHEt]LHRH and leuprolide in ovariectomized rats. However, only total radioactivity was measured in this study and possible formation of metabolites was not considered. The T 1/2 of buserelin in rats was also similar to that of LHRH [88], being 5 and 30 min, respectively, for the rapid and slow components. The biological half-lives of leuprolide in the rat were 4-8 min in the α phase and 33 min in the β phase [89]. In these studies on buserelin [88] and leuprolide [89], however, the methods for determining T 1/2 values were not specified, which makes comparison with data from other agonists difficult.

We studied the pharmacokinetics of radiolabeled nafarelin in different species after a single intravenous dose. Plasma samples were extracted with C-18 cartridges before determination of nafarelin concentrations by HPLC-radiochromatographic analysis. Plasma T 1/2 values were estimated from the terminal elimination phase over at least three half-lives. Table 2 compares the pharmacokinetic data among the various species. In the rhesus monkey, linear kinetics (AUC values proportional to dose) was demonstrated between the dose range of 7.5 to 75 µg/ kg. Data for nafarelin in rats and rhesus monkeys are also compared with those of LHRH. The longer duration of action of nafarelin relative to LHRH is evident from the much longer plasma T 1/2 values, lower metabolic clearance rates and a 6-8 fold increase in AUC values for approximately equal doses. Data for nafarelin in rats, mice and rabbits are very similar. The large volumes of distribution of nafarelin and LHRH in all animals studied imply that this type of drug is extensively distributed into body tissues. In cynomolgus monkeys, we showed that the plasma T 1/2 of nafarelin was independent of the route of dose administration. Detailed pharmacokinetic studies comparable to those for nafarelin are not available with other agonists.

Table 2. Pharmacokinetic data of radiolabeled nafarelin and LHRH after a single intravenous dose[a]

Species	Drug[b]	Dose (µg/kg)	Plasma[c] T 1/2 (min)	AUC$_{total}$[d] (ng/ml•hr)	Plasma Clearance (ml/min/kg)	VdB[d] (ml/kg)
Rhesus (F)[e]	Naf	6.4	108 ± 6	35.8 ± 0.6	3.0 ± 0.2	470 ± 23
		9.5	120 ± 6	62.4 ± 7.5	2.7 ± 0.3	441 ± 40
		73.5	120 ± 12	563 ± 32	2.2 ± 0.1	384 ± 30
	LHRH	7.7	33 ± 5	4.6 ± 1.0	31.4 ± 5.8	1529 ± 372
Rat (M)	Naf	495	48.6	788	10.5	734
(F)[e]	Naf	530	33.6	736	12.0	580
	LHRH	460	6.7	133	57.6	560
Mouse (M)	Naf	1150	40.8	3357	5.7	335
Rabbit (F)	Naf	94.6	34 ± 2	232 ± 31	7.0 ± 0.9	343 ± 51

[a]Values are mean ± SEM when n>3, [b]Naf = nafarelin, [c] Terminal elimination phase of plasma nafarelin concentration-time profiles, [d]AUC$_{total}$ = area under the plasma nafarelin concentration-time curves from 0 to infinity, VdB = apparent volume of distribution in the β phase, [e] Data from reference 12.

Antagonists. The long duration of action of the LHRH antagonist, detirelix, is reflected in its long plasma elimination half-lives in animals. Thus, after a single 0.3 mg/kg intravenous dose of ^{3}H-detirelix in the rat, the plasma T 1/2 was 96 min, which is 3 times as long as that of nafarelin. The metabolic clearance rate was correspondingly low, being 2.8 ml/min/kg. Mean plasma concentration profiles of detirelix in the cynomolgus monkeys given a single 80 µg/kg intravenous dose of ^{14}C-detirelix are shown in Figure 2. The plasma elimination T 1/2 in this study was at least 7 hr. Higher doses of detirelix (0.2 and 1.0 mg/kg) were also given to monkeys subcutaneously. T 1/2 values appeared to be dose-related, being 19 and 32 hr, respectively, for the 0.2 mg/kg and 1 mg/kg subcutaneous dose. A similar long T 1/2 (>21 hr) was observed in dogs after a 1.0 mg/kg subcutaneous dose of detirelix. Oral bioavailability of detirelix in the rhesus monkey was less than 2%, which agrees with the poor oral absorption estimated from biological activities reported for other antagonists [90-92]. Pharmacokinetic studies of other antagonists have not been reported.

Studies in Human

Agonists. Pharmacokinetic data of LHRH analogs in humans is very limited [93]. Post-infusion studies of tryptorelin in men [10,60] showed that this agonist is cleared from plasma at about one-third the rate of LHRH. Data from single-dose pharmaco-kinetic studies of leuprolide [94] are shown in Table 3 together with our data on nafarelin. Direct comparison of the two studies

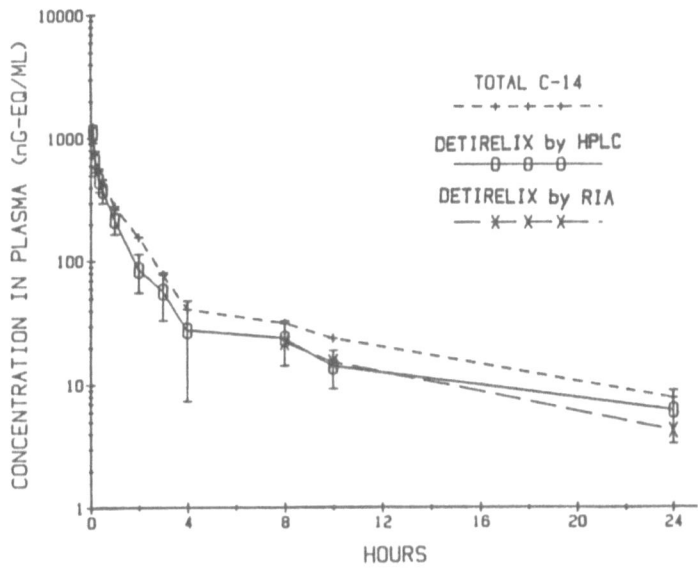

Figure 2   Mean plasma concentrations of total radioactivity and
detirelix in male cynomolgus monkeys after a single
80 µg/kg intravenous dose of ^{14}C-detirelix.   Concentrations are mean ± SEM, n = 3.

is complicated by the much larger dose of leuprolide
administered, which reflects the larger clinical dose required of
this compound.   Nafarelin nevertheless is cleared from the body
at a significantly (p<0.025) lower rate than leuprolide.
Subcutaneous doses of LHRH are associated with depot-like effects
[13], resulting in prolonged and delayed absorption by this route
of administration relative to intravenous administration.   With
nafarelin, such depot-like effects might well be enhanced by its
strong hydrophobic nature.

Table 3.   Pharmacokinetic data of single doses of leuprolide [94]
and nafarelin in human

Compound	Dose (mg)	Dose Route	T 1/2 (hr)	Vd$_{ss}$[a] (ℓ)	Plasma Clearance (ml/min)
Leuprolide[b]	1.0	iv	2.9 ± 0.5	26.5 ± 10.1	139 ± 30
	1.0	sc	3.6 ± 1.2	37.1 ± 16.8	151 ± 43
Nafarelin[c]	0.2	sc	4.3 ± 0.3	34.8 ± 7.3	97 ± 23

[a]Steady state volume of distribution, [b]Data are mean ± SD, n = 6,
[c]Mean ± SD, n = 3.

583

Antagonists. In a recent study on the hormonal (testosterone, LH, FSH) response in men after a single subcutaneous dose of the potent antagonist, detirelix, plasma elimination half-lives of this compound were 40 hr or greater for the three doses administered (Table 4). Maximum plasma concentrations (Cmax) were attained 1-2 hr after dose administration. Cmax values were proportional to dose (corr. coeff. = 0.995), indicating linear kinetics of detirelix in humans up to a 20 mg dose. Plasma disappearance T 1/2 of another antagonist, [N-acetyl-D-pCl-Phe^{1,2},D-Trp^3,D-Lys^6,D-Ala^{10}]-LHRH was 14-17 hr [86]. The long T 1/2 and low plasma clearance rates of detirelix (Table 4) and of other antagonists correlate well with their prolonged suppression of hormonal levels in men [86,95-97].

Table 4. Pharmacokinetic data of subcutaneous doses of detirelix in men[a]

Dose	Tmax (hr)	Cmax (ng/ml)	T 1/2[b] (hr)	Plasma Clearance (ml/min)
5	1.3 ± 0.5	37.9 ± 13.0	59.2 ± 21.9	58.6 ± 18.6
10	1.9 ± 0.9	67.1 ± 14.4	47.6 ± 15.3	65.0 ± 14.7
20	2.2 ± 1.2	117.5 ± 32.4	44.7 ± 8.1	74.1 ± 17.7

[a] Values are mean ± SD, n = 9. [b] Estimated from 8-96 hr postdose.

METABOLIC PROFILES

Sandow and Clayton [16] reported the 4-9 hexapeptide of buserelin to be the major urinary metabolite of ^{125}I-buserelin in rats. This metabolite could be formed by the action of pyroglutamate aminopeptidase [66,67] followed by aminopeptidases or more likely by the action of the non-chymotrypsin-like endopeptidase [56,57].

We determined the metabolic profile of ^{14}C-nafarelin in the urine of rats, monkeys, humans and rabbits and the bile of rats (Table 5). From the urine of rhesus monkeys given ^{14}C-nafarelin, we isolated and identified five major ^{14}C-labeled metabolites [98]: 6-10 pentapeptide amide, 5-10 hexapeptide amide, 6-7 dipeptide, 5-7 tripeptide and 2-naphthylacetic acid. Free 2-naphthylalanine was also present. Radiolabeled metabolites from other species were identified by comparison with HPLC retention times of nafarelin peptide fragments. Of particular interest is the finding that 2-naphthylacetic acid is a major metabolite of nafarelin in many species. Most of these metabolites were also present in the plasma of humans and other species shortly after administration of nafarelin.

An important step in the degradation of nafarelin _in vivo_ appears to be the cleavage of the Ser^4-Tyr^5 bond to yield the 5-10 hexapeptide amide. We observed a rapid cleavage of this bond when we incubated nafarelin with chymotrypsin _in vitro_. An aminopeptidase might then cleave the Tyr^5-D-Nal(2)^6 bond _in vivo_ to give the 6-10 pentapeptide amide. Cleavage of this

Table 5. Metabolic profiles of ^{14}C-nafarelin in human, monkeys, rabbit and rat

Metabolite	% of Radioactivity in Dose[a]				
	Human 0-2d urine	Cynomolgus 0-4d urine	Rabbit 0-3d urine	Rat 0-3d urine	Rat 0-1d bile
Naphthylalanine	8.3	1.5	7.7	1.0	—[b]
6-10 Pentapeptide amide	4.1	6.2	3.4	0.5	--
6-7 Dipeptide	7.4	3.9	11.1	1.4	3.1
5-10 Hexapeptide amide	9.1	10.9	6.1	2.1	27.7
2-Naphthylacetic acid	1.2	13.6	5.5	0.1	--
5-7 Tripeptide	2.7	1.4	4.3	0.7	5.2
1-7 Heptapeptide	--	--	--	0.1	8.8
1-9 Nonapeptide	--	--	--	--	7.8
Nafarelin	2.8	4.6	2.6	--	12.6
Total	35.6	42.1	40.7	5.9	65.2

[a]Recoveries of radioactivity in urine pool were: human, 38-48% (0-2d); cynomolgus, 45-72% (0-4d); rabbit, 57-64% (0-3d); rat, 13.1% (0-3d). Recovery in 0-1d rat bile was 83.4% of dose. Nafarelin was given subcutaneously to human and intravenously to all other species, [b]Below detection, [d]Below detection limit.

latter bond was probably slow due to the D-Nal(2)[6] residue. This explains the presence of the 5-10 and 6-10 peptide in urine or bile of most species that we have examined.

CONCLUDING REMARKS

Pharmacokinetic and metabolic studies of LHRH and its analogs are important in understanding the action of this class of compounds, for the evaluation of their therapeutic potentials and for designing new and potent analogs. We have shown here that increased biological activity of many agonists can be attributed, at least in part, to their enhanced resistance to enzymatic cleavage, stronger receptor or protein binding properties and prolonged plasma elimination half-lives. Limited data on antagonists indicate that the same physiological determinants are also important for the action of these compounds. The potential uses of the antagonists are probably much greater than were initially envisaged due to their very long half-lives in human.

ACKNOWLEDGMENTS

The authors are indebted to Su C. Hsieh, Austin S. Webb and JoAnn La Fargue for their assistance in some of the metabolic studies on nafarelin and detirelix.

REFERENCES

1. Miyachi, Y., Mecklenburg, R.S., Hansen, J.W. and Lipsett, M.B. Metabolism of ^{125}I-luteinizing hormone-releasing hormone. J. Clin. Endocrinol. Metab., 37, 63 (1973).

2. Redding, T.W., Kastin, A.J., Gonzalez-Barcena, D., Coy, D.H., Coy, E.J., Schalch, D.S. and Schally, A.V. The half-life, metabolism and excretion of tritiated luteinizing hormone-releasing hormone (LH-RH) in man. J. Clin. Endocrinol. Metab., 37, 626 (1973).

3. Redding, T.W. and Schally, A.V. The distribution, half-life and excretion of tritiated luteinizing hormone-releasing hormone (LH-RH) in rats. Life Sci., 12, 23 (1973).

4. Dupont, A., Labrie, F., Pelletier, G., Puviani, R., Coy, D.H., Coy, E.J. and Schally, A.V. Organ distribution of radioactivity and disappearance of radioactivity from plasma after administration of [^{3}H]-luteinizing hormone-releasing hormone to mice and rats. Neuroendocrinology, 16, 65 (1974).

5. Pimstone, B., Epstein, S., Hamilton, S.M., LeRoith, D. and Hendricks, S. Metabolic clearance and plasma half-disappearance time of exogenous gonadotropin releasing hormone in normal subjects and in patients with liver disease and chronic renal failure. J. Clin Endocrinol. Metab., 44, 356 (1977).

6. Chikamori, K., Suehiro, F., Ogawa, T., Sato, K., Mori, H., Oshima, I. and Saito, S. Distribution volume, metabolic clearance and plasma half-disappearance time of exogenous luteinizing hormone-releasing hormone in normal women and women with obesity and anorexia nervosa. Acta Endocrinol., 96, 1 (1981).

7. Fauconnier, J.P., Teuwissen, B. and Thomas, K. Rate of disappearance in plasma of synthetic LH-RH intravenously injected in man. Gynecol. Obstet. Invest., 9, 229 (1978).

8. Jeffcoate, S.L., Greenwood, R.H. and Holland, D.T. Blood and urine clearance of luteinizing hormone-releasing hormone in man measured by radioimmunoassay. J. Endocrinol., 60, 305 (1974).

9. Kelch, R.P., Clemens, L.E., Markovs, M., Westhoff, M.H. and Hawkins, D.W. Metabolism and effects of synthetic gonodotropin-releasing hormone (GnRH). J. Clin. Endocrinol. Metab., 40, 53 (1975).

10. Barron, J.L., Millar, R.P. and Searle, D. Metabolic clearance and plasma half-disappearance time of D-Trp^6 and exogenous luteinizing hormone-releasing hormone. J. Clin. Endocrinol. Metab., 54, 1169 (1982).

11. Swift, A.D. and Crighton, D.B. Relative activity, plasma elimination and tissue degradation of synthetic luteinizing hormone releasing hormone and certain of its analogues. J. Endocrinol., 80, 141 (1979).

12. Chu, N.I., Chan, R.L., Hama, K.M. and Chaplin, M.D. Disposition of nafarelin acetate, a potent agonist of luteinizing hormone-releasing hormone, in rats and rhesus monkeys. Drug Metab. Dispos., 13, 560 (1985).

13. Handelsman, D.J., Jansen, R.P.S., Boylan, L.M., Spaliviero, J.A. and Turtle, J.R. Pharmacokinetics of gonadotropin-releasing hormone: comparison of subcutaneous and intravenous routes. J. Clin. Endocrinol. Metab., 59, 739 (1984).

14. Tharandt, L., Rosanowski, C., Windeck, R., Benker, G., Hackenberg, K. and Reinwein, D. The metabolic serum clearance of GnRH. Relationship to age, sex and male puberty. Horm. Metab. Res., 13, 277 (1981).

15. Sandow, J.K., Jerabek-Sandow, G., Krauss, B. and Stoll, W. Metabolic and dispositional studies with LHRH analogs. In "LHRH Peptides as Female and Male contraceptives", G.I. Zatuchni, J.D. Shelton and J.J. Sciarra (Eds.), Harper & Row, New York, 1982, p. 338.

16. Sandow, J. and Clayton, R.N. The disposition, metabolism, kinetics and receptor binding properties of LHRH and its analogues. Prog. Horm. Biochem. Pharmacol., 2, 63 (1983).

17. Nikolics, K., Kéri, G., Szöke, B., Horváth, A. and Teplán, I. Biodegradation of luteinizing hormone-releasing hormone. In "Hormonally Active Brain Peptides. Structure and Function", K.W. McKerns and V. Pantić (Eds.), Plenum Press, New York, 1982, p. 427.

18. Bauer, K. and Horsthemke, B. Degradation of LH-RH. In "Hormonal control of the hypothalamo-pituitary-gonadal axis", K.W. McKerns and Z. Naor (Eds.), Plenum Press, New York, 1984, p. 101.

19. Flouret, G., Stetler-Stevenson, M.A., Carone, F.A. and Peterson, D.R. Enzymatic degradation of LHRH and analogs. In "LHRH and Its Analogs", B.H. Vickery, J.J. Nestor, Jr., and E.S.E. Hafez (Eds.), MTP Press, Boston, 1984, p. 397.

20. Clayton, R.N., Shakespear, R.A. and Marshall, J.C. Luteinizing hormone releasing hormone degrading activity associated with a purified pituitary plasma membrane fraction. J. Endocrinol., 73, 34P (1977).

21. Clayton, R.N., Shakespear, R.A., Duncan, J.A. and Marshall, J.C. Luteinizing hormone-releasing hormone inactivation by purified pituitary plasma membranes: effects on receptor-binding studies. Endocrinology, 104, 1484 (1979).

22. Baumann, R. and Kuhl, H. LH-RH receptors on isolated pituitary plasma membranes: an LH-RH degrading enzyme? Acta Endocrinol., 94 (Suppl. 234), 80 (1980).

23. Leblanc, P., Pattou, E., L'Heritier, A. and Kordon, C. Some properties of peptidasic activity bound to the anterior pituitary membranes. Biochem. Biophys. Res. Commun., 96, 1457 (1980).

24. Elkabes, S., Fridkin, M. and Koch, Y. Studies on the enzymic degradation of luteinizing hormone releasing hormone by rat pituitary plasma membranes. Biochem. Biophys. Res. Commun., 103, 240 (1981).

25. McDermott, J.R., Smith, A.I., Dodd, P.R., Hardy, J.A. and Edwardson, J.A. Mechanism of degradation of LH-RH and neurotensin by synaptosomal peptidases. Peptides, 4, 25 (1983).

26. Berger, H., Nikolics, K., Szöke, B. and Mehlis, B. Proteo-lytic degradation of gonadotropin-releasing hormone (GnRH) by rat ovarian fractions in vitro. Peptides, 4, 821 (1983).

27. Nikolics, K., Szöke, B., Kéri, G. and Teplán, I. Gonado-tropin releasing hormone (GnRH) is not degraded by intact

pituitary tissue in vitro. Biochem. Biophys. Res. Commun., 114, 1028 (1983).

28. Kéri, G., Szöke, B., Nikolics, K., Horvath, A., Teplan, I., Molnar, J. and Gyevai, A. GnRH secreting cultured fetal rat hypothalamic cells do not degrade GnRH. Biochem. Biophys, Res. Commun., 124, 87 (1984).

29. Hazum, E., Cuatrecasas, P., Marian, J. and Conn, P.M. Receptor-mediated internalization of fluorescent gonadotropin-releasing hormone by pituitary gonadotropes. Proc. Natl. Acad. Sci. USA, 77, 6692 (1980).

30. Naor, Z., Atlas, D., Clayton, R.N., Forman, D.S., Amsterdam, A. and Catt, K.J. Interaction of fluorescent gonadotropin-releasing hormone with receptors in cultured pituitary cells. J. Biol. Chem., 256, 3049 (1981).

31. Pelletier, G., Dubé, D., Guy, J., Séguin, C. and Lefebvre, F.A. Binding and internalization of a luteinizing hormone-releasing hormone agonist by rat gonadotrophic cells: A radioautographic study. Endocrinology, 111, 1068 (1982).

32. Hazum, E. and Nimrod, A. Photoaffinity-labeling and fluorescence-distribution studies of gonadotropin-releasing hormone receptors in ovarian granulosa cells. Proc. Natl. Acad. Sci. USA, 79, 1747 (1982).

33. Séguin, C., Pelletier, G., Dubé, D. and Labrie, F. Distribution of luteinizing hormone-releasing hormone receptors in the rat ovary. Regul. Pept., 4, 183 (1982).

34. Kuhl, H., Rosniatowski, C. and Taubert, H.-D. The activity of an LHRH-degrading enzyme in the anterior pituitary during the rat oestrus cycle and its alteration by injection of sex hormones. Acta Endocrinol., 87, 476 (1978).

35. Kuhl, H., Rosniatowski, C. and Taubert, H.-D. Effect of sex hormones on LH-RH-degrading hypothalamic enzyme system during estrus cycle in rats. Endocrinol. Exp., 13, 29 (1979).

36. Krause, J.E., Advis, J.P. and McKelvy, J.F. Characterization of the site of cleavage of luteinizing hormone-releasing hormone under conditions of measurement in which LHRH degradation undergoes physiologically related change. Biochem. Biophys. Res. Commun., 108, 1475 (1982).

37. O'Conner, J.L., Lapp, C.A. and Mahesh, V.B. Peptidase activity in the hypothalamus and pituitary of the rat: fluctuations and possible regulatory role of luteinizing hormone releasing hormone-degrading activity during the estrous cycle. Biol. Reprod., 30, 855 (1984).

38. Bauer, K., Beier, S., Horsthemke, B. Knisatschek, H., and Sievers, J. Estrogen effects on LH-RH degrading brain and pituitary enzymes. Exp. Brain Res. (Suppl. 3), 93 (1981).

39. Griffiths, E.C., Hooper, K.C., Jeffcoate, S.L. and Holland, D.T. The effects of gonadectomy and gonadal steroids on the activity of hypothalamic peptidases inactivating luteinizing hormone-releasing hormone (LH-RH). Brain Res., 88, 384 (1975).

40. Kuhl, H., Rosniatowski, C., Oen, S.A. and Taubert, H.-D. Sex steroids stimulate the activity of hypothalamic arylamidases in the rat. Acta Endocrinol., 76, 1 (1974).

41. Kuhl, H. and Taubert, H.-D. Short-loop feedback mechanism of luteinizing hormone: LH stimulates hypothalamic L-cystine arylamidase to inactivate LH-RH in the rat hypothalamus. Acta Endocrinol., 78, 649 (1975).

42. Advis, J.P., Krause, J.E. and McKelvy, J.F. Evidence that endopeptidase-catalyzed luteinizing hormone-releasing hormone cleavage contributes to the regulation of median eminence LHRH levels during positive steroid feedback. Endocrinology, 112, 1147 (1983).

43. König, W., Sandow, J. and Geiger, R. Structure-function relationships of LH-RH/FSH-RH. In "Peptides: Chemistry, Structure and Biology", R. Walter and J. Meienhofer (Eds.), Ann Arbor Science Publishers, Ann Arbor, 1975, p. 883.

44. Fujino, M., Shinagawa, S., Yamazaki, I., Kobayaski, S., Obayashi, M., Fukuda, T., Nakayama, R., White, W.F. and Rippel, R.H. [Des-Gly-NH$_2^{10}$,Pro-ethylamide^9]-LH-RH:A highly potent analog of luteinizing hormone-releasing hormone. Arch. Biochem. Biophys., 154, 488 (1973).

45. Nestor, J.J. Jr., Ho. T.L., Simpson, R.A., Horner, B.L., Jones, G.H., McRae, G.I. and Vickery, B.H. Synthesis and biological activity of some very hydrophobic superagonist analogues of luteinizing hormone-releasing hormone. J. Med. Chem., 25, 795 (1982).

46. Coy, D.H., Vilchez-Martinez, J.A., Coy, E.J. and Schally, A.V. Analogs of luteinizing hormone-releasing hormone with increased biological activity produced by D-amino acid substitutions in position 6. J. Med. Chem., 19, 423 (1976).

47. Nestor, J.J. Jr., Ho, T.L., Tahilramani, R., Horner, B.L., Simpson, R.A., Jones, G.H., McRae, G.I. and Vickery, B.H. In "LHRH and its Analogs", B.H. Vickery, J.J. Nestor, Jr. and E.S.E. Hafez (Eds.), MTP Press, Boston, 1984, p. 23.

48. Seyler, L.E. Jr. Disappearance of biologic activity of synthetic LRH in normal and hypogonadal men. J. Clin. Endocrinol. Metab., 41, 1155 (1975).

49. Dias, J.A. and Reeves, J.J. Disappearance of LHRH and D-Leu^6-des-GlyNH$_2^{10}$ LHRH ethylamide in ewes. J. Anim. Sci., 46, 1707 (1978).

50. Sandow, J. and König, W. Chemistry of the hypothalamic hormones. In "The Endocrine Hypothalamus," S.L. Jeffcoate and J.S.M. Hutchinson (Eds.), Academic Press, London, 1978, p. 149.

51. Yamazaki, I. and Okada, H. A radioimmunoassay for a highly active luteinizing hormone-releasing hormone analogue and relation between the serum level of the analogue and that of gonadotropin. Endocrinol. Jpn., 27, 593 (1980).

52. Barron, J., Millar, R.P. and Wegener, I. Radioimmunoassay of D-Trp^{6}LHRH: Investigation of the plasma elimination of the hormone analogue. In "Neuropeptides, Biochemical and Physiological Studies", R.P. Millar (Ed.), Churchill Livingstone, Edinburgh, 1981, p. 207.

53. Mason-Garcia, M., Vigh, S., Comaru-Schally, A.M., Redding, T.W., Somogyvari-Vigh, A., Horvath, J. and Schally, A.V. Radioimmunoassay for 6-D-Trytophan analog of luteinizing hormone-releasing hormone: Measurement of serum levels after administration of long-acting microcapsule formulations. Proc. Natl. Acad. Sci. USA, 82, 1547 (1985).

54. Nerenberg, C., Foreman, J., Chu, N., Chaplin, M.D. and Kushinsky, S. Radioimmunoassay of Nafarelin ([6-(3-(2-naphthyl)-D-alanine)]-luteinizing hormone-releasing hormone) in plasma or serum. Anal. Biochem., 141, 10 (1984).

55. Parnes, H. and Shelton, E.J. A potentially general synthesis of high specific activity specifically labelled tritiated peptides: synthesis of [D-3-(2-naphthyl-[2,3-^{3}H] alanine^6)]LHRH. J. Labelled Compd. Radiopharm., 21, 263 (1984).

56. Horsthemke, B. and Bauer, K. Characterization of a non-chymotrypsin-like endopeptidase from anterior pituitary that hydrolyzes luteinizing hormone-releasing hormone at the tyrosyl-glycine and histidyl-tryptophan bonds. Biochem., 19, 2867 (1980).

57. Horsthemke, B. and Bauer, K. Substrate specificity of an adenohypophyseal endopeptidase capable of hydrolyzing luteinizing hormone-releasing hormone: preferential cleavage of peptide bonds involving the carboxyl terminus of hydrophobic and basic amino acids. Biochem., 21, 1033 (1982).

58. Marks, N. and Stern, F. Enzymatic mechanisms for the inactivation of luteinizing hormone-releasing hormone (LH-RH). Biochem. Biophys. Res. Commun., 61, 1458 (1974).

59. Koch, Y., Baram, T., Hazum, E. and Fridkin, M. Resistance to enzymic degradation of LH-RH analogues possessing increased biological activity. Biochem. Biophys. Res. Commun., 74, 488 (1977).

60. Barron, J., Griffiths, E., Tsalacopoulos, G. and Millar, R.P. Metabolism of [D-Trp^6]LHRH. In "LHRH and Its Analogs", B.H. Vickery, J.J. Nestor, Jr., and E.S.E. Hafez (Eds.), MTP Press, Boston, 1984, p. 411.

61. Hersh, L.B. and McKelvy, J.F. Enzymes involved in the degradation of thyrotropin-releasing hormone (TRH) and luteinizing hormone releasing hormone (LH-RH) in bovine brain. Brain Res., 168, 553 (1979).

62. Knisatschek, H. and Bauer, K. Characterization of "Thyroliberin-deamidating enzyme" as a post-proline-cleaving enzyme. J. Biol. Chem., 254, 10936 (1979).

63. Orlowski, M., Wilk, E., Pearce, S. and Wilk, S. Purification and properties of a prolyl endopeptidase from rabbit brain. J. Neurochem., 33, 461 (1979).

64. Tate, S.S. Purification and properties of a bovine brain thyrotropin-releasing-factor deamidase. A post-proline cleaving enzyme of limited specificity. Europ. J. Biochem., 118, 17 (1981).

65. Camargo, A.C.M., Spadaro, A.C.C., Martins, A.R. and Greene, L.J. Brain endo-oligopeptidase B: Inactivation of LH-RH

by hydrolysis of the $Pro^9-Gly^{10}-NH_2$ peptide bond. Braz. J. Med. Biol. Res., <u>15</u>, 239 (1982).

66. Browne, P. and O'Cuinn, G. An evaluation of the role of a pyroglutamyl peptidase, a post-proline cleaving enzyme and a post-proline dipeptidyl amino peptidase, each purified from the soluble fraction of guinea-pig brain, in the degradation of thyroliberin in vitro. Europ. J. Biochem., <u>137</u>, 75 (1983).

67. Horsthemke, B., Knisatschek, H., Rivier, J., Sandow, J. and Bauer, K. Degradation of luteinizing hormone-releasing hormone and analogs by adenohypophyseal peptidases. Biochem. Biophys. Res. Commun., <u>100</u>, 753 (1981).

68. Clayton, R.N., Shakespear, R.A., Duncan, J.A. and Marshall, J.C. Radioiodinated nondegradable gonadotropin-releasing hormone analogs: New probes for the investigation of pituitary gonadotropin-releasing hormone receptors. Endocrinology, <u>105</u>, 1369 (1979).

69. Bienert, M., Albrecht, E., Berger, H., Klauschenz, E., Pleiss, U., Niedrich, H. and Mehlis, B. Direct tritium-labeling into histidine of luteinizing hormone-releasing hormone agonists and use of the tracers in studies on proteolytic breakdown. Biochem. Biophys. Acta, <u>761</u>, 183 (1983).

70. Clayton, R.N. and Shakespear, R.A. [D-Serine(Bu^t)^6] luteinizing hormone releasing hormone 1-9 ethylamide: enhanced biological activity because of resistance to degradation. J. Endocrinol., <u>77</u>, 34P (1978).

71. Sandow, J., Kuhl, H. and Krauss, B. Studies on enzyme stability of luteinizing hormone releasing hormone analogues. J. Endocrinol., <u>81</u>, 157P (1979).

72. Kelly, J.A., Griffiths, E.C., Jeffcoate, S.L. and Hopkinson, C.R.N. Hypothalamic inactivation of luliberin (luteinizing-hormone-releasing hormone). Biochem. Soc. Trans., <u>7</u>, 76 (1979).

73. Griffiths, E.C. and Hopkinson, C.R.N. Inactivation of two hyperactive LH-RH analogues by rat hypothalamic peptidases. Horm. Res., <u>10</u>, 233 (1979).

74. Bauer, K., Horsthemke, B., Knisatschek, H., Nowak, P. and Kleinkauf, H. Degradation of luliberin (LH-RF) by brain and pituitary tissue enzymes. Hoppe-Seyler's Z. Physiol. Chem., <u>360</u>, 229 (1979).

75. Hazum, E., Fridkin, M., Baram, T. and Koch, Y. Synthesis, biological activity and resistance to enzymic degradation of luteinizing hormone-releasing hormone analogues modified at position 7. FEBS Lett., <u>123</u>, 300 (1981).

76. Conn, P.M., Staley, D., Jinnah, H. and Bates, M. Molecular mechanism of gonadotropin releasing hormone action. J. Steroid Biochem., <u>23</u>, 703 (1985).

77. Pedroza, E., Vilchez-Martinez, J.A., Fishback, J., Arimura, A. and Schally, A.V.. Binding capacity of luteinizing hormone-releasing hormone and its analogues for pituitary receptor sites. Biochem. Biophys. Res. Commun., <u>79</u>, 234 (1977).

78. Heber, D. and Odell, W.D. Pituitary receptor binding activity of active, inactive, superactive and inhibitory analogs of gonadotropin-releasing hormone. Biochem. Biophys. Res. Commun., 82, 67 (1978).

79. Clayton, R.N. and Catt, K.J. Receptor-binding affinity of gonadotropin-releasing hormone analogs: Analysis by radioligand-receptor assay. Endocrinology, 106, 1154 (1980).

80. Reeves, J.J., Séguin, C., Lefebvre, F.-A., Kelly, P.A. and Labrie, F. Similar luteinizing hormone-releasing hormone binding sites in rat anterior pituitary and ovary. Proc. Natl. Acad. Sci. USA, 77, 5567 (1980).

81. Perrin, M.H., Rivier, J.E. and Vale, W.W. Radioligand assay for gonadotropin-releasing hormone: relative potencies of agonists and antagonists. Endocrinology, 106, 1289 (1980).

82. Loumaye, E., Naor, Z. and Catt, K.J. Binding affinity and biological activity of gonadotropin-releasing hormone agonists in isolated pituitary cells. Endocrinology, 111, 730 (1982).

83. Dayton, P.G., Israili, Z. H. and Perel, J.M. Influence of binding on drug metabolism and distribution. Ann. NY Acad. Sci, 226, 172 (1973)

84. Chan, R.L. and Chaplin, M.D. Plasma binding of LHRH and nafarelin acetate, a highly potent LHRH agonist. Biochem. Biophys. Res. Commun., 127, 673 (1985).

85. Tharandt, L., Schulte, H., Benker, G., Hackenberg, K. and Reinwein, D. Binding of luteinizing hormone releasing hormone to human serum proteins-influence of a chronic treatment with a more potent analogue of LH-RH. Horm. Metab. Res., 11, 391 (1978).

86. Davis, M., Veldhuis, J.D., Rogol, A.D., Dufau, M.L. and Catt, K.J. Sustained inhibitory actions of a novel antagonist of gonadotropin-releasing hormone (GnRH) in man. Clin. Res., 34, 423A (1986).

87. Reeves, J.J., Tarnavsky, G.K., Becker, S.R., Coy, D. and Schally, A.V. Uptake of iodinated luteinizing hormone releasing hormone analogs in the pituitary. Endocrinology, 101, 540 (1977).

88. Sandow, J., Eckert, H., Stoll, W. and von Rechenberg, W. The kinetics and organ distribution of a highly active analogue of luteinizing hormone releasing hormone. J. Endocrinol., 73, 33P (1977).

89. Okada, H., Yamazaki, I. Yashiki, T. Shimamoto, T. and Mima, H. Vaginal absorption of a potent luteinizing hormone-releasing hormone analogue (leuprolide) in rats IV: Evaluation of the vaginal absorption and gonadotropin responses by radioimmunoassay. J. Pharm. Sci., 73, 298 (1984).

90. Nekola, M.V., Horvath, A., Ge, L.J., Coy, D.H. and Schally, A.V. Suppression of ovulation in the rat by an orally active antagonist of luteinizing hormonereleasing hormone. Sci., 218, 160 (1982).

91. Folkers, K., Bowers, C.Y., Kubiak, T. and Stepinski, J. Antagonists of the luteinizing hormone releasing hormone with pyridyl-alanines which completely inhibit ovulation at nanogram dosage. Biochem. Biophys. Res. Commun., 111, 1089 (1983).

92. Rivier, C., Rivier, J., Perrin, M. and Vale, W. Comparison of the effect of several gonadotropin releasing hormone antagonists on luteinizing hormone secretion, receptor binding and ovulation. Biol. Reprod., 29, 374 (1983).

93. Handelsman, D.J. and Swerdloff, R.S. Pharmacokinetics of gonadotropin-releasing hormone and its analogs. Endocr. Rev., 7, 95 (1986).

94. Sennello, L.T., Finley, R.A., Chu, S.-Y., Jagst, C., Max, D., Rollins, D.E. and Tolman, K.G. Single-dose pharmaco-kinetics of leuprolide in humans following intravenous and subcutaneous administration. J. Pharm. Sci., 75, 158 (1986).

95. Wakefield, G.B., Kovacs, W.J., Island, D.P., Hoffman, P.G., LePage, M.E., Chan, R.L., Nerenberg, C.A. and Pavlou, S.N. Suppression of human pituitary-gonadal function by a potent new LHRH antagonist. Program and Abstracts, the Endocrine Society, 68th Annual Meeting, Anaheim, California, June 25-27, 1986, p.86.

96. Pavlou, S.N., Island, D.P., Wakefield, G.B., Hoffman, P.G., Chan, R.L., Nerenberg, C.A. and Kovacs, W.J. A potent new luteinizing hormone-releasing hormone antagonist is active in man. Clin. Res., 34, 432A (1986).

97. Pavlou, S.N., Wakefield, G.B. and Kovacs, W.J. LHRH antagonist in normal men. In "LHRH and Its Analogs, Part II", B.H. Vickery and J.J. Nestor, Jr. (Eds.), MTP Press, Boston, 1987, in press.

98. Chan, R.L. and Chaplin, M.D. Identification of major urinary metabolites of nafarelin acetate, a potent agonist of luteinizing hormone-releasing hormone in the rhesus monkey. Drug Metab. Dispos., 13, 566 (1985).

Epilog

B. H. VICKERY and J. J. NESTOR JR.

Institute of Biological Sciences and Bio-Organic Chemistry
Syntex Research, Palo Alto, CA 94304, USA

In the 3 years that have elapsed between the appearance of the first and second volume in this series interest in the field of LHRH analogs has continued unabated. Some of the promise of these agents as important therapeutic entities has now been fulfilled, and the therapeutic scope continues to expand. The innovative research into delivery of these agents will further increase the acceptability and compliance with this new class of drugs.

CHEMISTRY

Little new work has appeared in the chemistry of LHRH agonists, with the exception of the use of the N,N'-dialkyl-D-homoarginine substitutions [1]. Although there are theoretical advantages of the increased hydrophilicity of these analogs and they are of equivalent potency to the best of the previous hydrophobic analogs, no new agonist analog has proceeded to clinical evaluation.

Major strides have been made in LHRH antagonist chemistry. The development has involved the stepwise introduction of hydrophobic residues which block proteolysis, increase receptor affinity and prolong the pharmacokinetics [2]. The introduction of additional positively charged residues resulted in further increases in potency and extreme prolongation of action, measured in days in some species. This unfortunately turned out to be at the cost of increased mast cell degranulating activity and associated histamine release [3,4], the side effect of most concern for these agents. However, several of these analogs have been sufficiently well-tolerated in humans that their preliminary clinical pharmacology could be assessed [4-7]. The recent finding that shielding of the charge on the residues in positions 6 and 8 dramatically reduces the propensity for histamine release while retaining high LHRH competitiveness has breathed new life into this area [2,7]. We can look forward to the design of even more potent analogs with minimal histamine releasing activity.

Recombinant DNA methods were used to identify the precursor of LHRH [8]. This in turn has led to the discovery of an additional biologically active peptide, GAP, which is cosecreted with LHRH; they may be cooperative in their actions. The existence of another biologically active processed fragment with LHRH-like activity not mediated through LHRH receptors has also been suggested [9].

Control of gonadotropin release has taken a new turn, now that the long search for the elusive inhibin seems to have reached fruition [10,11]. The finding that dimeric recombination of inhibin subunits can give rise to a molecule with specific FSH releasing activity [12,13] has potentially important implications for profertility applications and exposes a whole new aspect of the modulation of hormone release.

A hypothalamic factor that inhibits LHRH-stimulated LH release but not basal release has been reported [14]. What role such a factor would play in control of gonadotrope secretion is not known.

MECHANISM OF ACTION

At the gonadotrope cellular level we are now beginning to understand the chain of events set in motion by receptor activation. A fascinating system of second and even third messenger molecules is emerging [15-19]. However our understanding of the control of pulsatile LHRH secretion by opioid or other factors [20] and how this mediates cyclic reproductive function and non-parallel secretion of FSH and LH [21] from cells which appear to be mostly bihormonal in content [22] is incomplete.

EXTRA-PITUITARY DISTRIBUTION OF LHRH-LIKE MATERIALS AND THEIR RECEPTORS

There is considerable evidence for the extrapituitary production and specific binding of LHRH-like molecules. In particular high affinity binding sites and direct interactions of LHRH and its analogs with the gonads in rats support important paracrine regulatory roles in this species [23,24]. The lower affinity of the binding sites, the large quantities of immunodetectable LHRH and the lack of correspondence of potency of LHRH analogs on human placental tissue relative to pituitary tissue caused doubts on such a role in this tissue [25]. However, the localization of the precursor for LHRH [26] and the numerous studies documenting in vitro and in vivo effects on specific placental functions now argue for at least a regulatory role in the production of chorionic gonadotropin. It is still not apparent why convincing effects have not been obtained in women [27-30], when human placental tissue in vitro clearly responds. Perhaps pharmacokinetic differences will ultimately explain the paradox. Although specific low affinity binding sites have been demonstrated in human corpora lutea and breast cancer cells [31], and some direct effects are claimed [32,33], local production of LHRH-like factors has not been demonstrated. It is difficult to account for the reported remission of postmenopausal breast cancer [34] without resorting to such a direct action, although not all investigators can confirm the activity [35]. Surprisingly large amounts of LHRH-like material are secreted in breast milk [36] arguing for local production. Presumably the cloned cDNA for the precursor for LHRH will be used to check these tissues using in situ hybridization for expression of the LHRH gene.

PHARMACOLOGY OF THE LHRH ANTAGONISTS

The LHRH antagonists, similarly to the agonists, are remarkably specific to the reproductive axis in their effects. All other pharmacological effects appear to be related to the propensity to degranulate mast cells, a propensity which was inadvertently enhanced in pursuit of greater potency. It should, however, be stressed that mast cell degranulation activity, a property which is shared by other peptides with positively charged amino acids [37], can be divorced from LHRH inhibitory activity.

It is now clear that rapid, specific and prolonged inhibition of pituitary/gonadal function can be achieved with LHRH antagonists [6]. Due to favorable pharmacokinetics both their potency and duration of action are greater in humans than in laboratory animals, for the analogs which have reached clinical evaluation.

From the preliminary studies several possible advantages of LHRH antagonists over the agonist analogs are suggested. The rapidity of inhibition and absence of early stimulation may make these analogs the agents of choice for a high risk subpopulation of metastatic breast and prostatic cancer patients.

An increased incidence of pituitary adenomas has been found in long-term carcinogenicity studies with LHRH agonists in rats and mice. This may be a result of long-term stimulation of the gonadotropes. Long-term gonadectomy also causes morphological changes resembling gonadotropic cell adenomas [22]. Similarly, acromegaly is associated with microadenomas of the somatotropes. Theoretically, the lack of activation of the LHRH receptors during inhibition with the LHRH antagonists would avoid this possibility.

In contrast to the agonist analogs, LHRH antagonists consistently result in azoospermia, even in primates. Although azoospermia can be achieved in man with the agonists, it requires heroic dosage schedules, particularly when the agonist is combined with testosterone supplementation to stop inhibition of libido and occurrence of hot flashes [38]. Therefore while the agonist approach to male contraception does still have its champions [39], the consensus discounts such use. The ease of induction of azoospermia in monkeys with the LHRH antagonists [40,41] and the degree of gonadal suppression achievable in man [42] leaves this possibility still open for the antagonists.

The requirement for a luteal component in the maintenance of pregnancy makes interception a possibility to be explored. The progressively increasing dependence of maintenance of pregnancy upon the corpus luteum/pituitary axis in dogs gives rise to a wide window of efficacy of the pregnancy terminating effects of LHRH antagonists in this species [43]. On the other hand the very small window of efficacy in primates (prior to the initiation of hCG production) suggests difficulty in finding an appropriate dosage regimen for women [44,45].

CLINICAL TRIALS WITH LHRH AGONISTS

The LHRH agonists have reached a mature stage of clinical evaluation [46-50]. Analogs are now marketed in several countries for treatment of prostatic cancer and at least one has received approval in France for the treatment of precocious puberty. Phase III trials are being completed in endometriosis patients and this indication will probably be the next one added to the approved list. However concerns over the effects of hypoestrogenism, particularly bone density changes, will probably result in initial regulatory restrictions on duration and repetition of therapy. It has been suggested that combination treatment with a progestogen might reduce the bone density changes [51]; clinical evaluation of this regimen is beginning. Exploration of the utility of LHRH agonists for treatment of metastatic breast cancer and for leiomyomata is in earlier stages [49,50,52]; it appears that because of rapid return in the latter indication the major use of the analogs would be in preparation for surgical myomectomy or hysterectomy [53]. In even earlier stages of evaluation are the benefits of LHRH agonist therapy in hirsutism [54], benign prostatic hypertrophy [55] and as an adjunctive treatment with clomiphene/gonadotropins in in vitro fertilization/egg transfer programs [56] or directly in infertility syndromes of variable etiology [57]. Case reports of treatment of other syndromes continue to appear [58-60] and depending upon the incidence of the condition, may proceed into clinical trial.
   Although some studies proceed in the area of female contraception it is not clear that combinations of LHRH agonist with progestogens have any advantage over available oral contraceptives [61]. Short term (3-6 month) use of LHRH agonist alone for post partum contraception may fulfill a useful role.

GONADAL PROTECTIVE PROSPECTS

Controversy still exists over the ability of LHRH analogs to protect against the gonadotoxic effects of cancer chemotherapeutic agents. The animal and clinical studies reported here [62,63] do not support the use of the agonists for this purpose. The reproducibility of the original finding of protection in mice has also been questioned [64]. However, investigations continue. Protection against radiation induced testicular damage has also been reported [65]. The different findings might arise from differences in dosage schedule or potency/dose of the agonist used. Studies with the LHRH antagonists may have a different outcome because of the more rapid and complete effect on gonadotropins/spermatogenesis.

DIAGNOSTIC UTILITY

A recent paper concluded that intravenous administration of 100 µg of LHRH to amenorrheic patients offered no help in their clinical classification and failed to assess the therapeutic potential of treatment with LHRH [66]. On the other hand a single subcutaneous injection of a potent LHRH agonist (nafarelin) was superior to intravenous LHRH as a rapid test for pituitary and gonadal function in cases of sexual precocity [67]. The use of an LHRH antagonist to cause acute estrogen deficiency in monkeys and the correlation of the calcium changes with those occurring after ovariectomy [68] is also novel, and may be of use in women to predict the predisposition to osteoporosis.

APPLICATIONS IN ANIMALS

It would appear that in food producing animals, such as cattle and fish, the major use of LHRH analogs is destined to be in the profertility mode [69,70]. In companion animals such as dogs and cats the use will be for fertility control: the agonists for long term suppression of reproductive function and behavior in both males and females and the antagonists for acute uses such as termination of heat and of pregnancy [43].

CONCLUDING REMARKS

The LHRH analogs are clearly destined to play a major role in reproductive medicine. In addition they may help in control of our pet population and be useful in increasing aspects of our food supply. A further spin-off of this research area will be the application of the novel amino acid substitutions to other synthetic peptides and the novel delivery routes and systems to other non-orally active agents. We look forward to the further maturation of this exciting research area.

REFERENCES

1. Nestor, J.J. Jr. and Vickery, B.H. Introduction, this volume
2. Nestor, J.J. Jr. Chapter 1, this volume
3. Karten, M., Hook, W.A., Siraganian, R.P., Coy, D.H., Folkers, K., Rivier, J.E. and Roeske, R.W. Chapter 11, this volume
4. Phillips, A., Hahn, D.W., Bishop, C., Capetola, R.J. and McGuire, J.L. Chapter 12, this volume
5. Mais, V., Kazer, R.R., Cetal, N.S, Rivier, J., Vale, W. and Yen, S.S.C. The dependency of folliculogenesis and corpus luteum function on pulsatile gonadotropin secretion in cycling women using a gonadotropin-releasing hormone antagonist as a probe. J. Clin. Endocrinol. Metab., 62, 1250 (1986)
6. Pavlou, S.N., Wakefield, G.B. and Kovacs, W.J. Chapter 16, this volume
7. Roeske, R., Chaturvedi, N.C., Hrinyo-Paulina, T. and Kowalczuk, M. Chapter 2, this volume
8. Nikolics, K. and Seeburg, P.H. Chapter 4, this volume
9. Millar, R.P., Wormald, P.J. and Milton, R.C. de L. Stimulation of gonadotropin release by a non-GnRH peptide sequence of the GnRH precursor. Science, 232, 68 (1986)

10. Mason, A.J., Hayflick, J.S., Ling, N., Esch, F., Ueno, N., Ying, S.Y., Guillenin, R., Niall, H. and Seeburg, P.H. Complementary DNA sequences of ovarian follicular inhibin show precursor structure and homology with transforming growth factor-β. Nature, 318, 659 (1985)

11. Rivier, J., Spiess, J., McClintock, R., Vaughan, J. and Vale, W. Purification and partial characterization of inhibin from porcine follicular fluid. Biochem. Biophys. Res. Commun., 133, 120 (1985)

12. Vale, W., Rivier, J., Vaughan, J., McClintock, R., Corrigan, A., Woo, W., Karr, D. and Spiess, J. Purification and characterization of an FSH-releasing protein from porcine ovarian follicular fluid. Nature, 321, 776 (1986)

13. Ling, N., Ying, S-Y., Ueno, N., Shimasaki, S., Esch, F., Hotta, M. and Guillemin, R. Pituitary FSH is released by a heterodimer of the β-subunits from the two forms of inhibin. Nature, 321, 779 (1986)

14. Hwan, J.-C. and Freeman, M. Partial purification of a hypothalamic factor that inhibits gonadotropin-releasing hormone-stimulated luteinizing hormone release. Endocrinology, 120, 483 (1987)

15. McArdle, C.A. and Conn, P.M. Chapter 6, this volume

16. Morgan, R.O., Chang, J.P. and Catt, K.J. Novel aspects of gonadotropin-releasing hormone action on inositol polyphosphate metabolism in cultured pituitary gonadotrophs. J. Biol. Chem., 262, 1166 (1987)

17. Ojeda, S.R., Capdevila, J., Snyder, G., McCann, S.M., Negro-Vilar, A. and Falck, J.R. Involvement of arachidonic acid metabolites in the control of hypothalamic-pituitary function. Adv. Prostag. Thrombox. Leuko. Res., 15, 559 (1985)

18. Naor, Z. and Childs, G.V. Binding and activation of gonadotropin-releasing hormone receptors in pituitary and gonadal cells. Int. Rev. Cytol., 103, 147 (1986)

19. Wisner-Provost, A., Gerozissis, K., Rommelaer, M.C., Renard, C.A., Rougeot, C., Levi, F.A. and Dray, F. Eicosanoids in relation with LHRH secretion. Adv. Prostag. Thrombox. Leuko. Res., 16, 235 (1986)

20. Barkan, A.L. and Marshall, J.C. Chapter 7, this volume

21. Gross, K.M., Matsumoto, A.M. and Bremner, W.J. Differential control of luteinizing hormone and follicle-stimulating hormone secretion by luteinizing hormone-releasing hormone pulse frequency in man. J. Clin. Endocrinol. Metab., 64, 675 (1987)

22. Childs, G.V. Functional ultrastructure of gonadotropes: a review. Curr. Top. Neuroendocrinol., 7, 49 (1986)

23. Clayton, R.N. and Catt, K.J. Gonadotropin-releasing hormone receptors: Characterization, physiological regulation and relationship to reproductive function. Endocr. Rev. 2, 186 (1981)

24. Jones, P.B.C. and Hsueh, A.J.W. Direct antigonadal actions of LHRH. In "LHRH and Its Analogs: Contraceptive and Therapeutic Applications", B.H. Vickery, J.J. Nestor, Jr. and E.S.E. Hafez (Eds.), MTP Press, Lancaster, p. 163, 1984

25. Siler-Khodr, T.M. Chapter 10, this volume
26. Adelman, J.P., Mason, A.J., Hayflick, J.S. and Seeburg, P.H. Isolation of the gene and hypothalamic cDNA for the common precursor of gonadotropin-releasing hormone and prolactin release-inhibiting factor in human and rat. Proc. Natl. Acad. Sci. U.S.A., 83, 179 (1986)
27. Tolis, G., Comraru-Schally, A.M., Mehta, A.E. and Schally, A.V. Failure to interrupt established pregnancy in humans by D-tryptophan-6-luteinizing-hormone-releasing-hormone. Fertil. Steril. 36, 241 (1981)
28. Casper, R.F., Sheehan, K.L. and Yen, S.S.C. Chorionic gonadotropin prevents LRF-agonist-induced luteolysis in the human. Contraception, 21, 471 (1980)
29. Skarin, G., Nillius, S.J. and Wide, L. Failure to induce abortion of early human pregnancy by high doses of a superactive LRH agonist contraception, 26, 457 (1982)
30. Rao, A.J., Mathialagan, N., Kotagi, S.G. and Moudgal, N.R. Studies on regulation of chorionic gonadotropin secretion in primates. J. Biosci., 6 (Suppl. 2), 97 (1984)
31. Bramley, T.A. Chapter 8, this volume
32. Miller, W.R., Scott, W.N., Morris, R., Fraser, H.M. and Sharpe, R.M. Growth of human breast cancer cells inhibited by a luteinizing hormone-releasing hormone agonist. Nature, 313, 231 (1985)
33. Eidne, K.A., Flanagan, C.A., Harris, N.S. and Millar, R.P. Gonadotropin-releasing hormone (GnRH)-binding sites in human breast cancer cell lines and inhibitory effects of GnRH antagonists. J. Clin. Endocrinol. Metab., 64, 425 (1987)
34. Plowman, P.H., Nicholson, R.I. and Walker, K.J. Remission of postmenopausal breast cancer during treatment with the luteinizing hormone releasing hormone agonist ICI 118630. Brit. J. Cancer, 54, 903 (1986).
35. Waxman, J.H., Harland, S.J., Coombes, R.C., Wrigley, P.F.M., Malpas, J.S., Powles, T. and Lister, T.A. The treatment of postmenopausal women with advanced breast cancer with buserelin. Cancer Chemother. Pharmacol., 15, 171 (1985)
36. Smith, S.S. and Ojeda, S.R. Maternal modulation of infantile ovarian development and available ovarian luteinizing hormone-releasing hormone (LHRH) receptors via milk LHRH. Endocrinology, 115, 1973 (1984)
37. Bouchard, P., Blondet, C., Spilz, I., Brailly, S., Jouannet, P. and Schaison, G. Sperm suppression by long acting GnRH agonist therapy in men: critical effect of testosterone substitution and duration of therapy. Endocrinology, 118, 155A (1986)
38. Foreman, J. and Jordan, C. Histamine release and vascular changes induced by neuropeptides. Agents and Actions, 13, 105 (1983)
39. Bhasin, S., Steiner, B.S. and Swerdloff, R.S. Chapter 28, this volume
40. Bremner, W.J., Adams, L.A. and Steiner, R.A. Chapter 14, this volume

41. Weinbauer, G.F., Surmann, F.J. and Nieschlag, E. Suppression of spermatogenesis in a non-human primate (Macaca fascicularis) by concomitant gonadotropin-releasing hormone antagonist and testosterone treatment. Acta Endocrinol. (Copenh.), 114, 138 (1987)

42. Pavlou, S.N., Wakefield, G.B. and Kovacs, W.J. Chapter 16, this volume

43. Vickery, B.H., McRae, G.I. and Goodpasture, J.C. Chapter 34, this volume

44. Fraser, H.M. Chapter 15, this volume

45. Van der Spuy, Z.M., Pillay, L., Hardie, F., van der Walt, M., de Chalain, T., Kaplan, H., Roeske, R. and Millar, R.P. Chapter 19, this volume

46. Henzl, M.R. and Monroe, S.E. Chapter 22, this volume

47. Kirkland, J.L. and Lin, T.H. Chapter 23, this volume

48. Sandow, J. and von Rechenberg, W. Chapter 24, this volume

49. Garnick, M.B., Lipton, A., Harvey, H.A., Max, D.T., Smith, J.A. and Glode, L.M. Chapter 25, this volume

50. Donnelly, R.J. and Milsted, R.A.V. Chapter 26, this volume

51. Meldrum, D.R. Clinical management of endometriosis with luteinizing hormone-releasing hormone analogues. Sem. Reprod. Endocrinol., 3, 371 (1985)

52. Healy, D.L., Lawson, S.R., Abbott, M., Baird, D.T. and Fraser, H.M. Toward removing uterine fibroids without surgery: subcutaneous infusion of a luteinizing hormone-releasing hormone agonist commencing in the luteal phase. J. Clin. Endocrinol. Metab., 63, 619 (1986)

53. Lumsdon, M.A., West, Christine P. and Baird, D.T. Goserelin therapy before surgery for uterine fibroids. Lancet, Jan. 3, 36 (1987)

54. Monroe, S., Andreyko, J.L. and Jaffe, R.B. Chapter 17, this volume

55. Schroeder, F.H., Westerhof, M., Bosch, R.J.L.H. and Kurth, K.H. Benign prostatic hyperplasia treated by castration or the LH-RH analogue buserelin: A report on 6 cases. Eur. Urol., 12, 318 (1986)

56. Lopes, P., Barriere, P., Charbonnel, B. and Paillard, B. Value of short-term use of a gonadorelin analog in an in vitro fertilization program. Presse Med., 15, 2074 (1986)

57. Jacobs, H.S., Porter, R., Eshel, A. and Craft, I. Chapter 20, this volume

58. Steingold, K.A., Judd, H.L., Neiberg, R.K., Lu, J.K.H. and Chang, R.J. Treatment of severe androgen excess due to ovarian hyperthecosis with a long-acting gonadotropin-releasing hormone agonist. Am. J. Obstet. Gynecol., 154, 1241 (1986)

59. Parmar, H., Nicoll, J., Stockdale, A., Cassoni, A., Phillips, R.H., Lightman, S.L. and Schally, A.V. Advanced ovarian carcinoma: response to the agonist D-Trp-6-LHRH. Cancer Treat. Rep., 69, 1341 (1985)

60. Vorobiof, D.A. and Falkson, G. Nasally administered buserelin inducing complete remission of lung metastases in male breast cancer. Cancer, 59, 688 (1987)

61. Lemay, A. and Faure, N. Chapter 27, this volume
62. Goodpasture, J.C. and Vickery, B.H. Chapter 29, this volume
63. Waxman, J. Chapter 30, this volume
64. Da Cunha, M.F., Meistrich, M.L. and Nader, S. Absence of testicular protection by a gonadotropin-releasing hormone analogue against cyclophosphamide-induced testicular cytotoxicity in the mouse. Cancer Res., 47, 1093 (1987)
65. Schally, A.V., Paz-Bouza, J.I., Schlosser, J.V., Karashima, T., Debeljuk, L., Candle, B. and Sampson, H. Protective effects of analogs of luteinizing hormone-releasing hormone against X-radiation-induced testicular damage in rats. Proc. Natl. Acad. Sci. U.S.A., 84, 851 (1987)
66. Adulwahid, N.A., Armar, N.A., Morris, D.V., Adams, J. and Jacobs, H.S. Diagnostic tests with luteinizing hormone releasing hormone should be abandoned. Brit. Med. J., 291, 1471 (1985)
67. Rosenfield, R.L., Garibaldi, L.R., Moll, G.W., Jr., Watson, A.C. and Burstein, S. The rapid ovarian secretory response to pituitary stimulation by the gonadotropin-releasing hormone agonist nafarelin in sexual precocity. J. Clin. Endocrinol. Metab., 63, 1386 (1986)
68. Hodgen, G.D., Kenigsberg, D. and Abbasi, R. Chapter 31, this volume
69. Crim, L.W. and Peter, R.E. Chapter 32, this volume
70. Garverick, R.A. and Stevenson, J.S. Chapter 33, this volume

Index

606

608

609